Board of Registry Study Guide
For Clinical Laboratory Certification Examinations

Board of Registry
Study Guide
For Clinical Laboratory Certification Examinations

Editor
Harriet B. Rolen, MA, MT(ASCP)

Associate Editors
Barbara M. Castleberry, PhD, MT(ASCP)
Mary E. Lunz, PhD

Research Associates
Barbara L. Grossklags, MT(ASCP)
Susan L. Wiseman, MT(ASCP)

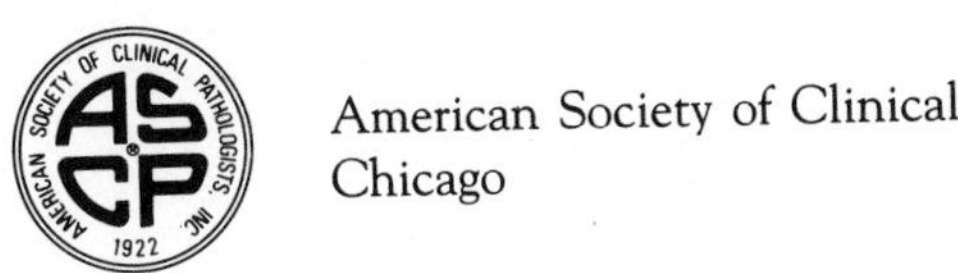

American Society of Clinical Pathologists Press
Chicago

Library of Congress Cataloging in Publication Data

Board of Registry study guide for clinical laboratory certification examinations.

Bibliography: p.
1. Medical technology--Examinations, questions, etc. I. Rolen, Harriet. II. Castleberry, Barbara M. III. Lunz, Mary E. IV. American Society of Clinical Pathologists. Board of Registry. [DNLM: 1. Allied Health Personnel--examination questions. 2. Certification. 3. Pathology, Clinical--examination questions. QY 18 B662]
RB37.B6 1986 616.07'5 86-1171
ISBN 0-89189-216-8

Copyright ©1986 by the American Society of Clinical Pathologists. All rights reserved. No part of this publication may be reproduced, stored in a retrieval system, or transmitted in any form or by any means, electronic, mechanical, photocopying, recording, or otherwise, without the prior written permission of the publisher. Printed in the United States of America.

93 92 91 90 89 8 7 6 5 4

Contents

To the Examinee

You have taken an important first step in your professional career by deciding to become certified. I wish you success as you prepare for these examinations.

Paul J. Cherney, M.D.

Chairman, Board of Registry

Introduction

Examination applicants have often expressed a need for a guide to help them prepare for the certification examinations. To respond to this need, the American Society of Clinical Pathologists (ASCP) Press and the Board of Registry of the American Society of Clinical Pathologists have produced this study guide for aspiring medical laboratory technicians and medical technologists. This guide contains background on the Board of Registry; guidelines for preparing for and taking the test; information on the development, content, structure, and scoring of the examinations; and practice questions and answers in the content areas covered by the examinations.

The practice questions are constructed in a format and style comparable to those on the Board of Registry certification examinations; however, none of these questions has ever appeared on a Board of Registry examination, and none of the questions will ever appear in future Board of Registry examinations. The practice questions were developed from previously published materials--including Continuing Education Update Examinations, Professional Self-Assessment Examinations Series III, Update/Educate, Audio-Visual Seminar Series in Immunology, and Tech Sample--which were prepared by the committees of the ASCP Commission on Continuing Education and the ASCP Commission on Associated Member Activities.

For applicants reading this book, taking the practice examination and answering the practice questions should help you prepare for the actual examinations. Use of this book, however, does not assure a passing score on the examinations. The Board of Registry's evaluation and credentialing process are entirely independent of this study guide.

For faculty, officials of clinical laboratory education programs, and examinees, this book provides information on how Board of Registry certification examinations are structured and scored. The technical summaries on these topics are designed to briefly explain the pertinent evaluation topics. Further information concerning evaluation techniques can be obtained from the books and articles noted in the education section of the reading list.

Reviewers of Questions

Our thanks to the following individuals who reviewed the questions contained in this book.

Blood Bank

Ann R. Hubbard, MT(ASCP)SBB
White Plains Hospital
White Plains, New York

Dee Simons, MT(ASCP)SBB
George Washington University Medical Center
Washington, DC

Graciela F. Taylor, MT(ASCP)SBB
University of Texas Health Science Center
Dallas, Texas

Candace K. Williams, MT(ASCP)SBB
University of Texas Health Science Center
Dallas, Texas

Chemistry

Mary G. Day, MT(ASCP)
George Washington University Medical Center
Washington, DC

Katherine G. Hardy, MT(ASCP)
George Washington University Medical Center
Washington, DC

Sharon A. Jackson, MEd, MT(ASCP)
University of Florida
Gainesville, Florida

Angela Jones, MT(ASCP)SC
Baptist Medical Center
Birmingham, Alabama

Chemistry (Continued)

Carol J. Pauley, MT(ASCP)
Geroge Washington University Medical Center
Washington, DC

Lynne F. Ross, PhD, MT(ASCP)SC
USDA, Southern Regional Research Center
New Orleans, Louisiana

Barbara Ward, MT(ASCP)SC
State University of New York
Syracuse, New York

Hematology

Judith Fincher, MT(ASCP)SH
University of Texas Health Science Center
Dallas, Texas

Jeanne Hitlan, MT(ASCP)SH
George Washington University Medical Center
Washington, DC

Janice Hundley, MS, MT(ASCP)SH
Medical University of South Carolina
Charleston, South Carolina

Pat Kellough, MT(ASCP)
Arlington Memorial Hospital Laboratory
Arlington, Texas

Janice H. Parrish, MEd, MT(ASCP)
University of Florida
Gainesville, Florida

Judy Varney, MS, MT(ASCP)SH
State University of New York
Syracuse, New York

Immunology

Steven A. Bryant, MS, MT(ASCP)SI
Wesley Medical Center
Wichita, Kansas

Immunology (Continued)

Cynthia K. Karr, PhD, MT(ASCP)
Medical University of South Carolina
Charleston, South Carolina

Raphael Yankey, MSc
George Washington University Medical Center
Washington, DC

Microbiology

Fran Fisher, MEd, MT(ASCP)
University of Florida
Gainesville, Florida

Barbara Jackson, MT(ASCP)
George Washington University Medical Center
Washington, DC

Aileen Janny, PhD
Charity Hospital
New Orleans, Louisiana

Frances Morgenstern, MS, MT(ASCP)SM
State University of New York
Syracuse, New York

Kim Watson, MT(ASCP)
Presbyterian Hospital of Dallas
Dallas, Texas

Body Fluids and Urinalysis

Mrs. Martha Fales
George Washington University Medical Center
Washington, DC

Reginaldo Lauzon, MS, MT(ASCP)
State University of New York
Syracuse, New York

Carolyn Sue Walters, MHS, MT(ASCP)
Louisiana State University
New Orleans, Louisiana

Management

Barbara Morris, MBA, MT(ASCP)
American Society of Clinical Pathologists
Chicago, Illinois

CHAPTER 1

Certification

The Importance of Certification

The practice of modern medicine would be impossible without the tests performed in the clinical laboratory. A medical team of pathologists, specialists, technologists, and technicians works together to determine the presence, extent, or absence of disease and provides data needed to evaluate the effectiveness of treatment.

Laboratory procedures require an array of complex precision instruments and a variety of automated and electronic equipment. However, men and women interested in helping others are the foundation of a successful laboratory. They must be accurate, reliable, have an interest in science, and be able to recognize their responsibility for human lives.

Critical to high-quality health care is the assurance that individuals performing laboratory tests are able to carry out their responsibilities in a proficient manner. Therefore, laboratory personnel of demonstrated competence are of prime importance.

Certification is the process by which a nongovernmental agency or association grants recognition of competence to an individual who has met certain predetermined qualifications, as specified by that agency or association. Certification affirms that an individual has demonstrated that he or she possesses the knowledge and skills to perform essential tasks in the medical laboratory.

Role of the ASCP Board of Registry

Founded in 1928 by the American Society of Clinical Pathologists (ASCP), the Board of Registry's mission is to develop and establish standards and procedures for individuals to enter, continue, or advance in a career in medical laboratory science, and to certify and register those individuals who meet the required criteria. This mission is accomplished through four major ongoing activities: (1) receiving and evaluating applications for examination and certification; (2) developing, administering, and scoring examinations; (3) conducting examination-related research to monitor and improve the quality of tests and testing methodologies; and (4) maintaining official records of all individuals certified by the Board.

The keystone of the Board of Registry is the team of approximately 100 volunteer technologists and technicians, laboratory scientists, physicians, and professional researchers in education, evaluation, and psychometrics who make up the Board of Governors, the Research and

Development Committee, and the examination committees. These individuals contribute their time and expertise to achievement of the goal of excellence in the certification process for medical laboratory personnel.

The Board of Governors is the policy-making body for the Board of Registry and is composed of twenty members. These twenty members include technologists, technicians, and pathologists nominated by the ASCP and representatives from the general public and the following societies: American Academy of Microbiology, American Association of Blood Banks, American Society of Cytology, American Society of Hematology, National Registry in Clinical Chemistry, and National Society of Histotechnology.

The Research and Development Committee's activities include the review of current methods and research related to competency definition, test development, validity and reliability assessment, examination performance, and standard setting.

The examination committees include technologists, technicians, laboratory scientists, and physicians. These committees are responsible for planning, development, and review of the examinations; determining the accuracy and relevancy of the examinations; and confirming the standard for each examination.

After Certification

Certification affirms that an individual has demonstrated that he or she possesses the knowledge and skills to perform essential tasks in the medical laboratory. The Board of Registry certifies individuals upon completion of academic prerequisites, clinical laboratory education or experience, and successful performance on a competency-based examination.

Registration is the process by which names of individuals certified by the Board of Registry are identified on an annual basis as being currently registered. Annual re-registration benefits include an identification card, registration seal, one-year subscription to Laboratory Medicine, eligibility for insurance programs, and upon request, written verification of certification.

Certification in a given category means that an individual has met all criteria for career entry in that category. As they continue on in their careers, many individuals who are certified at one professional level may work to obtain certification at a higher level to reflect their continued growth and development. Thus, a technician may move to the technologist level and even to the specialist level in a specific discipline.

The clinical laboratory sciences are among the fastest changing segments of the health care field. Therefore, each certificant should embrace a philosophy of life-long learning to remain current in a chosen discipline. This may be accomplished through formal course work, professional continuing education offerings, as well as individual regimens of journal reading and subscription to professional self-assessment examinations.

CHAPTER 2

The Three Levels of Certification

Three professional levels of practice have been established (Laboratory Medicine, 13:312-313, 1982) for which Board of Registry certification may be attained: technician, technologist, and specialist. These professional levels define in a general sense the skills and abilities that an individual is expected to have at career entry. The professional levels are considered hierarchical; that is, each level encompasses the knowledge and skill of the preceding levels.

There are several aspects of these definitions that should be noted. First, the roles are defined in a general sense. For example, Technologist describes the role of technologists in all categories, ie, general medical technology, chemistry, hematology, blood banking, immunology, microbiology, cytotechnology, and histotechnology. Second, the roles refer to skills and abilities that the individual is expected to have at career entry, not those that may be acquired with subsequent experience. Career entry is defined as the point in time when the individual meets all educational and/or experience requirements and is therefore eligible for Board certification. Thus, while supervision, management, and teaching are skills that technicians may possess and apply in the laboratory, they are not skills that the technician is expected to have learned prior to a career-entry examination.

The following sections describe each level, its roles and skills.

Technician

Knowledge. The technician has a working comprehension of the technical and procedural aspects of laboratory tests.

Technical Skills. The technician is able to read and follow directions and to perform those tests in a clinical laboratory that are considered to be of a straightforward nature. The technician has a practical understanding of quality control that is sufficient to enable him or her to determine whether or not tests are within control limits and to make the requisite adjustments according to specified procedures. The technician is capable of performing simple instrument maintenance.

Judgment and Decision Making. The technician is able to recognize the existence of common procedural and technical problems and to take corrective action according to predetermined criteria.

Communication. The technician communicates straightforward information, eg, reports test results and quotes normal ranges and specimen requirements.

Teaching and Training Responsibilities. The technician is capable of demonstrating learned technical skills.

Technologist

Knowledge. The technologist has an understanding of the underlying scientific principles, as well as of the technical and procedural aspects of laboratory testing. The technologist has a general comprehension of the physiologic, biochemical, immunologic, microbiologic, and genetic factors that affect health and disease; laboratory tests; and the importance of laboratory tests to medical care. The technologist is familiar with the various services available in the hospital and has an appreciation of the roles and interrelationships of paramedical and other health-related fields.

Technical Skills. The technologist is capable of performing technically demanding tests. The technologist has a theoretical understanding of quality assurance sufficient to enable him or her to monitor and to implement quality control programs. The technologist is able to participate in the introduction and implementation of new procedures and in the evaluation of new instruments. The technologist has a basic knowledge of accuracy, precision, normal ranges, and the ability to correlate this information with existing methods.

Judgment and Decision Making. The technologist has the ability to exercise initiative and independent judgment in dealing with the broad scope of procedural and technical problems. The technologist is able to participate in, and may be delegated, the responsibility for decisions involving quality control programs, instrument selection, preventative maintenance, safety test procedures, and reagent purchases.

Communication. The technologist communicates technical or general information to medical, paramedical, or lay persons. Information may include problems or matters of a scientific, technical, or administrative nature.

Supervision and Management. The technologist has a basic understanding of management theory and functions. The technologist is able to participate in and develop responsibility for establishment of technical and administrative procedures. The technologist can supervise technicians, aides, and clerical personnel as directed.

Teaching and Training Responsibilities. The technologist is able to provide instruction in the basic theory, technical skills, and application of laboratory test procedures. The technologist may participate in the evaluation of the effectiveness of educational programs.

Specialist

Knowledge. The specialist has knowledge of advanced scientific principles, as well as of the technical, procedural, and research aspects of laboratory testing in the specialty area and of factors that influence disease processes and laboratory tests. The specialist has knowledge of the structure and function of the organization, the principles of management and education, as well as the roles of other members of the health care team.

Technical Skills. The specialist is able to perform all laboratory tests and appropriate equipment maintenance in the specialty area. The specialist has the knowledge, ability, and technical skill to research, develop, implement, and evaluate new and existing methodologies, including instrumentation and quality assurance.

Judgment and Decision Making. The specialist is capable of implementing and delegating decisions regarding laboratory operation and of exercising independent judgment in problem solving. The specialist is able to anticipate and respond to unique situations regarding patients and/or samples in a laboratory setting. The specialist can participate in policy decisions affecting laboratory performance or laboratory personnel in the specialty area.

Communication. The specialist is able to communicate in depth with other health care personnel on the application and validity of laboratory data, as well as on the policies and operation of the specialty area. The specialist is capable of representing the specialty area to the community at large.

Supervision and Management. The specialist is capable of performing and directing administrative functions in the overall operation of the laboratory in the specialty area. Implicit is the capability to provide direct supervision of other personnel in that discipline.

Teaching and Training Responsibilities. The specialist has the ability to plan, implement, and evaluate effective educational programs.

CHAPTER 3

Applying for the Certification Examination

The Board of Registry administers examinations on the third Friday of February and August of each year.

Approximately one year before the date you wish to take the examination, you should contact the Board of Registry to obtain a current application packet. The application packet contains the following:

- examination announcement, indicating the examination dates, deadline dates, and examination categories offered;
- certification examination eligibility requirements;
- application form, including instructions for completion;
- rules and regulations;
- list of test centers.

Since the examination requirements, as well as other information included in the application packet, are periodically revised, be sure you have the most recent application packet available from the Board of Registry office. Once you have obtained these materials, it is important to review them to make sure that you have adequate time to obtain any required documents prior to the application deadline. Please contact the Board of Registry office at P.O. Box 12270, Chicago, Illinois 60612, for application forms and general information.

Application Deadlines

Your application and fee must be in the Board of Registry office by the first working day of October for the February examination and the first working day of April for the August examination.

Examination Eligibility

To be eligible to take the examination, you must (1) meet the current stated minimum requirements for a particular category or level of certification, and (2) submit a formal application form and pay the appropriate application fee.

Minimum requirements for the Medical Technologist examination are a baccalaureate degree including specific biology, chemistry, and mathematics credits and one of the following:

- completion of a CAHEA accredited Medical Technologist program,
- MLT(ASCP) certification and three years of acceptable clinical laboratory experience,
- five years of acceptable clinical laboratory experience.

Applicants for the Medical Laboratory Technician examination must meet the requirements of one of the following eligibility routes:

- an associate degree and completion of a CAHEA accredited Medical Laboratory Technician Associate Degree program or Military Medical Laboratory Specialist program,
- an associate degree and completion of five years of acceptable clinical laboratory experience,
- a high school diploma and completion of a CAHEA accredited Medical Laboratory Technician Certificate program and three years of acceptable clinical laboratory experience,
- a high school diploma and completion of a Military Medical Laboratory Specialist program and three years of acceptable clinical laboratory experience,
- 30 semester hours and completion of a CAHEA accredited Medical Laboratory Technician Certificate program,
- 60 semester hours and CLA(ASCP) certification.

Specific requirements vary. For complete information, refer to the current Board of Registry Certification Examination Eligibility Requirements.

CHAPTER 4

Preparing to Take the Examination

Begin early to prepare for the Certification Examination. Because of the broad range of knowledge and skills tested by the examination, even applicants with a great deal of college training and professional experience will probably find that some review is necessary, although the amount will vary from applicant to applicant. Generally, last-minute cramming is the least effective method for preparing for the examination. The earlier that you begin, the more time you will have to prepare; and the more you prepare, the better your chance of doing well on the examination.

The following are some guidelines for studying for the examination.

Diagnose Your Strengths and Weaknesses

Begin by taking the practice examination in this guide (Chapter 9) to assess your strengths and weaknesses. The practice test is based on the same distribution of questions across content and skill areas as are the Board of Registry examinations; however, none of the questions will appear on a Board of Registry examination. Try to take it under conditions similar to actual testing conditions. Find a quiet place and time yourself. Allow two hours to take the 100-question practice examination. Most Board of Registry examinations have slightly over 200 questions and four hours are allowed. Do not look up any answers while you are taking the practice examination and answer all the questions as best you can.

After you have taken the examination, use the directions provided to score it by total test and subtest (chemistry, microbiology, etc). Your scores on the subtests will give you an indication of your strengths and weaknesses. Because this practice examination is shorter than the actual Board of Registry examination and therefore provides a smaller sample of the information, you should supplement the practice test scores with other information that you have about your strengths and weaknesses. For example, if you currently work in the laboratory and do hematology tests, you may want to study the other laboratory areas more thoroughly. If you are a student and your lowest grades were in clinical chemistry, you may want to spend more time on that subject than the others. After you have diagnosed your weaknesses from several sources, such as the practice test, course grades, class tests, and laboratory experience, you are ready to begin studying.

Study for the Test

Plan a course of study that allows more time for your weaker areas. Although it is important to study your areas of weakness, be sure to allow enough time to review all areas.

It is better to spend a short time studying every day than to spend several hours every week or two. A regular time and special place to study will help because then study will become part of your daily routine.

Several resources can be used to help you to study. The reading lists at the end of this book identify many useful books and articles by subject area. The practice questions in this book provide an extensive overview of the content of medical technology. They can be used to test your knowledge in each subject area or they may be used to acquire experience in answering multiple-choice questions. You may also wish to consider the following.

Standard Textbooks. Textbooks tend to cover a broad range of knowledge in a given field and thus help you survey an entire field. An added benefit is that textbooks frequently have questions at the end of the chapters that you can use to test yourself.

Competency Statements, Content Outlines, and Item Descriptors. The Board of Registry has developed the competency statements and content outlines to delineate the content and tasks included in the test. These statements and outlines appear in Chapter 7, "Examination Content." The Board of Registry provides, as a part of score reporting, a list of item descriptors for each examination. An item descriptor is a shorthand method of describing the content and skill tested in a specific test question. The list of item descriptors shows the distribution of questions across content and skill areas by providing a description of each question (item). Item descriptors are explained in Chapter 8, "Examination Scoring." The lists of item descriptors for recent Board of Registry Examinations appear in Appendix A, "Item Descriptor Lists for Medical Laboratory Technician Examinations," and Appendix B, "Item Descriptor Lists for Medical Technologist Examinations."

Current Publications. It will be helpful to scan major journals from the past few years to keep up with the innovations in the field. Textbooks may be updated only every few years whereas new questions are added to the examinations every examination cycle. Therefore, it is possible that questions will be asked on content that is not yet in textbooks but has been added to the literature via journals and other periodicals.

Get Enough Rest Before the Examination

Ease up on your studying before the examination. Try to get plenty of rest and eat a good breakfast before going to take the examination. Most examinations are scheduled for a four-hour period.

Locate the Test Center

The authorization slip will have the room location of the examination test center, address, and proctor's name. Plan to arrive early at the test site to familiarize yourself with the area and locate the room in which the examination will be administered.

CHAPTER 5

Taking the Examination

Test Center Procedures

1. When you take the examination, you should bring with you at least two No. 2 soft lead pencils with good erasers.
2. Scratch paper will be provided for you. No books, dictionaries, or paper may be taken into the examination room.
3. Though they are not necessary, the Board of Registry does allow the use of slide rules and calculators during the test. They must be brought in without carrying cases.
4. You must present photo identification to the proctor along with your authorization slip (sent to you after your examination eligibility has been determined).
5. You will be required to sign the following: "I have read the Examination Instructions. I understand that if an applicant is caught cheating on a certifying examination, his/her results will be held until such time as the applicant appeals to the Board of Registry, at which time the Board will decide each individual case. I certify that I am the candidate whose signature appears below. I also certify that, because of the confidential nature of these copyright materials, I will not retain or copy any examination materials and I will not otherwise reveal the content of these materials."

Irregularities

If an examinee is suspected of cheating on a certifying examination, the results will be held until such time as the examinee appeals to the Board of Registry. If such an incident occurs, the examinee will be notified and informed of the appeals protocol. The Board will review each individual case and determine the appropriate consequences.

Suggestions for Taking the Test

1. Read the instructions carefully before beginning.
2. Read the stem (question) carefully looking for words such as best, most likely, least likely, and NOT.
3. Read all the answer choices before answering. Sometimes what initially appears to be a correct answer may not be the best answer.
4. Budget your time so you can answer each question. Do not spend an inordinate amount of time on any one question. If you are uncertain about the correct answer or it is taking a long time to get the correct answer (eg, in a calculation problem), it is best to skip it and return to it later if you have time.
5. Record your answers directly on the machine-scorable answer sheet to avoid transcription errors and conserve examination time.
6. Try to stay relaxed so that you can think through clearly and logically the problems presented on the examination.

Should You Guess

There is no built-in penalty for guessing on Board of Registry examinations. In other words, if you have some knowledge about the content of the question, it is advisable to select a response. If you can narrow the options to two answer choices, it is a good strategy to guess. However, an incorrect answer or no answer always results in the loss of the point value assigned to the question.

CHAPTER 6

Examination Development

Examination Committee

The Joint Generalist Examination Committee, which prepares the Medical Technologist and Medical Laboratory Technician examinations, is composed of medical technologists, medical laboratory technicians, and pathologists. The committee represents both diverse geographical areas and diverse types of practice. The responsibility of item writing, evaluation, and selection rests with the examination committee members. Question writing requires mastery of the subject as well as an understanding of the examination population and mastery of written communication skills. Question review by the entire committee ensures that the item adheres to appropriate technical and/or scientific principles. The committee is also responsible for maintaining the currency of the content of the examinations and writing item descriptors. It is supported by the Board of Registry staff which provides expertise in psychometrics and production.

Criterion-Referenced Testing

The Board of Registry's process of examination construction and analysis is based on the concept of criterion-referenced testing. Generally, a criterion-referenced examination is designed to ascertain an individual's knowledge as measured with respect to a set of previously defined competencies that summarize the domain of knowledge and skill represented on the examination. Each examination question is designed to test some aspect of the competencies that have been developed as criteria against which examinees are measured. Thus every question on an examination becomes a "criterion" against which the examinee is measured. If an examinee answers an item correctly, he or she has met the criterion; if an examinee answers incorrectly, he or she has not met the criterion. Since it is unlikely that one question would be the absolute measure of a competency, the Board of Registry examinations are carefully planned so that several items measure each competency. If an examinee answers a sufficient number of questions correctly, he or she has met the criterion for the test.

In criterion-referenced testing, the domain of practice of the Medical Technologist or Medical Laboratory Technician is delineated in the competency statements and content outlines (see Chapter 7, "Examination Content"). These competency statements are the basis for writing examination questions. Each examination question is a measure that impacts upon the minimum pass score, which is the ultimate criterion against which examinees are measured.

Purpose of the Examination

The Board of Registry certification examinations measure an examinee's level of skill and knowledge (competency) at a particular point in time. Each examination item, because it is tied to a competency statement, contributes to the pass/fail decision. Because items must accurately distinguish between qualified and unqualified candidates, each item is carefully written, reviewed, and evaluated. A very comprehensive process is used to assure that each item measures that which it is intended to measure.

Components of Competency

Examination items are written from competency statements. The Board of Registry competency statements were developed based on selected components of competence.

The three components are (1)knowledge, (2) technical skill, and (3) cognitive skill. The components expand into competency statements in which knowledge is represented in the content areas and technical skill is represented by task and task definitions (see Chapter 7).

Knowledge. This is the first dimension of competency and a criterion against which examinees are measured. Knowledge is the content base upon which the field of practice in Medical Technology is built. Content areas of Medical Technology typically include Blood Banking, Body Fluids including Urinalysis, Chemistry, Hematology, Immunology, and Microbiology.

Technical Skill. The second component of competency and a criterion against which the examinee is measured may be defined as the ability to complete an assigned activity or apply knowledge to a procedure. The implication is that laboratory tasks can be defined and that one's ability to perform them can be measured on a paper-and-pencil test. While these are not the only tasks completed by laboratory staff, they are the areas that are considered essential to test on the examinations.

Cognitive Skill. The third component of competence is the ability to deal with data at various cognitive skill levels. Cognitive skill refers to the cognitive or mental processes required to answer the question. Questions are classified into three cognitive skill levels, based on the structure of the question. The three cognitive skill levels used by the Board of Registry are defined as follows:

- Recall (level 1), the ability to recall or recognize previously learned (memorized) knowledge ranging from specific facts to complete theories;
- Interpretive skills (level 2), the ability to use recalled knowledge to interpret or apply verbal, numeric, or visual data;
- Problem solving (level 3), the ability to use recalled knowledge and the interpretation/application of distinct criteria to resolve a problem or situation and/or make an appropriate decision.

The cognitive skill level of a question is influenced by the construction of the stem in concert with the responses. Thus, a concept such as coagulation provides the content for the development of questions on all three cognitive skill levels. The sample questions in Figure 1 demonstrate this point.

All items appearing on a Board of Registry examination were written to test one of the competency statements listed in Chapter 7. Each question (item) in the examination is described by an item descriptor, which describes the content (knowledge), tasks (technical skills), and cognitive levels (also called taxonomy) covered in each question. The details about item descriptors appear in Chapter 8, "Examination Scoring."

Cognitive Skill Level 1: Recall

The prothrombin time test requires that the patient's citrated plasma be combined with:

a. platelet lipids
b. thromboplastin
c. Ca^{++} and platelet lipids
*d. Ca^{++} and thromboplastin

Cognitive Skill Level 2: Interpretation

A patient develops unexpected bleeding following three transfusions. The following test results were obtained:

Prolonged PT and APTT
Decreased fibrinogen
Increased fibrin split products
Decreased platelets

What is the most probable cause of these results?

a. familial afibrinogenemia
b. primary fibrinolysis
*c. DIC
d. liver disease

Cognitive Skill Level 3: Problem Solving

A patient develops severe unexpected bleeding following four transfusions. The following test results were obtained:

Prolonged PT and APTT
Decreased fibrinogen
Increased fibrin split products
Decreased platelets

Given these results, which of the following blood products should be recommended to the physician for this patient?

a. platelets
b. factor VIII
*c. cryoprecipitate
d. fresh frozen plasma

Figure 1. Sample questions that illustrate cognitive skill levels.

*Correct answer

Question Development

The Board of Registry examinations consist of objective multiple-choice items. A multiple-choice question may be defined as an objective measuring device that contains a STEM and four or five RESPONSES, one of which is the best answer. The form is flexible so that an item may ask a specific question, describe a situation, report laboratory results, etc.

The stem of a multiple-choice question (1) asks a question, (2) gives an incomplete statement, (3) states an issue, or (4) describes a situation. The content of the stem focuses on a central theme or problem, using clear and precise language, without excessive length that can confuse or distract examinees. The stem may describe clinical data and laboratory results that require interpretation or problem solving. The question or issue presented in the stem is relevant to the knowledge and task delineated in a competency statement.

The responses present the "best" answer and the "distractors." Each multiple-choice question has four or five independent responses. The best answer is the one agreed upon by the experts; however, the other three or four distractors may seem plausible to the examinee who has partial, incomplete, or inappropriate knowledge. The distractors may therefore be considered logical misconceptions of the best answer. The responses are written to be parallel in content, length, and category of information.

As you review the questions included in this book, it may be useful to note the construction of the item, carefully reviewing both the stem and responses as you practice selecting the best answer.

Color Plates and Other Visual Materials

Some of the questions on the examination will refer to color plates that contain photographs of clinical materials and other visual materials such as graphs or charts. Subject areas that may have color plates include Hematology, Urinalysis, and Microbiology (including Parasitology and Mycology). Although color plates are not provided in this book, you should study books containing color plates (often called atlases) as you prepare for this part of the examination. Some of these books are listed in the reading lists at the end of this book. In addition, many journals frequently contain photographs and graphs. One example is Laboratory Medicine, a monthly journal of the American Society of Clinical Pathologists. This and other journals are available in the laboratory or a medical library as well as by subscription.

To sharpen your ability to understand and analyze visual materials, a good exercise might be to look at an illustration and attempt to evaluate it without referring to the legend. Once you have analyzed the photograph, compare your analysis with the legend. Practice this exercise in your reading whenever the article or book contains photographic material.

Two examples of questions that contain visual materials appear in Figure 2.

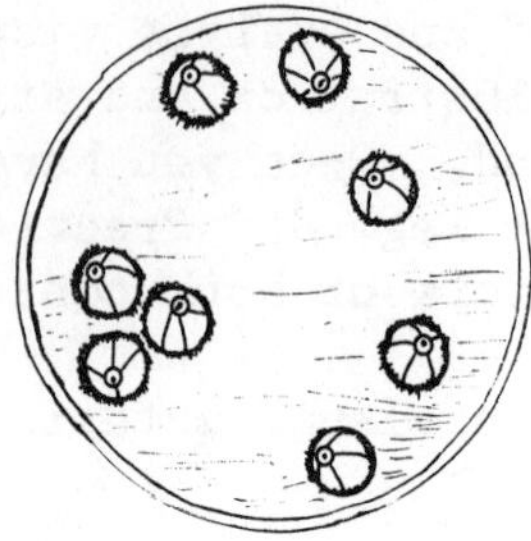

Trophozoites of the organism depicted above are likely to:

a. contain red blood cells
b. have clear, "pointed" pseudopodia
c. contain few, if any, vacuoles
*d. have slow, undefined motility

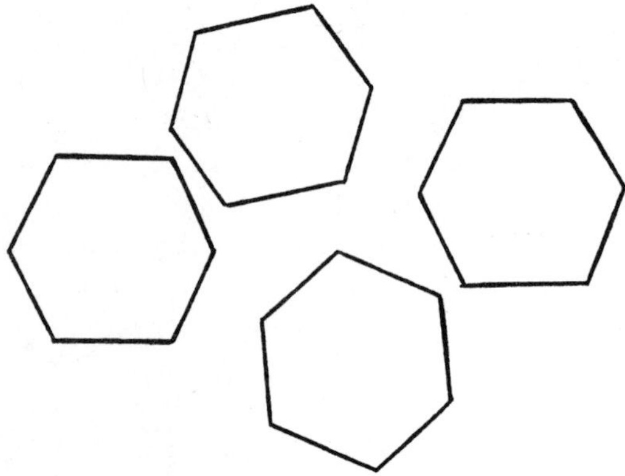

The crystals depicted above were seen in a urine specimen. This patient is most likely to have which of the following clinical conditions?

a. gout
b. renal damage
c. bilirubinuria
*d. cystinosis

Figure 2. Examples of questions containing visual material.

*Correct answer

Preparation of Examinations

The Board of Registry maintains databases containing more than 7,000 examination questions. This computerized database system has extensive identification and sorting capabilities. The number of multiple-choice questions in each Medical Laboratory Technician or Medical Technologist examination varies between 200 and 230. The average length of the examinations is 210 items.

Board of Registry examinations are carefully constructed according to the specific predetermined criteria summarized in the competency statements and content outlines. Each examination is constructed according to a "multidimensional examination blueprint." The blueprint delineates the number of questions that will be used to measure each competency statement and each content area. In this way the examination committee keeps the examination balanced in regard to knowledge, technical skills, and cognitive skills. The distribution of items across content areas, tasks, and cognitive skills on each examination is reflected in the item descriptor list that accompanies the Examinee Performance Report.

CHAPTER 7

Examination Content

The content of each examination is determined based on the competency statements and content outlines developed and published by the Board of Registry. These competency statements and content outlines are provided to show you what topics and tasks will be covered on the examinations.

COMPETENCY STATEMENTS
MEDICAL LABORATORY TECHNICIAN

In regard to Microbiology (M), Hematology (H), Chemistry (C), Body Fluids (BF), Immunology (I), and Blood Bank (BB), at career entry the Medical Laboratory Technician:

Task	Task Definitions	Content Areas
Defines and/or Identifies	- principles of basic laboratory procedures	M, H, C, BF, I, BB
	- basic procedures related to testing	*
	- fundamental biological characteristics as they pertain to laboratory testing	*
	- standard operating procedures	*
	- sources of error in laboratory testing	*
	- fundamental characteristics of laboratory operations	*
Selects and/or Prepares and/or Performs	- method	M, H, C, BF, I, BB
	- procedural course of action	*
	- reagents for test	*
	- instruments to perform test	*
	- controls for test	*
Calculates	- results from supplied data	M, H, C, BF, I, BB
	- results from obtained data	*
Associates	- laboratory findings and clinical data to assess test results and procedures	M, H, C, BF, I, BB
	- laboratory findings and quality control data to assess test results and procedures	*
	- laboratory findings and other laboratory data to assess test results and procedures	*
Analyzes and/or Evaluates	- laboratory findings to recognize common procedural problems	M, H, C, BF, I, BB
	- laboratory findings to recognize common technical problems	*
	- laboratory findings to take corrective action according to predetermined criteria	*
	- laboratory findings to check for common errors	*
	- laboratory findings to recognize and report the need for additional testing	*

CONTENT OUTLINE
MEDICAL LABORATORY TECHNICIAN

NOTE: Laboratory Operations is part of all content areas.

LABORATORY OPERATIONS

1. Quality assurance
2. Safety
3. Instruments
4. Laboratory mathematics

All percentages are approximate ranges to be included on the examination.

MICROBIOLOGY (20% OF TOTAL EXAMINATION)

1. Bacteria 75% of subtest
15% of total exam

A. Morphology, cultural and growth characteristics
B. Specimen and/or media selection, collection, transport, storage and processing
C. Laboratory examinations
  1. basic tests
  2. special tests
D. Infectious diseases
E. Laboratory operations

2. Fungi 5% of subtest
1% of total exam

A. Morphology, cultural and growth characteristics
B. Specimen and/or media selection, collection, transport, storage and processing
C. Laboratory examinations
  1. basic tests
  2. special tests
D. Infectious diseases
E. Laboratory operations

3. Mycobacteria 5% of subtest
1% of total exam

A. Morphology, cultural and growth characteristics
B. Specimen and/or media selection, collection, transport, storage and processing
C. Laboratory examinations
  1. basic tests
  2. special tests
D. Infectious diseases
E. Laboratory operations

4. Parasites 10% of subtest
2% of total exam

A. Morphology, cultural and growth characteristics
B. Specimen and/or media selection, collection, transport, storage and processing
C. Laboratory examinations
  1. basic tests
  2. special tests
D. Infectious diseases
E. Laboratory operations

5. Viruses, Rickettsiae and Other Microorganisms
5% of subtest
1% of total exam

A. Morphology, cultural and growth characteristics
B. Specimen and/or media selection, collection, transport, storage and processing
C. Laboratory examinations
  1. basic tests
  2. special tests
D. Infectious diseases
E. Laboratory operations

HEMATOLOGY (20% OF TOTAL EXAMINATION)

1. Erythrocytes 35% of subtest
7% of total exam

A. Anatomy and physiology of hematopoiesis
B. Specimen selection, collection, transport, storage and processing
C. Laboratory examinations
  1. basic tests
  2. special tests
D. Hematopoietic diseases
E. Laboratory operations

2. Leukocytes 35% of subtest
7% of total exam

A. Anatomy and physiology of hematopoiesis
B. Specimen selection, collection, transport, storage and processing
C. Laboratory examinations
  1. basic tests
  2. special tests
D. Hematopoietic diseases
E. Laboratory operations

3. Thrombocytes 10% of subtest
2% of total exam

A. Anatomy and physiology of hematopoiesis
B. Specimen selection, collection, transport, storage and processing
C. Laboratory examinations
   1. basic tests
   2. special tests
D. Hematopoietic disorders
E. Laboratory operations

4. Hemostasis 20% of subtest
4% of total exam

A. Physiology of hemostasis
B. Specimen selection, collection, transport, storage and processing
C. Laboratory examinations
   1. basic tests
   2. special tests
D. Hemostatic diseases
E. Laboratory operations

CHEMISTRY (20% OF TOTAL EXAMINATION)

1. Carbohydrates 10% of subtest
2% of total exam

A. Biochemical theory and physiology
B. Specimen selection, collection, transport, storage and processing
C. Laboratory examinations
   1. basic tests
   2. special tests
D. Biochemical manifestation of disease
E. Laboratory operations

2. Lipids and Lipoproteins 5% of subtest
1% of total exam

A. Biochemical theory and physiology
B. Specimen selection, collection, transport, storage and processing
C. Laboratory examinations
   1. basic tests
   2. special tests
D. Biochemical manifestation of disease
E. Laboratory operations

3. Heme Derivatives 5% of subtest
1% of total exam

A. Biochemical theory and physiology
B. Specimen selection, collection, transport, storage and processing
C. Laboratory examinations
   1. basic tests
   2. special tests
D. Biochemical manifestation of disease
E. Laboratory operations

4. Proteins and Enzymes 25% of subtest
5% of total exam

A. Biochemical theory and physiology
B. Specimen selection, collection, transport, storage and processing
C. Laboratory examinations
   1. basic tests
   2. special tests
D. Biochemical manifestation of disease
E. Laboratory operations

5. Acid Base-Electrolytes 25% of subtest
5% of total exam

A. Biochemical theory and physiology
B. Specimen selection, collection, transport, storage and processing
C. Laboratory examinations
   1. basic tests
   2. special tests
D. Biochemical manifestation of disease
E. Laboratory operations

6. Special Chemistry (Endocrinology, TDM and others) 10% of subtest
2% of total exam

A. Biochemical theory and physiology
B. Specimen selection, collection, transport, storage and processing
C. Laboratory examinations
D. Biochemical manifestation of disease
E. Laboratory operations

7. Instrumentation 20% of subtest
4% of total exam

A. Principles of operation
B. Essential components
C. Laboratory operations

BLOOD BANK (20% OF TOTAL EXAMINATION)

1. Red Blood Cells 60% of subtest
12% of total exam

A. Immunologic and genetic theory and principles
B. Specimen and component selection, collection, transport, storage and processing
C. Laboratory examinations
   1. basic tests
   2. special tests
D. Donor requirements
E. Laboratory operations

2. Platelets 5% of subtest
1% of total exam

A. Immunologic and genetic theory and principles

B. Specimen and component selection, collection, transport, storage and processing
C. Laboratory examinations
   1. basic tests
   2. special tests
D. Donor requirements
E. Laboratory operations

3. Other Components 10% of subtest
2% of total exam

A. Immunologic and genetic theory and principles
B. Specimen and component selection, collection, transport, storage and processing
C. Laboratory examinations
   1. basic tests
   2. special tests
D. Donor requirements
E. Laboratory operations

4. Hemotherapy 25% of subtest
5% of total exam

A. Transfusions
B. Phlebotomy
C. Apheresis
D. Adverse reactions
E. Clinical applications
F. Laboratory operations

IMMUNOLOGY (10% OF TOTAL EXAMINATION)

1. Humoral Immunity 65% of subtest
6.5% of total exam

A. Anatomy and physiology
B. Specimen selection, collection, transport, storage and processing
C. Laboratory examinations
   1. basic tests
   2. special tests
D. Immunologic manifestation of disease
E. Laboratory operations

2. Cellular Immunity 10% of subtest
1% of total exam

A. Anatomy and physiology
B. Specimen selection, collection, transport, storage and processing
C. Laboratory examinations
   1. basic tests
   2. special tests
D. Immunologic manifestation of disease
E. Laboratory operations

3. Autoimmunity 20% of subtest
2% of total exam

A. Anatomy and physiology
B. Specimen selection, collection, transport, storage and processing
C. Laboratory examinations
   1. basic tests
   2. special tests
D. Immunologic manifestation of disease
E. Laboratory operations

4. Allergy and Immediate Hypersensitivity
5% of subtest
0.5% of total exam

A. Anatomy and physiology
B. Specimen selection, collection, transport, storage and processing
C. Laboratory examinations
   1. basic tests
   2. special tests
D. Immunologic manifestation of disease
E. Laboratory operations

BODY FLUIDS (10% OF TOTAL EXAMINATION)

1. Urine 80% of subtest
8% of total exam

A. Anatomy and physiology
B. Specimen selection, collection, transport, storage and processing
C. Laboratory examinations
   1. basic tests
   2. special tests
   3. principles of microscopy
D. Related conditions and disorders
E. Laboratory operations

2. Other Body Fluids (CSF, feces, others)
20% of subtest
2% of total exam

A. Anatomy and physiology
B. Specimen selection, collection, transport, storage and processing
C. Laboratory examinations
   1. basic tests
   2. special tests
   3. principles of microscopy
D. Related conditions and disorders
E. Laboratory operations

COMPETENCY STATEMENTS
MEDICAL TECHNOLOGIST

In regard to Microbiology (M), Hematology (H), Chemistry (C), Body Fluids (BF), Immunology (I), and Blood Bank (BB), at career entry the Medical Technologist:

Task	Task Definitions	Content Areas
Defines and/or Identifies	- principles of basic laboratory procedures	M, H, C, BF, I, BB
	- principles of special laboratory procedures	*
	- basic procedures related to testing	*
	- special procedures related to testing	*
	- fundamental biological characteristics as they pertain to laboratory testing	*
	- standard operating procedures	*
	- sources of error in laboratory testing	*
	- fundamental characteristics of laboratory operations	*
Selects and/or Prepares and/or Performs	- method	M, H, C, BF, I, BB
	- procedural course of action	*
	- reagents for test	*
	- instruments to perform test	*
	- controls for test	*
Calculates	- results from supplied data	M, H, C, BF, I, BB
	- results from obtained data	*
	- statistics for quality assurance	*
Associates and/or Correlates	- laboratory findings and clinical data to assess test results and procedures	M, H, C, BF, I, BB
	- laboratory findings and quality control data to assess test results and procedures	*
	- laboratory findings with other laboratory data to assess test results and procedures	*
Analyzes and/or Evaluates	- laboratory findings to verify results	M, H, C, BF, I, BB
	- laboratory findings to check for possible source of errors	*
	- laboratory findings to take a course of action	*
	- laboratory findings to take corrective action	*
	- laboratory findings to determine possible inconsistent results	*
	- laboratory findings to assist in recognizing health and disease states	*
	- laboratory findings to verify quality assurance for a given test	*
	- laboratory findings to assess validity of a procedure for a given test	*
	- laboratory findings to determine appropriate instrument/instrument parameters for a given test	*
	- laboratory findings to assure laboratory safety	*

CONTENT OUTLINE
MEDICAL TECHNOLOGIST

> **NOTE:** Laboratory Operations is part of all content areas.
>
> **LABORATORY OPERATIONS**
> 1. Quality assurance
> 2. Safety
> 3. Management
> 4. Research and development
> 5. Instruments
> 6. Education
> 7. Laboratory mathematics

All percentages are approximate ranges to be included on the examination.

MICROBIOLOGY (20% OF TOTAL EXAMINATION)

1. **Bacteria 60% of subtest**
   12% of total exam
   A. Morphology, cultural and growth characteristics
   B. Specimen and/or media selection, collection, transport, storage and processing
   C. Laboratory examinations
      1. basic tests
      2. special tests
   D. Infectious diseases
   E. Laboratory operations

2. **Fungi 10% subtest**
   2% of total exam
   A. Morphology, cultural and growth characteristics
   B. Specimen and/or media selection, collection, transport, storage and processing
   C. Laboratory examinations
      1. basic tests
      2. special tests
   D. Infectious diseases
   E. Laboratory operations

3. **Mycobacteria 10% of subtest**
   2% of total exam
   A. Morphology, cultural and growth characteristics
   B. Specimen and/or media selection, collection, transport, storage and processing
   C. Laboratory examinations
      1. basic tests
      2. special tests
   D. Infectious diseases
   E. Laboratory operations

4. **Parasites 10% of subtest**
   2% of total exam
   A. Morphology, cultural and growth characteristics
   B. Specimen and/or media selection, collection, transport, storage and processing
   C. Laboratory examinations
      1. basic tests
      2. special tests
   D. Infectious diseases
   E. Laboratory operations

5. **Viruses, Rickettsiae and Other Microorganisms**
   10% of subtest
   2% of total exam
   A. Morphology, cultural and growth characteristics
   B. Specimen and/or media selection, collection, transport, storage and processing
   C. Laboratory examinations
      1. basic tests
      2. special tests
   D. Infectious diseases
   E. Laboratory operations

HEMATOLOGY (20% OF TOTAL EXAMINATION)

1. **Erythrocytes 35% of subtest**
   7% of total exam
   A. Anatomy and physiology of hematopoiesis
   B. Specimen selection, collection, transport, storage and processing
   C. Laboratory examinations
      1. basic tests
      2. special tests
   D. Hematopoietic diseases
   E. Laboratory operations

2. **Leukocytes 35% of subtest**
   7% of total exam
   A. Anatomy and physiology of hematopoiesis
   B. Specimen selection, collection, transport, storage and processing
   C. Laboratory examinations
      1. basic tests
      2. special tests
   D. Hematopoietic diseases
   E. Laboratory operations

3. **Thrombocytes 10% of subtest**
2% of total exam
   A. Anatomy and physiology of hematopoiesis
   B. Specimen selection, collection, transport, storage and processing
   C. Laboratory examinations
      1. basic tests
      2. special tests
   D. Hematopoietic disorders
   E. Laboratory operations

4. **Hemostasis 20% of subtest**
4% of total exam
   A. Physiology of hemostasis
   B. Specimen selection, collection, transport, storage and processing
   C. Laboratory examinations
      1. basic tests
      2. special tests
   D. Hemostatic diseases
   E. Laboratory operations

CHEMISTRY (20% OF TOTAL EXAMINATION)

1. **Carbohydrates 10% of subtest**
2% of total exam
   A. Biochemical theory and physiology
   B. Specimen selection, collection, transport, storage and processing
   C. Laboratory examinations
      1. basic tests
      2. special tests
   D. Biochemical manifestation of disease
   E. Laboratory operations

2. **Lipids and Lipoproteins 5% of subtest**
1% of total exam
   A. Biochemical theory and physiology
   B. Specimen selection, collection, transport, storage and processing
   C. Laboratory examinations
      1. basic tests
      2. special tests
   D. Biochemical manifestation of disease
   E. Laboratory operations

3. **Heme Derivatives 5% of subtest**
1% of total exam
   A. Biochemical theory and physiology
   B. Specimen selection, collection, transport, storage and processing
   C. Laboratory examinations
      1. basic tests
      2. special tests
   D. Biochemical manifestation of disease
   E. Laboratory operations

4. **Proteins and Enzymes 25% of subtest**
5% of total exam
   A. Biochemical theory and physiology
   B. Specimen selection, collection, transport, storage and processing
   C. Laboratory examinations
      1. basic tests
      2. special tests
   D. Biochemical manifestation of disease
   E. Laboratory operations

5. **Acid Base-Electrolytes 25% of subtest**
5% of total exam
   A. Biochemical theory and physiology
   B. Specimen selection, collection, transport, storage and processing
   C. Laboratory examinations
      1. basic tests
      2. special tests
   D. Biochemical manifestation of disease
   E. Laboratory operations

6. **Special Chemistry (Endocrinology, TDM and others) 10% of subtest**
2% of total exam
   A. Biochemical theory and physiology
   B. Specimen selection, collection, transport, storage and processing
   C. Laboratory examinations
   D. Biochemical manifestation of disease
   E. Laboratory operations

7. **Instrumentation 20% of subtest**
4% of total exam
   A. Principles of operation
   B. Essential components
   C. Laboratory operations

BLOOD BANK (20% OF TOTAL EXAMINATION)

1. **Red Blood Cells 60% of subtest**
12% of total exam
   A. Immunologic and genetic theory and principles
   B. Specimen and component selection, collection, transport, storage and processing

C. Laboratory examinations
   1. basic tests
   2. special tests
D. Donor requirements
E. Laboratory operations

2. Platelets 5% of subtest
1% of total exam

A. Immunologic and genetic theory and principles
B. Specimen and component selection, collection, transport, storage and processing
C. Laboratory examinations
   1. basic tests
   2. special tests
D. Donor requirements
E. Laboratory operations

3. Other Components 10% of subtest
2% of total exam

A. Immunologic and genetic theory and principles
B. Specimen and component selection, collection, transport, storage and processing
C. Laboratory examinations
   1. basic tests
   2. special tests
D. Donor requirements
E. Laboratory operations

4. Hemotherapy 25% of subtest
5% of total exam

A. Transfusions
B. Phlebotomy
C. Apheresis
D. Adverse reactions
E. Clinical applications
F. Laboratory operations

IMMUNOLOGY (10% OF TOTAL EXAMINATION)

1. Humoral Immunity 65% of subtest
6.5% of total exam

A. Anatomy and physiology
B. Specimen selection, collection, transport, storage and processing
C. Laboratory examinations
   1. basic tests
   2. special tests
D. Immunologic manifestation of disease
E. Laboratory operations

2. Cellular Immunity 10% of subtest
1% of total exam

A. Anatomy and physiology
B. Specimen selection, collection, transport, storage and processing
C. Laboratory examinations
   1. basic tests
   2. special tests
D. Immunologic manifestation of disease
E. Laboratory operations

3. Autoimmunity 20% of subtest
2% of total exam

A. Anatomy and physiology
B. Specimen selection, collection, transport, storage and processing
C. Laboratory examinations
   1. basic tests
   2. special tests
D. Immunologic manifestation of disease
E. Laboratory operations

4. Allergy and Immediate Hypersensitivity
5% of subtest
0.5% of total exam

A. Anatomy and physiology
B. Specimen selection, collection, transport, storage and processing
C. Laboratory examinations
   1. basic tests
   2. special tests
D. Immunologic manifestation of disease
E. Laboratory operations

BODY FLUIDS (10% OF TOTAL EXAMINATION)

1. Urine 80% of subtest
8% of total exam

A. Anatomy and physiology
B. Specimen selection, collection, transport, storage and processing
C. Laboratory examinations
   1. basic tests
   2. special tests
   3. principles of microscopy
D. Related conditions and disorders
E. Laboratory operations

2. Other Body Fluids (CSF, feces, others)
20% of subtest
2% of total exam

A. Anatomy and physiology
B. Specimen selection, collection, transport, storage and processing
C. Laboratory examinations
   1. basic tests
   2. special tests
   3. principles of microscopy
D. Related conditions and disorders
E. Laboratory operations

CHAPTER 8

Examination Scoring

Setting the Absolute Standard

Criterion-referenced testing is a form of measurement designed to measure an examinee's performance compared to a stated standard or criterion. For the Board of Registry examinations, the criterion is called the minimum pass score (MPS). Any individual who achieves the level of performance represented by the minimum pass score passes the examination. Those who do not meet this standard fail the examination.

In 1980, the Board of Registry adopted a policy of criterion-referenced testing. Absolute standards are established by a systematic evaluation of each item. The standard is equated from cycle to cycle to ensure that it is consistent from examination to examination.

Why Items Are Deleted from Scoring

The Board of Registry uses standard procedures for psychometric analysis to ensure that each examinee receives a fairly prepared and scored examination.

After a question is given on an examination it is subjected to rigorous statistical evaluation. Questions are evaluated through item analysis statistics, and tests are evaluated based on summary statistics. Item statistics are used to identify items that should be deleted from scoring. To ensure the continued quality of the examination, questions that prove unsatisfactory are excluded (by deletion) from the calculation of examination summary statistics and examinee scores.

Item (question) statistics include measures of difficulty and discrimination. Difficulty level is defined as the proportion or percentage of examinees selecting each response (p-value). The correct response or best answer should draw the highest proportion of the population while the distractors may draw a smaller percentage of the population. This provides an index of how easy or difficult the question was for a particular population.

Item discrimination provides an indication of how well the question differentiates between those examinees who did well on the total examination and those who did not. The computation compares or correlates the performance of candidates who selected the best answer on the question with the performance of those candidates who did well on the total examination. A positive correlation is anticipated for the correct response (best answer), and negative correlations are anticipated for the distractors. These expectations are based on the assumption that those who did well on the question should do well on the test.

The difficulty (percentage selecting the response) and discrimination (point biserial correlation) are considered simultaneously to meaningfully evaluate a question. Together, they indicate whether a question is measuring appropriately. Item analysis data do not reflect the value of the knowledge, task, or cognitive skill being tested, but rather suggest the potential contribution of the question toward making the decision to pass or fail an examinee.

After each item in the test has been carefully reviewed, the total test is analyzed. The summary statistics for the examination are critically reviewed. Typically, summary statistics include the number and percentage of passing and failing examinees; the number of questions scored on the test; and the mean, standard deviation, mode, range, and internal consistency values.

The examination mean, the sum of the scores on a test divided by the number of scores, is the most important measure of central tendency. The examination standard deviation is the measure of the variance of the scores around the mean. A large standard deviation indicates a lot of variance among the examination scores. The examination mode is the most frequent score on the test. The examination range is the number of points between the highest and lowest scores on the examination.

The internal consistency or internal reliability estimate assesses the consistency of measurement among items on an examination. A perfect reliability among questions would be a one-to-one relationship or 1.0. The difference between perfect reliability and calculated internal reliability indicates the potential amount of measurement error on the test. More information about the analysis of test items and tests may be obtained from the books and articles noted in the education section of the reading lists, "Education and Laboratory Operations."

Score Reporting

After the examination has been statistically evaluated, Examinee Performance Reports are generated and distributed to the candidates approximately six weeks following the date of test administration. (Test results are not released by telephone to anyone.) The purpose of the report is to provide examinees with specific information about their performance on the examination. The examinees can then use this information to analyze their performance. By using the subtest results to determine areas of weakness, the results of the test can be used to develop a course of study.

The following explanation refers to the sample Examinee Performance Report in Figure 3. The first paragraph provides an explanation of how to interpret the profile. Key information is presented under "YOUR

Figure 3. Sample Board of Registry Examinee Performance Report.

BOARD OF REGISTRY

EXAMINEE PERFORMANCE REPORT

MEDICAL TECHNOLOGIST EXAMINATION - AUGUST 1988

999999999
BARBARA JONES
ELM STREET
CHICAGO, IL 60606

THIS REPORT PROVIDES INFORMATION CONCERNING YOUR EXAMINATION PERFORMANCE. A SCALED MINIMUM PASS SCORE (MPS) OF 400 WAS REQUIRED TO PASS THE TEST. A REPORT OF YOUR SCORE ON THE TOTAL TEST AND STATUS IS SHOWN IN THE TABLE. FOLLOWING THE TABLE IS A LIST OF EXAMINATION ITEMS THAT YOU ANSWERED INCORRECTLY. INFORMATION CONCERNING THESE ITEMS IS SUMMARIZED IN AN ITEM DESCRIPTOR LIST ENCLOSED WITH THIS REPORT. THESE ITEM DESCRIPTORS IDENTIFY SUBJECT AREA, CONTENT AND TAXONOMY LEVEL OF EACH EXAMINATION ITEM AND SHOULD BE USEFUL TO YOU IN EVALUATING YOUR PERFORMANCE MORE SPECIFICALLY.

YOUR PERFORMANCE SUMMARY

MPS	YOUR SCORE	STATUS
400	702	PASS

LIST OF ITEMS WITH INCORRECT RESPONSES

1 8 9 15 17 25 28 29 44 63 68 88 97 110 134 135 138 161
181 182 187 190 193 195

PERFORMANCE SUMMARY." A scaled minimum pass score (MPS) of 400 is the criterion against which all examinees are measured. Individuals who achieve or exceed the MPS pass the examination; others fail. The decision to pass or fail is based on the total examination score. Pass or fail status is noted under STATUS. The LIST OF ITEMS WITH INCORRECT RESPONSES provides the sequence number of the items answered incorrectly on the examination.

The Medical Technologist and Medical Laboratory Technician examinations subtests are Microbiology, Blood Banking, Chemistry, Hematology, Immunology, and Body Fluids including Urinalysis. The item descriptor list details the subtest, tasks, and cognitive skill levels of all questions scored on the examination. Passing examinees can assess their level of knowledge in each area, and failing examinees can determine weaker areas by comparing the list of items with incorrect responses to the Item Descriptor list. This can provide specific information regarding areas of strength and weakness. For example, if an examinee found in reviewing the item descriptors for incorrectly answered questions that many of the missed questions related to "specimen processing" across content areas, it would then be possible to outline a course of study with this emphasis across all content areas.

Item Descriptors

An item descriptor is a shorthand method of describing the content and skill tested in a specific test question. Item descriptors specify the content, competency (task), and cognitive skill (taxonomy) necessary to answer a given question. Through this feedback, examinees should be able to identify the content and task areas tested as well as ascertain their strengths and weaknesses as measured by the examination.

The form of the item descriptors requires some explanation. Item descriptors are developed using the following sentence structure:

In regard to ________________________ the examinee will
1. Subtest Category

be able to ________________________
2. Task/Competence

concerning ________________________
3. Subject Content

for/of ________________________
4. Specifics

using the cognitive skill process of ________________.
5. Taxonomy

The first unit of the item descriptor indicates the SUBTEST or major content area in which the question is classified. The number of item descriptors with each of these first units matches the number of questions reported for the subtest. Subtests are listed on the Examinee Performance Report.

The TASK area is the second unit and relates directly to the competency statements found in Chapter 7, "Examination Content." The third and fourth units refer to CONTENT SPECIFICS. In many instances, these words can be traced to the content outlines found in Chapter 7. However, in an effort to be as specific as possible, the item descriptors are often more specific than the outlines and specify the specific tests, types of organisms, or quality control procedures covered in a question.

The fifth unit indicates the cognitive skill required to answer the question, typically called the TAXONOMY level (see description and examples of cognitive skill levels in Chapter 6, "Examination Development").

The following are examples of printed item descriptors:

	SUBTEST	TASK	CONTENT SPECIFICS	CONTENT SPECIFICS	TAXONOMY
1.	BF	CCLD	URINE	SPECIFIC GRAVITY	3
2.	HEMA	ELF	QC	PROTHROMBIN TIME	2

When translated from abbreviations, the item descriptors would read as follows:

1. In regard to body fluids, the examinee will be able to correlate clinical and laboratory data related to urine specimen, specific gravity test, at the taxonomy level 3 (problem-solving cognitive skill level).
2. In regard to hematology, the examinee will be able to evaluate laboratory findings related to performing quality control procedures on a prothrombin time test at the taxonomy level 2 (interpretative cognitive skill level).

The item descriptor list enables you to analyze each question on an examination in terms of its content, task, and cognitive skill. Lists of item descriptors for the Medical Laboratory Technician examinations from 1984 to 1987 are provided in Appendix A and for the Medical Technologist examinations from 1982 to 1987 in Appendix B.

Use the item descriptor lists to further structure your review for the certification examination. Each list represents the distribution of items on a particular examination and verifies the content, task, and cognitive skill distribution for each examination cycle.

CHAPTER 9

Practice Examination

Directions

There are 100 questions on this practice examination. Not only will this test give you the opportunity to simulate the test conditions, but it will also enable you to diagnose your strengths and weaknesses when you score the test. In addition, you will have the opportunity to indicate your answers on an answer sheet like the one used on examination day. Since some people find it useful to repeat a test at several points during their course of study, multiple copies of the answer sheets are provided at the back of the book.

Find a quiet place and allow yourself two hours of uninterrupted continuous time to complete the examination.

Choose the one best answer for each question and mark the appropriate response on the replica of the machine-scorable answer sheet by completely blackening the circle that corresponds to the response of your choice. Note that the questions are numbered consecutively DOWN (not across) the answer sheet. Be sure that the circle you mark on the answer sheet corresponds to the question on the test. DO NOT MAKE ANY MARKS ON YOUR ANSWER SHEET OTHER THAN YOUR IDENTIFICATION INFORMATION AND YOUR ANSWERS.

READ EACH QUESTION CAREFULLY. Pace yourself. Do not spend too much time on any one question. If a question is particularly time consuming or difficult, proceed to the next question. YOUR SCORE IS BASED UPON THE TOTAL NUMBER OF QUESTIONS YOU ANSWER CORRECTLY; therefore, it is to your advantage to record your best judgment for EVERY question, even if you are not completely sure of the answer.

On page 38 is a reproduction of the instructions for filling out examination answer sheets. It is not necessary to complete all of these instructions during the study process. After you have completed the examination, score it using the scoring instructions (in next section) and the answer key at the end of the test.

INSTRUCTIONS FOR FILLING OUT EXAMINATION ANSWER SHEET

CHECKING AND RECORDING IDENTIFICATION INFORMATION

ALL IDENTIFICATION INFORMATION AND ANSWERS MUST BE COMPLETED USING A NO. 1 OR 2 SOFT LEAD PENCIL. Answers marked with a hard pencil, ink or felt-tip pen cannot be scored. If you did not bring a No. 1 or 2 lead pencil, please ask your proctor for one.

Read these instructions carefully and fill out your answer sheet while you are waiting for the examination to begin. The answer sheet has two sides. Please turn to Side One.

YOU WILL NOTE THAT ON SIDE ONE IN THE GRID TO THE LEFT OF THE ANSWER SHEET YOUR EXAMINATION CODE HAS BEEN PRE-CODED AND PRE-PRINTED. Check to make certain that this code is for the examination for which you have applied and been determined eligible. EXAMPLE: MEDICAL TECHNOLOGIST - 01 (SEE LIST BELOW). You must complete this information if it has not been pre-printed and pre-coded. Answer sheets that do not contain this information cannot be scored.

INSTRUCTIONS FOR PRINTING AND CODING

Carefully print and code your Social Security Number (Personal Identification Number) in the designated area on Side One of the answer sheet. From left to right in the top row, print one number per space, and then code by filling in the corresponding circle in each column. Refer to your Authorization Slip for your personal Identification Number.

Check that both your Personal Identification Number and Exam Code have been entered correctly. SUGGESTION: Exchange your Authorization Slip and answer sheet with the person next to you to double check the information coded.

Record the test booklet number in the space provided below your Personal Identification Number on your answer sheet. Please be certain to include the letter that precedes this test booklet number (See example below).

The example given illustrates how the Identification Number and Exam Code should be printed and coded.

EXAMPLE: Identification Number 123456789 and Exam Code 01 - (Medical Technologist) are recorded in the example to the right. Note that the two digit Exam Code has been taken from the list below. USE your Personal Identification Number DO NOT use the number that appears in this example.

IDENTIFICATION									EXAM CODE	
1	2	3	4	5	6	7	8	9	0	1
0	0	0	0	0	0	0	0	0	●	0
●	1	1	1	1	1	1	1	1	1	●
2	●	2	2	2	2	2	2	2	2	2
3	3	●	3	3	3	3	3	3	3	3
4	4	4	●	4	4	4	4	4	4	4
5	5	5	5	●	5	5	5	5	5	5
6	6	6	6	6	●	6	6	6	6	6
7	7	7	7	7	7	●	7	7	7	7
8	8	8	8	8	8	8	●	8	8	8
9	9	9	9	9	9	9	9	●	9	9

TEST BOOKLET NUMBER				
A	0	5	2	6

	EXAM TYPE	EXAM CODE
Medical Technologist	MT	01
Medical Laboratory Technician	MLT	02
Histologic Technician	HT	04
Technologist in Chemistry	C	05
Specialist in Chemistry	SC	06
Technologist in Hematology	H	07
Specialist in Hematology	SH	08

	EXAM TYPE	EXAM CODE
Technologist in Microbiology	M	09
Specialist in Microbiology	SM	10
Cytotechnologist	CT	11
Specialist in Blood Banking	SBB	14
Histotechnologist	HTL	15
Technologist in Immunology	I	16
Specialist in Immunology	SI	17
Technologist in Blood Banking	BB	18

INDICATE YOUR NAME, EXAM TYPE AND EXAMINATION DATE IN THE SPACE PROVIDED ON SIDE ONE OF YOUR ANSWER SHEET.

WAIT FOR VERBAL INSTRUCTIONS FROM YOUR PROCTOR

NAME/ADDRESS CHANGES: Any change of name and/or address will not be made from the sign-in list or your answer sheet. Please indicate the change on the reverse side of your Authorization Slip supplied with your scheduling information.

Scoring Your Practice Examination

1. Compare your answer choices to the correct answers indicated in the practice test answer key. Circle the INCORRECT answers on the answer sheet.
2. Fill in the Performance Summary Sheet on page 40 and do the appropriate calculations to determine your TOTAL test and subtest scores.
3. Review the items you answered incorrectly to identify areas that you need to study. Develop a systematic pattern for studying these content areas and attempting the review questions in this guide.

****

PERFORMANCE SUMMARY SHEET

SUBTEST	ITEM NUMBERS	NUMBER OF ITEMS CORRECT	DIVIDE BY	PROPORTION CORRECT
Blood Bank	1-20		20	
Chemistry	21-40		20	
Hematology	41-60		20	
Immunology	61-70		10	
Microbiology	71-90		20	
Urinalysis (BF)	91-100		10	
TOTAL	1-100		100	

****

Practice Examination

FOR EACH QUESTION, CHOOSE THE ONE ANSWER THAT IS MOST CORRECT. MARK YOUR ANSWER ON YOUR ANSWER SHEET IN THE APPROPRIATE SPACE. ANSWERS INDICATED IN THIS EXAMINATION BOOKLET WILL NOT BE SCORED.

1. Proteolytic enzyme treatment of red cells usually destroys which of the following antigens?

   a. C
   b. E
   c. M
   d. Jk^a

2. When mixed field reactions with anti-A and anti-A,B and a negative reaction with anti-A_1 lectin (Dolichos biflorus) are observed, the only conclusion that can be reached without further testing is that the patient is presumptively group:

   a. A
   b. A_1
   c. A_2
   d. A_3

3. Following the second spin in the preparation of platelet concentrate to be stored at room temperature, the platelets should be:

   a. allowed to sit undisturbed for 1-2 hours
   b. agitated immediately
   c. pooled immediately
   d. transfused within 48 hours

4. Which one of the following histories represents an acceptable donor?

	HCT	BP	Temp	Pulse	Age	Sex
a.	39	110/70	99.8	75	40	F
b.	40	135/85	98.6	80	35	M
c.	41	90/50	99.4	65	65	M
d.	45	115/80	98.6	102	17	M

5. Hemoglobinuria, hypotension, and generalized bleeding are symptoms of which of the following transfusion reactions?

   a. allergic
   b. circulatory overload
   c. hemolytic
   d. anaphylactic

For questions 6 and 7, refer to the following panel:

Vial No.	Rh-hr								MNS				P		Lewis		Lutheran		Kell						Duffy		Kidd		Sex Linked	
	D	C	E	c	e	f	C^w	V	M	N	S	s	P_1	Tj^a	Le^a	Le^b	Lu^a	Lu^b	K	k	Kp^a	Kp^b	Js^a	Js^b	Fy^a	Fy^b	Jk^a	Jk^b	Xg^a	AG
1.	0	0	0	+	+	+	0	0	+	0	+	+	+	+	0	+	+	+	0	+	0	+	0	+	+	+	0	+	0	++
2.	0	0	0	+	+	+	0	0	0	+	0	+	+	+	+	0	0	+	+	+	0	+	0	+	0	+	+	0	+	++
3.	0	+	0	+	+	+	0	0	0	+	0	+	0	+	0	+	0	+	0	+	0	+	0	+	0	+	0	+	+	0
4.	0	0	+	+	0	0	0	0	+	+	+	+	+	+	0	+	0	+	0	+	0	+	0	+	+	+	+	+	0	++
5.	+	0	0	+	+	+	0	+	0	+	0	+	$+^s$	+	0	0	0	+	0	+	0	+	0	+	0	0	+	0	+	0
6.	+	0	0	+	+	+	0	0	+	+	0	0	+	+	0	+	0	+	0	+	0	+	+	+	0	0	+	+	+	0
7.	+	+	0	0	+	0	+	0	+	0	+	+	vw +	+	0	+	0	+	0	+	+	+	0	+	0	+	+	+	+	0
8.	+	+	0	0	+	0	0	0	+	0	0	+	$+^s$	+	0	+	0	+	+	+	0	+	0	+	0	+	0	+	+	++
9.	+	+	0	0	+	0	+	0	+	+	0	+	0	+	+	0	0	+	0	+	0	+	0	+	+	0	+	+	+	++
10.	+	0	+	+	0	0	0	0	0	+	0	+	+	+	0	+	0	+	0	+	0	+	0	+	+	0	0	+	+	++
11.	+	+	0	0	+	0	0	0	+	+	0	+	+	+	0	+	0	+	0	+	+	+	0	+	0	+	+	+	+	0
																									Autocontrol					0

6. Based on the results of the above panel, the patient most likely has antibodies:

   a. anti-M and anti-K

   b. anti-E, anti-Fy^a, and anti-K

   c. anti-Fy^a and anti-M

   d. anti-E and anti-Le^b

7. Based on the results of the above panel, which technique would be most helpful in determining antibody specificity?

   a. proteolytic enzyme treatment
   b. urine neutralization
   c. autoadsorption
   d. saliva inhibition

8. A unit of very rare cells has been deglycerolized for ten hours. The patient's condition has stabilized and transfusion of these cells is no longer necessary. Which of the following is the most appropriate course of action?

   a. Urge the attending physician to transfuse the patient due to the value of the rare cells.
   b. Discard the unit.
   c. Extend the expiration time and date an additional 24 hours.
   d. Document the value of the rare cells and refreeze before 20 hours have elapsed.

9. If the mother is DCe with anti-c (titer of 32 at AHG), the father is DCce, and the baby is D-negative and not affected with hemolytic disease of the newborn, what is the baby's most probable Rh genotype?

   a. r'r'

   b. r'r

   c. R_1R_1

   d. r"r

10. An assay of plasma from a bag of cryoprecipitate yields a concentration of 9 units of factor VIII per milliliter of cryoprecipitate. If the volume is 9 mL, what is the factor VIII content of the bag?

   a. 9
   b. 18
   c. 27
   d. 81

11. To confirm the specificity of a serum antibody identified as anti-P_1, a neutralization study was performed and the following results were obtained:

Neutralized serum	no reaction
Control - serum with saline	no reaction

What conclusion can be made from these results?

a. Anti-P_1 is confirmed.
b. Anti-P_1 is ruled out.
c. A second antibody is suspected due to the negative control.
d. Anti-P_1 cannot be confirmed due to the negative control.

12. When evaluating a suspected transfusion reaction, what is the ideal sample collection time for a bilirubin determination?

a. 5-7 hours posttransfusion
b. 12 hours posttransfusion
c. 24 hours posttransfusion
d. 48 hours posttransfusion

13. Results of a serum sample tested against a panel of reagent red cells provide presumptive evidence of an alloantibody directed against a high-incidence antigen. Further investigation to confirm the specificity should include which of the following?

a. Serum testing against red cells from random donors.
b. Serum testing against other examples of red cells known to lack high-incidence antigens.
c. Serum testing against enzyme-treated autologous cells.
d. Testing of an eluate prepared from the patient's red cells.

14. A 35-year-old woman, gravida 1, para 1, who never received a blood transfusion, has anti-C plus anti-D in her serum. Nine months ago, she received RhIG after delivery. Testing of the patient, her husband, and the child revealed the following:

	Anti-D	Anti-C	Anti-E	Anti-c	Anti-e
Patient	neg	neg	neg	+	+
Father	+	+	neg	+	+
Child	+	+	neg	+	+

What is the most likely explanation for these results?

a. Patient treatment with RhIG failed.
b. Patient has anti-D from RhIG dose.
c. Patient formed anti-G.
d. Patient has naturally occurring anti-D.

15. Tests on the supernatant of a deglycerolized unit of red blood cells yielded the following results:

Osmolality	350 mOsm
Red blood cell recovery	80%
Plasma hemoglobin	100 mg/dL

Which of the following actions is indicated?

a. rewash the unit
b. discard the unit
c. release the unit for transfusion
d. check the automated equipment

16. A temperature rise of 1°C or more occurring in association with a transfusion is usually indicative of which of the following transfusion reactions?

a. febrile
b. circulatory overload
c. hemolytic
d. anaphylactic

17. An adult patient who is actively bleeding has the following test results:

ABO	AB
Rh	positive
Screen	negative

Six units of blood are ordered STAT. The blood bank has the following packed red blood cell units available:

2 AB positive	12 A positive	2 B positive
1 AB negative	4 A negative	1 B negative

Which of the following should be crossmatched for this patient while more blood is being ordered?

a. A positive
b. AB positive
c. B positive
d. AB negative

18. The following phenotypes were determined for a patient's family:

Family Member	ABO	HLA			
Father	A	A3	A28	B18	B37
Mother	B	A2	A11	B7	B40
Patient	B	A3	A11	B7	B37
Sibling 1	AB	A3	A11	B7	B37
Sibling 2	B	A2	A3	B18	B40
Sibling 3	B	A3	A11	B7	B37
Sibling 4	A	A11	A28	B7	B18

On the basis of the information given, the best possible kidney donor for the patient would be:

a. mother
b. sibling 1
c. sibling 2
d. sibling 3

19. The following results were obtained:

	Anti-A	Anti-B	Anti-D	D^u	DAT	AB Screen
Infant	0	0	0	NT	4+	NT
Mother	4+	0	0	0	NT	Anti-D

NT = Not tested

Which of the following is the most probable explanation for these results?

a. ABO hemolytic disease of the newborn
b. Rh hemolytic disease of the newborn, infant has received intrauterine transfusions
c. Rh hemolytic disease of the newborn, infant has a false-negative Rh typing
d. large fetomaternal hemorrhage

20. A 24-year-old man with hemophilia is involved in an auto accident and is actively bleeding into his left knee joint. Factor VIII assay results are 8%. The blood product of choice is:

a. fibrinogen
b. fresh frozen plasma
c. whole blood
d. cryoprecipitate

21. In a specimen collected for plasma glucose analysis, sodium fluoride:

a. serves as a coenzyme of hexokinase
b. prevents reactivity of non-glucose reducing substances
c. precipitates proteins
d. inhibits glycolysis

22. A 2-year-old child is reported to have coarse features and is somewhat dwarfed. Laboratory results reveal a decreased serum T-4. Of the following, the most informative additional laboratory test would be the serum:

a. thyroxine-binding globulin (TBG)
b. thyroid-stimulating hormone (TSH)
c. triiodothyronine (T-3)
d. cholesterol

23. Which of the following occurs when serum is allowed to stand at room temperature for a period of time?

   a. pH decreases

   b. CO_2 content increases

   c. pCO_2 decreases

   d. bicarbonate increases

24. A solution contains 5.8 gm of NaCl (MW = 58) dissolved in 0.5 L of water. What is the molarity of this solution?

   a. 0.05 M
   b. 0.1 M
   c. 0.2 M
   d. 0.5 M

25. Coulometry is used to measure:

   a. chloride
   b. pH
   c. bicarbonate
   d. ammonia

26. A potassium level of 6.8 mmol/L is obtained. The technologist's next step should be to:

   a. check the serum for hemolysis
   b. rerun the test
   c. check the age of the patient
   d. report the result

27. A one-year-old girl with a lipoprotein lipase deficiency has the following lipid profile:

Cholesterol	300 mg/100 mL	LDL	increased
Triglycerides	200 mg/100 mL	HDL	decreased
Chylomicrons	present		

   A serum specimen from this patient that was refrigerated overnight would most likely be:

   a. clear
   b. cloudy
   c. cloudy with a creamy top layer
   d. clear with a creamy top layer

28. Amyloclastic methods for the determination of serum amylase activity measure the:

a. decrease in starch concentration
b. decrease in concentration of reducing compounds
c. amount of reducing compounds formed
d. amount of glucose formed

29. Carbon monoxide is toxic because it:

a. destroys lung tissue
b. is a strong enzyme inhibitor
c. prevents removal of CO_2 from cells
d. prevents binding of oxygen with hemoglobin

30. The illustration below represents a Lineweaver-Burk plot of 1/v versus 1/[S] in an enzyme reaction:

v = reaction rate
[S] = substrate concentration

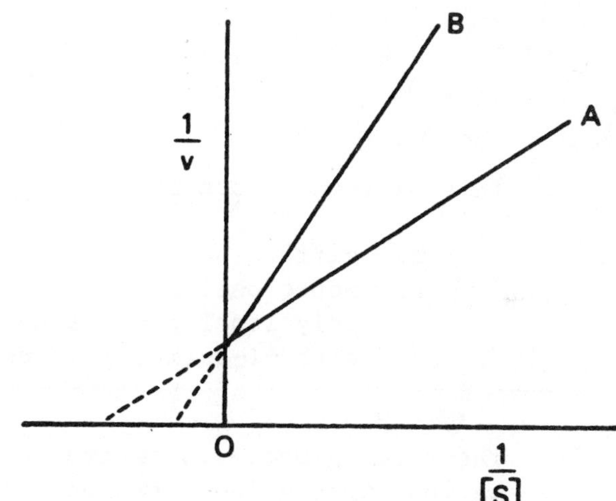

The following assumptions should be made:

The enzyme concentration was the same for reactions A and B.
The substrate concentration was in excess for reactions A and B.
Reaction A occurred under ideal conditions.

Which of the following statements about reaction B is true?

a. It illustrates noncompetitive inhibition.
b. It illustrates competitive inhibition.
c. It illustrates neither competitive nor noncompetitive inhibition.
d. It could be the result of heavy metal contamination.

For question 31, refer to the following serum protein electrophoresis pattern:

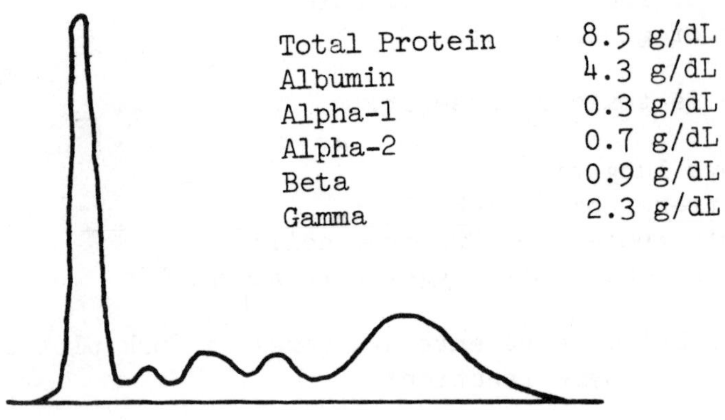

Total Protein 8.5 g/dL
Albumin 4.3 g/dL
Alpha-1 0.3 g/dL
Alpha-2 0.7 g/dL
Beta 0.9 g/dL
Gamma 2.3 g/dL

31. This pattern is consistent with:

    a. cirrhosis
    b. monoclonal gammopathy
    c. polyclonal gammopathy
    d. alpha-1-antitrypsin deficiency

---

32. The serum glucose concentration of a specimen from a diabetic patient undergoing a two-hour glucose tolerance test should return to the baseline (fasting level) after a minimum of:

    a. 30 minutes
    b. 60 minutes
    c. 90 minutes
    d. 120 minutes

33. A colorimetric method calls for the use of 0.1 mL serum, 5 mL of reagent, and 4.9 mL of water. What is the dilution of the serum in the final solution?

    a. 1 to 5
    b. 1 to 10
    c. 1 to 50
    d. 1 to 100

34. In the potentiometric measurement of hydrogen ion concentration, reference electrodes that may be used include:

a. silver-silver chloride
b. quinhydrone
c. hydroxide
d. hydrogen

35. In the sweat test, the sweating stimulant is introduced to the skin by application of:

a. filter paper moistened with pilocarpine nitrate
b. an electric current
c. copper electrodes
d. filter paper moistened with deionized water

36. Which of the following is used to verify wavelength settings for narrow bandwidth spectrophotometers?

a. didymium filter
b. prisms
c. holmium oxide glass
d. diffraction gratings

37. A 16-year-old boy is admitted to the hospital for hernia repair. A presurgical multichemistry screen reveals an alkaline phosphatase of 180 IU/L (180 U/L) and a serum bilirubin concentration of 1.9 mg/dL (32.5 μmol/L) total; 0.3 mg/dL (5.1 μmol/L) direct. History reveals that the patient has been in good health but has noted yellow sclera in times of stress. Which of the following explains these results?

a. The patient probably has a calculus of the biliary tract.
b. The elevated alkaline phosphatase and bilirubin are explained by the patient's age.
c. The patient may have constitution hyperbilirubinemia.
d. The patient probably has a pancreatic or biliary tract neoplasm.

38. The following results were obtained in a creatinine clearance evaluation:

Urine concentration	0.084 gm/dL (7.43 mmol/L)
Urine volume	1440 mL/24 hr
Serum concentration	1.4 mg/dL (124 µmol/L)
Body surface area	1.60 m^2 (average = 1.73 m^2)

The creatinine clearance in mL/min is:

a. 0.006
b. 0.022
c. 0.60
d. 64.9

39. In a continuous flow system, the pump tubing for the sample has a rating of 1.5 mL/min. The sampling rate is 90 samples/hr and the sample-to-wash ratio of the cam is 3:1. The minimum amount (mL) of serum necessary for analysis on the instrument is:

a. 0.5
b. 0.75
c. 1.0
d. 1.25

40. The following laboratory results were obtained:

Serum Electrolytes	Arterial Blood
Sodium 136 mEq/L	pH 7.32
Potassium 4.4 mEq/L	pCO_2 79 mm Hg (10.5 kPa)
Chloride 92 mEq/L	
Bicarbonate 40 mM/L	

These results are most compatible with:

a. respiratory alkalosis
b. respiratory acidosis
c. metabolic alkalosis
d. metabolic acidosis

41. Which of the following stains is closely associated with iron, ferritin, and hemosiderin?

   a. peroxidase
   b. Sudan black B
   c. periodic acid-Schiff (PAS)
   d. Prussian blue

42. On an electronic particle counter, hemoglobin determinations may be falsely elevated due to the presence of:

   a. lipemia or elevated bilirubin concentration
   b. a decreased WBC or lipemia
   c. an elevated bilirubin concentration or rouleaux
   d. rouleaux or lipemia

43. Multiple myeloma is generally characterized by:

   a. plasmacytic satellitosis in the bone marrow
   b. many plasma cells in the peripheral blood
   c. many Mott cells in the peripheral blood
   d. rouleaux formation

44. What is the mean corpuscular volume (MCV) if the hematocrit is 20%, the RBC is 1,500,000/μL, and the hemoglobin is 6 gm/dL?

   a. 68 fL
   b. 75 fL
   c. 115 fL
   d. 133 fL

For question 45, refer to the illustration below:

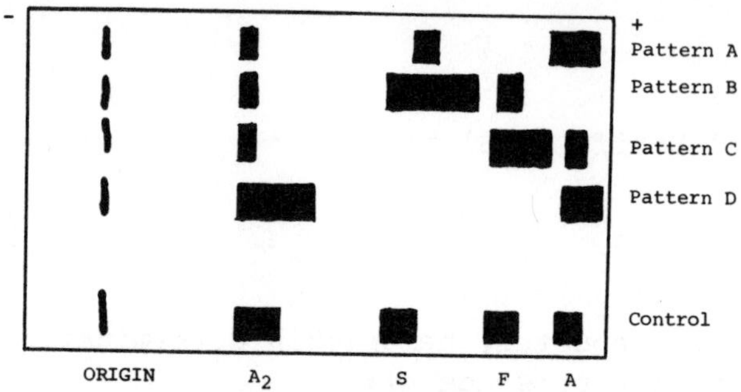

HEMOGLOBIN ELECTROPHORESIS PATTERNS AT pH 8.4
(CELLULOSE ACETATE STRIP)

45. Which of the following electrophoresis patterns is consistent with sickle cell trait?

    a. pattern A
    b. pattern B
    c. pattern C
    d. pattern D

---

46. The following results were obtained from a 35-year-old woman experiencing fatigue and weight loss:

    WBC 46,600/μL
    RBC 4,600,000/μL
    PLT 903,000/μL
    Differential 30% segs
    17% bands
    13% lymphs
    3% monos
    4% eos
    6% basos
    3% metamyelocytes
    20% myelocytes
    3% promyelocytes
    1% blasts
    4 NRBC
    Uric acid 6.4 mg/dL
    LAP 0
    Philadelphia chromosome-positive

    These results are consistent with:

    a. neutrophilic leukemoid reaction
    b. idiopathic thrombocythemia
    c. chronic granulocytic leukemia
    d. leukoerythroblastosis in myelofibrosis

47. A patient develops unexpected bleeding following three transfusions. The following test results were obtained:

Prolonged PT and APTT
Decreased fibrinogen
Increased fibrin split products
Decreased platelets

What is the most probable cause of these results?

a. familial afibrinogenemia
b. primary fibrinolysis
c. DIC
d. liver disease

48. A 56-year-old man was admitted to the hospital for treatment of a bleeding ulcer. The following laboratory data were obtained:

RBC	$4.2 \times 10^{12}/L$	Serum iron	40 µg/dL
Hct	30%	TIBC	460 µg/dL
Hgb	8.5 gm/dL	Serum ferritin	12 ng/mL
WBC	$5.0 \times 10^{9}/L$		

Examination of the bone marrow revealed the absence of iron stores. These data are most consistent with which of the following conditions?

a. iron deficiency anemia
b. anemia of chronic disease
c. hemochromatosis
d. acute blood loss

49. Which of the following stains is closely associated with the lysosomal enzyme in primary (azurophilic) granules?

   a. peroxidase
   b. Sudan black B
   c. periodic acid-Schiff (PAS)
   d. Prussian blue

50. The prothrombin time test requires that the patient's citrated plasma be combined with:

   a. platelet lipids
   b. thromboplastin
   c. Ca^{++} and platelet lipids
   d. Ca^{++} and thromboplastin

51. A total leukocyte count is 10,000/μL and 25 NRBCs are seen per 100 leukocytes on the differential. What is the corrected leukocyte count?

   a. 2,000/μL
   b. 8,000/μL
   c. 10,000/μL
   d. 12,000/μL

52. Blood collected in EDTA undergoes which of the following changes if kept at room temperature for 6-24 hours?

   a. increased hematocrit and MCV
   b. increased sedimentation rate and MCV
   c. increased MCHC and MCV
   d. decreased reticulocyte count and hematocrit

53. The following illustration presents composite displays of cellular size distribution histograms from an electronic cell counter:

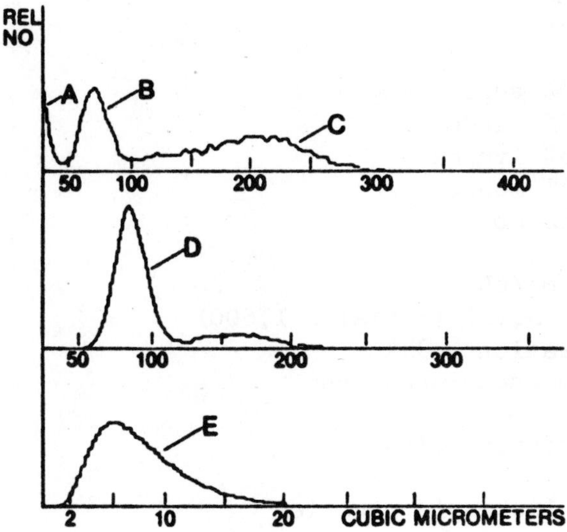

Which area of the above displays is appropriate for a lymphocyte population curve?

a. A
b. B
c. C
d. D

54. Which of the following laboratory procedures would be most helpful in differentiating between primary fibrinolysis and disseminated intravascular coagulation?

a. presence of fibrin split products
b. factor VIII activity
c. platelet count
d. fibrinogen level

55. The following results were obtained from a 55-year-old man experiencing headaches and blurred vision:

WBC 19,000/μL
RBC 7,200,000/μL
PLT 1,056,000/μL

Differential	84%	segs
	10%	bands
	3%	lymphs
	2%	monos
	1%	eos

LAP 320
Uric acid 13.0 mg/dL
Red cell volume 3,911 (normal = 1,600)
Arterial O_2 saturation 93%
Philadelphia chromosome-negative

These results are consistent with:

a. neutrophilic leukemoid reaction
b. polycythemia vera
c. chronic granulocytic leukemia
d. leukoerythroblastosis in myelofibrosis

56. Which of the following anomalies is an autosomal dominant disorder characterized by irregularly sized inclusions in polymorphonuclear neutrophils, abnormal giant platelets, and frequent thrombocytopenia?

a. Pelger-Huët
b. Chediak-Higashi
c. Alder-Reilly
d. May-Hegglin

57. The chamber counting method of platelet enumeration:

a. allows direct visualization of the particles being counted
b. has a high degree of precision
c. has a high degree of reproducibility
d. is the method of choice for the performance of 50-60 counts per day

58. A 53-year-old man was in recovery following a triple bypass operation. Oozing was noted from his surgical wound. The following laboratory data were obtained:

Hemoglobin	12.5 gm/dL
Hematocrit	37%
Prothrombin time	12.3 seconds (control 11.8)
APTT	38 seconds (control 36.5)
Platelet count	40,000/μL
Fibrinogen	250 mg/dL

The most likely cause of bleeding would be:

a. dilution of coagulation factors due to massive transfusion
b. intravascular coagulation secondary to microaggregates
c. hypofibrinogenemia
d. dilutional thrombocytopenia

59. The following results were obtained from a 45-year-old man experiencing chills and fever:

WBC 23,000/μL
Differential 60% segs
21% bands
11% lymphs
3% monos
2% metamyelocytes
3% myelocytes
toxic granulation, Döhle bodies, and vacuoles noted
LAP 200
Philadelphia chromosome-negative

These results are consistent with:

a. neutrophilic leukemoid reaction
b. polycythemia vera
c. chronic granulocytic leukemia
d. leukoerythroblastosis in myelofibrosis

60. A patient has a history of mild hemorrhagic episodes. Laboratory results include a prolonged prothrombin time and partial thromboplastin time. The abnormal prothrombin time was corrected by normal and adsorbed plasma, but not aged serum. Which of the following coagulation factors is deficient?

a. prothrombin
b. factor V
c. factor X
d. factor VII

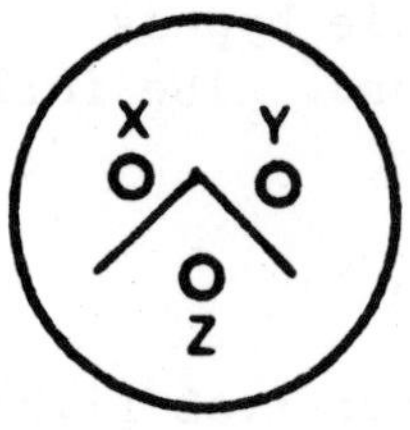

Figure #1

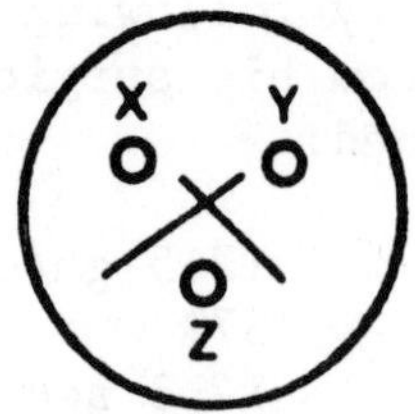

Figure #2

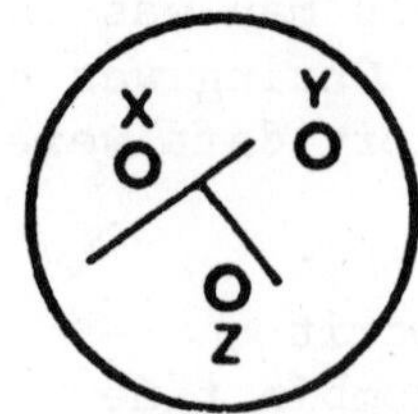

Figure #3

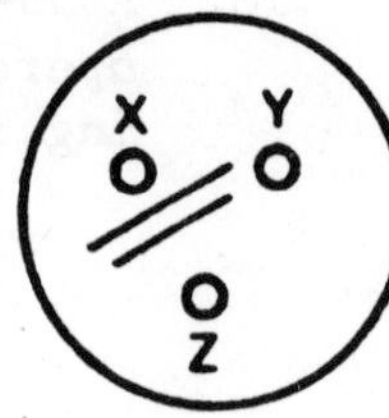

Figure #4

61. Which of the above figures demonstrates a reaction pattern of identity?

    a. Figure #1
    b. Figure #2
    c. Figure #3
    d. Figure #4

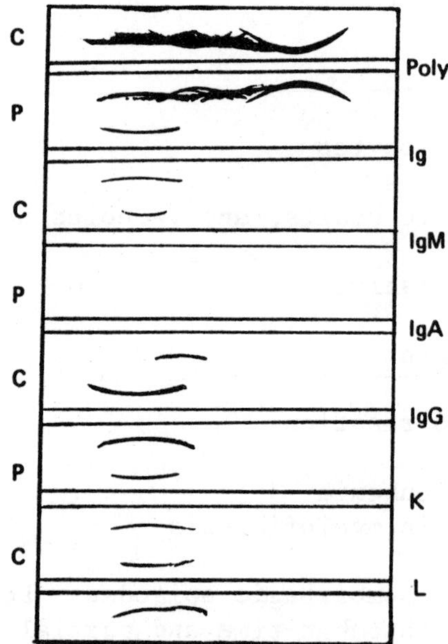

62. The serum immunoelectrophoretic pattern shown above is most likely associated with which of the following?

    a. IgG lambda myeloma
    b. IgA kappa myeloma
    c. light chain myeloma, lambda type
    d. light chain myeloma, kappa type

63. Which immunoglobulin is associated with allergic reactions?

   a. IgA
   b. IgE
   c. IgG
   d. IgM

64. A rapid indirect latex slide test showed no agglutination and was reported as negative on a woman who, on physical examination, was thought to be pregnant. A possible reason for the negative test result is:

   a. urine glucose was increased
   b. misinterpretation of the test
   c. urine specific gravity was greater than 1.015
   d. urine protein was greater than 100 mg/dL

65. In systemic lupus erythematosus, high levels of which of the following antibodies are seen?

   a. anti-mitochondrial
   b. anti-smooth muscle
   c. anti-DNA
   d. anti-parietal cell

66. A good way to monitor precision or reproducibility is by:

   a. duplicate assays
   b. repeated serial testing
   c. processing of unknown specimens
   d. running normal and abnormal controls

67. A patient's abnormal lymphocytes form rosettes with sheep red blood cells and lack C3 receptors and surface membrane immunoglobulin. This can be classified as a disorder of:

   a. T cells
   b. B cells
   c. monocytes
   d. null cells

68. A patient entered the hospital because of anemia and a facial rash. The antinuclear antibody and direct antiglobulin tests were positive. The following agarose-gel electrophoretic pattern was obtained (C = control, P = patient):

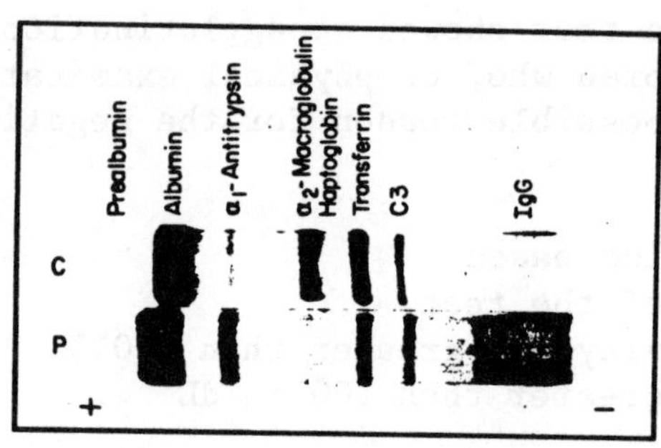

What abnormality does this pattern have that is consistent with the tentative diagnosis of systemic lupus erythematosus?

a. increased C3
b. increased albumin
c. increased alpha-1-antitrypsin
d. increased IgG

69. Immunoglobulin quantitation of a patient's serum was reported to show decreased concentrations of IgG, IgA, and IgM. Immunoelectrophoresis (IEP) of the same sample the next day showed an IgG kappa protein with decreased concentrations of IgA and IgM. Which of the following is the most appropriate course of action to resolve the discrepancy and minimize cost?

a. Repeat the IgG quantitation at dilutions of 1:2 and 1:4; run all future immunoglobulin quantitations at 1:2 and 1:4 dilutions.
b. Repeat the IgG quantitation at dilutions of 1:2 and 1:4; screen all future immunoglobulin quantitations with a serum protein electrophoresis to correlate results.
c. Repeat the IgG quantitation at dilutions of 1:2 and 1:4; screen all future immunoglobulin quantitations with IEP to correlate results.
d. Repeat the IgG, IgA, and IgM quantitations, protein electrophoresis, and IEP to determine which result was correct.

70. A 25-year-old woman is seen by a physician because of Raynaud's phenomemon, myalgias, arthralgias, and difficulty in swallowing. There is no evidence of renal disease. An ANA titer is 1:8,000 with a speckled pattern. Which of the following is also likely to be found in this patient?

a. high level nDNA antibody and a low CH50 level
b. high level Sm antibody
c. high titer rheumatoid factor
d. high level ribonucleoprotein (RNP) antibody

71. The stock culture needed for quality control testing of motility is:

a. Salmonella typhimurium/Escherichia coli
b. Escherichia coli/Pseudomonas aeruginosa
c. Serratia marcescens/Escherichia coli
d. Shigella sonnei/Escherichia coli

72. A 27-year-old scuba diver has an abrasion on his left thigh, which on culture grew an acid-fast organism at 30°C. This isolate most likely is:

a. Mycobacterium chelonei
b. Mycobacterium marinum
c. Mycobacterium tuberculosis
d. Mycobacterium xenopi

73. An unusual number of methicillin-resistant Staphylococcus aureus (determined by the Kirby-Bauer method) were isolated in the laboratory in the past month. Which of the following is the most likely explanation?

a. incubation of the susceptibility plates at 35°C
b. deterioration of the methicillin discs
c. inoculation of plates 10 minutes after standardizing the inoculum
d. standardization of the inoculum to a 0.5 McFarland turbidity standard

74. Which of the following sets of biochemicals best differentiates Salmonella and Citrobacter species?

a. KCN, malonate, β-galactosidase, lysine decarboxylase
b. dulcitol, citrate, indole, H_2S production
c. lactose, adonitol, KCN, motility
d. lysine decarboxylase, lactose, sucrose, malonate, indole

75. A fungal isolate from the sputum of a patient with a pulmonary infection is suspected to be Histoplasma capsulatum. Tuberculate macroconidia were seen on the hyphae of the mold phase, which was isolated at room temperature on Sabouraud's dextrose agar, containing chloramphenicol and cycloheximide (SDA-CC). A parallel set of cultures incubated at 35°C showed bacterial growth on SDA but no growth on SDA-CC. Which of the following is the appropriate course of action?

a. Repeat subculture of the mold phase to tubes of moist SDA-CC incubated at 35°C.
b. Subculture the mold phase to tubes of moist BHI-blood media incubated at 25°C.
c. Subculture the mold phase to tubes of moist BHI-blood media incubated at 35°C.
d. Perform animal inoculation studies.

76. Adenovirus infections primarily involve the:

a. respiratory tract
b. gastrointestinal tract
c. genital tract
d. urinary tract

77. A sputum Gram stain revealed 25 to 50 squamous epithelial cells and 25 to 50 polymorphonuclear leukocytes per low power field. Many lancet-shaped, gram-positive cocci; many gram-negative rods; and many gram-positive cocci in pairs, clumps, and long chains per oil immersion field were seen.

The technologist's best course of action would be to:

a. inoculate appropriate media and incubate aerobically
b. inoculate appropriate media and incubate anaerobically
c. call the physician and notify him of this "life-threatening" situation
d. call the nursing station and request a new specimen

78. A specimen of hair that fluoresced under a Wood's lamp was obtained from a child with low grade scaling lesions of the scalp. Cultures revealed a fungus with mycelium and very few macroconidia or microconidia. This fungus is most likely:

a. *Microsporum gypseum*
b. *Microsporum audouinii*
c. *Trichophyton tonsurans*
d. *Epidermophyton floccosum*

79. In a wet mount of sediment from formalin-ether concentrated material, protozoan cysts without peripheral chromatin on the nuclear membrane and four karyosomes (four nuclei) appearing as refractive dots were seen. These oval-shaped cysts are most likely:

a. *Endolimax nana*
b. *Chilomastix mesnili*
c. *Entamoeba histolytica*
d. *Entamoeba hartmanni*

80. Group B, β-hemolytic streptococci may be distinguished from other hemolytic streptococci by which of the following procedures?

a. Lancefield typing
b. growth in 6.5% NaCl broth
c. growth on bile esculin medium
d. bacitracin susceptibility

81. A 52-year-old woman was admitted for treatment of metastatic breast cancer. She became febrile and a chest radiograph revealed a left lower lobe infiltrate. Blood cultures were positive for an oxidase-negative, nonmotile organism that oxidized lactose. The antimicrobial susceptibility pattern of the organism was overall resistance except for the aminoglycosides. This organism is most likely:

a. *Pseudomonas maltophilia*
b. *Acinetobacter lwoffii*
c. *Pasteurella multocida*
d. *Acinetobacter anitratus*

82. Children with hemolytic streptococcal infections can develop:

a. acute pyelonephritis
b. acute glomerulonephritis
c. chronic glomerulonephritis
d. nephrosis

83. A jaundiced seven-year-old boy, with a history of playing in a pond in a rat-infested area, has a urine specimen submitted for a direct dark-field examination. Several spiral organisms are seen. Which of the following organisms would most likely be responsible for the patient's condition?

a. *Spirillum minor*
b. *Streptobacillus moniliformis*
c. *Listeria monocytogenes*
d. *Leptospira interrogans*

84. Which of the following organisms may exhibit a brick red fluorescence?

a. *Bacteroides melaninogenicus* and *Clostridium difficile*
b. *Clostridium difficile* and *Fusobacterium* sp.
c. *Veillonella parvula* and *Bacteroides melaninogenicus*
d. *Fusobacterium* sp. and *Veillonella parvula*

85. An acid-fast bacillus recovered from an induced sputum had the following characteristics: yellow pigmentation in the dark, turning a deeper yellow-orange after two weeks of light exposure; biochemicals were nitrate-negative, Tween hydrolysis-positive at 5-10 days, and urease-negative. Based on this information, the organism is most likely:

a. *Mycobacterium scrofulaceum*
b. *Mycobacterium gordonae*
c. *Mycobacterium kansasii*
d. *Mycobacterium fortuitum*

86. While checking the staining properties of an iodine solution as part of a routine quality control program, it is observed that the fecal suspension clumps in large aggregates. Which of the following is the most appropriate course of action?

a. Check the expiration date of the solution.
b. Centrifuge the solution and retest.
c. Dilute the solution and retest.
d. Prepare a fresh lot of iodine and retest.

87. A gram-negative diplococcus that grows on modified Thayer-Martin medium can be further confirmed as Neisseria gonorrhoeae if it is:

   a. oxidase-, glucose-, and maltose-positive
   b. oxidase- and glucose-positive, maltose-negative
   c. oxidase- and maltose-positive, glucose-negative
   d. glucose-positive, oxidase- and maltose-negative

88. In a disc diffusion susceptibility test, which of the following can result if discs are placed on the inoculated media and left at room temperature for an hour before incubation?

   a. The antibiotic would not diffuse into the medium, resulting in no zone.
   b. Zones of smaller diameter would result.
   c. Zones of larger diameter would result.
   d. There would be no effect on the final zone diameter.

89. A TSI tube inoculated with an organism gave the following reactions:

   Alkaline slant
   Acid butt
   No H_2S
   No gas produced

   This organism is most likely:

   a. Yersinia enterocolitica
   b. Salmonella typhi
   c. Salmonella enteritidis
   d. Shigella dysenteriae

90. Failure to obtain anaerobiosis in anaerobe jars is most often due to the:

   a. inactivation of palladium-coated alumina catalyst pellets
   b. condensation of water on the inner surface of the jar
   c. instability of reactants in the disposable hydrogen-carbon dioxide generator envelope
   d. expiration of the methylene blue indicator strip that monitors oxidation

91. Urine reagent strips should be stored in a(n):

   a. refrigerator (4 to 7°C)
   b. incubator (37°C)
   c. cool, dry area
   d. open jar exposed to air

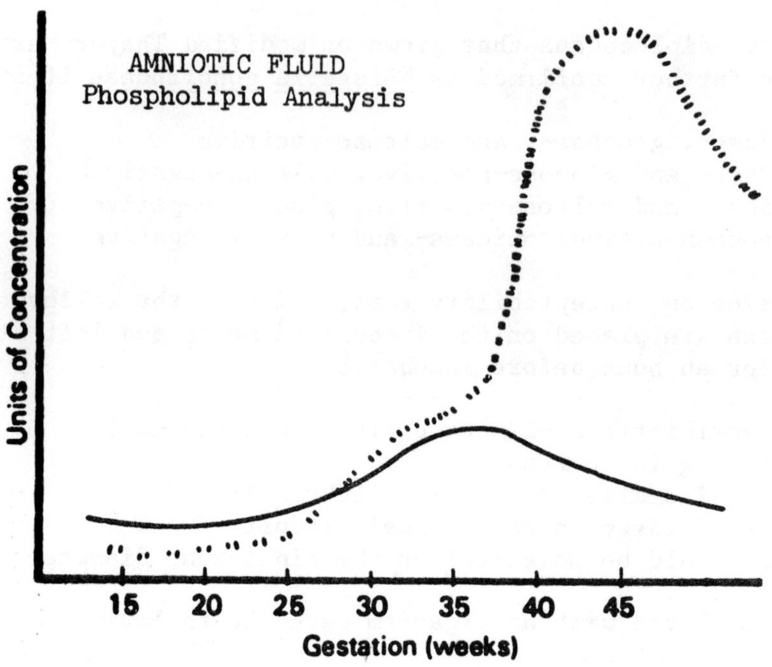

92. Which class of phospholipid surfactants associated with pulmonary maturity is represented by the dotted line on the amniotic fluid analysis shown above?

    a. sphingomyelin
    b. choline
    c. lecithin
    d. phosphatidic acid

---

93. A technologist performed a STAT microscopic urinalysis and reported the following:

WBCs	10 to 13
RBCs	2 to 6
Hyaline casts	2+
Bacteria	1+

The centrifuge tube was not discarded and the urine sediment was reevaluated microscopically five hours after the above results were reported. A second technologist reported the same results, except 2+ bacteria and no hyaline casts were found. The most probable explanation for the second technologist's findings is:

    a. Sediment was not agitated before inoculating microscope slide.
    b. Casts dissolved due to decrease in urine pH.
    c. Casts dissolved due to increase in urine pH.
    d. Casts were never present in this specimen.

94. The above symbol posted in an area would indicate which of the following hazards?

a. flammable
b. electrical
c. radiation
d. biohazard

---

95. A 27-year-old woman with severe lower back pain has the following urinalysis test results:

pH	5.5	Specific gravity		1.018
Protein	trace	Sulfosalicylic acid for protein		20 mg/dL
Glucose	negative			
Ketones	negative			
Blood	negative	Microscopic	WBC	3 to 5
Bilirubin	negative		RBC	25 to 50
Nitrite	negative		Epithelial cells	3 to 5
Urobilinogen	0.1 EU/dL		Mucous strands	moderate

Which of the following is the MOST likely explanation for the discrepancy in the blood portion of the urine reagent strip and the microscopic RBC finding?

a. Oxidizing contaminants are causing a false-negative blood on the urine reagent strip.
b. More red blood cells must be present in order for the blood portion to react.
c. Ascorbic acid is causing a false-negative reagent strip result.
d. The urine reagent strip is more sensitive to red blood cells than to hemoglobin.

96. A 62-year-old patient with hyperlipoproteinemia has a large amount of protein in his urine. Microscopic analysis yields moderate to many fatty, waxy, granular, and cellular casts. Many oval fat bodies are also noted. This is most consistent with:

a. nephrotic syndrome
b. viral infection
c. cystitis
d. acute glomerulonephritis

97. A urine specimen is analyzed for glucose by a glucose oxidase reagent strip and a copper reduction test. If both results are positive, which of the following interpretations is correct?

a. Only galactose is present.
b. Only glucose is present.
c. Only lactose is present.
d. Sugars other than glucose are present.

98. In patients with gout, the most characteristic microscopic finding in synovial fluid is:

a. calcium pyrophosphate crystals
b. cartilage debris
c. monosodium urate crystals
d. hemosiderin-laden macrophages

99. A urine specimen collected from an apparently healthy 25-year-old man shortly after he finished eating lunch was cloudy but showed normal results on a multiple reagent strip analysis. The most likely cause of the turbidity is:

a. fat
b. white blood cells
c. urates
d. phosphates

CHAPTER 10

Microbiology

1. *Haemophilus influenzae* becomes resistant to ampicillin when the organism develops a(n):

   a. capsule of polysaccharide material
   b. affinity for the β-lactam ring of the ampicillin
   c. requirement for hemin
   d. β-lactamase

2. Thioglycollate broth is stored at room temperature and in the dark so that:

   a. ureases are not formed
   b. the cysteine does not decompose
   c. sunlight does not hydrolyze the glucose in the medium
   d. there is a decreased absorption of oxygen by the medium

3. A liquid fecal specimen from a 3-month-old infant is submitted for microbiological examination. In addition to culture on routine media for *Salmonella* and *Shigella*, this specimen routinely should be:

   a. examined for the presence of *Entamoeba hartmanni*
   b. examined for the presence of *Campylobacter* sp.
   c. screened for the detection of enterotoxigenic *Escherichia coli*
   d. placed in thioglycollate broth to detect *Clostridium botulinum*

4. Which one of the following specimen requests is acceptable?

   a. feces submitted for anaerobic culture
   b. Foley catheter tip submitted for aerobic culture
   c. rectal swab submitted for direct smear for gonococci
   d. urine for culture of acid-fast bacilli

5. A gram-positive coccus isolated from a blood culture has the following characteristics:

Optochin sensitivity	negative
Bacitracin (0.04U) sensitivity	negative
Bile	no growth
Esculin hydrolysis	negative
Hippurate hydrolysis	positive
6.5% sodium chloride growth	positive
Catalase	negative

This organism is most likely:

a. Staphylococcus sp.
b. Streptococcus pneumoniae
c. Streptococcus pyogenes (group A)
d. Streptococcus agalactiae (group B)

6. A gram-negative rod was isolated from a wound infection caused by a bite from a pet rabbit. The following characteristic reactions were seen:

Oxidase production	positive
Glucose OF	fermentative
Catalase production	positive
Motility	negative
MacConkey agar	no growth

Which of the following is the most likely organism?

a. Pseudomonas aeruginosa
b. Pasteurella multocida
c. Aeromonas hydrophila
d. Vibrio albensis

7. A 10-year-old boy was admitted to the emergency room with lower right quadrant pain and tenderness. The following laboratory results were obtained:

	Patient	Normal	Range
% Segmented Neutrophils	75	38	16-60
White Cell Count			
per L	200×10^9	8.4×10^9	$4.0 \times 10^9 - 13 \times 10^9$
per µL	200×10^3	8.4×10^3	$4.0 \times 10^3 - 13 \times 10^3$

The admitting diagnosis was appendicitis. During surgery the appendix appeared normal; an enlarged node was removed and cultured. Small gram-negative rods were isolated from the room temperature plate. The organism most likely is:

a. *Bacteroides melaninogenicus*
b. *Shigella sonnei*
c. *Listeria monocytogenes*
d. *Yersinia enterocolitica*

8. The stock culture needed for quality control testing of deoxyribonuclease (DNAse) production is:

a. *Salmonella typhimurium/Escherichia coli*
b. *Escherichia coli/Pseudomonas aeruginosa*
c. *Proteus mirabilis/Escherichia coli*
d. *Serratia marcescens/Escherichia coli*

9. The stock culture needed for quality control testing of deamination activity is:

a. *Escherichia coli/Klebsiella pneumoniae*
b. *Salmonella typhimurium/Escherichia coli*
c. *Escherichia coli/Pseudomonas aeruginosa*
d. *Proteus mirabilis/Escherichia coli*

10. The stock culture needed for quality control testing of oxidase production is:

a. *Escherichia coli/Klebsiella pneumoniae*
b. *Salmonella typhimurium/Escherichia coli*
c. *Escherichia coli/Pseudomonas aeruginosa*
d. *Proteus mirabilis/Escherichia coli*

11. An antibiotic that inhibits cell wall synthesis is:

    a. chloramphenicol
    b. penicillin
    c. sulfonamide
    d. colistin

12. Quality control procedures in a microbiology laboratory must include checks on:

    1. sterility testing of all media
    2. monitoring of temperatures of each refrigerator, incubator, water bath, heat block, etc.
    3. antisera activity
    4. staining reagents

    a. only 1, 2 and 3 are correct
    b. only 1 and 3 are correct
    c. only 2 and 4 are correct
    d. only 4 is correct
    e. all are correct

13. The test NOT adequate for the definitive identification of *Neisseria gonorrhoeae* is:

    a. growth on Martin-Lewis medium
    b. coagglutination serology
    c. cystine trypticase agar carbohydrate utilization
    d. fluorescent antibody

14. Organisms that may be mistaken for *Neisseria gonorrhoeae* in Gram stained smears of uterine cervix exudates include:

    a. *Lactobacilli* sp.
    b. *Streptococcus agalactiae*
    c. *Pseudomonas aeruginosa*
    d. *Moraxella osloensis*

15. Specimens for which the use of modified Thayer-Martin or Martin-Lewis medium is mandatory for the optimal recovery of *Neisseria gonorrhoeae* include:

1. cervix
2. eye
3. oropharynx
4. joint fluid

a. only 1, 2 and 3 are correct
b. only 1 and 3 are correct
c. only 2 and 4 are correct
d. only 4 is correct
e. all are correct

16. Factors that limit the usefulness of counterimmunoelectrophoresis (CIE) in the diagnosis of meningitis include:

a. commercial antisera are not available for the detection of the organisms that commonly cause meningitis
b. cross-reactions commonly occur between *Streptococcus pneumoniae*, *Haemophilus influenzae*, and *Neisseria meningitidis*
c. antigens are detected in less than 50% of bacteriologically proven cases of meningitis
d. a concentration with 10^5 colony-forming units per milliliter is required before sufficient antigen can be detected

17. Coagglutination is associated with:

a. *Chlamydia trachomatis*
b. *Neisseria gonorrhoeae*
c. *Streptococcus pneumoniae*
d. *Klebsiella pneumoniae*

18. Pili antigens are associated with:

a. *Streptococcus pneumoniae*
b. *Neisseria gonorrhoeae*
c. *Chlamydia trachomatis*
d. *Pneumocystis carinii*

19. Omniserum is associated with:

    a. *Pneumocystis carinii*
    b. *Klebsiella pneumoniae*
    c. *Streptococcus pneumoniae*
    d. *Neisseria gonorrhoeae*

20. Chocolate agar base containing vancomycin, colistin, nystatin, and trimethoprim is also known as:

    a. EMB agar
    b. modified Thayer-Martin agar
    c. Columbia CNA agar
    d. KV-laked agar

21. Sodium bicarbonate and sodium citrate are components of which of the following?

    a. JEMBEC system
    b. modified Thayer-Martin agar
    c. NYC medium
    d. Martin-Lewis agar

22. One advantage of the antimicrobial dilution tests is that:

    a. they are based on a predetermined breakpoint
    b. contamination can be easily detected
    c. they provide categorical reports
    d. they can detect varying degrees of organism sensitivity and resistance

23. All of the following are advantages of automated susceptibility testing EXCEPT:

    a. endpoint objectivity
    b. greater sensitivity of readings
    c. cost reduction with small volumes
    d. reduction of experimental error

24. The minimal bacteriocidal concentration of a bacteriostatic agent is measured by performing a(n):

 a. MIC
 b. MBC
 c. antimicrobial dilution test
 d. antimicrobial diffusion test

25. Combining antibiotics in drug therapy can have a variety of results, the most desirable of which is:

 a. antagonistic
 b. synergistic
 c. indifferent
 d. additive

26. All of the following are in vitro methods of determining synergism EXCEPT:

 a. kill-curve method
 b. kill-curve using an MIC endpoint
 c. checkerboard using an MIC endpoint
 d. checkerboard using an MBC endpoint

27. Production of β-lactamase is inducible in which of the following:

 a. *Haemophilus influenzae*
 b. *Staphylococcus aureus*
 c. *Corynebacterium diphtheriae*
 d. *Streptococcus pyogenes*

28. Clinical resistance to penicillin dosages appears to correlate with β-lactamase production in:

 a. *Neisseria gonorrhoeae*
 b. *Neisseria meningitidis*
 c. *Streptococcus agalactiae*
 d. *Streptococcus pyogenes*

29. To date, which of the following remains fully susceptible to penicillin?

   a. _Haemophilus influenzae_
   b. _Neisseria gonorrhoeae_
   c. _Streptococcus pyogenes_
   d. _Corynebacterium diphtheriae_

30. First-generation cephalosporins can be adequately represented by:

   a. streptomycin
   b. chloramphenicol
   c. cephalothin
   d. colistin

31. Which of the following is used primarily for epidemiologic purposes:

   a. cephalothin
   b. chloramphenicol
   c. streptomycin
   d. kanamycin

32. Anaerobic susceptibility tests are helpful in the management of patients with:

   a. synovial infections
   b. rectal abscesses
   c. streptococcal pharyngitis
   d. pilonidal sinuses

33. When combination antibiotic therapy is used:

   a. antagonistic effects should exist between the antibiotics
   b. the combination effect of the drugs should be less than the sum of the independent effects of the two drugs
   c. the synergistic effects of the drugs should be assessed
   d. the killing power of the combination must be at least fourfold greater than the antimicrobic used alone

34. Valid reason(s) for using two or more antimicrobial agents is(are):

1. as initial therapy when the causative organism is not known
2. as treatment for mixed infections when the causative organisms are not susceptible to a single antimicrobic
3. to delay the development of organism resistance
4. to achieve a therapeutic result using nontoxic amounts of two antimicrobics when use of either one alone would require administration of unacceptably large doses

a. only 1, 2 and 3 are correct
b. only 1 and 3 are correct
c. only 2 and 4 are correct
d. only 4 is correct
e. all are correct

35. *Clostridium difficile*:

a. is associated with all cases of pseudomembranous colitis
b. is a likely pathogen in antibiotic-associated diarrhea
c. defines the colonic lesions
d. is the causative pathogen for many gastrointestinal diseases

36. The drug of choice for treating *Clostridium difficile* is:

a. chloramphenicol
b. colistin
c. penicillin
d. vancomycin

37. The most appropriate clinical test for the presence of *Clostridium difficile* is:

a. tissue culture toxin assay
b. gas-liquid chromatography
c. routine fecal cultures
d. anaerobic culture techniques

38. Which of the following media is routinely used to culture Campylobacter fetus subspecies jejuni?

    a. Skirrow's medium
    b. CIN agar
    c. anaerobic CNA agar
    d. bismuth sulfate

39. The tissue culture assay for Clostridium difficile toxin:

    a. is usually interpreted at 6-12 hours post-inoculation
    b. may show changes within four hours of inoculation
    c. shows a good correlation between the toxin titer and the severity of the disease
    d. is interpreted as positive when cytotoxicity affects at least 5% of the cell monolayer

40. Pseudomembranous colitis caused by Clostridium difficile toxin is confirmed by which of the following laboratory findings?

    a. isolation of the causative agent
    b. Gram stain showing many gram-positive rods
    c. gas production in chopped meat glucose
    d. presence of toxin in stool

41. Which one of the following results is typical of Campylobacter fetus subspecies jejuni?

    a. optimal growth at 42°C
    b. oxidase-negative
    c. catalase-negative
    d. nonmotile

42. Which one of the following results is typical of Campylobacter fetus subspecies intestinalis?

    a. optimal growth at 42°C
    b. oxidase-negative
    c. growth at 37°C
    d. catalase-negative

43. A presumptive identification of *Campylobacter fetus* subspecies *jejuni* can be made using a combination of which of the following?

    a. Gram stain, catalase and oxidase test reactions, phase-contrast microscopy
    b. Gram stain, catalase and oxidase test reactions, motility media
    c. catalase and oxidase test reactions, phase-contrast microscopy, motility media
    d. hematoxylin and eosin stain, catalase and oxidase test reactions, motility media

44. Which of the following organisms must be incubated in a microaerophilic environment for optimal recovery of the organism?

    a. *Campylobacter fetus* subspecies *intestinalis*
    b. *Escherichia coli*
    c. *Pseudomonas aeruginosa*
    d. *Proteus mirabilis*

45. Items to consider when using the staphylococcal CoA procedure include:

    a. Hyperproteinemia may cause autoagglutination and thus false-positive test results.
    b. Direct testing of group A, β-hemolytic streptococci isolates from agar plates results in pseudoagglutination.
    c. Gonococcal isolates must be cold-treated to avoid pseudoagglutination.
    d. Cerebrospinal fluid must be heated to 56°C for five minutes before testing.

46. Fluid from a cutaneous black lesion was submitted for routine bacteriological culture. After 18 hours of incubation at 35°C, there was no growth on MacConkey agar, but 3+ growth on sheep blood agar. The colonies were nonhemolytic, 4 to 5 mm in diameter, and off-white with a ground glass appearance. Each colony had an irregular edge with comma-shaped outgrowths that stood up like "beaten egg whites" when gently lifted with an inoculating needle. A Gram stained smear of a typical colony showed large, gram-positive, rectangular rods with central hyaline areas. This is consistent with:

    a. gas gangrene
    b. fish handler's disease
    c. malignant pustule
    d. swimming pool granuloma

47. A 25-year-old man who had recently worked as a steward on a transoceanic grain ship presented to the emergency room with high fever, diarrhea, and prostration. Axillary lymph nodes were hemorrhagic and enlarged. A Gram stained smear was prepared from a lymph node aspirate and many gram-negative bacilli were noted. The bacilli demonstrated a marked bipolar staining reaction described as a "safety-pin appearance" with Wayson's stain. The most likely identification of this organism is:

a. *Brucella melitensis*
b. *Streptobacillus moniliformis*
c. *Spirillum minor*
d. *Yersinia pestis*

48. An 8-year-old girl was admitted to the hospital with a three-day history of fever, abdominal pain, diarrhea, and vomiting. Stool occult blood was negative; stool culture grew many lactose-negative colonies that yielded the following test results:

Oxidase	negative
TSI	A/A
Indole	negative
Urease	positive
Ornithine decarboxylase	positive
Sucrose	positive
H_2S	negative
Motility at 22°C	positive

The most probable identification of this organism is:

a. *Providencia alcalifaciens*
b. *Providencia stuartii*
c. *Yersinia enterocolitica*
d. *Proteus rettgeri*

49. While swimming in a lake near his home, a young boy cut his foot as he stepped on a piece of glass from a broken bottle. An infection developed and the site was cultured. A nonfastidious gram-negative, oxidase-positive, β-hemolytic, motile bacillus was recovered. The organism produced deoxyribonuclease and was identified as:

a. *Enterobacter cloacae*
b. *Serratia marcescens*
c. *Aeromonas hydrophila*
d. *Escherichia coli*

50. An autopsy performed on an 8-year-old child revealed Waterhouse-Friderichsen syndrome. Blood and throat cultures taken just prior to death were positive for which of the following organisms?

a. Neisseria gonorrhoeae
b. Neisseria meningitidis
c. Haemophilus influenzae
d. Klebsiella pneumoniae

51. A culture from an infected animal bite on a small boy's finger yielded a small, gram-negative coccobacillus that was smooth, raised, and β-hemolytic on blood agar. The isolate was found to grow readily on MacConkey agar, forming colorless colonies. The organism was motile with peritrichous flagella, catalase-positive, oxidase-positive, reduced nitrate, utilized citrate, and was urease-positive within four hours. No carbohydrates were fermented.

The most likely identification of this isolate is:

a. Brucella canis
b. Yersinia pestis
c. Francisella tularensis
d. Bordetella bronchiseptica

52. An anaerobic gram-negative bacillus isolated from a blood culture following bowel surgery grew as 1 to 3 mm, smooth, white nonhemolytic colonies. A Gram stained smear showed a pale, bipolarly stained rod with rounded ends. Bile stimulated growth of the organism and catalase was produced. The isolate was not inhibited by colistin, kanamycin, or vancomycin; indole was not produced.

The most likely identification of this isolate is:

a. Bacteroides fragilis
b. Bacteroides melaninogenicus
c. Fusobacterium nucleatum
d. Fusobacterium varium

53. Multiple blood cultures from a patient presenting with endocarditis grew a facultatively anaerobic, pleomorphic gram-negative bacillus with the following characteristics:

Nonhemolytic	
Growth on blood and chocolate agar in 5% CO_2	enhanced
MacConkey agar	no growth
Catalase	negative
Oxidase	negative
X factor under 5-10% CO_2 atmosphere	required
Nitrate	positive, reduced to nitrites
Bile solubility	insoluble
Indole	negative
Glucose	acid and gas produced

The most likely identification is:

a. Brucella abortus
b. Actinobacillus actinomycetem-comitans
c. Haemophilus aphrophilus
d. Cardiobacterium hominis

54. Relapsing fever in humans is caused by:

a. Borrelia recurrentis
b. Brucella abortus
c. Leptospira icterohemorrhagiae
d. Spirillum minor

55. The most rapid and specific method of identifying Francisella tularensis is:

a. serological slide agglutination utilizing specific antiserum
b. dye-stained clinical specimens
c. fluorescent antibody staining techniques on clinical specimens
d. biotyping

56. The Schick test will:

   a. detect *Clostridium tetani* toxin
   b. identify *Bacillus anthracis*
   c. detect circulating antitoxin to *Corynebacterium diphtheriae*
   d. detect immunity to *Streptococcus pyogenes*

57. An organism isolated from a diarrheal stool produced the following reactions:

Oxidase	negative
Lactose	negative
Motility	negative
Urease	negative
LIA	K/K (alkaline slant/alkaline butt)
Glucose fermentation	no gas produced

A suspension of the organism did not agglutinate with *Shigella* antisera subgroups A, B, C, and D. You would conclude:

   a. this particular *Shigella* possesses a capsular antigen that blocks agglutination in O antiserum and must first be destroyed by heating
   b. this organism is not a *Shigella*
   c. the bacterial suspension was not dense enough, resulting in a false-negative reaction
   d. a rough colony was used for the serotyping procedure

58. The diagnosis of antibiotic-associated pseudomembranous colitis is best made by:

   a. isolation of *Clostridium difficile* from stool specimens
   b. demonstration of *Clostridium difficile* antitoxin in the serum
   c. prevention of CPE on a fibroblast monolayer by *Clostridium sordelii* antitoxin
   d. demonstration of CPE on a fibroblast monolayer

59. Which of the following tests is used to monitor bacteriocidal activity during antimicrobic therapy in cases of endocarditis?

a. Elek
b. tolerance
c. Sherris synergism
d. Schlicter

60. The macro-broth dilution method for determining antibiotic susceptibility of the Enterobacteriaceae cannot be used effectively for the sulfonamides or trimethoprim because:

a. misleading results can occur due to inadequate concentrations of Mg^{++} and Ca^{++}
b. organisms are resistant at 35°C; at 37°C endpoints are less clear unless incubated for 48 hours
c. definite endpoints have not yet been established
d. endpoints are difficult to determine as susceptible organisms can go through several generations before being inhibited

61. Which one of the following combinations of organisms would be appropriate as controls to test the reactions listed?

a. β-hemolysis: *Escherichia coli* and *Streptococcus pyogenes*
b. catalase: *Staphylococcus aureus* and *Staphylococcus epidermidis*
c. hydrogen sulfide production: *Proteus mirabilis* and *Salmonella typhi*
d. indole: *Escherichia coli* and *Proteus mirabilis*

62. Which one of the following organisms could be used as the positive quality control test for lecithinase on egg yolk agar?

a. *Bacteroides fragilis*
b. *Fusobacterium necrophorum*
c. *Clostridium perfringens*
d. *Clostridium sporogenes*

63. Which of the following is the most likely cause of a sharp increase in the minimal inhibitory concentration (MIC) of a quality control organism to ampicillin?

a. increase in the inoculum size from 10^5 to 10^6 organisms per mL
b. mutation of the organism to a more resistant strain
c. increased incubation time from 14 to 18 hours
d. instability of the antibiotic stock solution

64. The porphyrin test was devised to detect strains of Haemophilus capable of:

a. ampicillin degradation
b. capsule production
c. synthesis of porphobilinogen
d. chloramphenicol resistance

65. Which of the following is a true statement about collection of a stool specimen for suspected enteric disease?

a. Rectal swabs are equally as good as freshly passed stools.
b. Rectal swabs are very useful in surveying convalescent patients or screening for carriers.
c. Stool specimens should be collected early in the course of the disease before antibiotics are administered.
d. If the specimen cannot be cultured immediately, it should be placed in a suitable transport medium such as buffered glycerol-saline (pH 6.0).

66. A 1-2 mm translucent, nonpigmented colony, isolated from an anaerobic culture of a lung abscess after 72 hours, was found to fluoresce brick-red under ultraviolet light. A Gram stained smear of the organism revealed a coccobacillus that had the following characteristics:

Growth in bile	inhibited
Vancomycin	resistant
Catalase	negative
Esculin hydrolysis	positive
Indole	negative
Nitrate	negative
Glucose, lactose, and sucrose	acid produced

The most likely identification of this isolate is:

a. Bacteroides ovatus
b. Bacteroides oralis
c. Bacteroides melaninogenicus
d. Bacteroides asaccharolyticus

67. A thin, anaerobic gram-negative bacillus with tapered ends isolated from an empyema was found to be indole-positive, lipase-negative, and inhibited by 20% bile. Colonies were described as "speckled" or resembling "ground glass" and fluoresced weakly when exposed to ultraviolet light. The most probable identification of this isolate would be:

a. Bacteroides ureolyticus
b. Bacteroides melaninogenicus
c. Fusobacterium nucleatum
d. Fusobacterium mortiferum

68. An isolate of an anaerobic organism from a vaginal specimen was found to be a gram-positive bacillus with the following characteristics:

Catalase	negative
Glucose	positive
Trehalose	fermented

The gas-liquid chromatography (GLC) pattern revealed sizeable lactic, acetic, and formic acid peaks. The most likely identification is:

a. Eubacterium limosum
b. Propionibacterium acnes
c. Bifidobacterium eriksonii
d. Arachnia propionica

69. Which of the following anaerobes would be positive for indole?

a. *Bacteroides thetaiotaomicron*
b. *Bacteroides fragilis*
c. *Bacteroides distasonis*
d. *Bacteroides ureolyticus*

70. Which of the following anaerobes is inhibited by sodium polyanethole-sulfonate (SPS)?

a. *Peptococcus magnus*
b. *Peptococcus prevotii*
c. *Peptostreptococcus anaerobius*
d. *Veillonella parvula*

71. An aerobic, gram-negative coccobacillus was isolated on blood agar from a nasopharyngeal swab 48 hours after culture from a 6-month-old infant with suspected pertussis. The organism exhibited the following characteristics:

Urea	positive at 18 hours, negative at 4 hours
Oxidase	negative
Catalase	positive
Citrate	positive

Small zones of β-hemolysis
Slight brownish coloration of the medium

The most probable identification of this isolate is:

a. *Pasteurella multocida*
b. *Pasteurella ureae*
c. *Bordetella pertussis*
d. *Bordetella parapertussis*

72. A β-hemolytic, catalase-positive, gram-positive coccus is coagulase-negative by the slide coagulase test. Which of the following is the most appropriate action in identification of this organism?

a. report a coagulase-negative *Staphylococcus*
b. report a coagulase-negative *Staphylococcus aureus*
c. reconfirm the hemolytic reaction on a fresh 24-hour culture
d. do a tube coagulase test to confirm the slide test

73. Which of the following is the most reliable test to differentiate *Neisseria lactamicus* from *Neisseria meningitidis*?

    a. acid from maltose
    b. growth on modified Thayer-Martin
    c. lactose degradation
    d. nitrite reduction to nitrogen gas

74. Which feature distinguishes *Erysipelothrix rhusiopathiae* from other clinically significant nonspore-forming, gram-positive, facultatively anaerobic bacilli?

    a. "tumbling" motility
    b. β-hemolysis
    c. more pronounced motility at 25°C than 37°C
    d. H_2S production on TSI

75. Which of the following characteristics best differentiates *Bordetella bronchiseptica* from *Alcaligenes* species?

    a. flagellar pattern
    b. growth at 24°C
    c. oxidase activity
    d. rapid hydrolysis of urea

76. Which of the following results would you expect if motility agar was made with a 1% agar concentration?

    a. false-negative for *Acinetobacter lwoffii*
    b. false-positive for *Alcaligenes faecalis*
    c. false-positive for *Moraxella osloensis*
    d. false-negative for *Pseudomonas aeruginosa*

77. Which characteristic best differentiates between *Acinetobacter* species and *Moraxella* species?

    a. production of indophenol oxidase
    b. growth on MacConkey agar
    c. motility
    d. susceptibility of penicillin

78. The antibiotic used to suppress or kill contaminating fungi in media is:

 a. penicillin
 b. cycloheximide
 c. streptomycin
 d. amphotericin B

79. Which of the following would you least expect to culture from a case of otitis media?

 a. *Branhamella catarrhalis*
 b. *Neisseria meningitidis*
 c. *Haemophilus influenzae*
 d. *Streptococcus pneumoniae*

80. Each of the following statements about OF glucose medium is true EXCEPT:

 a. The semisolid agar gel localizes and prevents dispersion of the acid produced.
 b. The medium is used to differentiate streptococci.
 c. The medium supports the growth of all organisms.
 d. Due to the semisolid nature of the medium, bacterial motility can be accurately determined.

81. Which of the following organisms can grow in the small bowel and cause diarrhea in children, traveler's disease, or a severe cholera-like syndrome through the production of enterotoxins?

 a. *Yersinia enterocolitica*
 b. *Escherichia coli*
 c. *Salmonella typhi*
 d. *Shigella dysenteriae*

82. When combined antimicrobial drugs are clearly less effective than the most active drug alone, the condition is described as:

 a. minimal inhibitory concentration
 b. synergism
 c. minimal bacteriocidal concentration
 d. antagonism

83. The smallest concentration of antimicrobial agent which prevents growth in subculture or results in a 99.9% decrease of the initial inoculum, is the definition of:

a. minimal bacteriocidal concentration
b. indifference of additive
c. minimal inhibitory concentration
d. synergism

84. If the effect of combined antimicrobials is greater than the sum of the effects observed with the two drugs independently, the condition is described as:

a. indifference of additive
b. inhibition
c. synergism
d. antagonism

85. The amount of test antimicrobial that will inhibit visible growth of a microbe, is the definition of:

a. synergism
b. minimal inhibitory concentration
c. indifference of additive
d. minimal bacteriocidal concentration

86. If the combined effect of the antimicrobial is equal to the sum of the effect produced by the drugs independently, or equal to that of the most active drug in the combination, the condition is described as:

a. indifference of additive
b. synergism
c. antagonism
d. minimal bacteriocidal concentration

87. A β-hemolytic streptococcus which is bacitracin-resistant and CAMP-positive is:

a. group A or B
b. group A
c. group B
d. β-hemolytic, group D

88. A β-hemolytic streptococcus which is bacitracin-sensitive and CAMP-negative is:

a. group B
b. group A
c. β-hemolytic, not group A, B, or D
d. β-hemolytic, group D

89. Which of the following streptococci are β-hemolytic and CAMP-positive?

a. β-hemolytic, group D
b. β-hemolytic, not group A, B, or D
c. group B
d. group A

90. An organism was inoculated into a TSI tube and gave the following reactions:

Acid slant
Acid butt
No H_2S
Gas produced

This organism most likely is:

a. *Klebsiella pneumoniae*
b. *Shigella dysenteriae*
c. *Salmonella enteritidis*
d. *Salmonella typhi*

91. An organism was inoculated into a TSI tube and gave the following reactions:

Alkaline slant
Acid butt
H_2S produced
Gas produced

This organism most likely is:

a. *Klebsiella pneumoniae*
b. *Shigella dysenteriae*
c. *Salmonella enteritidis*
d. *Escherichia coli*

92. An organism was inoculated into a TSI tube and gave the following reactions:

Acid slant
Acid butt
No H_2S
No gas

This organism most likely is:

a. *Yersinia enterocolitica*
b. *Salmonella typhi*
c. *Salmonella enteritidis*
d. *Shigella dysenteriae*

93. A branching gram-positive, partially acid-fast organism is isolated from a bronchial washing from a 63-year-old woman receiving chemotherapy. The organism does NOT hydrolyze casein, tyrosine, or xanthine. The most likely identification is:

a. *Actinomadura madurae*
b. *Nocardia caviae*
c. *Streptomyces somaliensis*
d. *Nocardia asteroides*

94. An 18-year-old man from Mexico has had chronic infected lesions on his feet. Culture of the lesions reveals an organism which is a branching gram-positive rod that hydrolyzes casein and tyrosine. The most likely identification is:

a. *Nocardia caviae*
b. *Nocardia asteroides*
c. *Nocardia brasiliensis*

95. It is important to identify individual members of the group D streptococci because:

a. viridans streptococci are often confused with enterococci
b. several enterococci cause severe puerperal sepsis
c. nonenterococcal group D streptococci are avirulent
d. enterococci often show more resistance to penicillin than other group D streptococci

96. True statements about *Salmonella typhi* include:

   a. It does not invade the blood stream.
   b. It can be recovered easily from stool during the early stages of typhoid fever.
   c. It produces copious gas from glucose.
   d. It can be recovered from bile.

97. A false statement regarding surveillance of chronic nosocomial infection with *Klebsiella pneumoniae* is:

   a. As the incidence of infection increases, the organism may become resistant to gentamicin, tobramycin, and other aminoglycosides if these drugs are used extensively.
   b. Antibiotic susceptibility patterns (antibiograms) can be useful as epidemiological markers for documenting cross-infections.
   c. If only Bauer-Kirby disc diffusion testing is done, it is difficult to determine whether more than one strain is responsible.
   d. Commercially available identification panels (API-20Ek Micro-ID, Enterotube) provide reproducible differentiation of species into biotypes and can be routinely used in infection control.

98. When using cystine-trypticase agar (CTA) for carbohydrate tests of *Neisseria* species, one should not:

   a. use a heavy inoculum
   b. use reagent-grade carbohydrates
   c. work with pure subcultures
   d. store inoculated media in a CO_2 incubator

99. When testing for oxidase activity, for which of the following organisms is it recommended that a 5% aqueous solution of tetramethyl-phenylenediamine dihydrochloride be used, rather than commercially available strips?

   a. *Eikenella corrodens*
   b. *Haemophilus aphrophilus*
   c. *Flavobacterium meningosepticum*
   d. *Pasteurella multocida*

100. It has been recommended that cephalexin be incorporated into Bordet-Gengou agar instead of penicillin because:

 a. cephalexin is more stable at incubation temperature
 b. cephalexin inhibits organisms indigenous to the nasopharynx
 c. cephalexin may inactivate some inhibitory fatty acids and peroxides
 d. penicillin may inhibit some strains of *Bordetella pertussis*

101. Anaerobic infections differ from aerobic infections in which of the following?

 a. They usually respond favorably with aminoglycoside therapy.
 b. They usually arise from exogenous sources.
 c. They are usually polymicrobic.
 d. Gram stained smears of the specimens are less helpful in diagnosis.

102. The presence of 20% bile in blood agar would probably enhance the growth of:

 a. *Fusobacterium nucleatum* and *Bacteroides ovatus*
 b. *Bacteroides ovatus* and *Bacteroides fragilis*
 c. *Bacteroides melaninogenicus*
 d. *Bacteroides fragilis*

103. Two different-sized colonies are often observed on a chocolate agar plate subculture of *Neisseria gonorrhoeae* due to the:

 a. appearance of penicillin-resistant variants
 b. appearance of spontaneous lipopolysaccharide mutants
 c. presence of spontaneous auxotrophic mutants
 d. presence of both piliated (small) and nonpiliated (large) colonies

104. When a _Brucella_ species is suspected in a blood culture, the bottle should be held for a minimum of:

a. 5 days
b. 7 days
c. 14 days
d. 21 days

105. Once an organism has been identified as a member of the fluorescent group of _Pseudomonas_, which of the following tests must be performed to differentiate the species?

a. growth at 42°C, pyocyanin production, gelatinase production
b. pyocyanin production, gelatinase production, OF glucose reaction
c. growth at 52°C, pyocyanin production, OF glucose reaction
d. gelatinase production, growth at 52°C, H_2S production

106. _Eikenella_ _corrodens_ characteristically is:

a. identical to the organism known as _Bacteroides_ _corrodens_
b. dependent on factor X for initial aerobic growth
c. arginine dihydrolase- and lysine decarboxylase-positive
d. an obligate anaerobe

107. Cotton swabs submitted for culture of gonococci should be plated onto culture medium:

a. immediately
b. within 2 hours
c. within 4 hours
d. within 24 hours

108. The ONPG test allows organisms to be classified as a lactose fermenter by testing for which of the following?

a. permease
b. β-galactosidase
c. β-lactamase
d. phosphatase

109. For which of the following organisms is it important to test routinely for β-lactamase production?

   a. *Streptococcus pyogenes*
   b. *Klebsiella pneumoniae*
   c. *Haemophilus influenzae*
   d. *Escherichia coli*

110. Microorganisms resembling L-forms have been isolated from the blood of patients treated with antibiotics that:

   a. complex with flagellar protein
   b. interfere with cell membrane function
   c. inhibit protein synthesis
   d. interfere with cell wall synthesis

111. "Clue cells" are best seen in a:

   a. Gram stain of the vaginal discharge
   b. pelvic examination
   c. saline wet preparation of vaginal discharge material
   d. Gram stain of the typical colony of *Gardnerella vaginalis*

112. Tests for β-lactamase production in *Haemophilus influenzae*:

   a. are not commercially available
   b. include tests that measure a change to an alkaline pH
   c. should be performed on all blood and CSF isolates
   d. are not valid for any other bacterial species

113. Definitive identification of *Neisseria gonorrhoeae* is made based on the:

   a. Gram stain
   b. oxidase test
   c. degradation of amino acids
   d. hydrolysis of carbohydrates

114. *Listeria* can be confused with some streptococci because of its hemolysis and because it is:

   a. nonmotile
   b. catalase-negative
   c. oxidase-positive
   d. esculin-positive

115. Bacterial meningitis is not lethal when treated early with appropriate antimicrobials; therefore, it is important to:

   a. examine the Gram stained slide for purulent material
   b. select new slides for Gram stain
   c. evaluate morphology and Gram stain reaction
   d. perform catalase test on colonies

116. Clostridium difficile can best be recovered from feces on:

   a. enteric media and incubated aerobically
   b. blood agar incubated anaerobically
   c. CCFA incubated at 37°C under 5% CO_2
   d. CCFA incubated at 37°C anaerobically

117. At the present time Clostridium difficile toxin can be detected by:

   a. radioimmunoassays
   b. chromatographic procedures
   c. cytotoxicity
   d. high-pressure liquid chromatography

118. The most critical distinction between Staphylococcus aureus and other species of Staphylococcus is:

   a. phosphatase reaction
   b. DNA production
   c. coagulase production
   d. hemolysis

119. One of the enterotoxins produced by enterotoxigenic Escherichia coli in traveler's diarrhea is similiar to a toxin produced by:

   a. Clostridium perfringens
   b. Clostridium difficile
   c. Vibrio cholerae
   d. Yersinia enterocolitica

120. Optimum growth of *Campylobacter fetus* subspecies *jejuni* is obtained on suitable media incubated at 42°C in an atmosphere containing:

   a. 6% O_2, 10–15% CO_2, 85–90% N

   b. 10% H_2, 5% CO_2, 85% N

   c. 10% H_2, 10% CO_2, 80% N

   d. 25% O_2, 5% CO_2, 70% N

121. A 15-year-old girl was admitted to the hospital because of lower right quadrant pain and questionable rebound tenderness. The WBC was 12,000/mm^3 with 75% segmented neutrophils and 6% bands. The clinical diagnosis was probable appendicitis. At surgery the appendix was grossly normal, but several enlarged, red, mesenteric lymph nodes were observed. One of these was excised and cultured. The organism most likely to produce this clinical picture is:

   a. Enteropathogenic *Escherichia coli*
   b. *Listeria monocytogenes*
   c. *Salmonella enteritidis*
   d. *Yersinia pseudotuberculosis*

122. Which of the following statements regarding methods for the isolation of anaerobic bacteria is the most accurate?

   a. When properly performed, the use of the Gas Pak system is comparable to the roll tube or anaerobic chamber methods.
   b. The use of prereduced anaerobically sterilized (PRAS) media in roll tubes is the best and most practical method.
   c. The use of liquid media such as thioglycollate is comparable to other methods.
   d. The use of the anaerobic chamber is a most effective method because the growth of facultative organisms is inhibited.

123. A positive porphyrin production test indicates that the organism:

   a. requires both X and V factors
   b. requires X factor
   c. does not require X factor
   d. requires V factor

124. The epidemiologic investigation of a possible *Salmonella enteritidis* outbreak includes the documentation of single strain identity of:

a. bacteriocin typing
b. biotyping
c. phage typing
d. serologic typing

125. *Vibrio parahaemolyticus* can be isolated best from feces on:

a. eosin methylene blue (EMB) agar
b. Hektoen enteric (HE) agar
c. Salmonella-Shigella (SS) agar
d. thiosulfate citrate bile salts (TCBS) agar

126. Of the following bacteria, the most frequent cause of prosthetic heart valve infections occurring within two to three months after surgery is:

a. *Streptococcus pneumoniae*
b. *Streptococcus pyogenes*
c. *Staphylococcus aureus*
d. *Staphylococcus epidermidis*

127. The bacterium most often responsible for acute epiglottitis is:

a. *Bordetella pertussis*
b. *Haemophilus influenzae*
c. *Haemophilus aphrophilus*
d. β-hemolytic streptococcus group A

128. Which of the following is the most appropriate method for collecting a urine specimen from a patient with an indwelling catheter?

a. Remove the catheter, cut the tip, and submit it for culture.
b. Disconnect the catheter from the bag, and collect urine from the terminal end of the catheter.
c. Collect urine directly from the bag.
d. Aspirate urine aseptically from the catheter.

129. Diagnosis of typhoid fever during the first two days of illness can be confirmed best by:

   a. stool culture
   b. urine culture
   c. blood culture
   d. demonstration of antibodies against O antigen in the patient's serum

130. *Streptococcus pneumoniae* can be differentiated best from the viridans group of streptococci by:

   a. Gram stain
   b. the type of hemolysis
   c. colonial morphology
   d. bile solubility

131. Which of the two different antimicrobial agents listed below is commonly used and may result in synergistic action in the treatment of endocarditis caused by *Streptococcus faecalis*?

   a. an aminoglycoside and a macrolide
   b. a penicillin derivative and an aminoglycoside
   c. a cell membrane-active agent and nalidixic acid
   d. a macrolide and a penicillin derivative

132. A gram-negative, bipolar-staining bacillus isolated from an infected dog bite with a positive cytochrome oxidase and positive indole test is most likely to be:

   a. *Aeromonas hydrophila*
   b. *Pasteurella haemolytica*
   c. *Pasteurella multocida*
   d. *Vibrio parahaemolyticus*

133. The biochemical reactions of an organism are consistent with *Shigella*. A suspension is tested in polyvalent antiserum without resulting in agglutination. However, after 15 minutes of boiling, agglutination occurs in polyvalent and group D antisera. This indicates that the:

   a. organism contains a blocking O antigen
   b. antiserum is of low potency
   c. organism possesses capsular antigens
   d. antiserum is of low specificity

134. Which of the following would best differentiate *Streptococcus agalactiae* from *Streptococcus pyogenes*?

   a. ability to grow in sodium azide broth
   b. a positive bile-esculin reaction
   c. hydrolysis of sodium hippurate
   d. β-hemolysis on sheep blood agar

135. The most meaningful laboratory procedure in confirming the diagnosis of clinical botulism is:

   a. demonstration of toxin in the patient's serum
   b. recovery of *Clostridium botulinum* from suspected food
   c. recovery of *Clostridium botulinum* from the patient's stool
   d. Gram stain of suspected food for gram-positive, sporulating bacilli

136. Which one of the following organisms does not require susceptibility testing when isolated from a clinically significant source?

   a. *Staphylococcus aureus*
   b. *Proteus mirabilis*
   c. group A streptococcus
   d. *Escherichia coli*

137. Routine quality control tests revealed that a batch of chocolate agar was able to support the growth of *Haemophilus influenzae* only as satellite colonies around *Staphylococcus aureus*. The most likely source of difficulty is:

   a. excess heating in preparation of the medium
   b. dehydration during storage of the medium
   c. attenuation of the quality control organism
   d. use of improperly cleaned glassware

138. A 29-year-old urban businessman is seen for recurrence of a purulent urethral discharge ten days after the successful treatment of culture-proven gonorrhea. The most likely etiology of his urethritis is:

   a. *Mycoplasma hominis*
   b. *Chlamydia trachomatis*
   c. *Trichomonas vaginalis*
   d. *Neisseria gonorrhoeae*

139. _Shigella_ species characteristically are:

   a. urease-positive
   b. nonmotile
   c. oxidase-positive
   d. lactose fermenters

140. Characteristically group D enterococci are:

   a. unable to grow in 6.5% NaCl
   b. relatively resistant to penicillin
   c. sodium hippurate-positive
   d. members of the Enterobacteriaceae family

141. The best medium for culture of _Francisella tularensis_ is:

   a. Bordet-Gengou
   b. cystine blood agar
   c. Loeffler's medium
   d. Lowenstein-Jensen's medium

142. The best medium for culture of _Bordetella pertussis_ is:

   a. Bordet-Gengou
   b. cystine blood agar
   c. Thayer-Martin medium
   d. Loeffler's medium

143. _Haemophilus influenzae_ is most likely considered normal indigenous flora in the:

   a. oropharynx
   b. female genital tract
   c. large intestine
   d. small intestine

144. If all of the zone sizes are too small for the control strains in disc susceptibility tests, the most likely cause is that the:

   a. inoculum was too light
   b. inoculum was too heavy
   c. Mueller-Hinton agar is too acidic
   d. Mueller-Hinton agar had high calcium and magnesium levels

145. Quality control results for Kirby-Bauer sensitivity tests yield the aminoglycoside zones too small and the tetracycline zones too large. This is probably due to the:

a. inoculum being too heavy
b. inoculum being too light
c. pH of Mueller-Hinton agar being too low
d. calcium and magnesium concentrations in the agar being too high

146. When using control strains of Staphylococcus aureus and Streptococcus agalactiae, the technologist notices that the zones around the methicillin disc are too small. This is probably due to the use of:

a. too heavy an inoculum
b. too light an inoculum
c. Mueller-Hinton agar which is too acidic
d. outdated antibiotic discs

147. A characteristic helpful in separating Pseudomonas aeruginosa from other members of the Pseudomonas family is:

a. a positive test for cytochrome oxidase
b. oxidative metabolism in the O/F test
c. production of fluorescein pigment
d. production of pyocyanin pigment

148. An important cause of acute exudative pharyngitis is:

a. Staphylococcus aureus (β-hemolytic)
b. Streptococcus pneumoniae
c. Streptococcus agalactiae
d. Streptococcus pyogenes

149. How many hours after eating contaminated food do inital symptoms of staphylococcal food poisoning typically occur?

a. 5 to 7 hours
b. 12 to 18 hours
c. 24 to 48 hours
d. 72 hours to a week

150. A test that aids in differentiating between upper (kidney) and lower (bladder) urinary tract infection is:

a. luciferase assay of adenosine triphosphate
b. creatinine clearance
c. triphenyl tetrazolium chloride (TTC) test
d. demonstration of antibody-coated bacteria in the urine

151. The organism most commonly associated with neonatal purulent meningitis is:

a. *Neisseria meningitidis*
b. *Streptococcus pneumoniae*
c. group B streptococci
d. *Haemophilus influenzae*

152. Which of the following is a synergistic bacterial infection?

a. scarlet fever
b. strep throat
c. erythrasma
d. Vincent's angina

153. A catherized urine specimen from an 82-year-old woman with recurrent infections is submitted for culture. The Gram stain reveals:

Many WBCs
Many pleomorphic gram-negative rods
Many gram-positive cocci in chains
Few gram-positive rods

The physician requests that sensitivities be performed on all pathogens isolated. In addition to the sheep blood agar and EMB plates routinely used for urine cultures, the technologist should also process a(n):

a. CNA agar plate
b. chocolate agar plate
c. XLD agar plate
d. chopped meat glucose

154. A 73-year-old man diagnosed as having pneumococcal meningitis is not responding to his penicillin therapy. Which of the following tests should be performed on the isolate to best determine this organism's sensitivity?

a. β-lactamase
b. oxacillin disk diffusion
c. agar dilution
d. Schlichter test

155. Cerebrospinal fluid (CSF) from a febrile 25-year-old man with possible meningitis is rushed to the laboratory for a STAT Gram stain and culture. While performing the Gram stain, the technologist accidentally spills most of the spinal fluid. The smear shows many neutrophils and no microorganisms. Since there is only enough CSF to inoculate one plate, the technologist should use a:

a. blood agar plate
b. chopped meat glucose
c. chocolate agar plate
d. Thayer-Martin plate

156. A small gram-negative rod isolated from an eye culture has the following test results:

X Factor requirement	yes
V Factor requirement	yes
Hemolysis on rabbit blood agar	no

This organism should be identified as:

a. _Haemophilus influenzae_
b. _Haemophilus parainfluenzae_
c. _Haemophilus haemolyticus_
d. _Haemophilus parahaemolyticus_

157. When processing throat swabs for a "strep" screen, the medium of choice is:

a. sheep blood agar plates
b. rabbit blood agar plates
c. human blood agar plates
d. horse blood agar plates

158. When performing a Kovac's indole test, the inoculated media must contain:

a. indole
b. tryptophan
c. ornithine
d. para-dimethylaminobenzaldehyde

159. A throat swab is submitted for anaerobic culture. This specimen should be:

a. set up immediately
b. rejected
c. inoculated into thioglycollate broth
d. sent to a reference laboratory

160. A vaginal smear is submitted for a Gram stain for Neisseria gonorrhoeae. The technologist finds the following results on the Gram stain:

Many white blood cells
Few epithelial cells
Many gram-positive rods
Few gram-negative diplococci
Few gram-positive cocci in chains

The technologist should:

a. report that the smear is positive for gonorrhea
b. report that the smear is negative for gonorrhea
c. request a new specimen due to number of white blood cells
d. report that the smear is unacceptable for gonorrhea screen

161. A skin biopsy is submitted for routine, mycobacteria and mycology cultures. The best course of action is to:

a. grind tissue and inoculate all media
b. cut tissue into tiny pieces, inoculate mycology media, grind remaining tissue, and inoculate remaining media
c. cut tissue into tiny pieces, inoculate mycobacteria media, grind remaining tissue, and inoculate remaining media
d. vigorously rub the biopsy across appropriate media

162. A CSF is submitted for Gram stain and culture. The physician also requests that an aliquot of spinal fluid be saved for possible CIE. The microbiology laboratory is closing in five minutes. The technologist should:

a. inoculate culture, perform a Gram stain, and refrigerate remaining spinal fluid at 4°C
b. inoculate culture, perform a Gram stain, and incubate remaining spinal fluid at 36°C
c. incubate entire specimen at 36°C, perform culture and Gram stain the next day
d. refrigerate entire specimen, perform culture and Gram stain the next day

163. The optimal wound specimen for culture of anaerobic organisms should be:

a. a swab of lesion obtained before administration of antibiotics
b. a swab of lesion obtained after administration of antibiotics
c. a syringe filled with pus, obtained before administration of antibiotics
d. a syringe filled with pus, obtained after administration of antibiotics

164. Which of the following is most often used to prepare a slide from a plate culture for microscopic observation of a dermatophyte?

a. lactophenol cotton blue
b. potassium hydroxide
c. iodine solution
d. Gram stain

165. Which of the following is the most useful morphological feature in identifying the mycelial phase of _Histoplasma capsulatum_?

a. arthrospores every other cell
b. microspores 2-5 μm
c. tuberculate macrospores 8-14 μm
d. nonseptate macrospores of 5-7 cells

166. The recovery of some Cryptococcus species may be compromised if the isolation media contains:

   a. cycloheximide
   b. gentamicin
   c. chloramphenicol
   d. penicillin

167. The one characteristic by which an unknown Cryptococcus species can be identified as Cryptococcus neoformans is:

   a. appearance of yellow colonies
   b. positive urease test
   c. presence of a capsule
   d. positive bird seed agar test

168. The typical tissue inflammatory response to invasion with Cryptococcus is:

   a. polymorphonuclear
   b. lymphocytic
   c. monocytic
   d. minimal or absent

169. While reading the quality control smear for the periodic acid-Schiff (PAS) stain, you note the background and fungal elements appear pink. Which of the following is most likely?

   a. The periodic acid has deteriorated and is no longer able to oxidize the hydroxyl groups.
   b. The sodium meta-bisulfite solution is no longer stable and has lost its bleaching properties.
   c. The basic fuchsin solution is unstable and has deteriorated.
   d. The procedure is in control and all solutions are stable.

170. Pus from a draining fistula on a foot was submitted for culture. Gross examination of the specimen revealed the presence of a small (0.8 mm in diameter), yellowish, oval granule. Direct microscopic examination of the crushed granule showed hyphae 3-4 µm in diameter and the presence of chlamydospores at the periphery. After two days a cottony, white mold was seen that turned gray with a gray to black reverse after a few days. When viewed microscopically, moderately large hyaline septate hyphae with long or short conidiophores, each terminated by a single pear-shaped aleuiospore, 5-7 x 8-10 µm, were seen. The most likely identification is:

a. *Exophiala jeanselmei*
b. *Fonsecaea pedrosoi*
c. *Pseudallescheria boydii*
d. *Cladosporium carrionii*

171. Crust from a cauliflower-like lesion on the hand exhibited brown spherical bodies 6-12 µm in diameter when examined microscopically. After three weeks of incubation at room temperature, a slow-growing black mold grew on Sabouraud's dextrose agar. Microscopic examination revealed cladosporium, phialophora, and acrotheca types of sporulation. The probable identification of this organism is:

a. *Fonsecaea pedrosoi*
b. *Pseudallescheria boydii*
c. *Phialophora verrucosa*
d. *Cladosporium carrionii*

172. A fungus superficially resembles *Penicillium* species but may be differentiated because its sterigmata are long and tapering and bend away from the central axis. The sterigmata also arise singly from the hyphae. The most probable identification is:

a. *Exophiala* sp.
b. *Cephalosporium* sp.
c. *Cladosporium* sp.
d. *Paecilomyces* sp.

173. Culture of a strand of hair that fluoresced yellow-green when examined with a Wood's lamp produced a slow-growing, flat gray colony with a salmon-pink reverse. Microscopic examination demonstrated racquet hyphae, pectinate bodies, chlamydospores, and a few abortive or bizarre-shaped macroconidia.

The most probable identification of this isolate is:

a. *Microsporum gypseum*
b. *Microsporum canis*
c. *Microsporum audouinii*
d. *Trichophyton rubrum*

174. A mold grown at 25°C exhibited delicate, septate hyaline hyphae and many conidiophores extending at right angles from the hyphae. Oval, 2-5 µm conidia were formed at the end of the conidiophores, giving a flowerlike appearance. In some areas "sleeves" of spores could be found along the hyphae as well. A 37°C culture of this organism produced small, cigar-shaped yeast cells.

This organism is most likely:

a. *Histoplasma capsulatum*
b. *Sporothrix schenckii*
c. *Blastomyces dermatitidis*
d. *Cephalosporium falciforme*

175. Which of the following is the best aid in the identification of *Epidermophyton floccosum* macrospores?

a. parallel side walls with at least ten cells
b. spindle-shaped spore with thin walls
c. spindle-shaped spore, thick walls, and distinct terminal knob with echinulations
d. smooth walls, club-shaped

176. Which of the following statements concerning the germ tube test is true?

a. Using a heavy inoculum enhances the rapid production of germ tubes.
b. Germ tubes should be read after 2 hours incubation at 25°C.
c. *Candida albicans* and *Candida tropicalis* can be used as positive and negative control, respectively.
d. Prior to use, serum should be stored at 4°C, at which temperature it will be stable for one year.

177. Many fungal infections are the result of spore inhalation. Which of the following is usually NOT contracted in this manner?

a. histoplasmosis
b. blastomycosis
c. coccidioidomycosis
d. sporotrichosis

178. Skin scrapings obtained from the edge of a crusty wrist lesion were found to contain thick-walled, spherical yeast cells (8-15 μm in diameter) that had single buds with a wide base of attachment. Microscopic examination of the room temperature isolate from this specimen would probably reveal the presence of:

a. "rosette-like" clusters of pear-shaped conidia at the tips of delicate conidiophores
b. thick-walled, round to pear-shaped tuberculate macroconidia
c. numerous conidia along the length of hyphae in a "sleeve-like" arrangement
d. septate hyphae bearing round or pear-shaped small conidia attached to conidiophores of irregular lengths

179. *Trichophyton rubrum* characteristically:

a. gives a positive hair penetration test
b. has granular colonies
c. has a green reverse
d. has numerous small spherical to clavate microconidia

180. Which of the following fungi produce a positive nitrate assimilation test?

a. *Cryptococcus neoformans*
b. *Candida albicans*
c. *Candida tropicalis*
d. *Cryptococcus albidus*

181. Staib's medium (bird seed agar) is useful in the identification of which of the following?

a. *Candida albicans*
b. *Candida (Torulopsis) glabrata*
c. *Saccharomyces cerevisiae*
d. *Cryptococcus neoformans*

182. A urine culture from a patient with a urinary tract infection yields a yeast with the following characteristics: failure to produce germ tubes, hyphae not formed on cornmeal agar, urease-negative, assimilates trehalose.

The most likely identification is:

a. *Saccharomyces cerevisiae*
b. *Cryptococcus laurentii*
c. *Candida pseudotropicalis*
d. *Candida (Torulopsis) glabrata*

183. The serologic test most helpful in determining the prognosis of coccidioidomycosis is the:

a. precipitin test
b. complement fixation test
c. latex particle agglutination test
d. hemagglutination inhibition test

184. A major limitation of flucytosine (5-fluorocytosine) in the treatment of yeast infections is that:

a. absorption from the gastrointestinal tract is erratic and unpredictable
b. there is an antagonistic reaction when it is combined with amphotericin B
c. *Candida* and *Cryptococcus* develop resistance during therapy
d. penetration into cerebrospinal fluid is negligible in cryptococcal meningitis

185. False-positive reactions to the immunodiffusion test for histoplasmosis have been seen after:

a. amphotericin B therapy
b. skin testing with histoplasmin
c. cultures have reverted to negative
d. complement-fixing antibodies have disappeared

186. Which of the following is a dimorphic fungus?

a. *Sporothrix schenckii*
b. *Candida albicans*
c. *Cryptococcus neoformans*
d. *Aspergillus fumigatus*

187. Technologists should always work under a biological safety hood when working with cultures of:

a. *Streptococcus pyogenes*
b. *Staphylococcus aureus*
c. *Candida albicans*
d. *Coccidioides immitis*

188. The function of N-acetyl-L-cysteine, which is required in the NALC-NaOH reagent for acid-fast digestion-decontamination procedures, is to:

a. inhibit growth of normal respiratory flora
b. inhibit growth of fungi
c. neutralize the NaOH
d. liquify the mucus

189. Which of the following characteristics best distinguishes *Mycobacterium scrofulaceum* from *Mycobacterium gordonae*?

a. hydrolysis of Tween 80 and splitting of urea
b. no hydrolysis of Tween 80
c. good growth at 25°C
d. niacin production

190. Middlebrook 7H10 and 7H11 media must be refrigerated in the dark and incubated in the dark as well. If these conditions are not met, the media may prove toxic for *Mycobacteria* because:

a. carbon dioxide will be released, retarding growth
b. growth factors will be broken down
c. sunlight destroys the ammonium sulfate necessary in the mycobacterial metabolism
d. formaldehyde may be produced

191. A 2-week-old culture of a urine specimen produced a few colonies of acid-fast bacilli which were rough and nonpigmented. The niacin test was weakly positive and the nitrate test was positive. Which of the following is the most appropriate action when a presumptive identification has been requested as soon as possible?

   a. Report the organism as presumptive *Mycobacterium tuberculosis*.
   b. Wait a few days and repeat the niacin test; report presumptive *Mycobacterium tuberculosis* if the test is more strongly positive.
   c. Subculture the organism and set up the routine battery of biochemicals; notify the physician that results will not be available for three weeks.
   d. Set up a thiophene-2-carboxylic acid hydrazide (T_2H); if the organism is sensitive, report *Mycobacterium bovis*.

192. A nonpigmented, acid-fast organism was cultured in five days from a cutaneous infection aspirate. No branching filamentous extensions were noted on the Middlebrook 7H11 plate. The biochemical results were nitrate-negative, arylsulfatase (three days and two weeks)-positive, iron-uptake-negative, Tween 80 hydrolysis-negative. The organism most likely is:

   a. *Mycobacterium fortuitum*
   b. *Mycobacterium smegmatis*
   c. *Mycobacterium phlei*
   d. *Mycobacterium chelonei*

193. When staining acid-fast bacilli with Truant's auramine-rhodamine stain, potassium permanganate is used as a:

   a. decolorizing agent
   b. quenching agent
   c. mordant
   d. dye

194. Characteristics necessary for the definitive identification of *Mycobacterium tuberculosis* are:

  a. buff color, slow growth at 37°C, niacin production-positive, nitrate reduction-negative
  b. rough colony, slow growth at 37°C, nonpigmented
  c. rough, nonpigmented colony, cording positive, niacin production-negative, catalase-negative at pH 7/68°C
  d. rough, nonpigmented colony, slow growth at 37°C, niacin production-positive, nitrate reduction-positive

195. Which group of mycobacteria require an isolation temperature of 20-32°C?

  a. *M. chelonei, M. ulcerans, M. kansasii*
  b. *M. chelonei, M. ulcerans, M. haemophilum*
  c. *M. marinum, M. chelonei, M. ulcerans*
  d. *M. marinum, M. ulcerans, M. haemophilum*

196. Which of the following is a true statement about pigment production by *M. kansasii*?

  a. It is a result of β-carotene formation and accumulation.
  b. It can be an indication of virulence.
  c. It can be inhibited by inclusion of albumin in growth medium.
  d. It is increased at 30°C incubation.

197. Differentiation of *Mycobacterium avium* from *Mycobacterium intracellulare* can be accomplished by:

  a. nitrate reduction test
  b. Tween hydrolysis test
  c. resistance to 10 μg thiophene-2-carboxylic acid hydrazide
  d. gas liquid chromatography

198. Recent evidence has shown that specimens to be inoculated for the recovery of acid-fast bacilli should be centrifuged at approximately:

  a. 2000 X G
  b. 2500 X G
  c. 3000 X G
  d. 3500 X G

199. The most important constituent of the tubercle bacillus for the activity of the various tuberculins is the:

a. phospholipid
b. protein
c. wax D
d. polysaccharide

200. Differential skin testing for mycobacteriosis has diagnostic value in young children because:

a. immaturity of the immune system allows useful reactions
b. infections develop more slowly, yielding more definitive immune response
c. they have not yet become sensitized to many mycobacteria
d. they develop hypersensitivity at an early age

201. Which of the following test procedures lacks reproducibility?

a. niacin
b. catalase
c. Tween 80
d. nitrate

202. Because ultraviolet light is used to decontaminate the work surface inside a biological safety cabinet, the lamp should be replaced when the intensity compared to the original output reading differs by:

a. 10%
b. 20%
c. 30%
d. 40%

203. Which one of the following species of Mycobacterium does NOT usually fluoresce on fluorochrome stain?

a. Mycobacterium fortuitum
b. Mycobacterium tuberculosis
c. Mycobacterium ulcerans
d. Mycobacterium bovis

204. Which of the following reagents should be used as a mucolytic, alkaline reagent for digestion and decontamination of a sputum for mycobacterial culture?

   a. N-acetyl-L-cystine and NaOH
   b. NaOH alone
   c. zephiran-trisodium phosphate
   d. oxalic acid

205. The agent used for processing specimens for mycobacterial culture contaminated with *Pseudomonas* is:

   a. N-acetyl-L-cystine and NaOH
   b. NaOH alone
   c. zephiran-trisodium phosphate
   d. oxalic acid

206. Which of the following reagents is used only for decontamination of urine for mycobacterial culture?

   a. NaOH alone
   b. N-acetyl-L-cystine and NaOH
   c. sulfuric acid
   d. zephiran-trisodium phosphate

207. Which of the following mycobacterial species lack the enzyme to convert free niacin to niacin ribonucleotide?

   1. *Mycobacterium bovis*
   2. *Mycobacterium simiae*
   3. *Mycobacterium avium*
   4. *Mycobacterium tuberculosis*

   a. only 1, 2 and 3 are correct
   b. only 1 and 3 are correct
   c. only 2 and 4 are correct
   d. only 4 is correct
   e. all are correct

208. Mycobacterium szulgai characteristically:

a. produces niacin
b. is a low catalase producer (45 mm) and is nitrate-reduction positive
c. loses catalase after heating at 68°C, and has a negative Tween hydrolysis test at five days
d. is scotochromogenic at 37°C and photochromogenic at 25°C

209. Which of the following combinations of media provide an egg base, agar base, and a selective egg- or agar-base media?

a. Lowenstein-Jensen, American Thoracic Society (ATS), Middlebrook 7H11
b. Lowenstein-Jensen, Middlebrook 7H11, Lowenstein-Jensen (Gruft Modification)
c. Middlebrook 7H10, Petragnani, Lowenstein-Jensen
d. Middlebrook 7H10, Middlebrook 7H11, 7H11 (Mitchison's)

210. The rapid-growing mycobacteria can produce disease in humans. Therapy for this group of organisms should include:

1. isoniazid, ethambutol, and paraminosalicylic acid
2. rifampin, amikacin, and SCT/TMP
3. ampicillin, isoniazid, and rifampin
4. amikacin, doxycycline, and erythromycin

a. only 1, 2 and 3 are correct
b. only 1 and 3 are correct
c. only 2 and 4 are correct
d. only 4 is correct
e. all are correct

211. A FALSE statement about drug susceptibility testing of mycobacteria is:

a. It is difficult to standardize because of the variation in stability of drugs under different sterilization and storage methods.
b. It may be performed directly on a digested, concentrated specimen if acid-fast bacilli are seen on a prepared film.
c. Resistance is continued as 1% or more of the organisms that grow on the control quadrant also grow on a drug quadrant.
d. It requires the use of Mycobacterium tuberculosis H37Rv and known resistant strains as controls run on egg-base media.

212. The main reason for the administration of two or more drugs for the treatment of pulmonary tuberculosis is to:

a. obtain a greater therapeutic effect
b. prevent the emergence of bacilli resistant to the action of either or both drugs
c. reduce the toxicity of either drug if used alone
d. reduce the deleterious effect of tuberculin hypersensitivity

213. The disease-producing capacity of *Mycobacterium tuberculosis* depends primarily upon:

a. production of exotoxin
b. production of endotoxin
c. capacity to withstand intracellular digestion by macrophages
d. lack of susceptibility to the myeloperoxidase system

214. Assuming that the host has no known immunologic defect, which of the following is most likely to be associated with resistance to standard drug therapy?

a. *Mycobacterium tuberculosis*
b. *Mycobacterium bovis*
c. *Mycobacterium avium/intracellulare*
d. *Mycobacterium scrofulaceum*

215. The nitrate test for mycobacteria can be performed with a reagent-impregnated paper strip or by the use of standard reagents. In order to control the test properly, which of the following should be used for a positive control?

a. *Mycobacterium bovis*
b. *Mycobacterium gordonae*
c. *Mycobacterium tuberculosis*
d. *Mycobacterium intracellulare*

216. *Mycobacterium tuberculosis* can usually be distinguished from *Mycobacterium bovis* by positive tests for niacin accumulation and nitrate reductase. Occasional strains of *Mycobacterium bovis* may produce small amounts of both niacin and nitroreductase. In these strains, differentiation between the two species can best be accomplished by:

a. Tween 80 hydrolysis within ten days
b. demonstration of heat-stable catalase
c. a positive aryl sulfatase test within three days
d. growth inhibition by thiophene-2-carboxylic acid hydrazide

217. The best medium for culture of *Mycobacterium tuberculosis* is:

a. Bordet-Gengou
b. Loeffler's medium
c. Lowenstein-Jensen's medium
d. cystine blood agar

218. A nonphotochromogen which grows best at 42°C and is highly resistant to antibiotics is:

a. *Mycobacterium chelonei*
b. *Mycobacterium marinum*
c. *Mycobacterium tuberculosis*
d. *Mycobacterium xenopi*

219. A positive niacin test is most characteristic of:

a. *Mycobacterium chelonei*
b. *Mycobacterium marinum*
c. *Mycobacterium tuberculosis*
d. *Mycobacterium xenopi*

220. The organism, also known as the Battey bacillus, which can cause chronic pulmonary disease is:

a. *Mycobacterium tuberculosis*
b. *Mycobacterium bovis*
c. *Mycobacterium fortuitum/chelonei* complex
d. *Mycobacterium avium/intracellulare* complex

221. Which species of mycobacteria includes a BCG strain used for vaccination against tuberculosis?

   a. *Mycobacterium tuberculosis*
   b. *Mycobacterium bovis*
   c. *Mycobacterium kansasii*
   d. *Mycobacterium fortuitum/chelonei* complex

222. Which of the following organisms grows slowest?

   a. *Mycobacterium tuberculosis*
   b. *Mycobacterium bovis*
   c. *Mycobacterium kansasii*
   d. *Mycobacterium intracellulare*

223. A nonchromogen which grows unusually fast for the genus *Mycobacterium* is:

   a. *Mycobacterium bovis*
   b. *Mycobacterium kansasii*
   c. *Mycobacterium fortuitum*
   d. *Mycobacterium intracellulare*

224. A skin abcess is submitted for mycobacterial culture from a patient who scraped his hand while cleaning his fish aquarium. The technologist should:

   a. inoculate one tube of media at 30°C
   b. set up an anaerobic culture in addition to an acid-fast culture
   c. process the specimen immediately upon receipt
   d. keep inoculated media under a constant light source

225. Photochromogens produce pigment when:

   a. kept in the dark at 22°C
   b. exposed to light for one hour
   c. grown in the presence of CO_2
   d. incubated with x-ray film

226. Which of the following organisms may be mistaken for *Iodamoeba butschlii* due to the presence of an apparent large vacuole?

a. the pre-cyst of *Entamoeba histolytica*
b. vacuolated cyst of *Entamoeba coli*
c. *Endolimax nana*
d. *Blastocystis hominis*

227. The cyst stage can be recovered from formed fecal specimens submitted for parasitic examination if the specimen:

a. is incubated at 37°C for 24 hours
b. is the result of a saline enema
c. is stored at refrigerator temperature
d. contains barium

228. Primary amoebic-encephalitis may be caused by:

1. *Entabmoeba coli*
2. *Dientamoeba fragilis*
3. *Endolimax nana*
4. *Naegleria* sp.

a. only 1, 2 and 3 are correct
b. only 1 and 3 are correct
c. only 2 and 4 are correct
d. only 4 is correct
e. all are correct

229. The term "internal autoinfection" is generally used in referring to infections with:

a. *Ascaris lumbricoides*
b. *Necator americanus*
c. *Trichuris trichiura*
d. *Strongyloides stercoralis*

230. A 44-year-old man was admitted to the hospital following a two-week history of low-grade fever, malaise, and anorexia. Examination of a Giemsa stained blood film revealed many intraerythrocytic parasites. Further history revealed frequent camping trips near Martha's Vineyard and Nantucket Island, but no travel outside the continental United States. This parasite could easily be confused with:

   a. *Trypanosoma cruzi*
   b. *Trypanosoma rhodesiense/gambiense*
   c. *Plasmodium falciparum*
   d. *Leishmania donovani*

231. When stool examination is negative, the preferred specimen for the diagnosis of paragonimiasis is:

   a. bile drainage
   b. duodenal aspirate
   c. sputum
   d. rectal biopsy

232. A batch of trichrome-stained slides for ova and parasite examination contains numerous minute crystals which totally obscure the microscopic field. Which of the following measures is the most appropriate remedial action?

   a. Change the Schaudinn's fixative, remove coverslips, and restain.
   b. Change the acid alcohol and restain.
   c. Remove coverslips and remount using fresh Permount or similar medium.
   d. Change the iodine alcohol solution to obtain a strong tea-colored solution, restain.

233. In cases of suspected infection with *Pneumocystis carinii*, the preferred specimen for a methenamine silver stain is:

   a. lung biopsy
   b. sputum
   c. bronchial brushings
   d. tracheobronchial aspirate

234. A peripheral blood film differential was reported to have 20 to 70% eosinophilia. This is characteristic of:

1. schistosomiasis
2. strongyloides
3. trichinosis
4. cutaneous larva migrans

a. only 1, 2 and 3 are correct
b. only 1 and 3 are correct
c. only 2 and 4 are correct
d. only 4 is correct
e. all are correct

235. Pairs of organisms that can be easily differentiated and identified from ova in fecal specimens include:

a. *Metagonimus yokogawai*, *Heterophyes heterophyes*
b. *Taenia solium*, *Taenia saginata*
c. *Necator americanus*, *Ancylostoma duodenale*
d. *Paragonimus westermani*, *Hymenolepis nana*

236. A stool specimen for ova and parasite examination contained numerous rhabditiform larvae. Which factors do NOT aid in identification of larvae?

a. length of the buccal cavity
b. age of the specimen
c. appearance of the genital primordium
d. endemic area traveled

237. The causative agent of cysticercosis is:

a. *Taenia solium*
b. *Taenia saginata*
c. *Ascaris lumbricoides*
d. *Trichuris trichiura*

238. A liquid stool specimen is collected at 10:00 p.m. and brought to the laboratory for culture, and parasite and ova examination. It is refrigerated until 10:10 a.m. the next day when the physician requests that the technologist look for amoebic trophozoites. The best course of action would be to:

a. request a new specimen
b. proceed on the specimen from the previous evening
c. perform a trichrome stain on original specimen
d. perform a wet mount on original specimen

For questions 239 to 242, refer to the illustration pictured below:

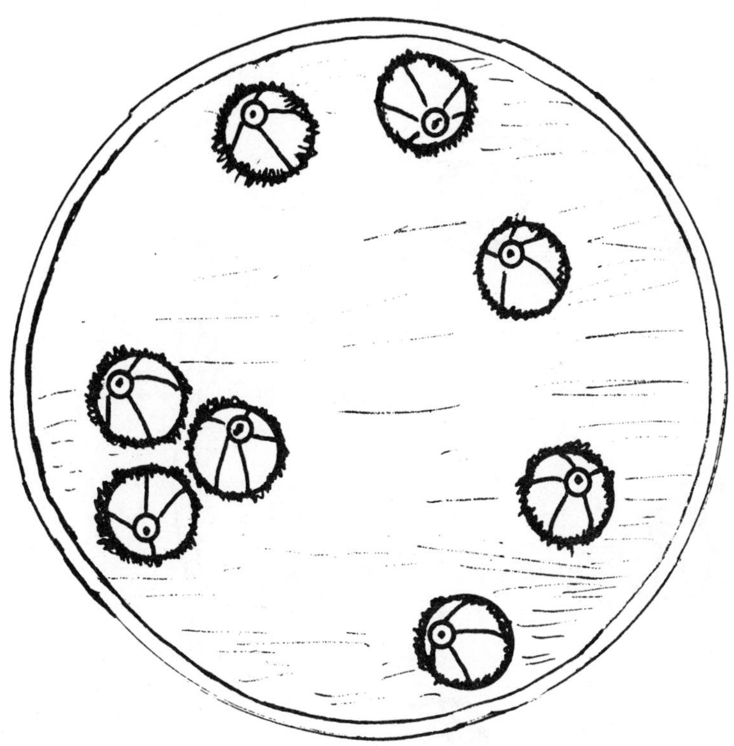

239. Trophozoites of the organism depicted above are likely to:

   a. contain red blood cells
   b. have clear, pointed pseudopodia
   c. contain few, if any, vacuoles
   d. have slow, undefined motility

240. Upon finding the above in a fecal concentrate, the technologist should:

   a. report this pathogen to the physician and begin patient isolation procedures
   b. review the fecal concentration carefully for the presence of other microorganisms which may be pathogenic
   c. look for motile trophozoites in the patient's sputum to better assess the patient's clinical condition
   d. request a new specimen because of the presence of excessive pollen grains

For questions 241 and 242, refer to the illustration pictured below:

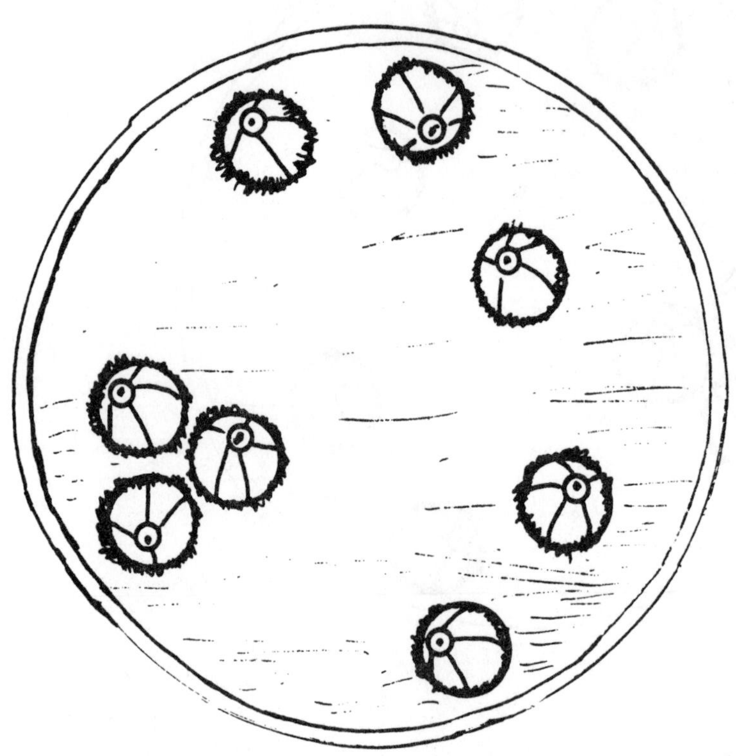

241. The above organism may easily be confused with:

   a. Entamoeba histolytica
   b. Iodamoeba butschlii
   c. Giardia lamblia
   d. Trichomonas vaginalis

242. The structure pictured above is a:

   a. cyst of a nonpathogenic amoeba
   b. trophozoite of a nonpathogenic amoeba
   c. cyst of a pathogenic amoeba
   d. trophozoite of a pathogenic amoeba

For questions 243 and 244, refer to the organism depicted below:

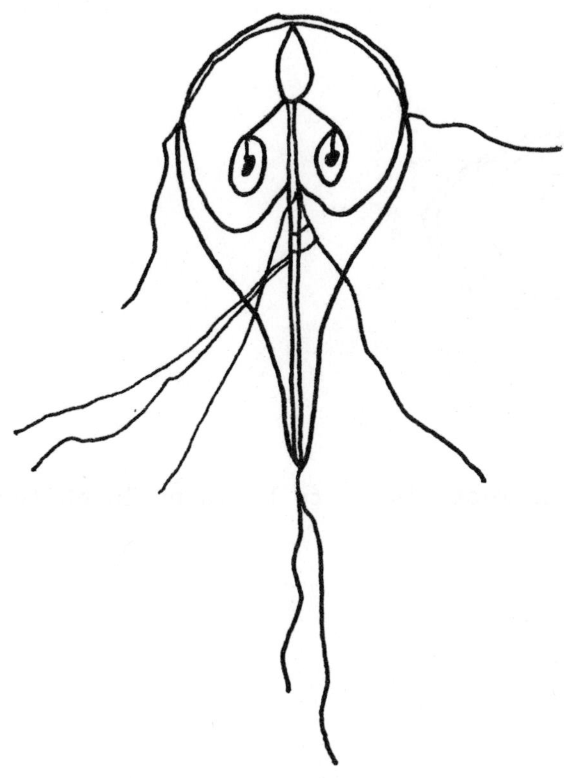

243. The organism depicted is a(n):

    a. amoeba
    b. flagellate
    c. trypanosoma
    d. sporozoan

244. A 24-year-old woman who just returned from vacationing in Russia became ill with steatorrheal diarrhea. The above organism was found in her stool. The patient most likely is suffering from:

    a. giardiasis
    b. amebiasis
    c. ascariasis
    d. balantidiasis

For questions 245 to 247, refer to the illustration below:

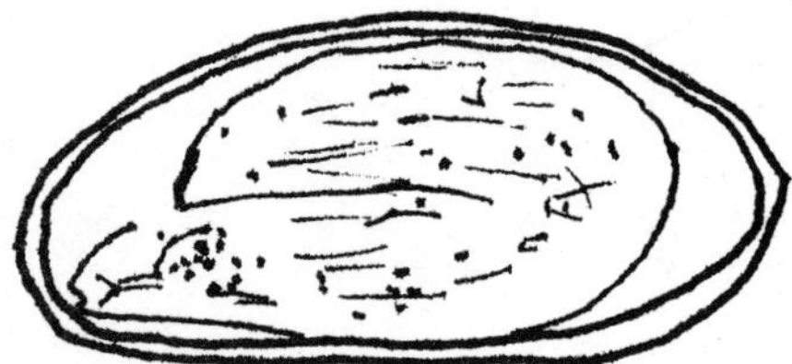

245. The egg depicted above is most likely to be found in children suffering from:

    a. diarrhea
    b. constipation
    c. perianal itching
    d. stomach pain

246. The specimen of choice for finding the above parasite is:

    a. stool
    b. duodenal washing
    c. rectal swab
    d. perianal Scotch-tape prep

247. A stool specimen from a 4-year-old boy is submitted for ova and parasite examination. The organism depicted above is suspected. The technologist should:

    a. perform a trichrome stain
    b. perform a wet mount
    c. request a Scotch-tape prep slide
    d. request a new stool specimen

248. *Mycoplasma* species are difficult to grow in the laboratory on routine media because of their requirement for:

a. sterols
b. horse blood
c. ferric pyrophosphate
d. surfactant such as Tween 80

249. In the first week of illness, leptospirosis may be detected by:

a. blood culture
b. urine culture
c. serum antibodies
d. spinal fluid culture

250. Microimmunofluorescence is associated with:

a. *Chlamydia trachomitis*
b. *Neisseria gonorrhoeae*
c. *Streptococcus pneumoniae*
d. *Klebsiella pneumoniae*

251. An RNA-containing virus is:

a. HAV
b. HBV
c. CMV
d. HSV

252. A DNA-containing virus is:

a. RSV
b. HBV
c. HAV
d. ECHO

253. The cell culture line most commonly used for the recovery of *Chlamydia trachomatis* from clinical specimens is:

a. HeLa 229
b. HEp-2
c. BHK-21
d. McCoy's

254. If gentamicin is incorporated into 2SP transport medium, there may be a compromise in the recovery of:

a. *Ureaplasma urealyticum*
b. *Chlamydia trachomatis*
c. *Chlamydia psittaci*
d. both *Chlamydia trachomatis* and *Chlamydia psittaci*

255. The serological test that is most sensitive for detecting all chlamydial infections is:

a. complement fixation (CF)
b. microimmunofluorescence (MIF)
c. single antigen immunofluorescence
d. indirect fluorescent antibody

256. Blood cultures from a case of suspected leptospiremia should be drawn:

a. between 10 p.m. and 2 a.m.
b. in the first 7-10 days of infection
c. during febrile periods, late in the course of the disease
d. after the first ten days of illness

257. Which of the following is a growth requirement for the isolation of *Leptospira*?

a. an atmosphere of 10% CO_2

b. an incubation temperature of 4°C

c. four- to five-day incubation

d. medium containing 10% serum plus fatty acids

258. The presence of actively motile spiral forms in a dark-field examination of an inflamed, ulcerating wound from a rat bite suggests a diagnosis of:

 a. sodoku
 b. plague
 c. tularemia
 d. leptospirosis

259. For direct smear examination either by special stains or FA technique for the detection of a virus, the material used to prepare the smears should contain:

 a. vesicular fluid
 b. leukocytes from the edge of the lesion
 c. the top portion of the vesicle
 d. epithelial cells from the base of the lesion

260. Which of the following is the single most important difference between viruses and chlamydia?

 a. obligate intracellular parasitism
 b. complex life cycle
 c. possession of mitochondria
 d. possession of a single type of nucleic acid

261. The most commonly used cell line in the clinical virus laboratory for viral propagation is the:

 a. KB cell
 b. HEp-2
 c. FL
 d. HeLa

262. Holding medium recommended for use in transporting urine or throat specimens for the recovery of cytomegalovirus contains:

 a. buffered tryptose phosphate broth
 b. sorbitol
 c. Hank's balanced salt solution
 d. 10% fetal albumin

263. In order to maintain virus recovery prior to inoculation, clinical material collected for viral culture should be:

 a. stored in the refrigerator
 b. maintained at room temperature
 c. frozen at -20°C
 d. frozen at 0°C

264. Inclusion blennorrhea, more commonly known as inclusion conjunctivitis of the newborn, may be acquired during birth when the mother is infected with:

 a. *Neisseria gonorrhoae*
 b. Herpes
 c. *Chlamydia trachomatis*
 d. *Treponema pallidum*

265. A whooping cough syndrome such as the one seen with infections caused by *Bordetella pertussis* can be seen in the infections due to:

 a. rhinovirus
 b. adenovirus
 c. coxsackie virus
 d. respiratory syncytial virus

266. Occasionally, Reye's syndrome appears as a severe complication of:

 a. poliomyelitis
 b. coxsackie B
 c. mumps encephalitis
 d. influenza

267. Which of the following viruses can only be detected by use of an electron microscope or ELISA methods?

 a. respiratory syncytial virus
 b. influenza A
 c. rotavirus
 d. herpes simplex 1

268. Throat swabs may be inoculated directly into the Bristol HeLa cell line when which of the following viruses is suspected?

    a. respiratory syncytial virus
    b. influenza A
    c. rotavirus
    d. herpes simplex 1

269. Humans commonly acquire leptospirosis by:

    a. ingestion of contaminated milk
    b. ingestion of contaminated salads
    c. inhalation of aerosol droplets from another person
    d. penetration through skin abrasions

270. *Legionella pneumophila* characteristically is:

    a. oxidase-positive
    b. gelatin-negative
    c. nonmotile
    d. gram-positive

271. Which of the following is characteristic of rickettsial disease testing?

    a. The Weil-Felix test is one of the most specific.
    b. Rickettsiae can be seen in infected tissue with immunofluorescent techniques.
    c. The complement fixation test is one of the least specific.
    d. Antibody to the Q fever agent will cross-react with the Rocky Mountain spotted fever agent.

272. Various *Chlamydia trachomatis* strains are capable of causing:

    1. nongonococcal ("nonspecific") urethritis
    2. pneumonia of newborns
    3. trachoma
    4. lymphogranuloma venereum

    a. only 1, 2 and 3 are correct
    b. only 1 and 3 are correct
    c. only 2 and 4 are correct
    d. only 4 is correct
    e. all are correct

273. The Epstein-Barr virus is associated with which of the following?

1. infectious mononucleosis
2. Hodgkin's lymphoma
3. Burkitt's lymphoma
4. chronic lymphocytic leukemia

a. only 1, 2 and 3 are correct
b. only 1 and 3 are correct
c. only 2 and 4 are correct
d. only 4 is correct
e. all are correct

274. Rickettsiae infecting man multiply preferentially within which of the following cells?

a. reticuloendothelial
b. hepatic
c. renal tubule
d. endothelial

275. Mycoplasmas differ from bacteria in that mycoplasmas:

a. do not cause disease in humans
b. cannot grow in artificial inanimate media
c. lack cell walls
d. are not serologically antigenic

276. The most reliable serologic test for the diagnosis of Q fever is the:

a. cold agglutinin test
b. heterophile antibody test
c. complement fixation test
d. Weil-Felix test

277. The preferred specimen for laboratory diagnosis of acquired cytomegalovirus infection is:

a. blood
b. urine
c. stool
d. cutaneous vesicular fluid

278. Leptospiremia is detectable:

a. for at least six months following infection
b. only when the patient becomes jaundiced
c. only during the first two weeks of acute illness
d. for at least one month following injection

279. Which of the following statements is true regarding the diagnosis of herpes simplex encephalitis caused by *Herpesvirus hominis*?

a. The virus can usually be recovered from fluid during the first week of illness.
b. The virus can usually be recovered from feces during the first week of illness.
c. The virus is rarely recoverable from either spinal fluid or feces during herpes encephalitis.
d. Cytopathic effects are slow to develop in cell cultures compared to those induced by mumps virus.

280. Psittacosis is transmissable to man via contact with:

a. insects
b. birds
c. cattle
d. dogs

281. Encephalitis is most commonly associated with which of the following viruses?

a. Epstein-Barr
b. herpes simplex
c. coxsackie B
d. varicella zoster

282. The causative agent of infantile myocarditis would most likely be:

a. herpes simplex
b. Epstein-Barr
c. coxsackie B
d. varicella zoster

283. Colds and other acute respiratory diseases are most often associated with:

a. Epstein-Barr virus
b. adenovirus
c. coxsackie B
d. reovirus

284. An example of a live attenuated vaccine used for human immunization is:

a. rabies
b. tetanus
c. influenza
d. measles (Edmonston)

285. Chlamydial infections have been implicated in:

a. urethritis and conjunctivitis
b. gastroenteritis and urethritis
c. neonatal pneumonia and gastroenteritis
d. neonatal meningitis and conjunctivitis

286. A jaundiced 7-year-old boy, with a history of playing in a pond in a rat-infested area, has a urine specimen submitted for a direct dark-field examination. No organisms are seen in the specimen. Which medium should be inoculated in an attempt to isolate the suspected organism?

a. blood cystine dextrose
b. PPLO agar
c. Fletcher's semisolid
d. chopped meat glucose

MICROBIOLOGY ANSWER KEY

1. d
2. d
3. b
4. d
5. d
6. b
7. d
8. d
9. d
10. c
11. b
12. e
13. a
14. d
15. a
16. d
17. b
18. b
19. c
20. b
21. a
22. d
23. c
24. b
25. b
26. b
27. b
28. a
29. c
30. c
31. c
32. a
33. c
34. e
35. b
36. d
37. a
38. a
39. b
40. d
41. a
42. c
43. a
44. a
45. a
46. c
47. d
48. c
49. c
50. b
51. d
52. a
53. c
54. a
55. c
56. c
57. b
58. c
59. d
60. d
61. d
62. c
63. d
64. c
65. c
66. c
67. c
68. c
69. a
70. c
71. d
72. d
73. c
74. d
75. d
76. d
77. a
78. b
79. b
80. d
81. b
82. d
83. a
84. c
85. b
86. a
87. c
88. b
89. c
90. a
91. c
92. a
93. d
94. c
95. d
96. d
97. d
98. d
99. d
100. d
101. c
102. b
103. d
104. d
105. a
106. b
107. a
108. b
109. c
110. d
111. c
112. c
113. d
114. d
115. c
116. d
117. c
118. c
119. c
120. a
121. d
122. a
123. c
124. d
125. d
126. d
127. b
128. d
129. c
130. d
131. b
132. c
133. c
134. c
135. a
136. c
137. a
138. b
139. b
140. b
141. b
142. a
143. a
144. b
145. c
146. d
147. d
148. d
149. a
150. d
151. c
152. d
153. a
154. b
155. c
156. a
157. a
158. b
159. b
160. d
161. b
162. b
163. c
164. a
165. c
166. a
167. d
168. a
169. a
170. c
171. a
172. d
173. c
174. b
175. d
176. c
177. d
178. d
179. d
180. d
181. d
182. d
183. b
184. c
185. b
186. a
187. d
188. d

MICROBIOLOGY ANSWER KEY (continued)

189. b
190. d
191. b
192. d
193. b
194. d
195. d
196. a
197. d
198. d
199. b
200. c
201. d
202. c
203. a
204. a
205. d
206. c
207. e
208. d
209. b
210. c
211. d
212. b
213. c
214. c
215. c
216. d
217. c
218. d
219. c
220. d
221. b
222. b
223. c
224. a
225. b
226. d
227. c
228. d
229. d
230. c
231. c
232. d
233. a
234. e
235. d
236. d
237. a
238. a
239. d
240. b
241. a
242. a
243. b
244. a
245. c
246. d
247. c
248. a
249. a
250. a
251. a
252. b
253. d
254. a
255. b
256. b
257. d
258. a
259. d
260. d
261. d
262. b
263. a
264. c
265. b
266. d
267. c
268. a
269. d
270. a
271. b
272. e
273. b
274. d
275. c
276. c
277. b
278. c
279. c
280. b
281. b
282. c
283. b
284. d
285. a
286. c

CHAPTER 11

Hematology

1. Which of the following should be used for calibration of hematology instruments?

    a. latex particles of known dimension
    b. stabilized red cell suspensions
    c. stabilized 7-parameter reference controls
    d. normal whole blood

2. Which of the following best describes the erythropoietin activity in patients with primary polycythemia?

    a. markedly increased
    b. absent or reduced
    c. normal
    d. slightly increased

3. Increased plasma iron turnover is a sign of:

    a. decreased red cell life span
    b. intravascular hemolysis
    c. increased heme catabolism
    d. increased erythropoiesis

4. A blood smear shows 80 nucleated red cells per 100 leukocytes. The total leukocyte count is 18 x 10^9/L or 18 x 10^3 μL. The true white cell count expressed in SI units is:

    a. 17.2 x 10^9/L
    b. 9.0 x 10^9/L
    c. 10.0 x 10^9/L
    d. 13.4 x 10^9/L

5. A Wright stained peripheral smear reveals the following: erythrocytes enlarged one-and-a-half to twice normal size with Schüffner's dots, parasites with irregular "spread out" trophozoites, golden-brown pigment, 12 to 24 merozoites, and a wide range of stages. This is consistent with Plasmodium:

   a. *falciparum*
   b. *malariae*
   c. *ovale*
   d. *vivax*

6. The values below were obtained from an automated blood count system on a blood sample from a 25-five-year-old man.

	Patient	Normal
WBC µL (per liter)	5.1×10^3 (5.1×10^9)	$5.0 - 10.0 \times 10^3$ $(5.0 - 10.0 \times 10^9)$
RBC µL (per liter)	2.94×10^6 (2.94×10^{12})	$4.6 - 6.2 \times 10^6$ $(4.6 - 6.2 \times 10^{12})$
Hb g/dL (mmol/L)	13.8 (2.14)	14 - 18 (2.0 - 2.8)
HCT %	35.4 0.354	40 - 54 (0.40 - 0.54)
MCV μ^3 (fL)	128 (128)	82 - 90 (82 - 90)
MCH pg	46.7	27 - 31
MCHC %	40 (0.40)	32 - 36 (0.32 - 0.36)

These results are most consistent with which of the following?

   a. megaloblastic anemia
   b. hereditary spherocytosis
   c. a high titer of cold agglutinins
   d. an elevated reticulocyte count

7. In an uncomplicated case of severe iron deficiency anemia, which of the following sets represents the typical pattern of results?

	Serum Iron	Serum TBIC	Saturation %	Marrow % Sideroblasts	Marrow Iron Stores	Serum Ferritin	Hgb A_2
a.	decreased	increased	decreased	decreased	decreased	increased	increased
b.	decreased	decreased	decreased	decreased	decreased	decreased	decreased
c.	decreased	increased	decreased	decreased	decreased	decreased	decreased
d.	decreased	decreased	increased	increased	decreased	increased	increased

8. On an electronic particle counter, if the MCV is erroneously increased, how will other parameters be affected?

   a. decreased RBC
   b. increased hemoglobin
   c. decreased MCH
   d. increased hematocrit

9. The most appropriate screening test for detecting hemoglobin F is:

   a. osmotic fragility
   b. dithionite solubility
   c. Kleihauer-Betke
   d. heat instability test

10. The most appropriate screening test for hemoglobin H is:

   a. dithionite solubility
   b. osmotic fragility
   c. sucrose hemolysis
   d. heat instability test

11. The most appropriate screening test for hemoglobin S is:

   a. Kleihauer-Betke
   b. dithionite solubility
   c. osmotic fragility
   d. sucrose hemolysis

12. The most appropriate screening test for hereditary spherocytosis is:

    a. osmotic fragility
    b. sucrose hemolysis
    c. heat instability test
    d. Kleihauer-Betke

13. The most appropriate screening test for paroxysmal nocturnal hemoglobinuria is:

    a. heat instability test
    b. sucrose hemolysis
    c. osmotic fragility
    d. dithionite solubility

14. The morphologic feature most characteristic of hemolytic anemia is:

    a. spherocytosis
    b. rouleaux formation
    c. basophilic stippling
    d. target cells (codocytes)

15. The characteristic morphologic feature in lead poisoning is:

    a. macrocytosis
    b. target cells (codocytes)
    c. basophilic stippling
    d. rouleaux formation

16. The characteristic morphologic feature in multiple myeloma is:

    a. basophilic stippling
    b. rouleaux formation
    c. spherocytosis
    d. macrocytosis

17. The characteristic morphologic feature in folic acid deficiency is:

    a. macrocytosis
    b. target cells (codocytes)
    c. basophilic stippling
    d. rouleaux formation

18. A characteristic morphologic feature in hemoglobin C disease is:

a. macrocytosis
b. spherocytosis
c. rouleaux formation
d. target cells (codocytes)

19. Which of the following are possible reasons for the quality control graph illustrated?

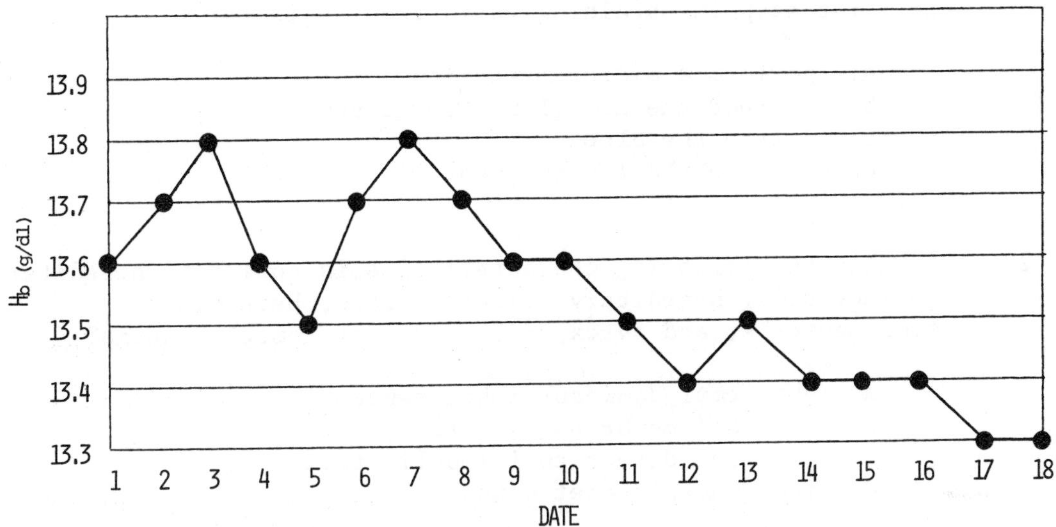

1. There is a gradual shift of the spectrophotometer.
2. The reagent is deteriorating.
3. The daily values show a downward trend.
4. The graph illustrates random error.

a. only 1, 2 and 3 are correct
b. only 1 and 3 are correct
c. only 2 and 4 are correct
d. only 4 is correct
e. all are correct

---

20. Hematological standards include:

a. stabilized RBC suspension
b. latex particles
c. stabilized avian RBCs
d. certified cyanmethemoglobin solution

21. The following results were obtained on an electronic particle counter:

WBC	$6.5 \times 10^3/\mu L$
RBC	$4.55 \times 10^6/\mu L$
HGB	18.0 g/dL
HCT	41.5%
MCV	90.1 fL
MCH	39.6 pg
MCHC	43.4%

The first step in obtaining valid results is to:

a. perform a microhematocrit
b. correct the hemoglobin for lipemia
c. dilute the blood
d. replace the lysing agent

22. Which of the following characteristics is common to hereditary spherocytosis, hereditary elliptocytosis, hereditary stomatocytosis, and paroxysmal nocturnal hemoglobinuria?

a. autosomal dominant inheritance
b. red cell membrane defects
c. positive direct antiglobulin test
d. measured platelet count

23. Which of the following tests is used to monitor red cell production?

a. packed cell volume (PCV)
b. total iron-binding capacity (TIBC)
c. Schilling test
d. reticulocyte count

24. The following results were obtained on an electronic particle counter:

WBC	$61.3 \times 10^3/\mu L$
RBC	$1.19 \times 10^6/\mu L$
HGB	9.9 g/dL
HCT	21%
MCV	125 fL
MCHC	54.1%

What action should be taken to obtain accurate results?

a. Dilute the specimen and recount.
b. Warm the specimen and recount.
c. Check the tube for clots.
d. Clean the aperture tubes and recount.

25. Thalassemias are characterized by:

a. structual abnormalities in the hemoglobin molecule
b. absence of iron in hemoglobin
c. decreased rate of heme synthesis
d. decreased rate of globin synthesis

26. A patient diagnosed with polycythemia vera five years ago now has a normal hematocrit, decreased hemoglobin, and microcytic, hypochromic red cells. What is the most probable cause for the current blood picture?

a. phlebotomy
b. myelofibrosis
c. preleukemia
d. aplastic anemia

27. Cells for the transport of O_2 and CO_2 are:

a. erythocytes
b. granulocytes
c. lymphocytes
d. thrombocytes

28. In polycythemia vera, the hemoglobin, hematocrit, red blood cell count, and red cell mass are:

    a. elevated
    b. normal
    c. decreased

29. A patient has been treated for polycythemia vera for several years. His blood smear now shows:

    Oval macrocytes
    Howell-Jolly bodies
    Hypersegmented neutrophils
    Large, agranular platelets

    The most probable cause of this blood picture is:

    a. iron deficiency
    b. alcoholism
    c. dietary B_{12} deficiency
    d. chemotherapy

30. The M:E ratio in polycythemia vera is usually:

    a. normal
    b. high
    c. low
    d. variable

31. Erythropoietin acts to:

    a. shorten the replication time of the granulocytes
    b. stimulate RNA synthesis of erythroid cells
    c. increase colony-stimulating factors produced by the B-lymphocytes
    d. decrease the release of marrow reticulocytes

32. The anemia in chronic renal failure is associated with ALL of the following <u>EXCEPT</u>:

    a. erythropoietin deficiency
    b. increased hemolysis of erythrocytes in the uremic environment
    c. blood loss
    d. elevated erythropoietin levels in tumor extracts

33. The anemia of chronic infection is characterized by:

    a. decreased iron stores in the reticuloendothelial system
    b. decreased serum iron levels
    c. macrocytic erythrocytes
    d. increased serum iron-binding protein levels

34. All of the following are characteristic of hemoglobin H <u>EXCEPT</u>:

    a. It is a tetramer of beta chains.
    b. It is relatively unstable and thermolabile.
    c. Electrophoretically, it represents a "fast" hemoglobin.
    d. Its oxygen affinity is lower than that of Hb A.

35. Hematologic findings associated with alcoholism include:

    1. megaloblastic anemia resulting from folate deficiency
    2. vacuolization of normoblasts in bone marrow
    3. increased number of sideroblasts and ringed sideroblasts
    4. transient stomatocytosis

    a. only 1, 2 and 3 are correct
    b. only 1 and 3 are correct
    c. only 2 and 4 are correct
    d. only 4 is correct
    e. all are correct

36. Which of the following is found in association with megaloblastic anemia?

a. neutropenia
b. decreased lactic dehydrogenase (LD) activity
c. increased erythrocyte folate levels
d. decreased plasma bilirubin levels

37. A patient's hemoglobin electrophoresis pattern suggests sickle cell trait, but the percentage of hemoglobin S is somewhat less than that usually seen in patients with sickle cell trait. The hemoglobin solubility test is positive. Which of the following could cause this type of pattern?

1. iron deficiency
2. alpha thalassemia
3. lead poisoning
4. previous transfusions

a. only 1, 2 and 3 are correct
b. only 1 and 3 are correct
c. only 2 and 4 are correct
d. only 4 is correct
e. all are correct

38. Which of the following is characteristic of polycythemia vera?

a. elevated urine erythropoietin levels
b. increased oxygen affinity of hemoglobin
c. "teardrop" poikilocytosis
d. decreased or absent bone marrow iron stores

39. A factor commonly involved in producing anemia in patients with chronic renal disease is:

a. marrow hypoplasia
b. ineffective erythropoiesis
c. vitamin B_{12} deficiency
d. increased erythropoietin production

40. Factor(s) implicated in the pathogenesis of anemia of chronic disease include:

    1. decreased erythrocyte survival time
    2. accelerated flow of iron from reticuloendothelial stores to plasma
    3. impaired bone marrow response
    4. accumulation of iron in mitochrondria or erythroblasts

    a. only 1, 2 and 3 are correct
    b. only 1 and 3 are correct
    c. only 2 and 4 are correct
    d. only 4 is correct
    e. all are correct

41. Correct technique(s) for obtaining blood specimens include:

    1. puncturing a vein 8 to 10 cm below an IV site
    2. using a syringe if the patient is elderly and has a low venous pressure
    3. massaging the vein toward the trunk to increase prominence after the tourniquet has been applied
    4. using the center of the finger tip as the puncture site for a capillary blood specimen

    a. only 1, 2 and 3 are correct
    b. only 1 and 3 are correct
    c. only 2 and 4 are correct
    d. only 4 is correct
    e. all are correct

42. The majority of the iron in an adult is found as a constituent of:

    a. hemoglobin
    b. hemosiderin
    c. myoglobin
    d. transferrin

43. A 20-year-old black man has peripheral blood changes suggesting thalassemia minor. The quantitative hemoglobin A_2 level is normal, but the hemoglobin F level is 5% (normal is less than 2%). This is most consistent with:

   a. alpha thalassemia minor
   b. beta thalassemia minor
   c. delta-beta thalassemia minor
   d. hereditary persistence of fetal hemoglobin

44. A native of Thailand has a normal hemoglobin level and the blood smear shows target cells. Hemoglobin cellulose electrophoresis on cellulose acetate shows 45% hemoglobin A and approximately 40% of a hemoglobin with the mobility of hemoglobin A_2. This is most consistent with:

   a. Hb C trait
   b. Hb E trait
   c. Hb O trait
   d. Hb D trait

45. A 20-year-old woman with sickle cell anemia whose usual hemoglobin concentration is 8 g/dL develops fever, increased weakness, and malaise. The hemoglobin concentration is 4 g/dL and the reticulocyte count is 0.1%. The most likely explanation for this clinical picture is:

   a. increased hemolysis due to hypersplenism
   b. aplastic crisis
   c. thrombotic crisis
   d. occult blood loss

46. Megaloblastic asynchronous development in the bone marrow indicates which one of the following?

   a. proliferation of erythrocyte precursors
   b. impaired synthesis of DNA
   c. inadequate production of erythropoietin
   d. deficiency of G-6-PD

47. A patient has the following blood values:

RBC	$6.5 \times 10^6/\mu L$
HGB	14.0 g/dL
HCT	42.0%
MCV	65 fL
MCH	21.5 pg
MCHC	33%

These results are compatible with:

a. iron deficiency
b. pregnancy
c. thalassemia minor
d. beta thalassemia major

48. On Monday a patient's hemoglobin determination was 11.3 g/dL and on Tuesday it measured 11.8 g/dL. The standard deviation of the method used is ± 0.2 g/dL. Which of the following can be concluded about the hemoglobin values given?

a. One value probably resulted from laboratory error.
b. There is poor precision; daily quality control charts should be checked.
c. The second value is out of range and should be repeated.
d. There is no significant change in the patient's hemoglobin concentration.

49. A patient has high cold agglutinin titer. Automated cell counter results reveal an elevated MCV, MCH, and MCHC. Individual erythrocytes appear normal on a stained smear, but agglutinates are noted. The appropriate course of action would be to:

a. Perform the RBC, Hb, and HCT determinations using manual methods.
b. Perform the RBC determination by a manual method; use the automated results for the Hb and HCT.
c. Repeat the determinations using a microsample of diluted blood.
d. Repeat the determinations using a prewarmed microsample of diluted blood.

50. The most common cause of error when using automated cell counters is:

    a. contamination of the diluent
    b. inadequate mixing of the sample prior to testing
    c. variation in voltage of the current supply
    d. a calibrating error

51. Many microspherocytes, schistocytes, and budding off of spherocytes can be seen on peripheral blood smears of patients with:

    a. hereditary spherocytosis
    b. disseminated intravascular coagulation (DIC)
    c. acquired autoimmune hemolytic anemia
    d. extensive burns

52. Hemolysis in paroxysmal nocturnal hemoglobinuria (PNH) is:

    a. temperature-dependent
    b. complement-independent
    c. antibody-mediated
    d. caused by a red cell membrane defect

53. In order for hemoglobin to combine reversibly with oxygen, the iron must be:

    a. complexed with haptoglobin
    b. freely circulating in the cytoplasm
    c. attached to transferrin
    d. in the ferrous state

54. The mean value of a reticulocyte count on specimens of cord blood from healthy, full-term newborns is about:

    a. 0.5%
    b. 2.0%
    c. 5.0%
    d. 8.0%

55. The most likely cause of the macrocytosis that often accompanies anemia of myelofibrosis is:

   a. folic acid deficiency
   b. increased reticulocyte count
   c. inadequate B_{12} absorption
   d. pyridoxine deficiency

56. Which one of the following is a true statement about Heinz bodies?

   a. They are readily identified with polychrome stains.
   b. They are rarely found in glucose-6-phosphate dehydrogenase-deficient erythrocytes.
   c. They are closely associated with spherocytes.
   d. They are denatured hemoglobin inclusions that are readily removed by the spleen.

57. Which of the following sets of laboratory findings is consistent with hemolytic anemia?

   a. normal or slightly increased erythrocyte survival; normal osmotic fragility
   b. decreased erythrocyte survival; increased catabolism of heme
   c. decreased serum lactate dehydrogenase activity; normal catabolism of heme
   d. normal concentration of haptoglobin; marked hemoglobinuria

58. Evidence indicates that the genetic defect in thalassemia usually results in:

   a. the production of abnormal globin chains
   b. a quantitative deficiency in RNA resulting in decreased globin chain production
   c. a structural change in the heme portion of the hemoglobin
   d. an abnormality in the alpha or beta chain binding or affinity

59. Hemoglobin H disease results from:

   a. absence of 3 of 4 alpha genes
   b. absence of 2 of 4 alpha genes
   c. absence of 1 of 1 alpha genes
   d. absence of all four alpha genes

60. Which of the following represents characteristic features of iron metabolism in patients with anemia of a chronic disorder?

   a. Serum iron is normal, transferrin saturation is normal, TBIC is normal.
   b. Serum iron is increased, transferrin saturation is increased, TBIC is normal or slightly increased.
   c. Serum iron is normal, transferrin saturation is markedly increased, TBIC is normal.
   d. Serum iron is decreased, transferrin saturation is decreased, TBIC is normal or decreased.

61. A patient with polycythemia vera who is treated by phlebotomy is most likely to develop a deficiency of:

   a. iron
   b. vitamin B_{12}
   c. folic acid
   d. erythropoietin

62. Hemorrhage in polycythemia vera is the result of:

   a. increased plasma viscosity
   b. persistent thrombocytosis
   c. splenic sequestration of platelets
   d. abnormal platelet function

63. Which of the following will distinguish early myeloid metaplasia from chronic granulocytic leukemia?

   a. bone marrow hyperplasia
   b. bone marrow fibrosis
   c. increased leukocytic alkaline phosphatase (LAP)
   d. megaloblastosis

64. Which of the following is a significant feature of erythroleukemia (Di Guglielmo's syndrome)?

   a. persistently increased M:E ratio
   b. megaloblastoid erythropoiesis
   c. marked thrombocytosis
   d. decreased stainable iron in the marrow

65. In an adult with rare homozygous delta-beta thalassemia, the hemoglobin produced is:

a. A
b. Bart's
c. F
d. H

66. A 40-year-old man had an erythrocyte count of $2.5 \times 10^6/\mu L$, hematocrit of 22%, and a reticulocyte count of 2.0%. Which of the following statements best describes his condition?

a. The absolute reticulocyte count is 50,000/µL, indicating that the bone marrow is not adequately compensating for the anemia.
b. The reticulocyte count is greatly increased, indicating an adequate bone marrow response for the anemia.
c. The absolute reticulocyte count is 500,000/µL, indicating that the bone marrow is adequately compensating for the anemia.
d. The reticulocyte count is slightly increased, indicating an adequate response to the slight anemia.

67. The following results were obtained from an osmotic fragility test:

Initial hemolysis - 0.4% NaCl
Complete hemolysis - 0.25% NaCl

The results indicate which of the following?

a. hemolytic uremic syndrome
b. hemolytic anemia
c. hereditary spherocytosis
d. thalassemia

68. When using an electronic cell counter, which of the following results can occur in the presence of a cold agglutinin?

a. increased MCV and decreased RBC
b. increased MCV and normal RBC
c. decreased MCV and increased MCHC
d. decreased MCV and RBC

69. A properly functioning electronic cell counter obtains the following results:

WBC	$5.1 \times 10^9/L$
RBC	$4.87 \times 10^{12}/L$
HGB	16.1 g/dL
HCT	39.3%
MCV	82.0 fL
MCH	33.1 pg
MCHC	41.3%

These results might be caused by:

a. lipemia
b. cold agglutinins
c. increased WBC
d. rouleaux

70. On setting up the electronic particle counter in the morning, one of the controls is slightly below the range for the MCV. Which of the following is indicated?

a. call for service
b. adjust the MCV up slightly
c. shut down the instrument
d. repeat the control

71. Decreased erythropoietin production is most likely to be associated with:

a. polycythemia vera
b. polycythemia, secondary to hypoxia
c. relative polycythemia associated with dehydration
d. polycythemia associated with renal disease

72. A patient has a tumor which concentrates erythropoietin. He is most likely to have which of the following types of polycythemia?

a. polycythemia vera
b. polycythemia, secondary to hypoxia
c. benign familial polycythemia
d. polycythemia associated with renal disease

For questions 73 to 77, refer to the following illustration:

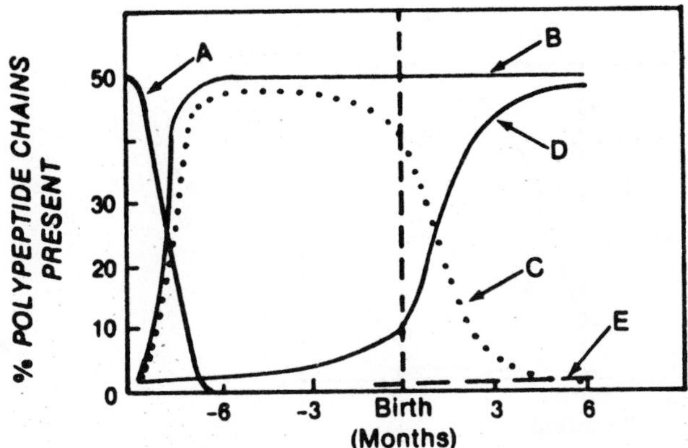

73. Which curve represents the production of alpha polypeptide chains of hemoglobin?

    a. A
    b. B
    c. C
    d. D

74. Which curve represents the production of beta polypeptide chains of hemoglobin?

    a. B
    b. C
    c. E
    d. D

75. Which curve represents the production of gamma polypeptide chains of hemoglobin?

    a. A
    b. B
    c. C
    d. D

76. Which curve represents the production of delta polypeptide chains of hemoglobin?

    a. B
    b. C
    c. D
    d. E

For question 77, refer to the following illustration:

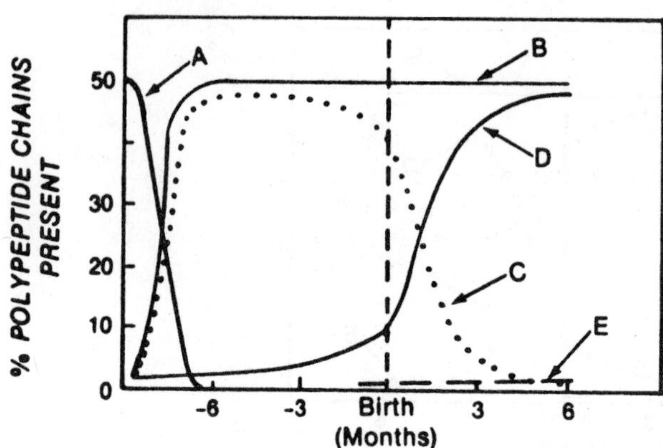

77. Which curve represents the production of epsilon polypeptide chains of hemoglobin?

    a. A
    b. B
    c. C
    d. D

---

78. Which of the following types of polycythemia is a severely burned patient most likely to have?

    a. polycythemia vera
    b. polycythemia, secondary to hypoxia
    c. relative polycythemia associated with dehydration
    d. polycythemia associated with renal disease

79. Which of the following types of polycythemia is most often associated with emphysema?

    a. polycythemia vera
    b. polycythemia, secondary to hypoxia
    c. relative polycythemia associated with dehydration
    d. polycythemia associated with renal disease

80. Which of the following is most closely associated with idiopathic hemochromatosis?

a. iron overload in tissue
b. codocytes
c. basophilic stippling
d. ringed sideroblast

81. Which of the following is most closely associated with iron deficiency anemia?

a. iron overload in tissue
b. codocytes
c. basophilic stippling
d. chronic blood loss

82. Which of the following is most closely associated with thalassemia?

a. chronic blood loss
b. codocytes
c. basophilic stippling
d. ringed sideroblast

83. Which of the following is most likely to be seen in lead poisoning?

a. iron overload in tissue
b. codocytes
c. basophilic stippling
d. ringed sideroblast

84. Which of the following is most closely associated with erythroleukemia?

a. ringed sideroblasts
b. disseminated intravascular coagulation
c. micromegakaryocytes
d. lysozymuria

For question 85, refer to the following illustration:

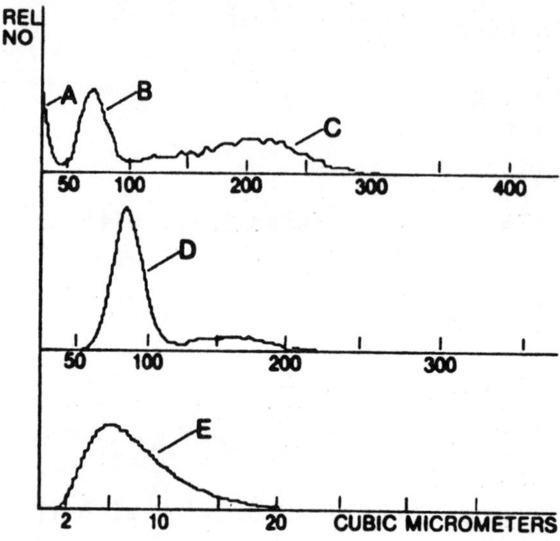

85. Which area of the above cell size distribution histograms from an electronic particle counter is appropriate for an RBC distribution curve?

a. A
b. B
c. C
d. D

---

86. Anaerobic glycolysis (Embden-Meyerhof pathway) in erythrocytes leads to the formation of which of the following products?

1. NADH (DPNH)
2. NADPH (TPNH)
3. ATP
4. gluthathione

a. only 1, 2 and 3 are correct
b. only 1 and 3 are correct
c. only 2 and 4 are correct
d. only 4 is correct
e. all are correct

87. True statements about evaluation of bone marrow films for the presence of iron include:

1. Only a few blue granules are seen in each sideroblast.
2. Twenty to sixty percent sideroblasts may be seen in normal bone marrow.
3. A film containing marrow particles must be used.
4. Storage iron in the marrow is located in macrophages.

a. only 1, 2 and 3 are correct
b. only 1 and 3 are correct
c. only 2 and 4 are correct
d. only 4 is correct
e. all are correct

88. Which of the following is NOT useful in distinguishing thalassemia minor from iron deficiency anemia?

a. free erythrocyte protoporphyrins (FEP)
b. serum ferritin
c. hemoglobin electrophoresis
d. osmotic fragility

89. An increased number of cells containing hemoglobin F can be observed by means of the Kleihauer-Betke stain in which of the following?

1. neonate
2. sickle cell anemia
3. thalassemia major
4. sickle cell trait

a. only 1, 2 and 3 are correct
b. only 1 and 3 are correct
c. only 2 and 4 are correct
d. only 4 is correct
e. all are correct

90. Heinz bodies are associated with:

1. May-Hegglin anomaly
2. favism and G-6-PD deficiency
3. Alder-Reilly anomaly
4. unstable hemoglobins

a. only 1, 2 and 3 are correct
b. only 1 and 3 are correct
c. only 2 and 4 are correct
d. only 4 is correct
e. all are correct

91. Laboratory findings in hereditary spherocytosis do NOT include:

a. decreased osmotic fragility
b. increased autohemolysis corrected by glucose
c. reticulocytosis
d. shortened erythrocyte survival

92. Patients with A-type G-6-PD deficiency are LEAST likely to have hemolytic episodes in which of the following situations?

a. following the administration of oxidizing drugs
b. the neonatal period
c. during infections
d. spontaneously

93. In most cases of hereditary persistence of fetal hemoglobin (HPFH):

1. Hb F is evenly distributed throughout the erythrocytes
2. the black heterozygote has 15% to 35% Hb F
3. beta and delta chain synthesis is decreased
4. gamma chain production equals alpha chain production

a. only 1, 2 and 3 are correct
b. only 1 and 3 are correct
c. only 2 and 4 are correct
d. only 4 is correct
e. all are correct

94. Which of the following is typical of polycythemia vera?

a. increased serum iron concentration
b. decreased thrombocyte count
c. increased erythropoietin
d. increased leukocyte alkaline phosphatase activity

95. Which of the following is increased in erythrocytosis secondary to a congenital heart defect?

a. arterial oxygen saturation
b. serum vitamin B_{12}
c. leukocyte alkaline phosphatase activity
d. erythropoietin

96. Biochemical abnormalities characteristic of polycythemia vera include:

a. increased serum B_{12}
b. hypouricemia
c. hypohistaminemia
d. decreased leukocyte alkaline phosphatase activity

97. Characteristics of senescent erythrocytes include an increase in:

a. enzymatic activity
b. ATP concentration
c. size
d. density

98. Abnormalities found in erythroleukemia include:

a. rapid DNA synthesis
b. decreased erythropoietin
c. megaloblastoid development
d. increased erythrocyte survival

99. A blood sample from a patient with a high-titer cold agglutinin, analyzed at room temperature with an electronic particle counter, would cause an error in the:

    a. hemoglobin and MCV
    b. MCHC and WBC
    c. WBC and RBC
    d. MCV and MCHC

100. Hematopoiesis is the formation of:

    1. erythrocytes
    2. granulocytes-monocytes
    3. megakaryocytes
    4. lymphocytes

    a. only 1, 2 and 3 are correct
    b. only 1 and 3 are correct
    c. only 2 and 4 are correct
    d. only 4 is correct
    e. all are correct

101. The anemia found in myeloproliferative disorders is usually:

    a. microcytic hypochromic
    b. macrocytic normochromic
    c. normocytic normochromic
    d. microcytic normochromic

102. Which one of the following hypochromic anemias is usually associated with a normal free erythrocyte protoporphyrin level?

    a. anemia of chronic disease
    b. iron deficiency
    c. lead poisoning
    d. thalassemia minor

103. Anemia secondary to uremia characteristically is:

a. microcytic hypochromic
b. hemolytic
c. normocytic normochromic
d. macrocytic

104. The hypoproliferative red cell population in the bone marrow of uremic patients is caused by:

a. infiltration of bone marrow by toxic waste products
b. decreased levels of circulating erythropoietin
c. defective globin synthesis
d. overcrowding of bone marrow space by increased myeloid precursors

105. A Kleihauer-Betke stain of a postpartum blood film revealed 0.3% fetal cells. What is the estimated volume (mL) of the fetomaternal hemorrhage expressed as whole blood?

a. 5
b. 15
c. 25
d. 35

106. A substance that has a greater affinity (210 times) than oxygen for binding to hemoglobin is:

a. carbon dioxide
b. carbon monoxide
c. cyanide
d. hydrogen sulfide

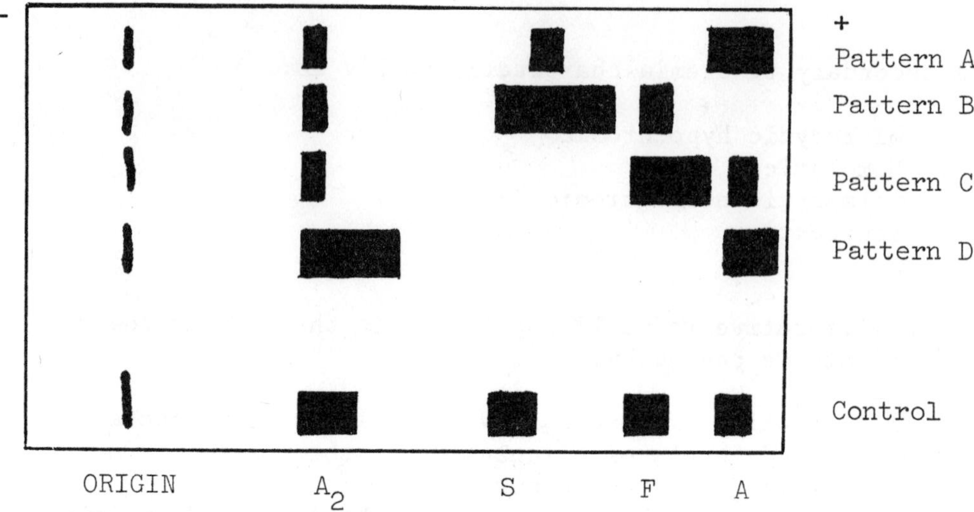

HEMOGLOBIN ELECTROPHORESIS PATTERNS AT pH 8.4
(CELLULOSE ACETATE STRIP)

107. Which of the above patterns is consistent with thalassemia major?

a. pattern A
b. pattern B
c. pattern C
d. pattern D

---

108. A 40-year-old white male was admitted to the hospital for treatment of anemia, lassitude, weight loss, and loss of libido. The patient presented with the following laboratory data:

RBC	$3.7 \times 10^{12}/L$	Serum iron	220 µg/dL
HCT	32%	TIBC	300 µg/dL
HGB	10.0 g/dL	Serum ferritin	2,800 ng/mL
WBC	$5.8 \times 10^{9}/L$		
MCV	86 fL		
MCH	26 pg		
MCHC	32%		

Examination of the bone marrow revealed erythroid hyperplasia with a shift to the left of erythroid precursors. Prussian blue staining revealed markedly elevated iron stores noted with occasional sideroblasts seen. These data are most consistent with which of the following conditions?

a. iron deficiency anemia
b. anemia of chronic disease
c. hemochromatosis
d. acute blood loss

109. An 89-year-old white female was transferred to the hospital from a nursing facility for treatment of chronic urinary tract infection with proteinuria. The patient presented with the following laboratory data:

RBC	3.1×10^{12}/L	Serum iron	29 µg/dL
HCT	24%	TIBC	160 µg/dL
HGB	7.2 g/dL	Serum ferritin	100 ng/mL
WBC	10.0×10^{9}/L		
MCV	78 fL		
MCH	23 pg		
MCHC	31%		

Examination of the bone marrow revealed a slightly fatty marrow with increased storage iron, as detected by the Prussian blue technique. These data are most consistent with which of the following conditions?

a. iron deficiency anemia
b. anemia of chronic disease
c. hemochromatosis
d. acute blood loss

110. The greatest activity of serum muramidase occurs with:

a. cancer of the prostate
b. myeloproliferative disease
c. myelomonocytic leukemia
d. Gaucher's disease

111. The most common form of childhood leukemia is:

a. acute lymphocytic
b. acute granulocytic
c. acute monocytic
d. chronic granulocytic

112. The following results were obtained on an electronic particle counter:

WBC	******
RBC	2.01×10^6
HGB	7.7 g/dL
HCT	28.2%
MCV	141 fL
MCH	38.5 pg
MCHC	23.3%

What step should be taken before recycling the sample?

a. Clean the apertures.
b. Warm the specimen.
c. Replace the lysing agent.
d. Dilute the specimen.

113. Of the following, the disease most closely associated with glucocerebrosidase deficiency is:

a. Gaucher's disease
b. Chediak-Higashi syndrome
c. Pelger-Huët anomaly
d. May-Hegglin anomaly

114. Of the following, the disease most closely associated with pale blue inclusions in granulocytes and giant platelets is:

a. Gaucher's disease
b. Alder-Reilly anomaly
c. May-Hegglin anomaly
d. Pelger-Huët anomaly

115. Which of the following tests can be useful in differentiating leukemoid reactions from chronic granulocytic leukemias?

a. peroxidase stain
b. Sudan black B stain
c. surface membrane markers
d. leukocyte alkaline phosphatase

116. A differential was performed on an asymptomatic patient. The differential included 60% neutrophils: 55 of which had 2 lobes and 5 had 3 lobes. There were no other abnormalities. This is consistent with which of the following anomalies?

a. Pelger-Huët
b. May-Hegglin
c. Alder-Reilly
d. Chediak-Higashi

117. T-cell acute lymphocytic leukemia (ALL) is closely related to:

a. chronic lymphocytic leukemia (CLL)
b. autoimmune disease
c. lymphoblastic lymphoma
d. acute granulocytic leukemia (AGL)

118. The stain that identifies intracellular carbohydrate, glycogen, mucopolysaccharide, mucoprotein, glycoprotein, and glycolipid is:

a. Sudan black B
b. leukocyte alkaline phosphatase (LAP)
c. periodic acid-Schiff (PAS)
d. peroxidase

119. The stain that selectively identifies phospholipid in the membranes of primary and secondary granules within myeloid cells is:

a. Sudan black B
b. leukocyte alkaline phosphatase (LAP)
c. perodic acid-Schiff (PAS)
d. peroxidase

120. The type of leukemia that is associated with severe coagulation abnormalities is:

a. acute myelogenous leukemia
b. erythroleukemia
c. acute promyelocytic leukemia
d. myelomonocytic leukemia

121. Cells for phagocytic defense are called:

   a. erythrocytes
   b. granulocytes
   c. lymphocytes
   d. thrombocytes

122. Cells that produce antibodies and lymphokines are:

   a. erythrocytes
   b. granulocytes
   c. lymphocytes
   d. thrombocytes

123. In polycythemia vera, the leukocyte alkaline phosphatase activity is:

   a. elevated
   b. normal
   c. decreased

124. Terminal deoxynucleotidyl transferase (TdT) is a marker found on:

   a. hairy cells
   b. myeloblasts
   c. monoblasts
   d. lymphoblasts

125. The M:E ratio in chronic granulocytic leukemia is usually:

   a. normal
   b. high
   c. low
   d. variable

126. The M:E ratio in erythroleukemia is usually:

   a. normal
   b. high
   c. low
   d. variable

127. The M:E ratio in acute granulocytic leukemia is usually:

   a. normal
   b. high
   c. low
   d. variable

128. In peripheral blood, 50% to 90% myeloblasts is typical of which of the following?

   a. chronic granulocytic leukemia
   b. myelofibrosis with myeloid metaplasia
   c. erythroleukemia
   d. acute granulocytic leukemia

129. Auer rods may be present in which of the following?

   a. chronic granulocytic leukemia
   b. myelofibrosis with myeloid metaplasia
   c. erythroleukemia
   d. acute granulocytic leukemia

130. Giant, bizarre-shaped, multinucleated erythroid precursors are present in which of the following?

   a. chronic granulocytic leukemia
   b. myelofibrosis with myeloid metaplasia
   c. erythroleukemia
   d. acute granulocytic leukemia

131. In the peripheral blood, all stages of neutrophilic development are likely to be seen in:

   a. chronic granulocytic leukemia
   b. myelofibrosis with myeloid metaplasia
   c. erythroleukemia
   d. acute granulocytic leukemia

132. In acute granulocytic leukemia, the myeloblasts stain positive with all of the following EXCEPT:

   a. specific esterase
   b. Sudan black B
   c. peroxidase
   d. PAS

133. In the French-American-British (FAB) classification, acute lymphocytic leukemia is divided into groups according to:

   a. prognosis
   b. immunology
   c. cytochemistry
   d. morphology

134. The LAP activity is increased in:

   a. paroxysmal nocturnal hemoglobinuria
   b. leukemoid reaction
   c. chronic granulocytic leukemia
   d. idiopathic thrombocytopenic purpura

135. In the immunologic classification of acute lymphocytic leukemia, the acid phosphatase stain is usually positive for:

   a. null cell
   b. T cell
   c. common
   d. B cell

136. The specimen of choice for preparation of blood films for manual differential leukocyte counts is whole blood collected in:

   a. EDTA
   b. oxalate
   c. citrate
   d. heparin

137. Elevation of the granulocyte percentage above 75% is termed:

   a. absolute lymphocytosis
   b. leukocytosis
   c. relative neutrophilic leukocytosis
   d. absolute neutrophilic leukocytosis

138. Elevation of the lymphocyte percentage above 47% is termed:

a. relative lymphocytosis
b. absolute lymphocytosis
c. leukocytosis
d. absolute neutrophilic leukocytosis

139. Elevation of the total granulocyte count above 9.0 X 10^9/L is termed:

a. relative lymphocytosis
b. leukocytosis
c. relative neutrophilic leukocytosis
d. absolute neutrophilic leukocytosis

140. Elevation of the total white cell count above 12 X 10^9/L is termed:

a. relative lymphocytosis
b. absolute lymphocytosis
c. leukocytosis
d. relative neutrophilic leukocytosis

141. Clinical uses of differential leukocyte counts include:

1. screening of normal populations for occult disease
2. definitive diagnosis of both hematologic and nonhematologic diseases
3. monitoring of patients' response to therapy
4. following the course of a disease

a. only 1, 2 and 3 are correct
b. only 1 and 3 are correct
c. only 2 and 4 are correct
d. only 4 is correct
e. all are correct

142. A neutropenic leukocyte reaction can be caused by:

1. marrow failure
2. immunodeficiency
3. megaloblastic anemia
4. lymphoma

a. only 1, 2 and 3 are correct
b. only 1 and 3 are correct
c. only 2 and 4 are correct
d. only 4 is correct
e. all are correct

143. The accuracy of automated differential leukocyte counts can be determined by:

1. cell-by-cell comparisons
2. slide-by-slide comparisons
3. specimen-by-specimen comparisons
4. case-by-case comparisons

a. only 1, 2 and 3 are correct
b. only 1 and 3 are correct
c. only 2 and 4 are correct
d. only 4 is correct
e. all are correct

144. The peripheral blood monocyte is an intermediate stage in the formation of the:

a. plasmacyte
b. Turk irritation cell
c. bone marrow histiocyte
d. large atypical cell present in infectious mononucleosis

145. Specific (secondary) granules of the neutrophilic granulocyte:

a. appear first at the myelocyte stage
b. contain lysosomal enzymes
c. are formed on the mitochondria
d. are derived from azurophil (primary) granules

146. Which of the following has a B cell origin?

a. Sezary syndrome
b. malignant lymphoma, lymphoblastic type
c. Sternberg sarcoma
d. Waldenström's macroglobulinemia

147. Which of the following is characteristic of Auer rods?

a. They contain lactoferrin.
b. They are lysosomes and stain acid phosphatase-positive.
c. They are found in the leukemic phase of lymphoma.
d. They are found in acute lymphocytic leukemia.

148. Mechanism of cortisol-induced neutrophilia includes:

a. an acute shift in granulocytes from the marginating pool to the circulating pool
b. an increased egress of granulocytes from the circulation
c. a decreased egress of granulocytes from the bone marrow
d. granulocyte return from the tissues to the circulating pool

149. A characteristic of cyclic neutropenia is:

a. episodes of neutropenia beginning in infancy and recurring at three-week intervals
b. presence of leukoagglutinins in the serum
c. presence of serum neutropenic factors
d. production of neutropenia in persons transfused with plasma from an affected patient

150. Thrombocytopenia is a characteristic of:

a. classic von Willebrand's disease
b. hemophilia A
c. Glanzmann's thrombasthenia
d. May-Hegglin anomaly

151. A leukocyte count and differential on a 40-year-old white man revealed:

5,400/µL (5.4 x 10^9/L)
20% polymorphonuclear neutrophils
58% lymphocytes
20% monocytes
2% eosinophils

This represents:

a. relative lymphocytosis
b. absolute lymphocytosis
c. relative neutrocytosis
d. leukopenia

152. A leukocyte count and differential on a 40-year-old white man revealed:

5,400/µL (5.4 x 10^9/L)
20% polymorphonuclear neutrophils
58% lymphocytes
20% monocytes
2% eosinophils

This represents:

a. absolute lymphocytosis
b. relative neutrocytosis
c. absolute neutropenia
d. leukopenia

153. On an electronic particle counter, if a leukocyte count is reported as 50,000/µL (50.0 x 10^9/L) or greater, the blood should be diluted and the count repeated because:

1. coincidence error will cause factitiously low leukocyte counts
2. carryover will produce an erroneous elevation of the leukocyte count in the next specimen counted
3. the hemoglobin determination will be affected
4. the aspirating apparatus will become clogged

a. only 1, 2 and 3 are correct
b. only 1 and 3 are correct
c. only 2 and 4 are correct
d. only 4 is correct
e. all are correct

154. Precursors of tissue macrophages of the reticuloendothelial system most likely are:

   a. T lymphocytes
   b. B lymphocytes
   c. monocytes
   d. mast cells

155. Which of the following cells are most likely identified in lesions of mycosis fungoides?

   a. T lymphocytes
   b. B lymphocytes
   c. monocytes
   d. mast cells

156. Which of the following most likely contain receptors for the Epstein-Barr virus?

   a. T lymphocytes
   b. B lymphocytes
   c. monocytes
   d. mast cells

157. In which of the following cells is the atypical lymphocyte seen on the peripheral blood smear of patients with infectious mononucleosis?

   a. T lymphocytes
   b. B lymphocytes
   c. monocytes
   d. mast cells

158. The type of leukemia seen most commonly as a terminal event in plasma cell myeloma is:

   a. acute lymphoblastic leukemia
   b. acute monocytic leukemia
   c. acute myelomonocytic leukemia
   d. chronic myelogenous leukemia

159. An automated leukocyte count is 22,500/μL (22.5 x 10^9/L). The differential reveals 200 normoblasts/100 leukocytes. What is the actual leukocyte count per microliter?

a. 7,500
b. 11,500
c. 14,400
d. 22,300

160. A 50-year-old woman who has been receiving busulfan for three years for chronic granulocytic leukemia becomes anemic.

Laboratory tests reveal:

Thrombocytopenia
Many peroxidase-negative blast cells in the peripheral blood
Bone marrow hypercellular in blast transformation
Markedly increased bone marrow TdT

Which of the following complications is this patient most likely to have?

a. acute lymphocytic leukemia
b. acute granulocytic leukemia
c. acute myelomonocytic leukemia
d. busulfan toxicity

161. Which of the following is associated with May-Hegglin anomaly?

a. membrane defect of lysosome
b. Döhle bodies and giant platelets
c. chronic granulocytic leukemia
d. mucopolysaccharidosis

162. Which of the following is associated with Chediak-Higashi syndrome?

a. membrane defect of lysosome
b. Döhle bodies and giant platelets
c. two-lobed neutrophils
d. mucopolysaccharidosis

163. Which of the following is associated with pseudo-Pelger-Huët anomaly?

    a. aplastic anemia
    b. iron deficiency anemia
    c. granulocytic leukemia
    d. Chediak-Higashi syndrome

164. Which of the following is associated with Alder-Reilly inclusions?

    a. membrane defect of lyosome
    b. Döhle bodies and giant platelets
    c. two-lobed neutrophils
    d. mucopolysaccharidosis

165. Cytochemical stains were performed on bone marrow smears from an acute leukemia patient. All blasts were periodic acid-Schiff (PAS)-negative. The majority of the blasts showed varying amounts of Sudan black B positivity. Some of the blasts stained positive for naphthol AS-D acetate esterase, some were positive for naphthol AS-D chloroacetate esterase, and some blasts stained positive for both esterases. What type of leukemia is indicated?

    a. lymphocytic
    b. granulocytic
    c. myelomonocytic
    d. erythroleukemia

166. Which substrate is used for the detection of specific esterase?

    a. acetate
    b. chloroacetate
    c. pararosaniline acetate
    d. phenylene diacetate

167. Which one of the following is <u>NOT</u> a possible cause of neutropenia?

    a. viral infections
    b. Hodgkin's disease
    c. select antibiotics
    d. chemotherapy

168. Long-term exposure to certain antibiotics such as penicillin has been found to result in:

   a. leukopenia
   b. thrombocytosis
   c. lymphocytosis
   d. polycythemia

169. Which one of the following cell types shows the most intense staining with peroxidase?

   a. segmented neutrophil
   b. eosinophil
   c. band
   d. monocyte

170. Muramidase (lysozyme) is present in:

   a. granulocytes and their precursors
   b. monocytes and their precursors
   c. granulocytes, monocytes, and their precursors
   d. lymphocytes and their precursors

171. In normal adult bone marrow, the most common granulocyte is the:

   a. basophil
   b. myeloblast
   c. eosinophil
   d. metamyelocyte

172. Which one of the following is a true statement about megakaryocytes in a bone marrow aspirate?

   a. An average of 1 to 3 should be found in each low power field (10 x).
   b. The majority of forms are the MK_1 stage.
   c. Morphology must be determined from the biopsy section.
   d. Quantitative estimation is done using the 100 x oil immersion lens.

173. In addition to a Romanowsky stain, routine evaluation of a bone marrow should include which of the following stains?

    a. chloroacetate esterase
    b. PAS
    c. Prussian blue
    d. Sudan black B

174. A hypercellular marrow with an M:E ratio of 6:1 is most commonly due to:

    a. lymphoid hyperplasia
    b. granulocytic hyperplasia
    c. normoblastic hyperplasia
    d. myeloid hypoplasia

175. In chronic myelocytic leukemia, blood histamine concentrations tend to reflect the:

    a. number of platelets present
    b. serum uric acid concentrations
    c. number of basophils present
    d. total number of granulocytes

176. The primary use of the toluidine blue stain is to distinguish between:

    a. myeloblasts and lymphoblasts
    b. "hairy cells" and lymphocytes
    c. leukemoid reactions and chronic granulocytic leukemia
    d. progranulocytes and basophils

177. The Philadelphia chromosome is formed by a translocation between the:

    a. long arm of chromosome 22 and long arm of chromosome 9
    b. long arm of chromosome 21 and long arm of chromosome 9
    c. long arm of chromosome 21 and short arm of chromosome 6
    d. long arm of chromosome 22 and short arm of chromosome 6

178. The absence of intermediate maturing cells between the blast and mature neutrophil commonly seen in acute myelocytic leukemia and preleukemic states is called:

    a. subleukemia
    b. aleukemic leukemia
    c. leukemic hiatus
    d. leukemoid reaction

179. A 30-year-old man who had been diagnosed as having leukemia two years previously was readmitted because of cervical lymphadenopathy. Laboratory findings included the following:

CBC		Differential	
WBC	39.6×10^9/L	Polys	7
RBC	3.25×10^{12}/L	Lymph	4
HGB	9.4 g/dL (1.46 mmol/L)	Mono	2
HCT	28.2% (0.28)	Eos	3
MCV	86.7 fL	Baso	48
MCH	29.0 pg	Myelo	13
MCHC	33.4% (0.33)	Promyelo	2
PLT	53×10^9/L	Meta	8
		Blast	13
		NRBC	11
		Megakaryoblast	3

Bone marrow: 95% cellularity, 50% blast cells (some with peroxidase and Sudan black B positivity)
Neutrophil alkaline phosphatase (NAP): 11 (15 to 100)
Ph^1 chromosome: positive

These results are most consistent with:

a. acute myeloid leukemia
b. erythroleukemia
c. chronic granulocytic leukemia
d. chronic granulocytic leukemia in blast transformation

180. Which of the following leukemias is characterized by immature cells that are Sudan black B-positive with discrete fine granules, peroxidase-negative, PAS-variable, strongly alpha-naphthyl acetate esterase-positive, and muramidase-positive?

a. acute lymphocytic
b. chronic lymphocytic
c. acute granulocytic
d. acute myelomonocytic

181. A 30-year-old woman was admitted to the hospital for easy bruising and menorrhagia. Laboratory findings included the following:

CBC		Differential		Coagulation	
WBC	$3.5 \times 10^9/L$	Polys	3	PT	34.0 (control 11.5)
RBC	$2.48 \times 10^{12}/L$	Lymph	2	APTT	62.5 (control 35.0)
HGB	8.6 g/dL	Mono	2	TT	20.0 (control 20.0)
HCT	25.0%	Myelo	4	Fibrinogen	315 (200-400)
MCV	100.7 fL	Abnormal immature	58	FSP	greater than 40
MCH	34.7 pg	Blasts	31		
MCHC	34.3%	NRBC	1		
PLT	$30 \times 10^9/L$				

Auer bodies,
1+ macrocytes,
1+ polychromasia

The cells identified as abnormal immature were described as having lobulated nuclei with prominent nucleoli; the cytoplasm had intense azurophilic granulation over the nucleus, with some cells containing 1 to 20 Auer bodies frequently grouped in bundles.

A 15:17 chromosomal translocation was noted.

Cells were Sudan black B-, peroxidase, and NAS-D-chloroacetate-positive; PAS-negative.

Which of the following types of acute leukemia is most likely?

a. myeloblastic
b. promyelocytic
c. myelomonocytic
d. monocytic

182. The bone marrow in the terminal stage of erythroleukemia is indistinguishable from that seen in:

a. myeloid metaplasia
b. polycythemia vera
c. acute granulocytic leukemia
d. aplastic anemia

183. A 50-year-old man was admitted into the hospital with acute leukemia. Laboratory findings included the following:

Myeloperoxidase stain - blast cells negative
PAS stain - blast cells demonstrate a punctate pattern of positivity
TdT - blast cells positive
Surface immunoglobulin - blast cells negative
E rosettes - blast cells negative
Philadelphia chromosome - positive

These results are most consistent with:

a. acute myelogenous leukemia
b. chronic lymphocytic leukemia in lymphoblastic transformation
c. T cell acute lymphocytic leukemia
d. chronic myelogenous leukemia in lymphoblastic transformation

184. A bone marrow report described cells containing 1 to 2 nucleoli, moderately coarse nuclear chromatin, a high N/C ratio, and a coarse staining pattern with PAS. These cells are most likely:

a. myeloblasts
b. lymphocytes
c. monoblasts
d. lymphoblasts

185. In which of the following disease states are dacryocytes and abnormal platelets most characteristically seen?

a. chronic myelocytic leukemia
b. multiple myeloma
c. thalassemia
d. myeloid metaplasia

186. In the FAB classification, myelomonocytic leukemia would be:

a. M1 and M2
b. M3
c. M4
d. M5

187. A bone marrow shows foam cells ranging from 20 to 100 μm in size, with vacuolated cytoplasm containing sphingomyelin, only faintly PAS-positive. This cell type is most characteristic of:

a. Gaucher's disease
b. myeloma with Russell bodies
c. Di Guglielmo disease
d. Niemann-Pick disease

188. Patients with chronic granulomatous disease suffer from frequent pyogenic infections due to the inability of:

a. lymphocytes to produce bacterial antibodies
b. eosinophils to degranulate in the presence of bacteria
c. neutrophils to kill phagocytized bacteria
d. basophils to release histamine in the presence of bacteria

189. Which of the following cells contains hemosiderin?

a. megakaryocyte
b. osteoclast
c. histiocyte
d. mast cell

190. Which of the following cells contains granules that stain with toluidine blue?

a. megakaryocyte
b. osteoclast
c. histiocyte
d. mast cell

191. Which of the following cells is the largest cell in the bone marrow?

a. megakaryocyte
b. histiocyte
c. osteoblast
d. mast cell

192. Which of the following is most closely associated with chronic granulocytic leukemia?

   a. ringed sideroblasts
   b. disseminated intravascular coagulation
   c. micromegakaryocytes
   d. Philadelphia chromosome

193. Which of the following is most closely associated with chronic monocytic leukemia?

   a. Philadelphia chromosome
   b. disseminated intravascular coagulation
   c. micromegakaryocytes
   d. lysozymuria

194. Which of the following is most closely associated with acute promyelocytic leukemia?

   a. ringed sideroblasts
   b. disseminated intravascular coagulation
   c. micromegakaryocytes
   d. Philadelphia chromosome

195. Which of the following stains is closely associated with glycogen, polysaccharides, mucopolysaccharides, and glycoproteins?

   a. peroxidase
   b. Sudan black B
   c. PAS
   d. nitroblue tetrazolium (NBT)

196. Which of the following stains is closely associated with neutral fats, phospholipids, and sterols?

   a. peroxidase
   b. Sudan black B
   c. PAS
   d. Prussian blue

For question 197, refer to the following illustration:

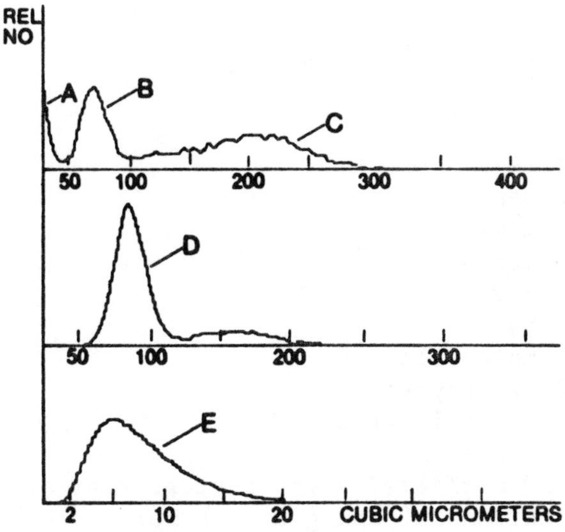

197. Which area of the above cell size distribution histograms from an electronic cell counter is appropriate for a non-lymphocyte leukocyte population curve?

a. A
b. B
c. C
d. D

---

198. Leukocyte alkaline phosphatase activity is decreased in:

1. myeloid metaplasia
2. polycythemia vera
3. reactive neutrophilia
4. paroxysmal nocturnal hemoglobinuria

a. only 1, 2 and 3 are correct
b. only 1 and 3 are correct
c. only 2 and 4 are correct
d. only 4 is correct
e. all are correct

199. The following results were obtained:

WBC 5.0 x $10^3/\mu L$
RBC 1.7 x $10^6/\mu L$
MCV 84 mm^3
PLT 89,000/μL

Differential - 16% segs
22% bands
28% lymphs
16% monos
1% eos
1% baso
4% metamyelocytes
3% myelocytes
4% promyelocytes
5% blasts

1 megakaryoblast, 30 nucleated erythrocytes, tear drops, schistocytes, polychromasia, and giant, bizarre platelets noted

LAP 142
Philadelphia chromosome - negative

This is consistent with:

a. idiopathic thrombocythemia
b. polycythemia vera
c. chronic granulocytic leukemia
d. leukoerythroblastosis in myelofibrosis

200. Conditions that may predispose to a "dry tap" from bone marrow aspirations include:

1. myelofibrosis
2. metastatic carcinoma
3. acute leukemia
4. leukemic reticuloendotheliosis (hairy cell leukemia)

a. only 1, 2 and 3 are correct
b. only 1 and 3 are correct
c. only 2 and 4 are correct
d. only 4 is correct
e. all are correct

201. Sections of bone marrow aspirate or biopsy are essential in the diagnosis of:

1. aplastic anemia
2. granulomatous disease
3. metastatic carcinoma
4. myelofibrosis

a. only 1, 2 and 3 are correct
b. only 1 and 3 are correct
c. only 2 and 4 are correct
d. only 4 is correct
e. all are correct

202. Which of the following conditions is <u>NOT</u> associated with a high incidence of leukemia?

a. paroxysmal nocturnal hemaglobinuria
b. Fanconi's anemia
c. aplastic anemia
d. megaloblastic anemia

203. Acquired autoimmune hemolytic anemias are generally secondary to which of the following conditions?

1. lymphoma
2. macroglobulinemia
3. leukemia
4. viral infections

a. only 1, 2 and 3 are correct
b. only 1 and 3 are correct
c. only 2 and 4 are correct
d. only 4 is correct
e. all are correct

204. Auer bodies are:

a. a normal aggregation of lysosomes or primary (azurophilic) granules
b. predominately found in acute myelogenous leukemia
c. peroxidase-negative
d. alkaline phosphatase-positive

205. True statements about blood monocytes include:

1. They are the precursors of tissue macrophages.
2. They produce interferon.
3. They are increased in number in many malignancies.
4. They are derived from promonocytes.

a. only 1, 2 and 3 are correct
b. only 1 and 3 are correct
c. only 2 and 4 are correct
d. only 4 is correct
e. all are correct

206. True statements about basophils include:

1. Their major function involves histamine release.
2. Stages of maturation are difficult to identify.
3. They are often increased in myeloproliferative disorders.
4. They are capable of phagocytosis.

a. only 1, 2 and 3 are correct
b. only 1 and 3 are correct
c. only 2 and 4 are correct
d. only 4 is correct
e. all are correct

207. A 10-year-old patient's bone marrow is classified morphologically by the FAB system as an L3 acute lymphocytic leukemia. Which of the following results supports this diagnosis?

a. TdT-positive
b. Pelger-Huët-like neutrophils are found
c. surface immunoglobulin-positive
d. E-rosette-positive

208. The absence of the Philadelphia chromosome in granulocytic leukemia suggests:

a. rapid progression of the disease
b. a polyclonal origin to the disease
c. excellent response to therapy
d. conversion from another myeloproliferative disorder

209. In myelofibrosis, extramedullary hematopoiesis may develop in the:

1. lungs
2. liver
3. kidney
4. spleen

a. only 1, 2 and 3 are correct
b. only 1 and 3 are correct
c. only 2 and 4 are correct
d. only 4 is correct
e. all are correct

210. Morphologic variants of plasma cells do NOT include:

a. flame cells
b. thesaurocytes
c. grape cells
d. Gaucher's cells

211. Which of the following bone marrow findings favors the diagnosis of multiple myeloma?

a. presence of Reed-Sternberg cells
b. sheaths of immature plasma cells
c. presence of flame cells and Russell bodies
d. presence of plasmacytic satellitosis

212. Leukocyte alkaline phosphatase activity is decreased in:

a. patients with acute infections
b. pregnant women
c. patients with polycythemia vera
d. patients with paroxysmal nocturnal hemoglobinuria

213. Pluripotent stem cells are capable of producing:

a. daughter cells of only one cell line
b. only T-lymphocytes and B-lymphocytes
c. erythropoietin, thrombopoietin, and leukopoietin
d. lymphoid and myeloid stem cells

214. All of the following conditions are myeloproliferative disorders <u>EXCEPT</u>:

   a. granulocytic leukemia
   b. lymphocytic leukemia
   c. polycythemia vera
   d. idiopathic thrombocythemia

215. A term that means varying degrees of leukocytosis with a "shift to the left" and occasional nucleated red cells in the peripheral blood is:

   a. polycythemia vera
   b. erythroleukemia
   c. leukoerythroblastosis
   d. megaloblastoid

216. Which of the following is true of acute lymphoblastic leukemia?

   a. occurs most commonly in children 1 to 2 years of age
   b. patient is asymptomatic
   c. massive accumulation of primitive lymphoid-appearing cells in bone marrow occurs
   d. children under 1 year of age have a good prognosis

217. The most frequent type of acute lymphocytic leukemia is:

   a. T cell
   b. common
   c. B cell
   d. undifferentiated

218. True Auer bodies stain negative with which one of the following cytochemical stains?

   a. peroxidase
   b. Sudan black B
   c. alkaline phosphatase
   d. specific esterase

219. Bone marow examination reveals a hypercellular marrow consisting of probable lymphoblasts with receptors for sheep rosettes and TdT; however, the lymphoblasts are negative for SMIgs, Ia antigen, CALLA, Fc, and complement receptors. The most likely diagnosis is:

a. null-cell acute lymphocytic leukemia (non-B, non-T cell)
b. chronic lymphocytic leukemia
d. T-cell leukemia
d. hairy cell leukemia

220. Chronic lymphocytic leukemia is defined as:

a. a malignancy of the thymus
b. an accumulation of prolymphocytes
c. an accumulation of hairy cells in the spleen
d. an accumulation of monoclonal B cells with a block in cell maturation

221. The most characteristic morphologic features of "atypical lymphocytes" include:

a. the nuclear chromatin and mitochondria
b. cytoplasmic RNA and indentation by erythrocytes
c. nucleoli and deep blue RNA-rich cytoplasm
d. a stretched nucleus and cytoplasmic indentations

222. In comparison to malignant lymphoma cells, reactive lymphocytes:

a. have a denser nuclear chromatin
b. are known to be T cells
c. have more cytoplasm and more mitochondria
d. are morphologically more variable throughout the smear

223. In patients with atypical lymphocytosis and persistently negative tests, the disease most frequently present is:

a. toxoplasmosis
b. cytomegalovirus (CMV) infection
c. herpes virus infection
d. viral hepatitis

224. In an uncomplicated case of infectious mononucleosis, which of the following cells are affected?

a. erythrocytes
b. lymphocytes
c. monocytes
d. thrombocytes

225. Hairy cell leukemia (leukemic reticuloendotheliosis) is:

a. an acute myelocytic leukemia
b. a chronic leukemia of myelocytic origin
c. a chronic leukemia of mononuclear origin
d. an acute myelocytic monocytic-type leukemia

226. Which of the following is NOT a characteristic usually associated with hairy cell leukemia?

a. pancytopenia
b. mononuclear cells with ruffled edges
c. splenomegaly
d. increased resistance to infection

227. A useful chemical test for the diagnosis of hairy cell leukemia is the:

a. peroxidase test
b. Sudan black B test
c. tartrate-resistant alkaline phosphatase test
d. tartrate-resistant acid phosphatase test

228. What feature would NOT be expected in pseudo-Pelger-Huët cells?

a. hyperclumped chromatin
b. decreased granulation
c. normal peroxidase activity
d. normal neutrophils

229. The most characteristic cell type in the Pelger-Huët anomaly is the:

a. band form
b. pince-nez form
c. normal neutrophil
d. myelocyte

230. The cytoplasmic abnormality of the white blood cell of Alder-Reilly anomaly is found in the:

a. endoplasmic reticulum
b. lysosomes
c. mitochondria
d. ribosomes

231. The cytochemical stain that is positive for the granules of Alder-Reilly anomaly is:

a. Sudan black B
b. PAS
c. myeloperoxidase
d. naphthol-AS-D chloroacetate esterase

232. TdT is an enzyme associated with:

a. RNA
b. cytoplasm
c. Golgi bodies
d. DNA

233. Increased levels of TdT activity are indicative of:

a. Burkitt's lymphoma
b. acute granulocytic leukemia
c. acute lymphocytic leukemia
d. eosinophilia

234. Which of the following properties of neutrophils allow them to be physically separated from lymphocytes?

1. adherence to various surfaces
2. phagocytic activity
3. density in comparison to lymphocytes
4. presence of Fc receptors on the neutrophil cell membrane

a. only 1, 2 and 3 are correct
b. only 1 and 3 are correct
c. only 2 and 4 are correct
d. only 4 is correct
e. all are correct

235. The isoimmunization for platelet antigen (P1A1) and the placental transfer of maternal antibodies would be expected to preclude which one of the following effects in a newborn?

a. erythroblastosis
b. leukocytosis
c. leukopenia
d. thrombocytopenia

236. Which of the following detects or measures platelet function?

a. bleeding time
b. prothrombin time
c. thrombin time
d. partial thromboplastin time

237. Of the following, the disease most closely associated with granulocyte hyposegmentation is:

a. May-Hegglin anomaly
b. Pelger-Huët anomaly
c. Chediak-Higashi syndrome
d. Gaucher's disease

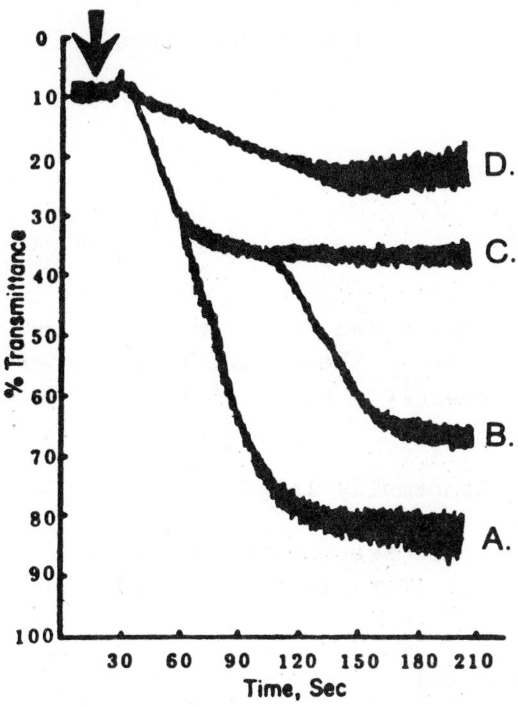

238. In the platelet aggregation curves shown above, the aggregating agent was added at the point indicated by the arrow. Select the appropriate aggregation curve for recent aspirin ingestion. (Aggregating agent is ADP or epinephrine.)

   a. A
   b. B
   c. C
   d. D

---

239. Of the following, the disease most closely associated with cytoplasmic granule fusion is:

   a. Chediak-Higashi syndrome
   b. Pelger-Huët anomaly
   c. May-Hegglin anomaly
   d. Alder-Reilly anomaly

240. Of the following, the disease most closely associated with mucopolysaccharidosis is:

   a. Pelger-Huët anomaly
   b. Chediak-Higashi syndrome
   c. Gaucher's disease
   d. Alder-Reilly anomaly

241. A platelet determination was performed on an automated instrument and a very low value was obtained. The platelets appeared adequate when estimated from the stained blood film. A possible explanation for this discrepancy is that:

   a. many platelets are abnormally large
   b. the blood sample was hemolyzed
   c. white cell fragments are present in the blood
   4. red cell fragments are present in the blood

242. Cells involved in hemostasis are:

   a. erythrocytes
   b. granulocytes
   c. lymphocytes
   d. thrombocytes

243. In polycythemia vera, the platelet count is:

   a. elevated
   b. normal
   c. decreased

244. When platelets concentrate at the edges and feathered end of a blood smear, it is usually due to:

   a. abnormal proteins
   b. inadequate mixing of blood and anticoagulant
   c. hemorrhage
   d. poorly made wedge smear

245. Irregular clumping of platelets is usually due to:

a. inadequate mixing of blood and anticoagulant
b. hemorrhage
c. poorly made wedge smear
d. hypersplenism

246. Platelet satellitosis is usually due to:

a. abnormal proteins
b. inadequate mixing of blood and anticoagulant
c. hemorrhage
d. poorly made wedge smear

247. Before an interpretation of thrombocytopenia is rendered from a peripheral blood smear examination, the entire smear should be scanned for platelet distribution, because:

1. smears of skin-puncture blood may show irregular platelet distribution and clumping
2. platelets are sometimes concentrated in the feathered end or edges of the smear
3. platelets may clump spontaneously in EDTA
4. patient hemorrhage may cause platelet clumping

a. only 1, 2 and 3 are correct
b. only 1 and 3 are correct
c. only 2 and 4 are correct
d. only 4 is correct
e. all are correct

248. Which of the following platelet responses is most likely associated with Glanzmann's thrombasthenia?

a. decreased platelet aggregation to ristocetin
b. defective ADP release; normal response to ADP
c. decreased amount of ADP in platelets
d. markedly decreased aggregation to epinephrine, ADP, and collagen

249. Erratic counting of platelets by instruments that use platelet-rich plasma can be caused by:

    1. improperly sedimented blood
    2. multiple myeloma and paraproteinemia
    3. aspiration of leukocytes with the clear plasma layer
    4. severe hypolipoproteinemia

    a. only 1, 2 and 3 are correct
    b. only 1 and 3 are correct
    c. only 2 and 4 are correct
    d. only 4 is correct
    e. all are correct

250. What is the effect of aspirin on platelets?

    1. It blocks aggregation to collagen.
    2. It blocks the release of adenosine diphosphate.
    3. It blocks the constriction phase of the release reaction.
    4. It causes decreased platelet survival time.

    a. only 1, 2 and 3 are correct
    b. only 1 and 3 are correct
    c. only 2 and 4 are correct
    d. only 4 is correct
    e. all are correct

251. Decreased platelet retention in glass-bead columns is associated with:

    1. Bernard-Soulier disease
    2. uremia
    3. von Willebrand's disease
    4. Addison's disease

    a. only 1, 2 and 3 are correct
    b. only 1 and 3 are correct
    c. only 2 and 4 are correct
    d. only 4 is correct
    e. all are correct

252. Characteristics of classic von Willebrand's disease include:

1. prolonged bleeding time
2. abnormal aggregation response of platelets to ADP
3. abnormal aggregation response of platelets to ristocetin
4. normal platelet adhesiveness

a. only 1, 2 and 3 are correct
b. only 1 and 3 are correct
c. only 2 and 4 are correct
d. only 4 is correct
e. all are correct

253. Which of the following platelet responses is most likley associated with classic von Willebrand's disease?

a. decreased platelet aggregation to ristocetin
b. normal platelet aggregation to ristocetin
c. absent aggregation to epinephrine, ADP, and collagen
d. decreased amount of ADP in platelets

254. Which of the following platelet responses is most likely associated with hemophilia A (factor VIII deficiency)?

a. defective ADP release; normal response to ADP
b. decreased amount of ADP in platelets
c. absent aggregation to epinephrine, ADP, and collagen
d. normal platelet aggregation

255. Platelet aggregation will occur with the production of:

a. cyclo-oxygenase
b. arachidonic acid
c. prostacyclin
d. thromboxane A_2

256. A 60-year-old man has a painful right knee and a slightly enlarged spleen. Hematology results include:

Hemoglobin	15 g/dL
Absolute neutrophil count	10,000/μL
Platelet count	900,000/μL
Reticulocyte count	1%

Red cell morphology and indices were normal. A slight increase in bands, rare metamyelocyte and myelocyte, and giant and bizarre-shaped platelets were observed in the blood smear.

This is most compatible with:

a. congenital spherocytosis
b. rheumatoid arthritis with reactive thrombocytosis
c. myelofibrosis
d. idiopathic thrombocythemia

257. Abnormal platelet retention in von Willebrand's disease is:

a. due to defective nucleotide release
b. related to a plasma factor deficiency
c. one of the most important criteria in making the diagnosis
d. improved following aspirin ingestion

258. Which of the following is characteristic of platelet disorders?

a. deep muscle hemorrhages
b. retroperitoneal hemorrhages
c. mucous membrane hemorrhages
d. severely prolonged clotting times

259. Which of the following is a true statement about acute idiopathic thrombocytopenic purpura (ITP)?

a. It is found primarily in adults.
b. Spontaneous remission usually occurs within several weeks.
c. Women are more commonly affected.
d. Peripheral destruction of platelets is decreased.

260. In an electronic or laser particle cell counter, clumped platelets may interfere with which of the following parameters?

   a. WBC count
   b. RBC count
   c. Hb
   d. HCT

261. Which of the following is associated with Glanzmann's thrombasthenia?

   a. normal bleeding time
   b. normal ADP aggregation
   c. abnormal ristocetin aggregation
   d. absence of clot retraction

262. Which of the following is characteristic of Bernard-Soulier syndrome?

   a. giant platelets
   b. normal bleeding time
   c. abnormal aggregation with ADP
   d. increased platelet count

263. Using a dark-field optical system for enumerating platelets, each of the following usually causes erroneous results <u>EXCEPT</u>:

   a. incipient clotting
   b. decreased HCT
   c. Howell-Jolly bodies
   d. leukocyte cytoplasmic fragments

264. Platelet aggregation is dependent in vitro on the presence of:

   a. calcium ions
   b. sodium citrate
   c. sodium chloride
   d. potassium

For question 265, refer to the following illustration:

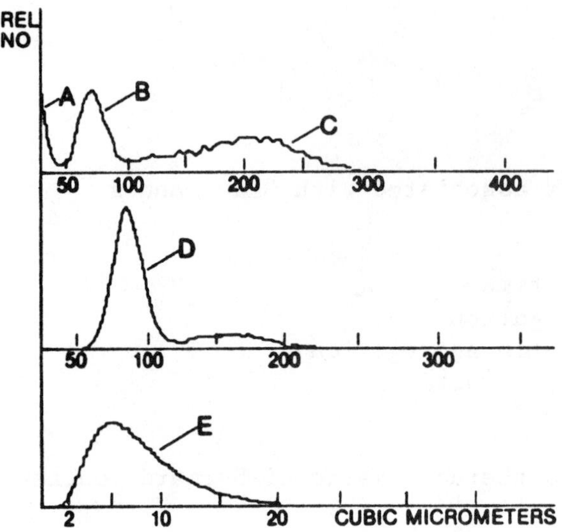

265. Which area of the above cell size distribution histograms from an electronic particle counter is appropriate for a platelet distribution curve?

a. A
b. B
c. C
d. E

---

266. Thrombocytopenia in a newborn can be due to:

1. maternal platelet antibody
2. DIC
3. sepsis
4. leukemia

a. only 1, 2 and 3 are correct
b. only 1 and 3 are correct
c. only 2 and 4 are correct
d. only 4 is correct
e. all are correct

267. The following results were obtained:

WBC 1.8 x $10^3/\mu L$
HGB 8.9 g/dL
HCT 27.4%
PLT 2,300,000/µL
Differential - 70% segs
10% bands
18% lymphs
2% monos

Giant, bizarre platelets, rare megakaryocyte, 4+ poikilocytosis, 3+ anisocytosis, 4+ echinocytosis, and 2+ schistocytes noted

LAP 90

This is consistent with:

a. neutrophilic leukemoid reaction
b. polycythemia vera
c. leukoerythroblastosis in myelofibrosis
d. idiopathic thrombocythemia

268. Following aspirin ingestion, abnormal platelet aggregation results are expected with:

1. ADP
2. ristocetin
3. arachidonic acid
4. collagen

a. only 1, 2 and 3 are correct
b. only 1 and 3 are correct
c. only 2 and 4 are correct
d. only 4 is correct
e. all are correct

269. On electronic particle counters, the platelet count can be falsely elevated due to:

1. debris in the diluent
2. electronic noise
3. microcytic erythrocytes
4. leukocyte fragments

a. only 1, 2 and 3 are correct
b. only 1 and 3 are correct
c. only 2 and 4 are correct
d. only 4 is correct
e. all are correct

270. A 33-year-old woman has recurrent thrombocytopenia. Examination revealed mucous membrane bleeding, an ecchymotic area over the right hip, and extensive bruising. There was no previous history of bleeding or bruising. Laboratory tests revealed:

Platelet count	5.5×10^9/L	Factor activities	(1:5/1:10 dilution)	
PT	11.8 seconds (control, 11.5)		VIII	25/64%
			IX	38/62%
APTT	58 seconds (control, 32)		XI	64/83%
			XII	58/79%
APTT with 50/50 normal plasma	48 seconds	Tissue thromboplastin inhibition test	1.6 (1:100) and 1.8 (1:1,000)	
Bleeding time	21 minutes (normal, 3-10)			
ANA	positive at 1:320; speckled pattern			

These results are most consistent with:

a. "lupus-like" inhibitor
b. thrombocytopenia secondary to systemic lupus erythematosus
c. combined thrombocytopenia and "lupus-like" inhibitor
d. specific coagulation factor inhibitors

271. Which of the following can cause false prolongation of prothrombin times (PT)?

1. temperatures above 38°C
2. plasma pH of 6.6
3. calcium concentration above normal
4. insufficient blood sample collected

a. only 1, 2 and 3 are correct
b. only 1 and 3 are correct
c. only 2 and 4 are correct
d. only 4 is correct
e. all are correct

272. Which of the following are likely to be found in a woman who is a carrier of hemophilia A (factor VIII deficiency)?

1. factor VIII coagulant activity about 50%
2. factor VIII antigenic activity about 100%
3. normal APTT
4. bleeding problems with major surgery

a. only 1, 2 and 3 are correct
b. only 1 and 3 are correct
c. only 2 and 4 are correct
d. only 4 is correct
e. all are correct

273. Antithrombin III deficiency is associated with:

1. an increased incidence of deep vein thrombosis
2. impaired clinical response to heparin
3. use of oral contraceptives
4. disseminated intravascular coagulation

a. only 1, 2 and 3 are correct
b. only 1 and 3 are correct
c. only 2 and 4 are correct
d. only 4 is correct
e. all are correct

274. Normal and abnormal control values for the activated partial thromboplastin time (APTT) are both greater than the established two standard deviations above the mean. Values obtained on patients are also higher than expected. What steps should be taken to resolve the problem?

1. Check the incubation chamber temperature of the coagulation instrument.
2. Check the timing device of the coagulation instrument.
3. Check the delivery calibration of pipettes being used.
4. Replace the calcium chloride.

a. only 1, 2 and 3 are correct
b. only 1 and 3 are correct
c. only 2 and 4 are correct
d. only 4 is correct
e. all are correct

275. Which of the following is the most common cause of an abnormality in hemostasis?

a. decreased plasma fibrinogen level
b. decreased factor VIII level
c. decreased factor IX level
d. qualitative abnormality of platelets

276. A hemophiliac male and a normal female can produce a:

a. female carrier
b. male carrier
c. male hemophiliac
d. normal female

277. A patient has a normal PT and a prolonged APTT using a kaolin activator. The APTT corrects to normal when the incubation time is increased. These results suggest that the patient has:

a. hemophilia A (factor VIII deficiency)
b. Hageman factor (XII) deficiency
c. Fletcher factor deficiency (prekallikrein)
d. factor V deficiency

278. Acute disseminated intravascular coagulation is characterized by:

a. hypofibrinogenemia
b. thrombocytosis
c. negative plasma protamine paracoagulation test (PPP test)
d. shortened thrombin time

279. Coagulation factors affected by coumarin drugs are:

a. VIII, IX, and X
b. I, II, V, and VII
c. II, VII, IX, and X
d. II, V, and VII

280. The following results were obtained on a patient:

PT	20 seconds (normal, 12-14)
Thrombin time	21 seconds (normal, 20-24)
APTT	55 seconds (normal, less than 40)
APTT plus aged serum	corrected
APTT plus adsorbed plasma	not corrected
Circulatory inhibitor	none present

Which of the following coagulation factors is deficient?

a. factor V
b. factor VIII
c. factor X
d. factor XI

281. A prolonged thrombin time and a normal reptilase-R time are characteristic of:

a. dysfibrinogenemia
b. increased fibrin split products
c. fibrin monomer-split product complexes
d. therapeutic heparinization

282. Which of the following laboratory findings is associated with factor XIII deficiency?

a. prolonged APTT
b. clot solubility in a 5 molar urea solution
c. prolonged thrombin time
d. prolonged PT

283. The preferred blood product for a bleeding patient with von Willebrand's disease is transfusion with:

a. factor II, VII, IX, X concentrates
b. factor VIII concentrates
c. fresh frozen plasma and platelet concentrates
d. cryoprecipitate

284. An abnormal Stypven time is associated with deficiency of factor:

a. VII
b. X
c. XI
d. XIII

285. The anticoagulant of choice for routine coagulation procedures is:

a. sodium oxalate
b. sodium citrate
c. heparin
d. sodium fluoride

286. Hageman factor (XII) is involved in each of the following reactions <u>EXCEPT</u>:

a. activation of C1 to C1 esterase
b. activation of plasminogen
c. activation of factor XI
d. transformation of fibrinogen to fibrin

287. Which of the following is most useful in differentiating hemophilias A and B?

a. pattern of inheritance
b. clinical history
c. whole blood clotting time and APTT
d. mixing studies (correction studies)

288. A 56-year-old woman was admitted to the hospital with a history of a moderate to severe bleeding tendency of several years' duration. Epistaxis and menorrhagia were reported. Prolonged APTT was corrected with fresh normal plasma, adsorbed plasma, and aged serum. Deficiency of which of the following abnormalities is most likely?

a. factor XII
b. factor VIII
c. factor XI
d. factor IX

289. Which of the following is a characteristic of factor XII deficiency?

a. negative bleeding history
b. normal clotting times
c. decreased risk of thrombosis
d. epistaxis

290. Which of the following is most closely associated with vitamin dependency?

a. factor XII
b. fibrinogen
c. antithrombin III
d. factor VII

291. Which of the following is present in the highest concentration of any clotting factor in blood?

a. factor XII
b. fibrinogen
c. Fitzgerald factor
d. antithrombin III

292. Which of the following are true statements about laboratory findings in acute disseminated intravascular coagulation?

1. Fibrinogen concentration progressively decreases.
2. Clot retraction shows increased erythrocyte fallout.
3. APTT, PT, and thrombin time are prolonged.
4. Rate of clot lysis is increased.

a. only 1, 2 and 3 are correct
b. only 1 and 3 are correct
c. only 2 and 4 are correct
d. only 4 is correct
e. all are correct

293. Conditions that may trigger disseminated intravascular coagulation include:

1. incomplete abortions
2. damage to endothelial surfaces
3. stagnation of blood flow
4. gram-negative endotoxin

a. only 1, 2 and 3 are correct
b. only 1 and 3 are correct
c. only 2 and 4 are correct
d. only 4 is correct
e. all are correct

294. Which of the following are inhibited by antithrombin III (AT-III)?

1. IXa
2. Xa
3. XIa
4. thrombin

a. only 1, 2 and 3 are correct
b. only 1 and 3 are correct
c. only 2 and 4 are correct
d. only 4 is correct
e. all are correct

295. Factor VIII activity following cryoprecipitate therapy of patients with von Willebrand's disease is best described by which of the following statements?

a. The activity is higher than would be predicted.
b. An immediate response is seen.
c. The activity disappears quickly.
d. The pattern is similar to that seen in hemophiliacs.

296. In the investigation of coagulation defects, enzymatic reactions in synthetic substrate assays may be evaluated by:

1. spectrophotometry
2. clot formation
3. fluorometry
4. densitometry

a. only 1, 2 and 3 are correct
b. only 1 and 3 are correct
c. only 2 and 4 are correct
d. only 4 is correct
e. all are correct

297. Which one of the following factors typically shows the least reduction in liver disease?

a. factor IX
b. factor X
c. factor VII
d. factor V

298. Which one of the following statements concerning vitamin K is <u>NOT</u> true?

a. There are two sources of vitamin K: vegetable and bacterial.
b. Vitamin K converts precursor molecules into active coagulation factors.
c. Heparin inhibits the action of vitamin K.
d. Vitamin K is fat soluble.

299. A blood sample was received in the Transfusion Service for a "type and cross" for two units of whole blood. After 20 minutes the technologist noticed that the sample had not clotted, and added thrombin. After an additional 10 minutes, the sample clotted. Possible explanations for this occurrence include:

1. factor II (prothrombin) deficiency
2. circulating anticoagulant
3. hemophilia A (factor VIII deficiency)
4. hypofibrinogenemia

a. only 1, 2 and 3 are correct
b. only 1 and 3 are correct
c. only 2 and 4 are correct
d. only 4 is correct
e. all are correct

300. A patient develops severe unexpected bleeding following four transfusions. The following test results were obtained:

Prolonged PT and APTT
Decreased fibrinogen
Increased fibrin split products
Decreased platelets

Given these results, which of the following blood products should be recommended to the physician for this patient?

a. platelets
b. factor VIII
c. cryoprecipitate
d. fresh frozen plasma

301. In manual or visual endpoint coagulation tests, duplicates are needed because:

a. reagents and samples must be paired
b. coagulation controls are expensive
c. high precision is unattainable in manual methodology
d. the CAP requires duplicate testing

302. Using automated coagulation instruments, duplication of normal tests is no longer appropriate because:

   a. the laboratory can document precision by collecting data to reflect precision performance
   b. all technologists on all shifts can be taught quality control
   c. it is difficult to have duplicates done in a blind fashion
   d. one technologist can monitor quality control

303. Of the following, the most potent plasminogen activator in the contact phase of coagulation is:

   a. kallikrein
   b. streptokinase
   c. factor XIIa
   d. fibrinogen

304. A test used to monitor streptokinase therapy is:

   a. reptilase time
   b. euglobulin clot lysis
   c. staphylococcal clumping test
   d. thrombin generation time

305. The most accurate bedside test used to monitor heparin activity is the:

   a. activated clotting time
   b. Stypven time
   c. reptilase time
   d. partial thromboplastin time

HEMATOLOGY ANSWER KEY

1. d
2. b
3. d
4. c
5. d
6. c
7. c
8. d
9. c
10. d
11. b
12. a
13. b
14. a
15. c
16. b
17. a
18. d
19. a
20. d
21. b
22. b
23. d
24. b
25. d
26. a
27. a
28. a
29. d
30. a
31. b
32. d
33. b
34. d
35. e
36. a
37. e
38. d
39. b
40. b
41. a
42. a
43. c
44. b
45. b
46. b
47. c
48. d
49. d
50. b
51. d
52. d
53. d
54. c
55. a
56. d
57. b
58. b
59. a
60. d
61. a
62. d
63. c
64. b
65. c
66. a
67. d
68. a
69. a
70. d
71. a
72. d
73. b
74. d
75. c
76. d
77. a
78. c
79. b
80. a
81. d
82. b
83. c
84. a
85. d
86. b
87. e
88. d
89. a
90. c
91. a
92. d
93. e
94. d
95. d
96. a
97. d
98. c
99. d
100. e
101. c
102. d
103. c
104. b
105. b
106. b
107. c
108. c
109. b
110. c
111. a
112. d
113. a
114. c
115. d
116. a
117. c
118. c
119. a
120. c
121. b
122. c
123. a
124. d
125. b
126. c
127. b
128. d
129. d
130. c
131. a
132. d
133. d
134. b
135. b
136. a
137. c
138. a
139. d
140. c
141. e
142. a
143. e
144. c
145. a
146. d
147. b
148. a
149. a
150. d
151. a
152. c
153. b
154. c
155. a
156. b
157. a
158. c
159. a
160. a
161. b
162. a
163. c
164. d
165. c
166. b
167. b
168. a
169. b
170. c
171. d
172. a
173. c
174. b
175. c
176. d
177. a
178. c
179. d
180. d
181. b
182. c
183. d
184. d
185. d
186. c
187. d
188. c

HEMATOLOGY ANSWER KEY (continued)

189. c
190. d
191. a
192. d
193. d
194. b
195. c
196. b
197. c
198. d
199. d
200. e
201. e
202. d
203. e
204. b
205. e
206. e
207. c
208. a
209. e
210. d
211. b
212. d
213. d
214. b
215. c
216. c
217. b
218. c
219. c
220. d
221. a
222. d
223. b
224. b
225. c
226. d
227. d
228. c
229. b
230. b
231. b
232. d
233. c
234. a
235. d
236. a
237. b
238. c
239. a
240. d
241. a
242. d
243. a
244. d
245. a
246. a
247. e
248. d
249. e
250. a
251. a
252. b
253. a
254. d
255. d
256. d
257. b
258. c
259. b
260. a
261. d
262. a
263. b
264. a
265. d
266. e
267. d
268. e
269. e
270. c
271. e
272. a
273. e
274. e
275. d
276. a
277. c
278. a
279. c
280. c
281. d
282. b
283. d
284. b
285. b
286. d
287. d
288. c
289. a
290. d
291. b
292. e
293. e
294. e
295. a
296. b
297. a
298. c
299. a
300. c
301. c
302. a
303. a
304. b
305. a

CHAPTER 12

Chemistry

1. In a laboratory quality control program where the range of acceptability for a value of an assayed control serum is the mean ± 2 standard deviations, the probability of a value falling inside this range is approximately:

   a. 50%
   b. 64%
   c. 90%
   d. 95%

2. Which of the following hormones can influence blood glucose concentration?

   1. insulin
   2. adrenocorticotropic hormone (ACTH)
   3. glucagon
   4. epinephrine

   a. only 1, 2 and 3 are correct
   b. only 1 and 3 are correct
   c. only 2 and 4 are correct
   d. only 4 is correct
   e. all are correct

3. Which of the following serum constituents is unstable if a blood specimen is left standing at room temperature for eight hours before processing?

   a. cholesterol
   b. triglyceride
   c. creatinine
   d. glucose

4. A series of glucose measurements obtained on a lyophilized quality control serum yields the following:

Mean	100 mg/dL	(5.6 mmol/L)
Standard deviation	4 mg/dL	(0.2 mmol/L)

Assuming that the data are normally distributed, approximately 95% of the results would be between:

a. 90-110 mg/dL (5.0-6.1 mmol/L)
b. 92-108 mg/dL (5.2-6.0 mmol/L)
c. 96-104 mg/dL (5.3-5.8 mmol/L)
d. 98-102 mg/dL (5.5-5.7 mmol/L)

5. Two standard deviations is the acceptable limit of error in the chemistry laboratory. If you run the normal control 100 times, how many of the values would be out of control due to random error?

a. 20
b. 5
c. 1
d. 10

6. Results of oral glucose tolerance tests that mimic diabetes mellitus may also be caused by:

1. prolonged inactivity (eg, hospitalization and bed rest)
2. obesity
3. administration of thiazide diuretics
4. administration of oral contraceptive agents

a. only 1, 2 and 3 are correct
b. only 1 and 3 are correct
c. only 2 and 4 are correct
d. only 4 is correct
e. all are correct

7. Total glycosylated hemoglobin levels in a hemolysate reflect the:

a. average blood glucose levels of the past 2-3 months
b. average blood glucose levels for the past week
c. blood glucose level at the time the sample is drawn
d. hemoglobin A_{1c} level at the time the sample is drawn

8. The conversion of glucose or other hexoses into lactate or pyruvate is called:

   a. glycogenesis
   b. glycogenolysis
   c. gluconeogenesis
   d. glycolysis

9. The different water content of erythrocytes and plasma makes true glucose concentrations in whole blood a function of the:

   a. hematocrit
   b. leukocyte count
   c. erythrocyte count
   d. erythrocyte indices

10. Which of the following inhibits glycolysis and glucose uptake by muscle cells, and causes a rise in blood glucose concentration?

    a. parathyroid hormone
    b. calcitonin
    c. growth hormone
    d. gastrin

11. In the fasting state, the arterial and capillary blood glucose concentration varies from the venous glucose concentration by approximately how many mg/dL?

    a. 2 mg/dL higher
    b. 5 mg/dL higher
    c. 10 mg/dL lower
    d. 12 mg/dL lower

12. Which of the following hemoglobins has glucose-6-phosphate on the amino terminal valine of the beta chain?

    a. S
    b. C
    c. A_2
    d. A_{1c}

13. Increased concentrations of ascorbic acid inhibit chromogen production in which of the following glucose methods?

    a. ferricyanide
    b. ortho-toluidine
    c. glucose oxidase (peroxidase)
    d. oxidase-oxygen

14. A mean value of 100 and a standard deviation of 1.8 mg/dL were obtained from a set of glucose measurements on a control solution. The 95% confidence interval in mg/dL would be:

    a. 94.6 to 105.4
    b. 96.4 to 103.6
    c. 97.3 to 102.7
    d. 98.2 to 101.8

15. Which of the following hormones is <u>NOT</u> important in the regulation of blood glucose concentration?

    a. insulin
    b. hydrocortisone
    c. thyroxine
    d. prolactin

16. Which of the following hormones that regulate blood glucose concentration are secreted by the pancreas?

    1. glucagon
    2. epinephrine
    3. insulin
    4. growth hormone

    a. only 1, 2 and 3 are correct
    b. only 1 and 3 are correct
    c. only 2 and 4 are correct
    d. only 4 is correct
    e. all are correct

17. True statements about insulin include:

    1. It increases cell permeability to glucose.
    2. It promotes glycogenesis.
    3. It promotes lipogenesis.
    4. It promotes glycogenolysis.

    a. only 1, 2 and 3 are correct
    b. only 1 and 3 are correct
    c. only 2 and 4 are correct
    d. only 4 is correct
    e. all are correct

18. Type 1 hyperlipoproteinemia (based on Fredrickson's classification) is characterized by high concentrations of exogenous triglycerides. This is due to:

    a. absence of pre-β lipoprotein
    b. absence of β lipoprotein
    c. absence of lipoprotein lipase
    d. presence of excess low density lipoprotein

19. The Liebermann-Burchard reagent for the determination of cholesterol in serum contains:

    1. acetic anhydride
    2. acetic acid
    3. concentrated sulfuric acid
    4. potassium hydroxide

    a. only 1, 2 and 3 are correct
    b. only 1 and 3 are correct
    c. only 2 and 4 are correct
    d. only 4 is correct
    e. all are correct

20. A cholesterol quality control chart has the following data for the normal control:

$\bar{X}$	137 mg/dL	ΣX	1,477 mg/dL
2SD	6 mg/dL	N	14

The coefficient of variation for this control is:

    a. 1.14
    b. 2.28
    c. 4.38
    d. 9.49

21. The moiety that is measured to estimate the serum concentration of triglycerides by most methods is:

    a. phospholipids
    b. glycerol
    c. fatty acids
    d. pre-β lipoprotein

22. Storage of serum at low temperatures or in a lyophilized condition usually ensures the stability of each of the following EXCEPT:

    a. serum lipoprotein
    b. cholinesterase
    c. gamma globulin
    d. alanine aminotransferase

23. With which of the following methods for measuring serum triglycerides is use of lyophilized quality control materials LEAST satisfactory?

    a. nephelometry following ultrafiltration of diluted serum
    b. alkaline saponification, periodate oxidation, and condensation with acetylacetone
    c. alkaline saponification, with enzymatic analysis of liberated glycerol
    d. enzymatic hydrolysis, with enzymatic analysis of liberated glycerol

24. A blood sample from a 32-year-old man was sent to the laboratory for lipoprotein phenotyping. The results were:

Triglyceride	340 mg/dL	β	normal
Cholesterol	180 mg/dL	Chylomicrons	absent
Pre-β	increased	Serum	turbid

Considering the results, what is the lipoprotein phenotype?

    a. type I
    b. type II
    c. type III
    d. type IV

25. A serum sample, examined after 18 hours at 4°C, shows a creamy layer floating on the surface with a clear layer underneath. This finding:

    a. clearly indicates an abnormality of lipid metabolism
    b. is characteristic of hypercholesterolemia
    c. suggests an α-lipoprotein deficiency
    d. may be seen in specimens collected from normal patients, in a nonfasting state

26. A patient in her thirty-third week of pregnancy is hospitalized with toxemia. Her doctor would like to deliver the baby early because the toxemia is becoming more severe. The baby's best chance of delivery without respiratory distress due to lung immaturity is if:

    a. the lecithin/sphingomyelin (L/S) ratio is greater than 4
    b. the L/S ratio is greater than 3
    c. PE is present
    d. creatinine is 1.3 mg/dL

27. The function of the major lipid components of the very low density lipoproteins is to transport:

    a. cholesterol from peripheral cells to the liver
    b. cholesterol and phospholipids to peripheral cells
    c. exogenous triglycerides
    d. endogenous triglycerides

28. The most common type of primary hyperlipoproteinemia is Frederickson, Levy, and Lee's type:

    a. I
    b. II
    c. III
    d. IV

29. Which of the following diseases results from a familial high density lipoprotein deficiency?

    a. Krabbe's
    b. Gaucher's
    c. Tangier
    d. Tay-Sachs

30. Types I and V hyperlipoproteinemia are characterized by massive increases in:

    a. chylomicrons
    b. low density lipoproteins
    c. very low density lipoproteins
    d. high density lipoproteins

31. The most widely used media for electrophoretic separation of lipoproteins are:

    a. starch gel and paper
    b. cellulose acetate and paper
    c. starch gel and agar gel
    d. paper and agarose gel

32. Sixty to seventy-five percent of the plasma cholesterol is transported by:

    a. chylomicrons
    b. very low density lipoprotein
    c. low density lipoprotein
    d. high density lipoprotein

33. In type II-A hyperlipidemia (Fredrickson), which of the following lipids is ALWAYS present in abnormal amounts:

    a. β lipoproteins
    b. chylomicrons
    c. pre-β lipoproteins
    d. α lipoproteins

34. Which of the following is <u>NOT</u> a stain for lipids?

    a. congo red
    b. Sudan IV
    c. oil red O
    d. osmium tetroxide

35. Serum from an individual with a type IV hyperlipoprotein phenotype would best be described as:

    a. being cloudy; chylomicron layer absent
    b. being cloudy; chylomicron layer present
    c. being clear; chylomicron layer present
    d. being clear; chylomicron layer absent

36. A 23-year-old healthy pregnant female has serum submitted for lipoprotein electrophoresis. Which type of secondary hyperlipoproteinemia would this woman most likely have?

    a. type I
    b. type II
    c. type III
    d. type IV

37. In the liver, bilirubin is converted to:

    a. urobilinogen
    b. urobilin
    c. bilirubin-albumin complex
    d. bilirubin glucuronide

38. In the Evelyn-Malloy method for the determination of serum bilirubin concentration, quantitation is obtained by measuring the purple color of:

    a. azobilirubin
    b. bilirubin glucuronide
    c. urobilin
    d. urobilinogen

39. The fast hemoglobin fraction is:

    a. Hb A
    b. Hb A_2
    c. Hb A_1
    d. Hb F

40. A patient with hemolytic anemia will:

    a. show a decrease in glycosylated Hb values
    b. show an increase in glycosylated Hb values
    c. show little or no change in glycosylated Hb values
    d. demonstrate an elevated Hb A_1

41. In using the chromatographic methods, falsely decreased levels of Hb A_{1c} will be demonstrated in the presence of:

    a. Hb F
    b. pernicious anemia
    c. thalassemia
    d. Hb S

42. Which of the following methods measures total glycosylated Hb?

    a. high-performance liquid chromatography
    b. colorimetric
    c. electrophoresis
    d. chromatography

43. Which of the following allows separation of Hb A_{1a} and A_{1b}?

 a. high-performance liquid chromatography
 b. electrophoresis
 c. chromatography
 d. spectrophotometry

44. The photometric procedure for plasma hemoglobin determination is based upon the property of hemoglobin to function as a:

 a. reductase
 b. protease
 c. peroxidase
 d. dehydrogenase

45. The urinary excretion of porphobilinogen is increased in patients with:

 a. erythropoietic protoporphyria
 b. porphyria cutanea tarda
 c. hemolytic anemia
 d. acute intermittent porphyria

46. Conditions associated with increased erythrocyte protoporphyrin include each of the following <u>EXCEPT</u>:

 a. anemia of chronic blood loss
 b. lead intoxication
 c. acute intermittent porphyria
 d. erythrocytic protoporphyria

47. Kernicterus is an abnormal accumulation of bilirubin in:

 a. heart tissue
 b. brain tissue
 c. liver tissue
 d. kidney tissue

48. Amniotic fluid scans are generally made to evaluate impending fetal distress from:

 a. maternal diabetes
 b. immature fetal lung
 c. respiratory distress syndrome
 d. hemolytic disease of the newborn

49. In the total bilirubin assay, bilirubin reacts with diazotized sulfanilic acid to form:

    a. diazo bilirubin
    b. biliverdin
    c. azobilirubin
    d. bilirubin glucuronide

50. In which of the following conditions does decreased activity of glucuronyl transferase cause an increase in unconjugated bilirubin concentration sufficient to cause kernicterus in neonates?

    a. Gilbert's disease
    b. Rotor's syndrome
    c. Dubin-Johnson syndrome
    d. Crigler-Najjar syndrome

51. The hemoglobin that is resistant to alkali denaturation is:

    a. A
    b. A_2
    c. C
    d. F

52. In the Evelyn-Malloy method for the determination of bilirubin, the reagent that is reacted with bilirubin to form a purple azobilirubin is:

    a. dilute sulfuric acid
    b. diazonium sulfate
    c. sulfobromophthalein
    d. diazotized sulfanilic acid

53. Fasting and postprandial bile acid concentrations are useful to assess:

    a. diabetes mellitus
    b. hepatobiliary disease
    c. intestinal malabsorption
    d. kidney function

54. In which of the following disease states is conjugated bilirubin a major serum component?

    a. biliary obstruction
    b. hemolysis
    c. neonatal jaundice
    d. erythroblastosis fetalis

55. True statements about haptoglobin include:

    1. It is an α-2 protein.
    2. Plasma concentrations are decreased in chronic hepatocellular disease.
    3. It binds with hemoglobin.
    4. Plasma concentrations are increased in infections.

    a. only 1, 2 and 3 are correct
    b. only 1 and 3 are correct
    c. only 2 and 4 are correct
    d. only 4 is correct
    e. all are correct

56. If the total bilirubin is 4.3 mg/dL and the conjugated bilirubin is 2.1 mg/dL, the unconjugated bilirubin in mg/dL is:

    a. 1.1
    b. 2.2
    c. 4.2
    d. 6.3

57. The Bessey-Lowry-Brock unit for the assay of alkaline phosphatase is defined as one millimole of substrate (p-nitrophenylphosphate) hydrolyzed in 60 minutes. This is the same as:

    a. 0.0167 IU
    b. 1 IU
    c. 16.7 IU
    d. 1,000 IU

58. The normal concentration of proteins in cerebrospinal fluid, relative to serum protein, is:

    a. 50-60%
    b. 25-30%
    c. 5-10%
    d. less than 1%

59. The electrophoretic pattern of a plasma sample as compared to a serum sample shows a:

   a. broad prealbumin peak
   b. sharp fibrinogen peak
   c. diffuse pattern because of the presence of anticoagulants
   d. decreased globulin fraction

60. The biuret reaction for the analysis of serum protein depends on the number of:

   a. free amino groups
   b. free carboxyl groups
   c. peptide bonds
   d. tyrosine residues

61. The urea nitrogen concentration of a serum sample was measured to be 15 mg/dL (5.36 mmol/L). The urea concentration of the same sample, in mg/dL, is:

   (Atomic weights: C = 12, O = 16, N = 14, H = 1)

   a. 15
   b. 24
   c. 32
   d. 40

62. In an alkaline picrate procedure to measure creatinine concentration in serum, the sodium hydroxide solution used contains 30 g NaOH/L. One milliliter of this solution is added to 1.5 mL water, 1.5 mL serum, and 1 mL picric acid. The concentration of NaOH in the final solution is equivalent to:

   (Atomic weights: Na = 23, H = 1, O = 16)

   a. 1.5 mol/L
   b. 0.75 mol/L
   c. 0.3 mol/L
   d. 0.15 mol/L

63. Below are the results of a protein electrophoresis:

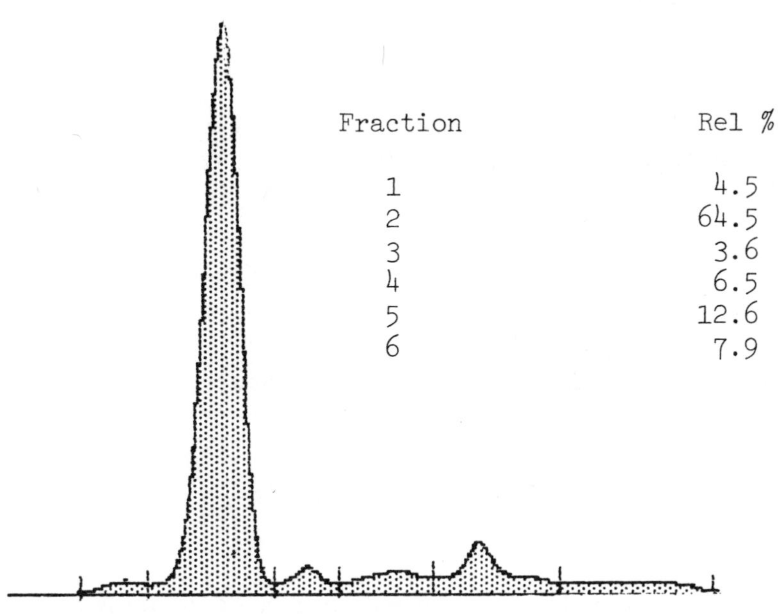

Fraction	Rel %
1	4.5
2	64.5
3	3.6
4	6.5
5	12.6
6	7.9

These results are consistent with a(n):

a. normal serum protein pattern
b. normal cerebrospinal fluid (CSF) protein pattern
c. abnormal serum protein pattern
d. abnormal CSF protein pattern

---

64. At a pH of 8.6 the gamma globulins move toward the cathode, despite the fact that they are negatively charged. What is this phenomenon called?

a. reverse migration
b. molecular sieve
c. endosmosis
d. migratory inhibition factor

65. Aspartate aminotransferase (AST) and alanine aminotransferase (ALT) are both elevated in which of the following diseases?

a. muscular dystrophy
b. viral hepatitis
c. pulmonary emboli
d. myocardial infarction

66. Isoenzymes of alkaline phosphatase occur in:

    a. kidney and bone
    b. bone and brain
    c. liver and pancreas
    d. brain and liver

67. The buffer pH most effective at allowing amphoteric proteins to migrate toward the cathode in an electrophoretic system would be:

    a. 4.5
    b. 7.5
    c. 8.6
    d. 9.5

68. The protein that has the highest dye-binding capacity is:

    a. albumin
    b. α globulin
    c. β globulin
    d. gamma globulin

69. The property most responsible for the migration of proteins in an electrical field is:

    a. molecular weight
    b. net surface charge
    c. endosmotic flow
    d. protein:lipid ratio

70. The electrophoretic resolution of serum globulins can be improved by:

    a. using high ionic strength buffer
    b. using a buffer with high osmolality
    c. adding calcium ions to the buffer
    d. using TRIS rather than barbital buffer

71. In an electrophoretic separation, the zones appear artifactually crescent-shaped. The most likely cause is:

    a. insufficient amount of sample
    b. overload of sample
    c. use of phosphate-borate buffer
    d. inadequate fixation prior to staining

72. In electrophoresis of serum proteins, artifacts at the application point are most frequently caused by:

    a. endosmosis
    b. prestaining with tracer dye
    c. overloading of serum sample
    d. dirty applicators

73. On electrophoresis, distorted zones of protein separation are usually due to:

    a. presence of therapeutic drugs in serum sample
    b. dirty applicators
    c. overloading of serum sample
    d. prestaining with tracer dye

74. On electrophoresis, spurious bisalbuminemia is associated with:

    a. dirty applicators
    b. presence of therapeutic drugs in serum sample
    c. endosmosis
    d. prestaining with tracer dye

75. On electrophoresis, protein migration forced toward the cathode indicates:

    a. endosmosis
    b. prestaining with tracer dye
    c. overloading of serum sample
    d. dirty applicators

76. On electrophoresis, distortion of albumin concentration may be obtained due to:

a. overloading of serum sample
b. prestaining with tracer dye
c. endosmosis
d. presence of therapeutic drugs in serum sample

77. Which of the following is characteristic of ammonia?

a. a waste product of amino acid and protein metabolism
b. obtained from hydrolysis of urea in the kidney
c. obtained from ingested carbohydrates
d. found in low concentrations in red blood cells

78. Erroneous ammonia levels can be eliminated by all of the following EXCEPT:

a. checking water and reagents to ensure they are ammonia-free
b. separating plasma from cells and performing test analysis as soon as possible
c. drawing the specimen in a prechilled tube and immersing the tube in ice
d. storing the specimen at room temperature until the analysis is done

79. Ammonia measurement is helpful in the diagnosis of:

1. Reye's syndrome
2. the underlying cause of some mental retardation
3. encephalopathy in patients without liver disease
4. urea cycle disorders

a. only 1, 2 and 3 are correct
b. only 1 and 3 are correct
c. only 2 and 4 are correct
d. only 4 is correct
e. all are correct

80. In the urea cycle:

a. mitochondria carbamyl phosphate is activated by N-acetyl glutamate
b. cytoplasmic carbamyl phosphate is activated by N-acetyl glutamate
c. hepatic ornithine levels are determined by ornithine transcarbamylase
d. ammonia, CO_2, and ATP are unnecessary for the first step of the urea cycle

81. A critically ill patient becomes comatose. The physician believes the coma is due to hepatic failure. The assay <u>most</u> <u>helpful</u> in this diagnosis is:

a. ammonia
b. ALT
c. AST
d. gamma-glutamyl transferase (GGT)

82. Gout is a pathologic condition that is characterized by the accumulation of which of the following in joints and other body tissues?

a. calcium
b. phosphorous
c. blood urea nitrogen (BUN)
d. uric acid

83. The degree to which the kidney concentrates the glomerular filtrate can be determined by:

a. urine creatine
b. serum creatinine
c. creatinine clearance
d. urine to serum osmolality ratio

84. High alkaline phosphatase activity is found mainly in:

a. hyperthyroidism
b. heart disease
c. liver disease
d. pancreatic carcinoma

85. The Jaffe reaction is used in the measurement of:

a. bilirubin
b. ammonia
c. BUN
d. creatinine

86. A physician suspects his patient has pancreatitis. Which test would be most indicative of this disease:

a. creatinine
b. LD isoenzymes
c. β-hydroxybutyrate
d. amylase

87. Fluoride ion usually influences the results of which of the following analyses?

a. sodium by flame photometry
b. urease method for urea
c. atomic absorption spectroscopy for calcium
d. atomic absorption spectroscopy for lithium

88. In the International System of Units, serum urea is expressed in millimoles per liter. A serum urea nitrogen concentration of 28 mg/dL would be equivalent to what concentration of urea (not urea nitrogen)?

(Urea: NH_2CONH_2; atomic weights: N = 14, C = 12, O = 16, H = 1)

a. 4.7 mmol/L
b. 5.0 mmol/L
c. 10.0 mmol/L
d. 20.0 mmol/L

89. Which of the following combinations in a base two number system represents the number "nine" in a base ten number system?

a. 1001
b. 11001
c. 12003_3
d. $1 + 2^3$

90. Erythrocytes contain approximately 73 mL of water per 100 mL of cells; plasma contains approximately 93 mL of water per 100 mL of plasma. Urea is distributed uniformly throughout the water phase in both cells and plasma. The whole blood urea nitrogen concentration in a specimen is 30 mg/dL (10.7 mmol/L); hematocrit is 40%. What is the calculated urea nitrogen concentration in plasma water?

   a. 26.7 mg/dL (9.5 mmol/L)
   b. 30.0 mg/dL (10.7 mmol/L)
   c. 23.3 mg/dL (11.5 mmol/L)
   d. 35.3 mg/dL (12.6 mmol/L)

91. One international unit of enzyme activity is the amount of enzyme that will, under specified reaction conditions of substrate concentration, pH, and temperature, cause utilization of substrate at the rate of:

   a. 1 mol/min
   b. 1 mmol/min
   c. 1 μmol/min
   d. 1 nmol/mil

92. In the "reverse reaction" of creatine kinase (CK) (Creatine Phosphate + ADP - Creatine + ATP), thiol compounds such as cysteine, glutathione, and dithiothreitol serve to:

   a. predictably inhibit enzyme activity
   b. enhance enzyme activity
   c. bind ADP
   d. precipitate proteins

93. For valid performance of a first-order (rate) determination of a substrate using an enzyme as a specific catalyst, which of the following relationships must be true?

([S] = substrate concentration, Km = Michaelis constant, Vm = maximal enzyme velocity)

ILLUSTRATION

a. [S] << Vm

b. [S] >> Vm

c. [S] << Km

d. [S] >> Km

94. Which of the following statements about immunoassays using enzyme-labeled antibodies or antigens is correct?

    a. Inactivation of the enzyme is required.
    b. The enzyme label is less stable than an isotopic label.
    c. Quantitation of the label can be carried out with a spectrophotometer.
    d. The enzyme label provides a high specificity for the substance being quantitated.

95. Which of the following chemical determinations may be of help in establishing the presence of seminal fluid?

    a. lactic dehydrogenase (LD)
    b. isocitric dehydrogenase (ICD)
    c. acid phosphatase
    d. alkaline phosphatase

96. Which of the following serum protein fractions is most likely to be elevated in patients with nephrotic syndrome?

    a. alpha-1 globulin
    b. alpha-1 globulin and alpha-2 globulin
    c. alpha-2 globulin and beta globulin
    d. beta globulin and gamma globulin

97. Which of the following enzyme substrates for acid phosphatase determination results in the highest specificity for prostatic acid phosphatase?

    a. phenol-phosphate
    b. thymolphthalein monophosphate
    c. α-naphthyl-phosphate
    d. β-glycerophosphate

98. Decreased concentrations of red blood cell 2,3-diphosphoglycerate (2,3-DPG) are found in which of the following?

    a. iron deficiency anemia
    b. chronic pulmonary disease
    c. uremia
    d. hexokinase deficiency

99. Increased total serum lactic dehydrogenase activity, confined to fractions 4 and 5, is most likely to be associated with:

    a. pulmonary infarction
    b. hemolytic anemia
    c. myocardial infarction
    d. acute viral hepatitis

100. The isoenzyme(s) of creatine kinase found in the myocardium is(are):

    a. MB
    b. MB and BB
    c. MM and BB
    d. MM and MB

101. Regan isoenzyme has the same properties as alkaline phosphatase that originates in the:

    a. skeleton
    b. kidney
    c. intestine
    d. placenta

102. Assay of transketolase activity in blood is used to detect deficiency of:

    a. thiamine
    b. folic acid
    c. ascorbic acid
    d. riboflavin

103. The most sensitive enzymatic indicator for liver damage from ethanol intake is:

    a. ALT
    b. AST
    c. GGT
    d. alkaline phosphatase

For question 104, refer to the following illustration:

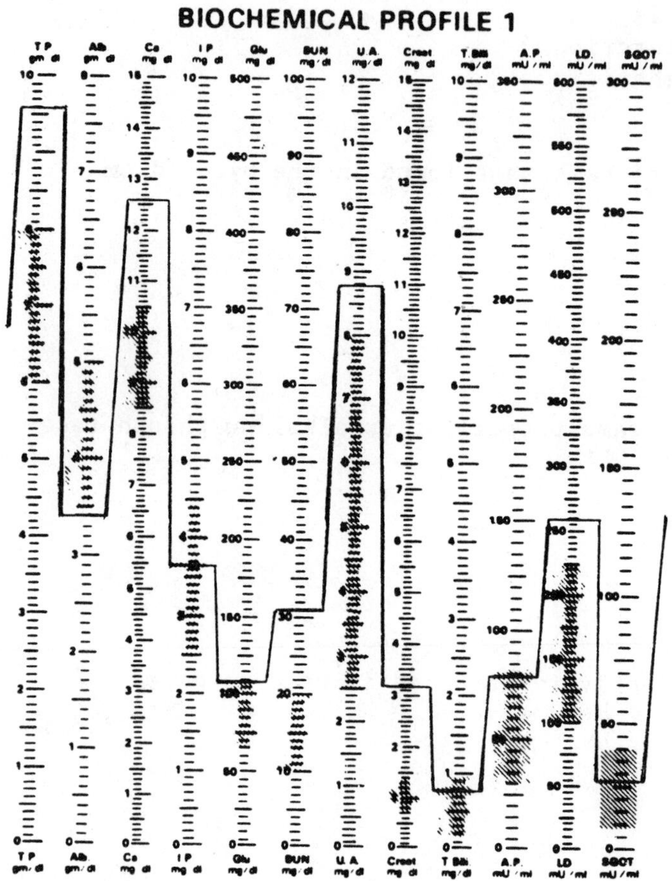

104. The elevated urea nitrogen concentration shown in biochemical profile 1 is most likely to have been caused by:

   a. dehydration
   b. thiazide diuretic therapy
   c. gastrointestinal hemorrhage
   d. renal insufficiency

For question 105, refer to the following illustration:

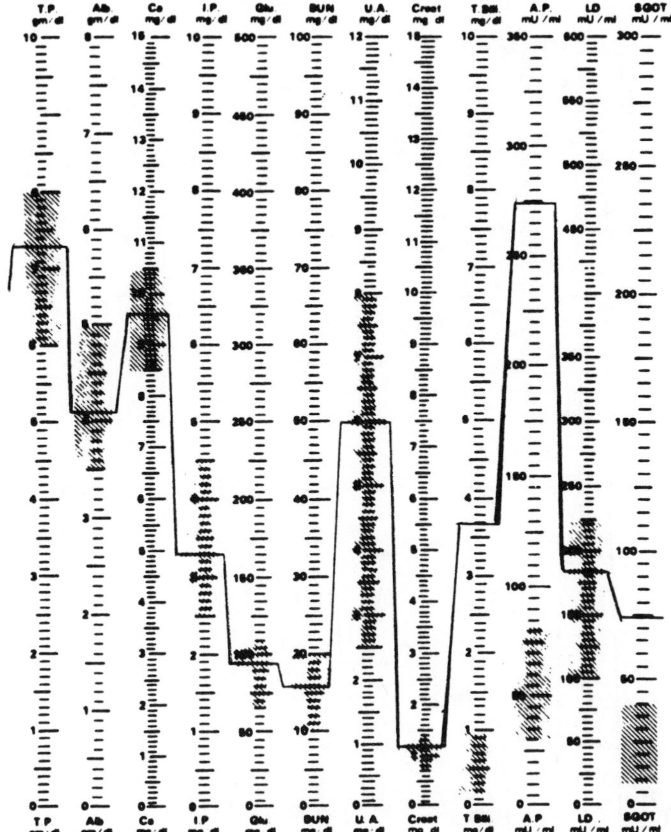

105. The results in biochemical profile 2 are most consistent with:

   a. viral hepatitis
   b. hemolytic anemia
   c. common bile duct stone
   d. chronic active hepatitis

For question 106, refer to the following illustration:

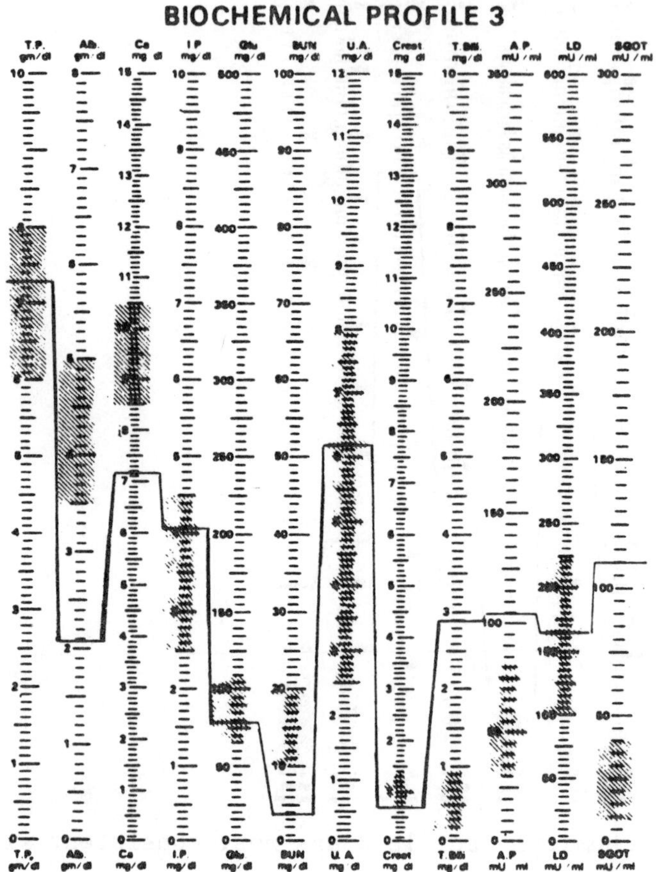

106. The results shown in biochemical profile 3 are most consistent with:

  a. acute viral hepatitis
  b. Laennec's cirrhosis
  c. eclampsia
  d. metastatic carcinoma

For question 107, refer to the following illustration:

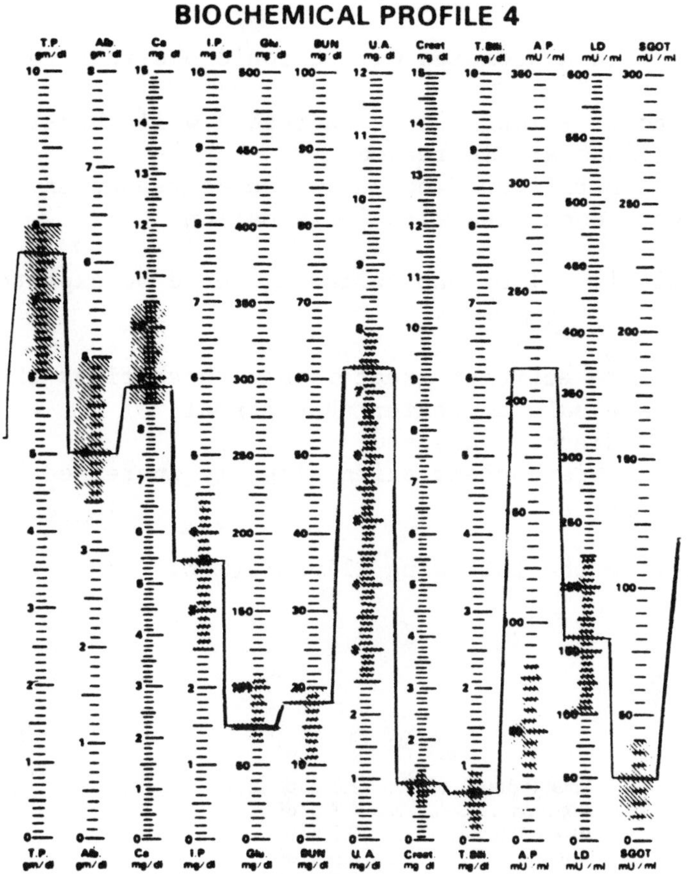

107. The results shown in biochemical profile 4 are <u>LEAST</u> consistent with:

   a. normal pregnancy
   b. secondary hyperparathyroidism
   c. carcinoma metastatic to liver
   d. Paget's disease of bone

108. Each of the following statements about alpha-1-antitrypsin is true <u>EXCEPT</u>:

a. it constitutes the major portion of the alpha-1 globulin fraction
b. deficiency is associated with chronic obstructive lung disease
c. serum concentrations can be decreased while hepatocyte concentrations are increased
d. serum concentrations frequently are decreased in conditions associated with inflammation

109. In acute pancreatitis, all of the following would be expected <u>EXCEPT</u>:

a. serum amylase activity greater than three times the normal
b. serum lipase values greater than normal
c. amylase clearance decreased
d. serum bilirubin concentration slightly increased

For question 110, refer to the following illustration:

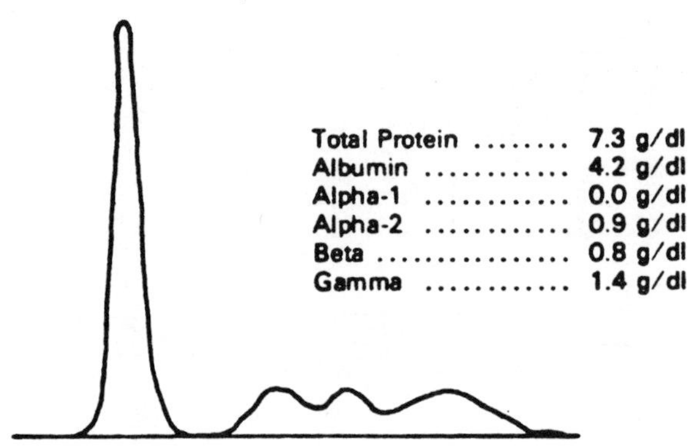

Total Protein .... 7.3 g/dl
Albumin .... 4.2 g/dl
Alpha-1 .... 0.0 g/dl
Alpha-2 .... 0.9 g/dl
Beta .... 0.8 g/dl
Gamma .... 1.4 g/dl

110. This pattern is consistent with:

a. cirrhosis
b. monoclonal gammopathy
c. polyclonal gammopathy (eg, chronic inflammation)
d. alpha-1-antitrypsin deficiency; severe emphysema

For question 111, refer to the following illustration:

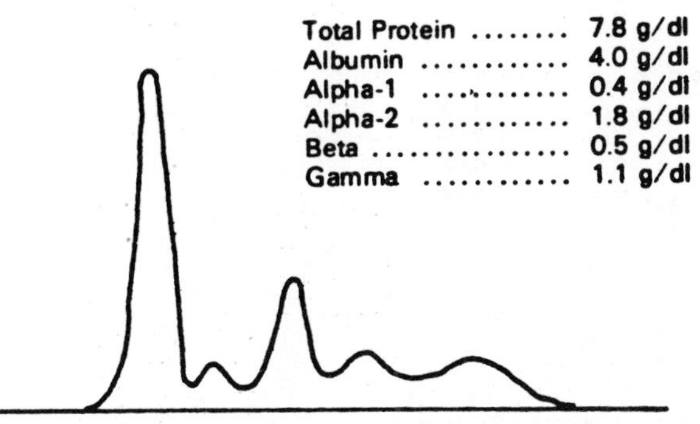

Total Protein .... 7.8 g/dl
Albumin .... 4.0 g/dl
Alpha-1 .... 0.4 g/dl
Alpha-2 .... 1.8 g/dl
Beta .... 0.5 g/dl
Gamma .... 1.1 g/dl

111. This pattern is consistent with:

a. cirrhosis
b. acute inflammation
c. polyclonal gammopathy (eg, chronic inflammation)
d. alpha-1-antitrypsin deficiency; severe emphysema

For question 112, refer to the following illustration:

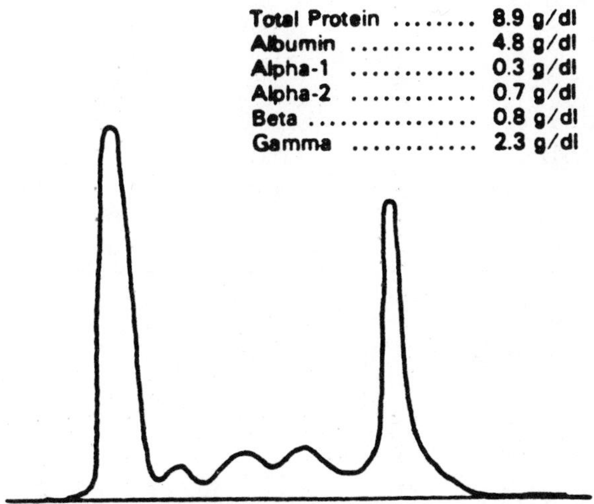

Total Protein .... 8.9 g/dl
Albumin .... 4.8 g/dl
Alpha-1 .... 0.3 g/dl
Alpha-2 .... 0.7 g/dl
Beta .... 0.8 g/dl
Gamma .... 2.3 g/dl

112. This pattern is consistent with:

a. cirrhosis
b. acute inflammation
c. monoclonal gammopathy
d. polyclonal gammopathy (eg, chronic inflammation)

For question 113, refer to the following illustration:

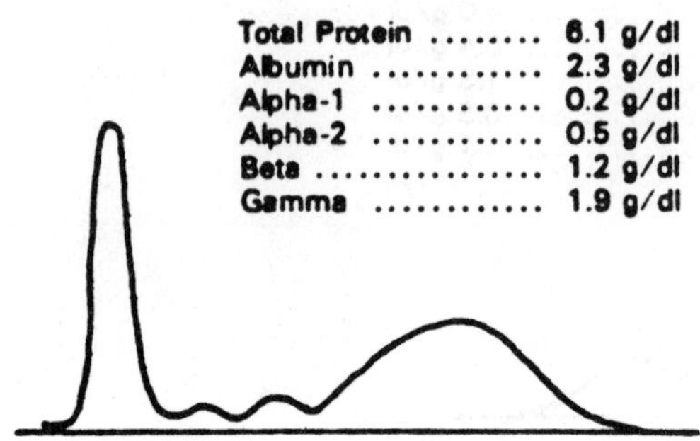

113. This pattern is consistent with:

a. cirrhosis
b. acute inflammation
c. polyclonal gammopathy (eg, chronic inflammation)
d. alpha-1-antitrypsin deficiency; severe emphysema

---

114. Given the following results:

Alkaline Phosphatase	Aspartate amino transferase	Alanine amino transferase	γ - Glutamyl transpeptidase
Slight Increase	Marked Increase	Marked Increase	Slight Increase

This is most consistent with:

a. acute hepatitis
b. chronic hepatitis
c. obstructive jaundice
d. liver hemangioma

115. Given the following results:

Alkaline Phosphatase	Aspartate amino transferase	Alanine amino transferase	γ - Glutamyl transpeptidase
Marked Increase	Slight Increase	Slight Increase	Marked Increase

This is most consistent with:

a. acute hepatitis
b. osteitis fibrosa
c. chronic hepatitis
d. obstructive jaundice

---

116. Given the following results:

Alkaline Phosphatase	Aspartate amino transferase	Alanine amino transferase	γ - Glutamyl transpeptidase
Slight Increase	Slight Increase	Slight Increase	Slight Increase

This is most consistent with:

a. acute hepatitis
b. chronic hepatitis
c. obstructive jaundice
d. liver hemangioma

117. A serum sample drawn in the emergency room from a 42-year-old man yielded the following laboratory results:

CK	185 units (normal = 15-160)
AST	123 units (normal = 0-48)

Which of the following conditions might account for these values?

a. crush injury to the thigh
b. cerebrovascular accident
c. pulmonary infarction
d. early acute hepatitis

118. In competitive inhibition of an enzyme reaction, the:

a. inhibitor binds to the enzyme at the same site as does the substrate
b. inhibitor often has a chemical structure different to that of the substrate
c. activity of the reaction can be decreased by increasing the concentration of the substrate
d. activity of the reaction can be increased by decreasing the temperature

For questions 119 to 121, refer to the following illustration:

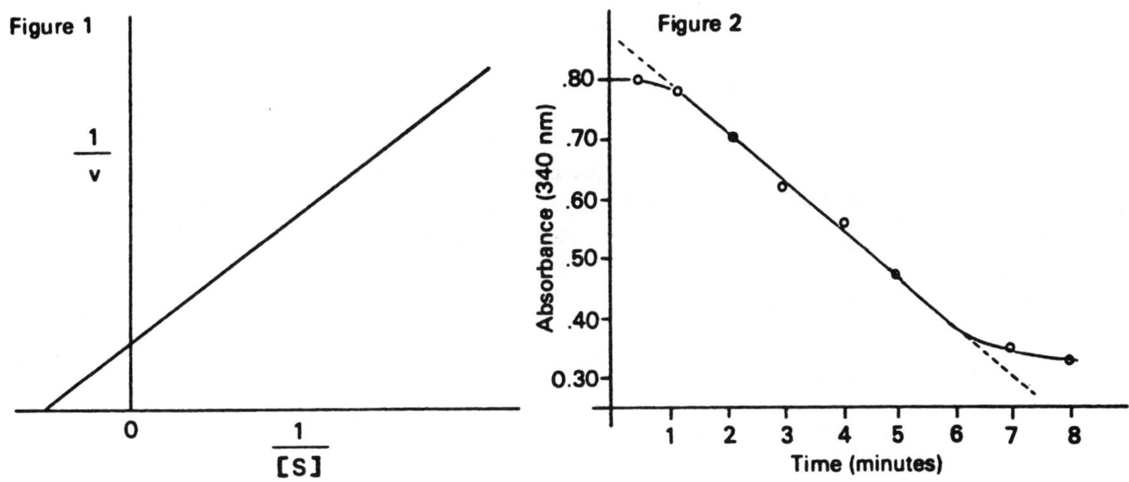

119. Figure 1 shows the reciprocal of the measured velocity of an enzyme reaction plotted against the reciprocal of the substrate concentration. A true statement about this figure is:

   a. the intercept of the line on the abscissa (x axis) can be used to calculate the V_{max}
   b. the straight line indicates that the enzyme reaction proceeds according to zero order kinetics
   c. the intercept on the abscissa (x axis) can be used to calculate the Michaelis-Menten constant
   d. the fact that the substrate concentration is plotted on both sides of the zero point indicates that the reaction is reversible

120. Figure 1 shows the reciprocal of the measured velocity of an enzyme reaction plotted against the reciprocal of the substrate concentration. A true statement about this figure is:

   a. the intercept of the line on the ordinate (y axis) can be used to calculate the V_{max}
   b. the straight line indicates that the enzyme reaction proceeds according to zero order kinetics
   c. the intercept on the ordinate (y axis) can be used to calculate the Michaelis-Menten constant
   d. the fact that the substrate concentration is plotted on both sides of the zero point indicates that the reaction is reversible

For question 121, refer to the following illustration:

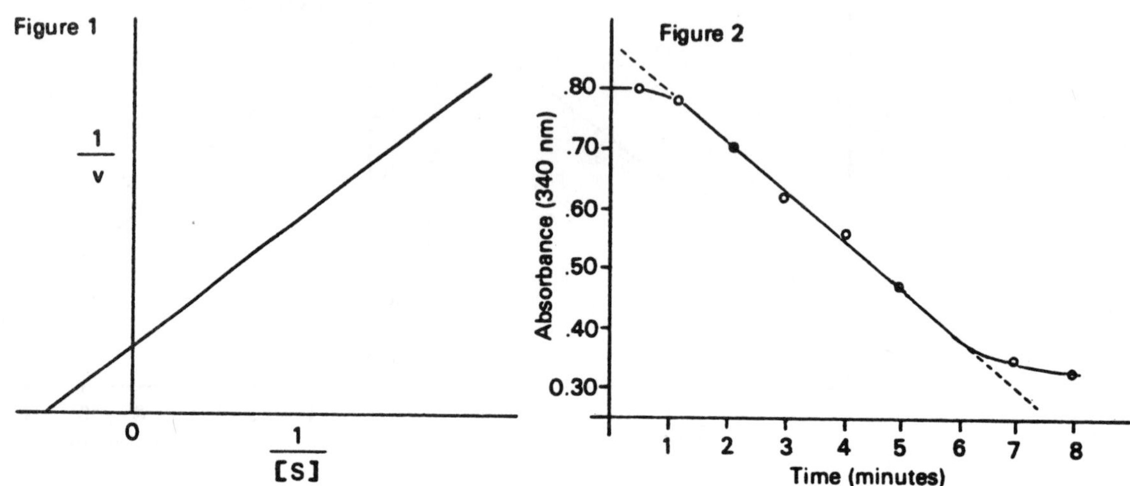

121. Figure 2 represents the change in absorbance at 340 nm over a period of 8 minutes in an assay for lactate dehydrogenase. A true statement about this figure is:

a. the reaction follows zero order kinetics between 5 and 8 minutes
b. the reaction is proceeding from lactate to pyruvate
c. non-linearity after 6 minutes is due to substrate exhaustion
d. the change in absorbance is due to reduction of NAD to NADH

---

122. Serum haptoglobin:

a. is decreased in patients with tissue injury and neoplasia
b. is increased in patients with prosthetic heart valves
c. can be separated into distinct phenotypes by starch-gel electrophoresis
d. binds heme

123. Which of the following serum proteins migrates in the beta-globulins on cellulose acetate at pH 8.6?

a. ceruloplasmin
b. hemoglobin
c. haptoglobin
d. C3 component of complement

124. Which of the following are associated with a serum albumin concentration less than 2 g/dL (20 g/L)?

1. advanced cirrhosis of the liver
2. protein-losing enteropathy
3. nephrotic syndrome
4. hereditary analbuminemia

a. only 1, 2 and 3 are correct
b. only 1 and 3 are correct
c. only 2 and 4 are correct
d. only 4 is correct
e. all are correct

125. Creatinine metabolism in patients with decreased renal function is characterized by:

a. linear increase in serum concentrations (mg/dL) as creatinine clearance (in mL/min) decreases
b. decreased excretion into the gut
c. enzymatic conversion of creatine to creatinine
d. increased renal tubular secretion of creatinine

126. Increased serum lactic dehydrogenase activity due to elevation of fast fractions (1 and 2) on electrophoretic separation is caused by:

a. nephrotic syndrome
b. hemolytic anemia
c. pancreatitis
d. hepatic damage

127. In acute pancreatitis, the relative increase in urinary amylase activity is greater than that of serum amylase activity because:

a. salivary isoamylases are increased
b. there are fewer inhibitors of amylase in urine
c. there is an increased renal clearance of amylase
d. measurements exhibit greater linearity in urine

128. CSF and serum specimens were sent to the lab for protein electrophoresis. On the CSF pattern, the technologist notes a fast-moving peak anodic to albumin. This peak is not seen on the corresponding serum pattern. How can this apparent discrepancy be explained?

    a. Bence Jones protein peak
    b. monoclonal spike
    c. pre-albumin peak
    d. samples are not from the same patient

129. Which of the following enzymes of heme biosynthesis is inhibited by lead?

    a. aminolevulinate synthetase
    b. porphobilinogen synthetase
    c. uroporphyrinogen synthetase
    d. bilirubin synthetase

130. In a severely hemolyzed specimen, the fluorescence observed cathodal to the CK-MM isoenzyme is caused by:

    a. hemoglobin
    b. adenylate kinase
    c. CK-BB
    d. CK-MB

131. The presence of increased CK-MB activity on a CK electrophoresis pattern is most likely found in a patient suffering from:

    a. acute muscular stress following strenuous exercise
    b. malignant liver disease
    c. myocardial infarction
    d. severe head injury

132. The identification of Bence Jones protein is best accomplished by:

    a. a sulfosalicylic acid test
    b. urine reagent strips
    c. immunoelectrophoresis
    d. electrophoresis

133. In the immuno-inhibition phase of the CK-MB procedure:

a. CK-MM is inactivated
b. CK-MB is activated
c. CK-BB is inactivated
d. B subunits are activated

134. Analysis of CSF for oligoclonal bands is used to screen for which of the following disease states?

a. multiple myeloma
b. multiple sclerosis
c. myesthenia gravis
d. von Willebrand's disease

135. When myocardial infarction occurs, the first enzyme to become elevated is:

a. CK
b. LD
c. AST
d. ALT

136. In the determination of lactate dehydrogenase at 340 nm, using pyruvate as the substrate, one actually measures the:

a. decrease in pyruvate
b. decrease in NADH
c. increase in lactate
d. increase in NADH

137. In the Bessey-Lowry-Brock method for determining alkaline phosphatase activity, the substrate used is:

a. monophosphate
b. phenylphosphate
c. disodium phenylphosphate
d. para-nitrophenyl phosphate

138. Which of the following structures reacts with biuret in the measurement of protein?

a. tripeptides or larger chains
b. primary amino acids
c. amine terminal of the protein
d. carboxyl terminal of the protein

139. In the Jaffe reaction, creatinine reacts with:

  a. alkaline sulfasalazine solution to produce an orange-yellow complex
  b. potassium iodide to form a reddish-purple complex
  c. sodium nitroferricyanide to yield a reddish-brown color
  d. alkaline picrate solution to yield an orange-red complex

140. Which of the following represents the end product of nucleic acid and purine metabolism in man?

  a. AMP and GMP
  b. DNA and RNA
  c. allantoin
  d. uric acid

141. In electrophoresis of proteins, when the sample is placed in an electric field connected to a buffer of pH 8.6, all of the proteins:

  a. have a positive charge
  b. have a negative charge
  c. are electrically neutral
  d. migrate toward the cathode

142. The classic method for determining protein is the Kjeldahl technique, which is based on the oxidation of organic protein using:

  a. heat (350°C) and H_2SO_4
  b. phosphotungstic-phosphomolybdic acid reagent in the presence of KOH
  c. phenol reagent in the presence of cupric ions
  d. heat (180°C) and NaOH

143. Maple syrup urine disease is characterized by an increase in which of the following urinary amino acids?

  a. phenylalanine
  b. tyrosine
  c. valine, leucine, and isoleucine
  d. cystine and cysteine

144. Enzyme studies on an inpatient give the following results:

CK	93 U/L
CK-MB	30 U/L
Heated CK-MB	6 U/L

The results indicate:

a. patient may have a myocardial infarction
b. patient has CK-BB
c. patient has macro-CK interference
d. patient has macro-CK and a myocardial infarction

145. A 24-hour urine specimen (total volume = 1,136 mL) is submitted to the laboratory for quantitative urine protein. Calculate the amount of protein excreted <u>per day</u>, if the total protein is 52 mg/dL.

a. 591 mg
b. 487 mg
c. 220 mg
d. 282 mg

146. A characteristic of the Bence Jones protein that is used to distinguish it from other urinary proteins is its solubility:

a. in ammonium sulfate
b. in sulfuric acid
c. at 40-60°C
d. at 100°C

147. Which of the following is an example of a peptide bond?

a. $R_1\text{—}C(H)(NH_2)\text{—}C(=O)\text{—}NH_2$

b. $R\text{—}CH(NH_2)\text{—}C(=O)\text{—}N(H)\text{—}CH(R_1)\text{—}C(=O)\text{—}OH$

c. $HO\text{—}C(=O)\text{—}CH{=}CH\text{—}C(=O)\text{—}OH$

d. $COOH\text{—}C(=O)\text{—}CH_2\text{—}COOH$

148. The principle excretory form of nitrogen is:

    a. amino acids
    b. creatinine
    c. urea
    d. uric acid

149. A 45-year-old male of average height and weight was admitted to the hospital for renal function studies. His serum creatinine was 1.5 mg/dL and urine creatinine was 120 mg/dL; the total volume of urine collected over a 24-hour period was 1,800 mL. Calculate the creatinine clearance for this patient, in mL/min.

    a. 100
    b. 144
    c. 156
    d. 225

150. An international unit of enzyme activity is defined as that amount of enzyme which will catalyze the transformation or the conversion of one of which of the following units of substrate to product per minute, per milliliter of serum at 25°C?

    a. mole
    b. millimole
    c. micromole
    d. micromillimole

151. Which of the following enzymes catalyzes the conversion of starch to glucose and maltose?

    a. malate dehydrogenase (MD)
    b. amylase
    c. CK
    d. ICD

152. A scanning of a CK isoenzyme fractionation revealed two peaks: a slow cathodic peak (CK-MM) and an intermediate peak (CK-MB).

A possible interpretation for this pattern is:

a. brain tumor
b. muscular dystrophy
c. myocardial infarction
d. viral hepatitis

153. Which of the following enzymes are used in the diagnosis of acute pancreatitis?

a. amylase and lipase
b. AST and ALT
c. 5'-Nucleotidase (5'N) and GGT
d. AST and LD

154. Which of the following glycolytic enzymes catalyzes the cleavage of fructose-1, 6-diphosphate to glyceraldehyde-3-phosphate and dihydroxyacetone phosphate?

a. aldolase
b. phosphofructokinase
c. pyruvate kinase
d. fumarase

155. The greatest activities of serum AST and ALT are seen in:

a. acute hepatitis
b. primary biliary cirrhosis
c. metastatic hepatic carcinoma
d. alcoholic cirrhosis

156. An electrophoretic separation of lactate dehydrogenase isoenzymes that demonstrates an elevation in LD-1 and LD-2 is indicative of:

a. myocardial infarction
b. viral hepatitis
c. pancreatitis
d. renal failure

157. Which of the following is a characteristic shared by lactate dehydrogenase, malate dehydrogenase, isocitrate dehydrogenase, and hydroxybutyric dehydrogenase (HBD)?

   a. They are liver enzymes.
   b. They are cardiac enzymes.
   c. They catalyze oxidation-reduction reactions.
   d. They are class III enzymes.

158. The protein portion of an enzyme complex is called the:

   a. apoenzyme
   b. coenzyme
   c. holoenzyme
   d. proenzyme

159. The prostatic fraction of acid phosphatase is inhibited by:

   a. acetic acid
   b. citric acid
   c. sodium nitrite
   d. tartrate

160. The most heat labile fraction of alkaline phosphatase is obtained from:

   a. liver
   b. bone
   c. intestine
   d. placenta

161. A 10-year-old child was admitted to pediatrics with an initial diagnosis of skeletal muscle disease. The best confirmatory tests would be:

   a. CK and ICD
   b. GGT and alkaline phosphatase
   c. aldolase and CK
   d. LD and MD

162. Which of the following is the most likely interpretation of the LD isoenzyme scan illustrated?

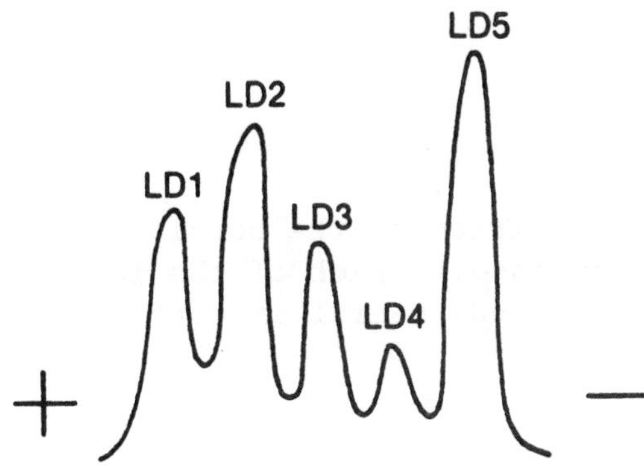

a. myocardial infarction
b. megaloblastic anemia
c. acute pancreatitis
d. viral hepatitis

163. Patients who have a certain defective enzyme are unable to hydrolyze succinyl choline and may suffer from respiratory paralysis for up to 24 hours after administration of the muscle relaxant. This phenomenon is referred to as:

a. pharmacogenetic variability
b. enzyme induction
c. drug-protein interaction
d. drug-drug interaction

164. Malic dehydrogenase is added to the transaminase reaction (AST) to catalyze the conversion of:

a. alpha-ketoglutarate to aspartate
b. alpha-ketoglutarate to malate
c. aspartate to oxalacetate
d. oxalacetate to malate

165. Loss of renal function is demonstrated by high serum concentrations in each of the following analytes EXCEPT:

a. creatinine
b. phosphate
c. protein
d. uric acid

166. Decreased serum albumin concentrations are seen in each of the following conditions <u>EXCEPT</u>:

    a. malnutrition
    b. acute hepatitis
    c. chronic inflammation
    d. dehydration

167. A 36-week-pregnant woman was admitted to the hospital with a diagnosis of possible liver disease. Which of the following enzyme determinations would be <u>LEAST</u> useful in confirming the diagnosis?

    a. alkaline phosphatase
    b. ALT
    c. GGT
    d. ICD

168. Each of the enzymes listed is included in the hepatobiliary panel for assessing liver function <u>EXCEPT</u>:

    a. alkaline phosphatase
    b. gamma-glutamyltransferase
    c. aldolase
    d. 5'-Nucleotidase

169. Which of the following amino acids is associated with the sulfhydryl group?

    a. cysteine
    b. glycine
    c. serine
    d. tyrosine

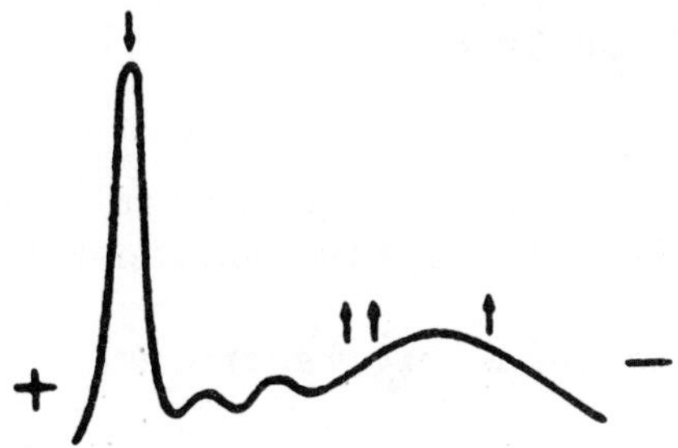

170. The serum protein electrophoretic pattern illustrated is consistent with which of the following diseases?

a. hepatic cirrhosis
b. monoclonal gammopathy
c. nephrotic syndrome
d. infection

---

171. A patient with glomerulonephritis would present the following serum results:

a. creatinine decreased
b. calcium increased
c. phosphorous decreased
d. BUN increased

172. True statements about ceruloplasmin include:

1. It is an alpha-2 protein.
2. It is decreased in Wilson's disease.
3. It transports copper.
4. It is increased in chronic hepatocellular disease.

a. only 1, 2 and 3 are correct
b. only 1 and 3 are correct
c. only 2 and 4 are correct
d. only 4 is correct
e. all are correct

173. True statements about transferrin include:

1. It is a β-protein
2. It is decreased in chronic hepatocellular disease.
3. It transports iron from absorptive surfaces to bone marrow.
4. It is increased in inflammatory reactions.

a. only 1, 2 and 3 are correct
b. only 1 and 3 are correct
c. only 2 and 4 are correct
d. only 4 is correct
e. all are correct

174. The serum protein electrophoresis pattern shown below was obtained on cellulose acetate at pH 8.6.

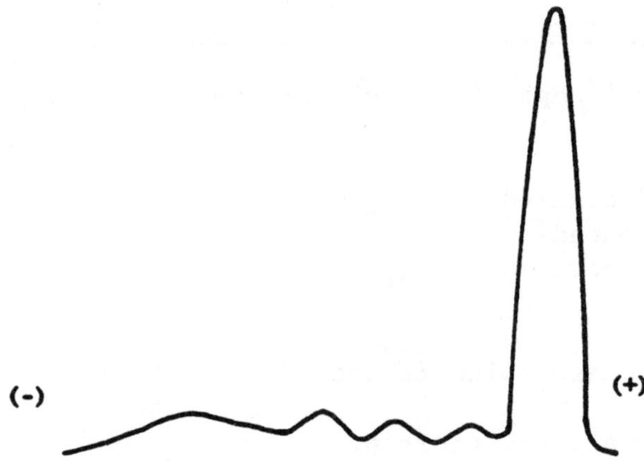

Identify the serum protein fraction on the far right of the illustration.

a. gamma globulin
b. albumin
c. alpha-1 globulin
d. alpha-2 globulin

175. A patient was admitted to the hospital with a liver involvement disease. A protein electrophoresis was performed with the following pattern:

Albumin	moderately decreased
Alpha-1	normal
Alpha-2	normal
Beta	marginal increase
Gamma	moderately increased

The beta and gamma fractions showed no distinct separation. The most likely pathologic condition would be:

a. chronic infection
b. obstructive jaundice
c. hepatic cirrhosis
d. nephrotic syndrome

176. Once technical artifact is eliminated, beta-gamma bridging on a serum protein electropherogram is indicative of:

a. viral pneumonia
b. chronic liver disease
c. acute renal disease
d. multiple myeloma

177. The creatinine clearance (mL/min) is equal to:

a. $$\frac{\text{urinary creatinine (mg/L)}}{\text{volume of urine (mL/min)} \times \text{plasma creatinine (mg/L)}}$$

b. $$\frac{\text{urinary creatinine (mg/L)} \times \text{volume (mL/min)}}{\text{plasma creatinine (mg/L)}}$$

c. $$\frac{\text{urinary creatinine (mg/L)}}{\text{volume of urine (mL/hour)} \times \text{plasma creatinine (mg/L)}}$$

d. $$\frac{\text{urinary creatine (mg/L)} \times \text{volume (mL/hour)}}{\text{plasma creatinine (mg/L)}}$$

178. The following results were obtained:

Urine creatinine	90 mg/100 mL
Serum creatinine	0.90 mg/100 mL
Patient's total body surface	1.73 m^2 (average = 1.73 m^2)
Total urine volume in 24 hours =	1,500 mL

Given the above data, calculate the patient's creatinine clearance.

a. 104 mL/min
b. 124 mL/min
c. 144 mL/min
d. 150 mL/min

179. Total iron-binding capacity measures the serum iron transporting capacity of:

a. hemoglobin
b. ceruloplasmin
c. transferrin
d. ferritin

180. In respiratory acidosis, a compensatory mechanism is the decrease in:

a. respiration rate
b. ammonia formation
c. blood pCO_2
d. plasma bicarbonate concentration

181. Calcium concentration in the serum is regulated by:

a. insulin
b. parathyroid hormone
c. thyroxine
d. vitamin C

182. In blood, pCO_2 may be measured by:

a. direct colorimetric measurement of dissolved CO_2

b. calculations of blood pH and total CO_2 concentration

c. measurement of CO_2-saturated hemoglobin

d. a silver-silver chloride electrode

183. The stimulant of localized sweating for the sweat test is:

a. polyvinyl alcohol
b. lithium sulfate
c. potassium sulfate
d. pilocarpine nitrate

184. Osmometry can be used to:

1. evaluate hypo- or hypernatremia
2. evaluate metabolic disturbances resulting from liver disease
3. evaluate solutes in the urine of patients with renal disease
4. check the chemical purity of solutions

a. only 1, 2 and 3 are correct
b. only 1 and 3 are correct
c. only 2 and 4 are correct
d. only 4 is correct
e. all are correct

185. The formula for calculating serum osmolality that incorporates a correction for the water content of plasma is (BS = blood sugar; UN = urea nitrogen):

a. $2\text{Na} \times \frac{\text{BS}}{20} \times \frac{\text{UN}}{3}$

b. $\text{Na} + \frac{2 \times \text{BS}}{20} \times \frac{\text{UN}}{3}$

c. $2\text{Na} + \frac{\text{BS}}{20} + \frac{\text{UN}}{3}$

d. $2\text{Na} + \frac{\text{BS}}{3} + \frac{\text{UN}}{20}$

186. Δ - osmolality (Δ - osmol) is:

a. the difference between the ideal and real osmolality values
b. the difference between the calculated and determined osmolality values
c. the difference between plasma and water osmolality values
d. the difference between molality and molarity at 4°C

187. In the sweat test, after the removal of the electrodes, what is the NEXT step for sweat collection?

   a. cleaning the "stimulated" area with pilocarpine-soaked gauze
   b. placing the filter paper on the stimulated area
   c. removing the filter paper from the forearm and weighing
   d. allowing the sweat to collect for 10 minutes

188. A sweat chloride result of 55 mmol/L and a sweat sodium of 52 mmol/L were obtained on a patient who has a history of respiratory problems. The best interpretation of these results is:

   a. normal
   b. normal sodium and abnormal chloride; test should be repeated
   c. abnormal
   d. borderline; the test should be repeated

189. The method in which ammonia is eluted and measured colorimetrically with the phenol-hypochlorite reaction is:

   a. ammonia electrode method
   b. enzymatic method
   c. diffusion method
   d. resin absorption method

190. The correct procedure for sweat sodium analysis is:

   a. Add 4 ml of lithium diluent to the vial containing the filter paper and elute for 15-30 minutes.
   b. Using your fingers, remove the filter paper from the vial and squeeze the excess liquid from the paper into the vial.
   c. The flame photometer is standardized using a 1:200 dilution of a 100 mmol/L NaCL standard solution.
   d. Results of the sweat Na are taken directly from the reading obtained from the flame photometer.

191. The method by which ammonia is converted to glutamate and changes NADH to NAD^+ is:

a. ammonia electrode method
b. enzymatic method
c. diffusion method
d. resin absorption method

192. A fire victim is being treated in the emergency room for smoke inhalation. No other injuries are noted. Which of the following tests would be most helpful in the treatment of this patient?

a. hemoglobin
b. pH
c. base excess
d. pO_2

193. Most of the carbon dioxide present in blood is in the form of:

a. dissolved CO_2
b. carbonate
c. bicarbonate ion
d. carbonic acid

194. In various colorimetric methods for determining inorganic phosphorus concentrations, reagents such as stannous chloride, ferrous sulfate, and ascorbic acid function as:

a. oxidizing agents
b. reducing agents
c. stabilizing agents
d. catalysts

195. The following laboratory results were obtained:

	Calcium	Phosphate	Alkaline Phosphatase
Serum	increased	decreased	normal or increased
Urine	increased	increased	

These results are most compatible with:

a. multiple myeloma
b. milk-alkali syndrome
c. sarcoidosis
d. primary hyperparathyroidism

196. A 57-year-old man with congestive heart failure has a serum potassium of 2.6 mEq/L (mmol/L). Twelve hours later, the serum potassium is 2.3 mEq/L. Assuming the laboratory coefficient of variation for potassium is 1.5%, which of the following is applicable?

a. The difference in the determinations confirms a labeling error.
b. The standard deviation is approximately 0.015 mEq/L for the 2.6 mEq/L concentration.
c. The values are not significantly different.
d. The change is greater than 3 standard deviations and is significant.

197. A low concentration of serum phosphorus is commonly found in:

a. patients who are receiving carbohydrate hyperalimentation
b. chronic renal disease
c. hypoparathyroidism
d. patients with pituitary tumors

198. A patient with metabolic acidosis has the following arterial blood values:

pH 7.1, pCO_2 20 mmHg.

If pK (H_2CO_3 - HCO_3)= 6.1, and $[H_2CO_3]$ = 0.03 X pCO_2, what is the bicarbonate concentration of the sample?

a. 0.6 mEq/L
b. 1.67 mEq/L
c. 6.0 mEq/L
d. 16.7 mEq/L

199. Fasting serum phosphate concentration is controlled primarily by the:

a. pancreas
b. skeleton
c. parathyroid glands
d. small intestine

200. Serum "anion gap" is increased in patients with:

a. renal tubular acidosis
b. diabetic alkalosis
c. metabolic acidosis due to diarrhea
d. lactic acidosis

201. Serum iron concentration is increased in:

1. hemolytic anemia
2. lead poisoning
3. massive lobular necrosis of the liver
4. nephrosis

a. only 1, 2 and 3 are correct
b. only 1 and 3 are correct
c. only 2 and 4 are correct
d. only 4 is correct
e. all are correct

For question 202, refer to the following illustration:

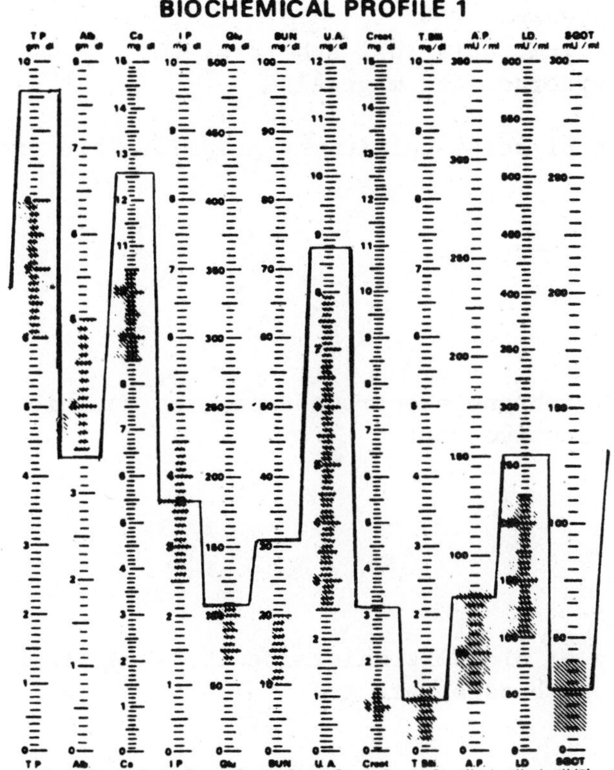

202. The results in the biochemical profile 1 are most consistent with:

a. primary hyperparathyroidism
b. multiple myeloma
c. dehydration
d. thiazide diuretic therapy

203. In establishing a normal range of values for serum iron, which of the following should be taken into consideration?

   a. All specimens should be obtained at approximately the same time of day.
   b. Procedures that employ a protein precipitation step may yield higher iron concentrations.
   c. Iron values are lower in women taking oral contraceptives.
   d. Late afternoon serum iron concentrations may be as much as 40% higher than morning serum iron concentrations in the same patient.

204. The anion gap is useful for quality control of laboratory results for:

   a. amino acids and proteins
   b. blood gas analyses
   c. sodium, potassium, chloride, and total CO_2
   d. calcium, phosphorus, and magnesium

205. Which percentage of total serum calcium is nondiffusible protein-bound?

   a. 80-90%
   b. 51-60%
   c. 40-50%
   d. 10-30%

206. A liquid ion-exchange membrane electrode using the antibiotic valinomycin is most selective for:

   a. sodium
   b. glucose
   c. chloride
   d. potassium

207. The buffering capacity of blood is maintained by a reversible exchange process between bicarbonate and:

   a. sodium
   b. potassium
   c. calcium
   d. chloride

208. Which of the following electrolytes is the chief plasma base whose main function is maintaining osmotic pressure?

a. chloride
b. calcium
c. potassium
d. sodium

209. A reciprocal relationship exists between:

a. sodium and potassium
b. calcium and phosphorus
c. chloride and CO_2
d. calcium and magnesium

210. Which of the following calcium procedures utilizes lanthanum chloride to eliminate interfering substances?

a. o-cresolphthalein complexone
b. precipitation with chloranilic acid
c. chelation with EDTA
d. atomic absorption spectrophotometry

211. At blood pH 7.40, what is the ratio between bicarbonate and carbonic acid?

a. 15:1
b. 20:1
c. 25:1
d. 30:1

212. The bicarbonate and carbonic acid ratio is calculated from an equation by:

a. Siggaard-Andersen
b. Bohr
c. Natelson
d. Henderson-Hasselbalch

213. Acidosis and alkalosis are best defined as fluctuations in blood pH and CO_2 content due to changes in:

a. Bohr's effect
b. O_2 content
c. bicarbonate buffer
d. carbonic anhydrase

214. A common cause of respiratory alkalosis is:

a. vomiting
b. starvation
c. asthma
d. hyperventilation

215. Metabolic acidosis is described as a(n):

a. increase in CO_2 content and pCO_2 with a decreased pH
b. decrease in CO_2 content with an increased pH
c. increase in CO_2 with an increased pH
d. decrease in CO_2 content and pCO_2 with a decreased pH

216. Respiratory acidosis is described as a(n):

a. increase in CO_2 content and pCO_2 with a decreased pH
b. decrease in CO_2 content with an increased pH
c. increase in CO_2 content with an increased pH
d. decrease in CO_2 content and pCO_2 with a decreased pH

217. Normally the bicarbonate concentration is about 24 mmol/L and the carbonic acid concentration is about 1.2; pK = 6.1, log 20 = 1.3. Using the equation $pH = pK + \log \frac{[salt]}{[acid]}$, calculate the pH.

a. 7.28
b. 7.38
c. 7.40
d. 7.42

218. The normal range for the pH of arterial blood measured at 37°C is:

a. 7.28–7.34
b. 7.33–7.37
c. 7.35–7.45
d. 7.45–7.50

219. Unless blood gas measurements are made immediately after sampling, *in vitro* glycolysis of the blood causes a:

a. rise in pH and pCO_2

b. fall in pH and a rise in pO_2

c. rise in pH and a fall in pO_2

d. fall in pH and a rise in pCO_2

220. Hydrogen ion concentration (pH) in blood is usually determined by means of which of the following electrodes?

a. silver
b. glass
c. platinum
d. platinum-lactate

221. A 68-year-old man arrives in the emergency room with a glucose level of 722 mg/dL and serum acetone of 4+ undiluted. An arterial blood gas from this patient is likely to indicate which of the following?

a. low pH
b. high pH
c. low pO_2
d. high pO_2

222. A hospitalized patient is experiencing increased neuromuscular irritability (tetany). Which of the following tests should be ordered immediately?

a. calcium
b. phosphorus
c. BUN
d. potassium

223. A blood gas was sent to the lab on ice, but there was no cap on the syringe. The blood had been exposed to room air for at least 30 minutes. The following change in blood gases occurred:

a. CO_2 content increased/ pCO_2 decreased

b. CO_2 content and pO_2 increased/ pH increased

c. CO_2 content and pCO_2 decreased/ pH decreased

d. pO_2 increased/ HCO_3 decreased

224. Decreased serum iron associated with increased total iron binding capacity (TIBC) is compatible with which of the following disease states?

a. anemia of chronic infection
b. iron deficiency anemia
c. chronic liver disease
d. nephrosis

225. Calculate the serum osmolality in mOsmol/kg H_2O, based on the following serum data:

Sodium	140 mmol/L
Potassium	4.0 mmol/L
Glucose	120 mg/dL
BUN	60 mg/dL

a. 234
b. 252
c. 289
d. 320

226. Serum and urine copper levels are run on a hospital patient with the following results:

Serum Cu	58 µg/dL
Urine Cu	83 µg/dL

This is most consistent with:

a. normal copper levels
b. Wilm's tumor
c. Wilson's disease
d. Addison's disease

227. The regulation of calcium and phosphorus metabolism is accomplished by the:

   a. thyroid
   b. parathyroid
   c. adrenal glands
   d. pituitary

228. An arterial blood specimen is submitted for blood gas analysis. The specimen was obtained at 8:30 a.m. but was not received in the laboratory until 11:00 a.m. The technologist should:

   a. perform the test immediately upon receipt
   b. perform the test only if the specimen was submitted in ice water
   c. request a venous blood specimen
   d. request a new arterial specimen be obtained

229. Specimens for blood gas determination should be drawn into a syringe containing:

   a. nothing
   b. heparin
   c. EDTA
   d. oxalate

230. A patient has the following test results:

   Increased serum calcium levels
   Decreased serum phosphorus levels
   Increased levels of parathyroid hormone

   This patient most likely has:

   a. hyperparathyroidism
   b. hypoparathyroidism
   c. nephrosis
   d. steatorrhea

231. The urinary excretion product measured as an indicator of epinephrine production is:

   a. dopamine
   b. dihydroxyphenylalanine (DOPA)
   c. homovanillic acid
   d. vanillylmandelic acid

232. The presence of formaldehyde and formic acid in the blood results in:

   a. increased serum activity of hepatic enzymes
   b. elevated serum concentrations of urea nitrogen and creatinine
   c. low serum concentrations of total CO_2
   d. low serum activity of pseudocholinesterase

233. The T-3 resin uptake test is a measure of:

   a. circulating T-3
   b. bound T-3
   c. binding capacity of thyroxine-binding globulin
   d. total thyroxine-binding globulin

234. During an evaluation of adrenal function, a patient had plasma cortisol determinations in the morning after awakening and in the evening. Laboratory results indicated that the morning value was higher than the evening concentration. This is indicative of:

   a. a normal finding
   b. Cushing's syndrome
   c. Addison's disease
   d. hypopituitarism

235. Absorption of vitamin B_{12} requires the presence of:

   a. intrinsic factor
   b. gastrin
   c. secretin
   d. folic acid

236. The Porter-Silber reaction measures:

   a. androgen steroids
   b. 17-ketosteroids
   c. 17-hydroxysteroids
   d. cortisol specifically

237. Each of the following is a tropic hormone <u>EXCEPT</u>:

   a. thyroid-stimulating hormone (TSH)
   b. follicle-stimulating hormone (FSH)
   c. luteinizing hormone (LH)
   d. growth hormone (GH)

238. Which of the following steroids is an adrenal cortical hormone?

a. angiotensinogen
b. corticosterone
c. progesterone
d. pregnanetriol

239. The pH that is most suitable for storing urine for porphyrin analysis is:

a. 2
b. 5
c. 7
d. 9

240. The method of choice for diagnosis of a protracted attack of porphyria is:

a. screening a fresh morning urine for porphobilinogen
b. analysis of delta-aminolevulinic acid in a morning urine
c. screening a fresh morning urine for porphyrin
d. ion-exchange analysis of porphobilinogen in a fresh morning urine

241. The screening test for urine porphyrin becomes positive at concentrations of:

a. 1 µmol/L
b. 10 µmol/L
c. 30 µmol/L
d. 50 µmol/L

242. When clinical response does not agree with total drug concentration, free drug levels may be of clinical use in all of the following cases EXCEPT:

a. uremia
b. hypoalbuminemia
c. ingestion of other drugs
d. patient noncompliance

243. Screening of freshly voided urine for porphobilinogen is done when which of the following is suspected?

a. lead poisoning
b. acute porphyric attack
c. erythrocytic protoporphyria
d. carrier state of acute intermittent porphyria

244. Fecal porphyrin analysis by talc thin-layer chromatography will reveal:

a. hereditary coproporphyria
b. carrier state of acute intermittent porphyria
c. erythrocytic protoporphyria
d. acute porphyric attack

245. Quantitative analysis of urine for delta-aminolevulinic acid is associated with:

a. lead poisoning
b. hereditary coproporphyria
c. carrier state of acute intermittent porphyria
d. erythrocytic protoporphyria

246. Analysis of erythrocytes for uroporphyrinogen synthetase detects:

a. acute porphyric attack
b. lead poisoning
c. hereditary coproporphyria
d. carrier state of acute intermittent porphyria

247. Pharmacologically active drugs are:

a. always nonlinear in their level-dose relationship
b. always linear in their level-dose relationship
c. protein bound
d. not protein bound

248. A fresh urine sample is received for analysis for "porphyrins" or "porphyria" without further information or specifications. Initial analysis should include:

a. porphyrin screen and quantitative total porphyrin
b. quantitative total porphyrin and porphobilinogen screen
c. porphyrin and porphobilinogen screen
d. porphobilinogen screen and ion-exchange analysis for porphobilinogen

249. A test request slip indicates that an acute porphyric attack is suspected clinically. Analysis should include:

a. quantitative delta-aminolevulinic acid
b. porphyrin screen
c. quantitative 24-hour porphobilinogen
d. porphobilinogen screen

250. Testing for the diagnosis of lead poisoning should include:

a. ion-exchange analysis of urine for porphobilinogen
b. analysis of morning urine for delta-aminolevulinic acid
c. analysis of feces for porphyrin
d. ion-exchange analysis of feces for protoporphyrin

251. A urine screening test for porphobilinogen is positive. Likely disease states include:

a. lead poisoning
b. porphyria cutanea tarda
c. acute porphyric attack
d. erythrocytic protoporphyria

252. Detection of carriers of hereditary coproporphyria should include analysis of:

a. 24-hour urine for porphobilinogen
b. fresh morning urine for delta-aminolevulinic acid
c. erythrocyte protoporphyrin
d. 24-hour urine for porphyrin

253. Screening tests for porphyrin in feces may be of value in diagnosing:

1. porphyria cutanea tarda
2. variegate porphyria
3. erythropoietic protoporphyria
4. lead poisoning

a. only 1, 2 and 3 are correct
b. only 1 and 3 are correct
c. only 2 and 4 are correct
d. only 4 is correct
e. all are correct

254. Conditions in which erythrocyte protoporphyrin is increased include:

a. acute intermittent porphyria
b. iron deficiency anemia
c. porphyria cutanea tarda
d. acute porphyric attack

255. The main reason for suboptimal drug levels in therapeutic drug monitoring is:

a. renal failure
b. liver failure
c. improper dosage prescribed
d. patient noncompliance with dosage regimen

256. Currently, the most common method for specific identification and quantitation of serum barbiturates is:

a. immunoassay
b. thin-layer chromatography (TLC)
c. gas-liquid chromatography (GLC)
d. ultraviolet absorption spectroscopy

257. Gas-liquid chromatography is the current method of choice for qualitative and quantitative analysis of:

a. benzodiazepines
b. barbiturates
c. antibiotics
d. drugs of abuse

258. Phenobarbital is toxic above the level of:

a. 30 mg/L
b. 40 mg/L
c. 60 mg/L
d. 80 mg/L

259. The normal range for methanol is:

a. 0
b. 2-4 mg/dL
c. 5-9 mg/dL
d. greater than 10 mg/dL

260. Acidification of the urine specimen (to pH 2) is essential during 24-hour collection for which one of the following compounds?

a. ketosteroids
b. hydroxycorticosteroids
c. catecholamines
d. calcium

261. Most drugs and intracellular metabolites measured by radioimmunoassay have molecular weights between 200 and 1,000 and can be made immunogenic by:

   a. attaching them to protein molecules
   b. frequent injections of the compound mixed with Freund's adjuvant
   c. sensitizing the animal with another antigen first before injection
   d. treating the animals with glucocorticoids before injection

262. The Porter-Silber method for determining urinary 17-hydroxycorticosteroids (phenylhydrazine in alcohol and sulfuric acid) involves which part of the steroid molecule?

   a. ketone group
   b. hydroxyl group
   c. dihydroxyacetone side chain
   d. steroid ring

263. Which family of steroid hormones is characterized by an unsaturated A ring?

   a. progestins
   b. estrogens
   c. androgens
   d. glucocorticoids

264. The concentration of serum carotene is affected MOST by which of the following?

   a. diet
   b. hepatic function
   c. time of drawing the specimen
   d. age

265. A patient with malabsorption receives 25 g of d-xylose orally. During the subsequent five-hour period, the urine excretion of d-xylose is less than 3 g. This would indicate:

   a. pancreatic malabsorption
   b. chronic pancreatitis
   c. intestinal malabsorption
   d. absence of disease

266. The most common type of congenital adrenal hyperplasia associated with increased plasma concentrations of 17 α-hydroxyprogesterone and increased urinary excretion of pregnanetriol is:

a. 17 α-hydroxylase deficiency
b. 11 β-hydroxylase deficiency
c. 21-hydroxylase deficiency
d. 18-hydroxysteroid dehydrogenase deficiency

267. A patient has signs and symptoms suggestive of acromegaly. The diagnosis would be confirmed if the patient had which of the following?

a. an elevated serum phosphate concentration
b. a decreased serum growth hormone-releasing factor concentration
c. no decrease in serum growth hormone concentration 90 minutes after oral glucose administration
d. an increased serum somatostatin concentration

268. Oral administration of L-dopa in children provokes stimulation of:

a. insulin
b. growth hormone
c. estrogen
d. pituitary gonadotropin

269. In a normal individual, injection of thyrotropin-releasing hormone (TRH) causes an increase in blood concentrations of which of the following hormones?

a. growth hormone
b. prolactin
c. ACTH
d. insulin

270. The thyrotropin-releasing hormone stimulation test rules out the diagnosis of mild or subclinical hyperthyroidism if TRH infusion causes:

a. a rise in plasma TSH
b. no rise in plasma TSH
c. a rise in plasma growth hormone concentration
d. no rise in plasma growth hormone concentration

271. A 33-year-old patient who developed diabetes as a child complains of heat intolerance. Triiodothyronine (T-3) resin uptake and thyroxine (T-4) concentrations are within normal limits. The 24-hour ^{131}I uptake is 34% (normal is 10-30%). Which of the following statements about this patient is true?

a. The patient is hyperthyroid.
b. The patient has iodine deficiency rather than thyrotoxicosis.
c. The possibility of T-3 toxicosis exists in this patient.
d. The patient is hypothyroid.

272. The test for adrenal cortical hyperfunction that has the greatest diagnostic sensitivity is measurement of:

a. urinary-free cortisol
b. plasma cortisol
c. urinary 17-hydroxycorticosteroids
d. plasma corticosterone

273. The definitive diagnosis of primary adrenal insufficiency requires demonstration of:

a. decreased urinary 17-keto- and 17-hydroxysteroids
b. decreased cortisol production
c. impaired response to ACTH stimulation
d. increased urinary cortisol excretion after metyrapone

274. Urinary estrogen in pregnant women consists chiefly of:

a. estradiol
b. estriol
c. estrone
d. pregnanediol

275. Serum concentrations of vitamin B_{12} are elevated in:

a. pernicious anemia in relapse
b. patients on chronic hemodialysis
c. chronic granulocytic leukemia
d. Hodgkin's disease

276. A gamma scintillation counter with a sodium iodide crystal would be suitable for counting each of the following EXCEPT:

a. ^{57}Co
b. ^{14}C
c. ^{24}Na
d. ^{59}Fe

277. Patients with Cushing's syndrome exhibit:

a. decreased plasma 17-hydroxysteroid concentration
b. decreased urinary 17-hydroxysteroid excretion
c. serum cortisol concentrations greater than 15 mg/dL
d. decreased cortisol secretory rate

278. Which of the following might contribute to signs and symptoms of digoxin toxicity in a patient with a serum digoxin concentration of 1.9 ng/mL (therapeutic range, 0.5-2.0 ng/mL)?

1. serum potassium 1.2 mEq/L
2. serum calcium 16.9 mEq/L
3. serum thyroxine 0.6 μg/dL
4. plasma quinidine 5 μg/dL

a. only 1, 2 and 3 are correct
b. only 1 and 3 are correct
c. only 2 and 4 are correct
d. only 4 is correct
e. all are correct

279. Characteristics of malabsorption syndrome due to pancreatic insufficiency include:

a. fecal fat excretion greater than 10 g/day
b. urinary excretion of 2.0 g of d-xylose within five hours after the patient has received 24 g orally
c. marked changes of secretion into the duodenum following injection of secretin
d. normal or elevated serum carotene concentration

280. When taken by a euthyroid individual, oral contraceptives containing estrogens will have which of the following effects on the thyroid function studies?

a. increase total circulating T-4
b. increase T-3 resin uptake
c. decrease thyroxine-binding globulin
d. decrease circulating T-3

281. In the normal person, which of the following increases in the peripheral circulation during the "insulin tolerance test"?

a. growth hormone
b. luteinizing hormone
c. follicle-stimulating hormone
d. thyroid-stimulating hormone

282. Major actions of angiotensin II include:

a. increased pituitary secretion of renin
b. increased vasoconstriction
c. increased parathormone secretion by the parathyroid
d. decreased adrenal secretion of aldosterone

283. The color reagent for the determination of 17-ketosteroids by the Zimmerman reaction is:

a. dihydroxyacetone
b. phenylhydrazine
c. m-dinitrobenzene
d. m-dinitrophenol

284. In the uncontrolled diabetic patient, urine glucose may give false elevations in the colorimetric assay of:

a. androgens
b. estrogens
c. 17-hydroxycorticosteroids
d. estriol

285. Which one of the following statements about triiodothyronine (T-3) is NOT true?

a. It is thought to be the active thyroid hormone.
b. It may be elevated to a greater extent than (T-4) in hyperthyroidism.
c. It is not bound to serum proteins.
d. It is commonly decreased in patients with nonthyroidal illness.

286. Which one of the following statements about thyroid-stimulating hormone is true?

a. TSH is increased in primary and secondary hypothyroidism.
b. When TSH is increased, the total concentration of thyroid hormone-binding proteins increases.
c. TSH accelerates the thyroid gland to produce and secrete thyroid hormones.
d. TSH is produced by the thyroid gland.

287. Iron deficiency would be consistent with which pattern below? (N=normal, I=increased, D=decreased)

	Serum	Iron	TIBC	Saturation	Stores
a.	D	D,N	D		I,N
b.	I,N	D,N	I		I
c.	D	I	D		D
d.	I,N	D,N	I		I

288. The major fraction of organic iodine in the circulation is in the form of:

a. thyroglobulin
b. thyroxine
c. triiodothyronine
d. diiodotyrosine

289. Total T-4 by competitive protein binding or displacement is based on the specific binding properties of:

a. thyroxine-binding prealbumin
b. albumin
c. thyroxine-binding globulin
d. thyroid-stimulating hormone

290. Which of the following methods employs a highly specific antibody to thyroxine?

a. total T-4 by competitive protein binding
b. T-4 by radioimmunoassay (RIA)
c. T-4 by column
d. T-4 by equilibrium dialysis

291. The triiodothyronine uptake ratio is used in the estimation of:

a. T-3 by RIA
b. T-4 by column
c. T-4 by displacement analysis
d. free thyroxine

292. The secretin stimulation test is often used to diagnose which of the following conditions?

a. Hollander's syndrome
b. perforated peptic ulcer
c. Chiari's syndrome
d. pancreatic carcinoma

293. The parent substance in the biosynthesis of androgens and estrogens is:

    a. cortisol
    b. catecholamines
    c. progesterone
    d. cholesterol

294. The biologically most active, naturally occurring androgen is:

    a. androstenedione
    b. dehydroepiandrosterone
    c. epiandrosterone
    d. testosterone

295. Which of the following is a true statement about progesterone?

    a. It is produced by Leydig's cells of the adult testes and is responsible for genital development, beard growth, muscle development, and sexual drive.
    b. It is produced by the placenta during pregnancy; the highest concentration is seen at the time of conception and then steadily decreases to nondetectable levels at term.
    c. Plasma concentrations are lowest during the luteal phase of the menstrual cycle and highest during the follicular phase.
    d. It parallels the activity of the corpus luteum by rapidly increasing following ovulation and then abruptly falling to initial low concentrations prior to the onset of menstruation.

296. Androgen secretion by the testes is stimulated by:

    a. interstitial cell-stimulating hormone
    b. follicle-stimulating hormone
    c. testosterone
    d. gonadotropins

297. Which of the following is secreted by the placenta and used for the early detection of pregnancy?

    a. follicle-stimulating hormone
    b. human chorionic gonadotropin
    c. luteinizing hormone
    d. progesterone

298. Chronic fetal metabolic distress is demonstrated by:

a. decreased estrogen concentrations in maternal plasma and increased estriol concentrations in amniotic fluid
b. increased estradiol concentrations in maternal plasma with a corresponding increase of estriol in amniotic fluid
c. increased urinary estriol excretion and increased maternal serum estriol concentrations
d. decreased urinary estriol excretion and decreased maternal serum estriol concentrations

299. Blood specimens for digoxin assays should be obtained between six to eight hours after drug administration because:

a. adequate time for tissue distribution and equilibration with serum levels must be allowed
b. serum digoxin concentration will be falsely low prior to six hours
c. all of the digoxin is in the cellular fraction prior to six hours
d. digoxin protein-binding interactions are minimal prior to six hours

300. About 90% of phenytoin is excreted in the urine as:

a. phenobarbital
b. para-hydroxyphenyl hydantoin
c. primidone
d. procainamide

301. Bioavailability of a drug refers to the:

a. availability for therapeutic administration
b. availability of the protein-bound fraction of the drug
c. drug transformation
d. extent and rate at which the active drug reaches target tissues

302. Most drug assays should NOT be performed during the first two hours after oral administration because:

a. plasma concentration does not reflect tissue concentration
b. all the drug will be in free form
c. drug-metabolite interactions will occur
d. tissue concentration exceeds plasma concentration during absorption

303. The trade name for chlordiazepoxide is:

   a. Librium
   b. Valium
   c. Tegretol
   d. Luminal

304. The tricyclic antidepressants are:

   a. basic drugs
   b. neutral drugs
   c. acidic drugs
   d. structurally cycloparaffinic

305. Certain enzymes are activated to metabolize drugs as a result of another drug action. This is referred to as:

   a. substrate depletion
   b. enzyme depletion
   c. enzyme induction
   d. enzyme inhibition

306. Zinc protoporphyrin or free erythrocyte protoporphyrin measurements are useful to assess blood concentrations of:

   a. lead
   b. mercury
   c. arsenic
   d. beryllium

307. Gas chromatography with the nitrogen-sensitive detector is most sensitive for the analysis of:

   a. digoxin
   b. acetyl salicylic acid
   c. ethyl alcohol
   d. tricyclic antidepressants

308. The most widely employed screening technique for drug abuse is:

   a. high-performance liquid chromatography
   b. gas-liquid chromatography
   c. thin-layer chromatography
   d. UV spectrophotometry

309. Nortriptyline is a metabolite of:

a. amitriptyline
b. protriptyline
c. butriptyline
d. norbutriptyline

310. Cocaine is metabolized to:

a. carbamazepine
b. codeine
c. hydrocodone
d. benzoylecgonine

311. In acid solution, 5,5-disubstituted barbiturates exist in which state of ionization?

a. first ionized species
b. second ionized species
c. non-ionized
d. an equilibrium mixture of non-ionized and the first species

312. If a drug has a half-life of seven hours, how many doses given at seven-hour intervals does it usually take to achieve a steady state or plateau level?

a. one
b. three
c. five
d. eight

313. Both phenobarbital and phenylethylmalonimide (PEMA) are metabolites of:

a. primidone
b. phenytoin
c. amobarbital
d. secobarbital

314. Each of the following factors influences the serum calcium concentration <u>EXCEPT</u>:

a. vitamin D
b. calcitonin
c. proteins
d. tyrosine

315. Alcohol and drug screens were run on samples from a comatose patient in the emergency room: Methanol = negative, Ethanol = 450 mg/dL, Isopropanol = 29 mg/dL, Acetone = present, Gastric drug screen = + for caffeine, Serum drug screen = none detected. Considering these results, what is the <u>most likely</u> cause(s) for the coma?

1. too much ethanol
2. acetone metabolized to isopropanol
3. isopropanol ingestion
4. overdose of caffeine

a. only 1, 2 and 3 are correct
b. only 1 and 3 are correct
c. only 2 and 4 are correct
d. only 4 is correct
e. all are correct

316. Hyperthyroidism has been associated with each of the following <u>EXCEPT</u>:

a. increased T-4
b. increased T-3
c. decreased serum cholesterol
d. decreased serum calcium

317. Which of the following vitamins is <u>NOT</u> fat-soluble?

a. A
b. B complex
c. D
d. E

318. An obese 15-year-old girl with excessive facial hair presented for evaluation of possible hirsutism. To confirm this diagnosis, each of the following should be ruled out <u>EXCEPT</u>:

a. the adrenogenital syndrome
b. diabetes mellitus
c. heredity
d. ovarian tumors

319. Precursors in the synthesis of estrogen include each of the following <u>EXCEPT</u>:

a. acetate
b. cholesterol
c. cortisol
d. progesterone

320. Toxic effects of lead poisoning are manifested by each of the following <u>EXCEPT</u>:

   a. increased excretion of delta-aminolevulinic acid
   b. increased excretion of coproporphyrins
   c. increased excretion of porphyrins
   d. increased erythrocyte protoporphyrins

321. Beriberi is associated with deficiency of vitamin:

   a. A
   b. B_1
   c. C
   d. niacin

322. Night blindness is associated with deficiency of vitamin:

   a. niacin
   b. C
   c. B_1
   d. A

323. Scurvy is associated with deficiency of vitamin:

   a. A
   b. B_1
   c. C
   d. niacin

324. Pellagra is associated with deficiency of vitamin:

   a. A
   b. B_1
   c. C
   d. niacin

325. Rickets is associated with deficiency of vitamin:

   a. B_1
   b. C
   c. niacin
   d. D

326. The anticonvulsant used to control tonoclonic (grand mal) seizures is:

    a. digoxin
    b. acetaminophen
    c. lithium
    d. phenytoin

327. A drug that relaxes the smooth muscles of the bronchial passages is:

    a. acetaminophen
    b. lithium
    c. phenytoin
    d. theophylline

328. A cardiac glycoside that is used in the treatment of congenital heart failure and arrhythmias by increasing the force and velocity of myocardial contraction is:

    a. digoxin
    b. acetaminophen
    c. lithium
    d. phenytoin

329. A carbonate salt used to control manic-depressive disorders is:

    a. digoxin
    b. acetaminophen
    c. lithium
    d. phenytoin

330. An analgesic that alleviates pain without causing loss of consciousness is:

    a. digoxin
    b. acetaminophen
    c. lithium
    d. phenytoin

331. It is preferable to draw a blood sample for analysis at a standardized time during the day, usually early in the morning, because concentrations of some body constituents fluctuate during the day. Which of the following blood constituent(s) concentrations vary during the time of the day?

1. sodium, potassium, and chloride
2. hormones
3. enzymes
4. plasma protein

a. only 1, 2 and 3 are correct
b. only 1 and 3 are correct
c. only 2 and 4 are correct
d. only 4 is correct
e. all are correct

332. A psychiatric patient was experiencing severe depression, but responded to treatment with amitriptylene with no apparent side effects. A blood sample was sent to the laboratory for therapeutic monitoring. Which of the following drug levels would be MOST reflective of this patient's condition?

a. amitriptylene = 237 μg/L
b. amitriptylene = 104 μg/L
c. protriptylene = 76 μg/L
d. imipramine = 103 μg/L

333. In a flame photometer, the concentration of sodium is determined by measuring the light:

a. absorbed by the atoms
b. emitted by the atoms
c. transmitted by the atoms
d. absorbed by the sodium atoms and water vapor

334. In thin-layer chromatography, the R_f value for a compound is given by the:

a. ratio of distance moved by compound:distance moved by solvent
b. rate of movement of compound through the adsorbent
c. distance between the compound spot and solvent front
d. distance moved by compound from the origin

335. Absorbance (A) of a solution may be converted to percent transmittance (%T) using the formula:

a. 1 + log %T
b. 2 + log %T
c. 1 - log %T
d. 2 - log %T

336. In a spectrophotometer, light of a specific wavelength can be isolated from white light with a(n):

a. double beam
b. diffraction grating
c. aperture
d. slit

337. The osmolality of a urine or serum specimen is measured by a change in the:

a. vapor pressure
b. boiling point
c. midpoint
d. osmotic pressure

338. Instruments suitable for use in reading quantitative porphyrin analyses include:

a. UV spectrophotometer
b. colorimeter
c. nephelometer
d. filter photometer

339. In electrophoretic analysis, buffers:

a. stabilize electrolytes
b. maintain basic pH
c. act as a carrier for ions
d. produce an effect on protein configuration

340. The results from a densitometer tracing of a serum protein electrophoretic separation appear to be too low. Possible explanations include:

1. lack of agitation of the dye during staining
2. inadequate fixation of the strip prior to staining
3. washing of the strip to eliminate background
4. presence of detergents in the buffer

a. only 1, 2 and 3 are correct
b. only 1 and 3 are correct
c. only 2 and 4 are correct
d. only 4 is correct
e. all are correct

341. Which of the following statements is NOT true of vapor pressure osmometers:

a. The change in the resistance of the thermistors is measured.
b. The sample and a pure solvent each are placed on separate thermistors in a temperature-controlled chamber that is saturated with the solvent vapor.
c. The "water potential" is determined by a dew-point hygrometer.
d. The change in vapor pressure of the serum is directly proportional to the osmolality of the sample.

342. Which of the following applies to cryoscopic osmometry?

a. The temperature of the sample rises to the freezing point of the solution.
b. The temperature plateau for a solution is horizontal.
c. The freezing point of a sample is absolute.
d. The initial freezing of a sample produces an immediate solid state.

343. Which of the following is very sensitive to pH and ionic strength of eluting buffers?

a. chromatography
b. spectrophotometry
c. HPLC
d. colorimetry

344. The first step to be taken when attempting to repair a piece of electronic equipment is:

a. check all the electronic connections
b. reseat all the printed circuit boards
c. turn the instrument off
d. replace all the fuses

345. Which of the following does not detect volatiles such as alcohol?

a. vapor pressure osmometry
b. ideal osmolality values
c. cryoscopic osmometry
d. true vapor pressure osmometry

346. In which of the following techniques is the induced temperature change directly proportional to the osmolality:

a. vapor pressure osmometry
b. ideal osmolality value
c. cryoscopic osmometry
d. true vapor pressure osmometry

347. A temperature plateau is obtained by use of:

a. vapor pressure osmometry
b. ideal osmolality values
c. cryoscopic osmometry
d. true vapor pressure osmometry

348. Which of the following operates based on a principle of the evaporation of the solvent?

a. vapor pressure osmometry
b. ideal osmolality values
c. cryoscopic osmometry
d. true vapor pressure osmometry

349. The blood gas analyzer had been calibrating well all day. However, the last two patient blood gases had pH readings of 6.843 and 6.992. You immediately run a control--the pH is reading low and on the next calibration the pH has ???? on the printout. All other parameters of the calibration and control are acceptable. What is the MOST LIKELY cause of the problem?

a. protein on the pH electrode tip
b. low level of salt bridge solution
c. low level of rinse solution
d. patient syringe contained too much heparin

350. The osmolal gap is defined as measured Osm/kg minus the calculated Osm/kg. The average osmolal gap is near:

a. 0
b. 2
c. 4
d. 6

351. Light intensity in the crystal of a scintillation system is proportional to the:

a. amount of voltage applied to the photomultiplier tube
b. energy level of the gamma radiation
c. penetration strength of the β particle
d. geometry of the crystal

352. The function of lithium in the flame emission method for sodium analysis is to:

a. enhance dialysis
b. act as an internal standard
c. stabilize electrode potential
d. act as a quality control precision check

353. The usual radiation source in atomic absorption instruments is the:

a. xenon arc
b. deuterium lamp
c. tungsten lamp
d. hollow cathode lamp

354. To be analyzed by gas-liquid chromatography, a compound must:

a. be volatile or made volatile
b. not be volatile
c. be water-soluble
d. contain a nitrogen atom

355. The solute that contributes the most to the total serum osmolality is:

a. glucose
b. sodium
c. chloride
d. urea

356. Mass spectrometry:

a. does not require a pure sample for analysis
b. is a useful method for identifying and quantitating compounds with molecular weights less than 1,500
c. requires a large sample for analysis
d. permits the recovery of the material after it has been analyzed

357. In mass spectrometry, the "appearance potential" is defined as the:

a. minimum energy required to produce a molecular ion
b. maximum energy required to produce a molecular ion
c. minimum energy required for the appearance of a particular fragment ion in the mass spectrum
d. maximum energy required for the appearance of a particular fragment ion in the mass spectrum

358. A radioactive sample is decaying at an average rate of 250 cpm. How long must the sample be counted so that the standard deviation will be 1%?

a. 20 min
b. 40 min
c. 50 min
d. 60 min

359. In automated methods utilizing a bichromatic analyzer, dual wavelengths are employed to:

a. minimize the effect of interference (eg, from turbidity)
b. improve precision
c. facilitate dialysis
d. monitor temperature changes

360. The centrifugal fast analyzer:

a. employs the concept of sequential analysis
b. employs the concept of discrete sample analysis
c. is limited to kinetic analyses
d. is limited to endpoint analyses

361. Which of the following electrodes is based on the principle of amperometric measurement?

a. pCO_2 electrode
b. pO_2 electrode
c. pH electrode
d. ionized calcium electrode

362. Which of the following statements about fluorometry is true?

a. A compound is said to fluoresce when it absorbs light at one wavelength and emits light at a second wavelength.
b. Detectors in fluorometers are plated at 180° from the excitation source.
c. It is less sensitive than spectrophotometry.
d. It avoids the necessity for complexing of components because fluorescence is a native property.

363. A true statement about high-performance liquid chromatography is that it:

a. utilizes a flame ionization detector
b. requires derivation of non-volatile compounds
c. can be used to separate gases, liquids, or soluble solids
d. can be used for adsorption, partition, ion exchange, and gel permeation chromatography

364. In mass spectrometry:

1. most ion sources produce more positive ions than negative ions
2. both molecular and fragment ions are produced
3. organic compounds are identified by fragmentation patterns
4. fragmentation requires less energy than single ionization

a. only 1, 2 and 3 are correct
b. only 1 and 3 are correct
c. only 2 and 4 are correct
d. only 4 is correct
e. all are correct

365. True statements about centrifugal fast analyzers include:

1. Upon rotation, cuvettes pass sequentially through the light beam of the photometer.
2. Transmittance of each reaction mixture is referenced against a reagent blank.
3. Light passes through the cuvettes perpendicularly to the transfer disc.
4. Serum and reagents are placed in the outermost wells of the transfer disc.

a. only 1, 2 and 3 are correct
b. only 1 and 3 are correct
c. only 2 and 4 are correct
d. only 4 is correct
e. all are correct

366. The nanometer is used as a measure of:

a. absorbance
b. % transmittance
c. intensity of radiant energy
d. wavelength of radiant energy

367. In addition to its use as an internal standard in the flame emission method for sodium and potassium analyses, lithium:

a. minimizes interference
b. improves precision
c. increases flame temperature
d. acts as a radiation buffer

368. The three general types of interference in atomic absorption spectrophotometry:

a. are chemical, ionization, and matrix interference
b. only occur in organic solvents
c. can all be overcome by the addition of certain competing cations
d. significantly hinder method specificity

369. Reverse phase high-performance liquid chromatography is being increasingly utilized in therapeutic drug monitoring. The term "reverse phase" implies that the column eluent is:

a. pumped up the column
b. more polar than the stationary phase
c. always nonpolar
d. less polar than the stationary phase

370. In gas-liquid chromatography, actual separation of compounds occurs in the column by the:

a. inert phase
b. solid phase
c. liquid phase
d. mobile phase

371. Lithium therapy is widely used in the treatment of:

a. depression
b. hyperactivity
c. aggression
d. manic-depression

372. True statements about electrophoretic mobility include:

1. It is directly proportional to the net charge of the molecule.
2. It is inversely proportional to the size of the molecule.
3. It is inversely proportional to the viscosity of the buffer.
4. The rate of migration is independent of time.

a. only 1, 2 and 3 are correct
b. only 1 and 3 are correct
c. only 2 and 4 are correct
d. only 4 is correct
e. all are correct

373. True statements about electrophoresis include:

1. It can be conducted under varying voltage AND constant current.
2. Support media used include cellulose acetate and paper.
3. It can be conducted under constant voltage AND varying current.
4. Increasing distance between electrodes has no effect on the migration rate.

a. only 1, 2 and 3 are correct
b. only 1 and 3 are correct
c. only 2 and 4 are correct
d. only 4 is correct
e. all are correct

374. Spectrophotometers isolate a narrow band pass by means of:

a. filters and prisms
b. prisms and grating
c. barrier layer cells and filters
d. gratings and lanier layer cells

375. Photomultiplier tubes:

1. have extremely rapid response times
2. are very sensitive
3. do not show as much fatigue as other detectors
4. cannot be used in double-beam-in-time spectrophotometers

a. only 1, 2 and 3 are correct
b. only 1 and 3 are correct
c. only 2 and 4 are correct
d. only 4 is correct
e. all are correct

376. Wetting agents in flame photometry:

1. are frequently recommended for inclusion in standards and sample dilutions
2. minimize changes in atomizer flow rates due to differences in sample viscosity
3. provide more uniform flow rates
4. minimize fluctuations in gas pressure

a. only 1, 2 and 3 are correct
b. only 1 and 3 are correct
c. only 2 and 4 are correct
d. only 4 is correct
e. all are correct

377. The measurement of light scattered by particles in the sample is the principle of:

a. spectrophotometry
b. fluorometry
c. nephelometry
d. atomic absorption

378. The measurement of the amount of electricity passing between two electrodes in an electrochemical cell is the principle of:

a. electrophoresis
b. amperometry
c. nephelometry
d. coulometry

379. Thin-layer chromatography is of particular use in the identification of:

a. amino acids
b. drugs
c. inorganic ions
d. enzyme inhibitors

Chemistry Answer Key

1. d
2. e
3. d
4. b
5. b
6. e
7. a
8. d
9. a
10. c
11. b
12. d
13. c
14. b
15. d
16. b
17. a
18. c
19. a
20. c
21. b
22. a
23. a
24. d
25. d
26. a
27. d
28. d
29. c
30. a
31. d
32. c
33. a
34. a
35. a
36. d
37. d
38. a
39. c
40. a
41. d
42. b
43. a
44. c
45. d
46. c
47. b
48. d
49. c
50. d
51. d
52. d
53. b
54. a
55. e
56. b
57. c
58. d
59. b
60. c
61. c
62. d
63. b
64. c
65. b
66. a
67. a
68. a
69. b
70. c
71. b
72. d
73. c
74. b
75. a
76. b
77. a
78. d
79. e
80. a
81. a
82. d
83. d
84. c
85. d
86. d
87. b
88. c
89. a
90. d
91. c
92. b
93. c
94. c
95. c
96. c
97. b
98. d
99. d
100. d
101. d
102. a
103. c
104. d
105. c
106. b
107. b
108. d
109. c
110. d
111. b
112. c
113. a
114. a
115. d
116. b
117. a
118. a
119. c
120. a
121. c
122. c
123. d
124. e
125. d
126. b
127. c
128. c
129. b
130. b
131. c
132. c
133. a
134. b
135. a
136. b
137. d
138. a
139. d
140. d
141. b
142. a
143. c
144. a
145. a
146. d
147. b
148. c
149. a
150. c
151. b
152. c
153. a
154. a
155. a
156. a
157. c
158. a
159. d
160. b
161. c
162. d
163. a
164. d
165. c
166. d
167. a
168. c
169. a
170. a
171. d
172. a
173. a
174. b
175. c
176. b
177. b
178. a
179. c
180. c
181. b
182. b
183. d
184. e
185. c
186. b
187. b
188. d

Chemistry Answer Key (continued)

189. d
190. c
191. b
192. d
193. c
194. b
195. d
196. d
197. a
198. c
199. c
200. d
201. a
202. b
203. a
204. c
205. c
206. d
207. d
208. d
209. b
210. d
211. b
212. d
213. c
214. d
215. d
216. a
217. c
218. c
219. d
220. b
221. a
222. a
223. d
224. b
225. c
226. c
227. b
228. d
229. b
230. a
231. d
232. c
233. c
234. a
235. a
236. c
237. d
238. b
239. c
240. d
241. a
242. d
243. b
244. a
245. a
246. d
247. c
248. c
249. d
250. b
251. c
252. b
253. a
254. b
255. d
256. c
257. b
258. c
259. a
260. c
261. a
262. c
263. b
264. a
265. c
266. c
267. c
268. b
269. b
270. a
271. c
272. a
273. c
274. b
275. c
276. b
277. c
278. a
279. a
280. a
281. a
282. b
283. c
284. c
285. c
286. c
287. c
288. b
289. c
290. b
291. d
292. d
293. d
294. d
295. d
296. a
297. b
298. d
299. a
300. b
301. d
302. a
303. a
304. a
305. c
306. a
307. d
308. c
309. a
310. d
311. c
312. c
313. a
314. d
315. a
316. d
317. b
318. b
319. c
320. c
321. b
322. d
323. c
324. d
325. d
326. d
327. d
328. a
329. c
330. b
331. c
332. b
333. b
334. a
335. d
336. b
337. a
338. a
339. c
340. e
341. d
342. a
343. a
344. c
345. a
346. a
347. c
348. d
349. a
350. a
351. b
352. b
353. d
354. a
355. b
356. b
357. c
358. b
359. a
360. b
361. b
362. a
363. d
364. a
365. a
366. d
367. d
368. a
369. b
370. c
371. d
372. a

Chemistry Answer Key (continued)

373. a
374. b
375. a
376. a
377. c
378. d
379. b

CHAPTER 13

Blood Bank

1. Which one of the following immunizations would be cause for donor deferment for four weeks?

   a. rubeola
   b. yellow fever
   c. mumps
   d. rubella

2. Following plasmapheresis, how long must a person wait before being eligible to donate a unit of whole blood?

   a. eight weeks
   b. two weeks
   c. 48 hours
   d. 24 hours

3. Tetany in donors is usually due to:

   a. blood loss
   b. hyperventilation
   c. hypoventilation
   d. fall in blood pressure

4. Addition of which one of the following will enhance the shelf life of blood?

   a. heparin
   b. adenine
   c. hydroxyethyl starch
   d. lactated Ringer's solution

5. Pretransfusion compatibility testing must include:

   a. absolute patient identification
   b. syphilis serology on recipient
   c. minor crossmatch
   d. hepatitis testing on recipient

6. Severe intravascular hemolysis is most likely caused by antibodies of which blood group system?

   a. ABO
   b. Rh
   c. Kell
   d. Duffy

7. Under extreme emergency conditions, when there is no time to determine ABO group for transfusion, the technologist should:

   a. refuse to release any blood until the patient's sample has been typed

   b. release O Rh_o-negative whole blood

   c. release O Rh_o-negative red blood cells

   d. release O Rh_o-positive red blood cells

8. An obstetrical patient has had three previous pregnancies. Her first baby was healthy, the second was jaundiced at birth and required an exchange transfusion, while the third was stillborn. Which of the following is the most likely cause?

   a. ABO incompatibility
   b. immune deficiency disease
   c. congenital spherocytic anemia
   d. Rh incompatibility

9. Which of the following medications is most likely to cause production of antibodies having Rh specificity?

   a. penicillin
   b. Keflin
   c. Aldomet
   d. tetracycline

10. With regard to inheritance, most blood group systems are:

    a. sex-linked dominant
    b. sex-linked recessive
    c. autosomal recessive
    d. autosomal codominant

11. Leukocyte-poor red blood cells, prepared by the washing technique, are indicated for patients with:

    a. febrile transfusion reaction
    b. iron deficiency anemia
    c. hemophilia A
    d. von Willebrand's disease

12. The optimum storage temperature for frozen red cells is:

    a. 4°C
    b. -12°C
    c. -20°C
    d. -80°C

13. The optimum storage temperature for whole blood is:

    a. 4°C
    b. -12°C
    c. -20°C
    d. -80°C

14. Quality control tests must be performed daily on:

    a. reagent RBCs
    b. oral thermometers
    c. banked whole blood
    d. centrifuge timers

15. A patient has become refractory to platelet transfusion. Which of the following is the probable cause?

    a. transfusion of Rh_o-incompatible platelets
    b. decreased pH of the platelet concentrates
    c. development of an alloantibody with anti-D specificity
    d. development of platelet antibodies

16. Which of the following constitutes permanent rejection status of a donor?

    a. A tattoo five months previously.
    b. Close contact with a patient with viral hepatitis.
    c. Two units of blood transfused four months previously.
    d. Confirmed positive test for HB_sAg ten years previously.

17. Which of the following is a cause for temporary deferment of a blood donor?

    a. Aspirin ingestion 12 hours previously.
    b. Antibiotics taken four weeks previously.
    c. Oral polio vaccine four weeks previously.
    d. Rubella injection one week previously.

18. A way in which a weak subgroup of A in a recipient may manifest itself includes:

    a. positive autocontrol
    b. heavy rouleaux in the serum
    c. positive antibody screening test
    d. discrepancy between cell and serum ABO grouping

19. The major crossmatch will detect a(n):

    a. group A patient mistyped as group O
    b. irregular antibody in the donor unit
    c. Rh_o-negative donor unit mislabeled as Rh_o-positive
    d. recipient antibody directed against antigens on the donor red cells

20. Cells of the A_3 subgroup:

    a. will react with <u>Dolichos</u> <u>biflorus</u>
    b. will not be agglutinated by anti-A
    c. will give a mixed-field reaction with anti-A,B
    d. will not be agglutinated by anti-H

21. Transfusion of Ch(a+) blood to a patient with anti-Ch^a has been reported to cause:

    a. no clinically significant red cell destruction
    b. clinically significant immune red cell destruction
    c. decreased ^{51}Cr red cell survivals
    d. febrile transfusion reactions

22. Which of the following occurs to the patient's antibody in an in vitro neutralization study when a soluble antigen preparation is added?

    a. inhibition
    b. dilution
    c. complement fixation
    d. hemolysis

23. Anti-Fy^a is:

    a. usually a cold-reactive agglutinin
    b. more reactive when tested with enzyme-treated RBCs
    c. capable of causing hemolytic transfusion reactions
    d. an autoagglutinin

24. Which one of the following is NOT an indicator of polyagglutination?

    a. positive minor crossmatch
    b. positive reactions with certain lectins
    c. decreased bilirubin
    d. agglutination with normal adult ABO compatible sera

25. Anti-Sd^a is strongly suspected if:

    a. the patient has been previously transfused
    b. the agglutinates are mixed-field and refractile
    c. the patient is group A or B
    d. panel results show varying strengths of reactions

26. Mixed-field agglutination at the antihuman globulin phase of a crossmatch may be attributed to:

    a. recently transfused cells
    b. intrauterine exchange transfusion
    c. an antibody such as anti-Sd^a
    d. fetal maternal hemorrhage

27. In suspected hemolytic disease of the newborn cases, what significant information can be obtained from a blood smear?

    a. Estimation of WBC and platelets.
    b. Shift to the left.
    c. A differential to estimate the absolute number of lymphocytes present.
    d. Determination of the presence of spherocytes and elevated numbers of nucleated RBCs.

28. A panel of tests composed of HB_sAg, HAVAb-IgM, and HB_cAb is designed to:

   a. indicate immunity to hepatitis
   b. estimate the degree of inactivity
   c. aid in the diagnosis of past hepatitis infection
   d. aid in the diagnosis of acute viral hepatitis

29. One of the most useful techniques in the identification and classification of high-titer, low-avidity (HTLA) antibodies is:

   a. reagent red cell panels
   b. adsorption and elution
   c. titration and inhibition
   d. cold autoadsorption

30. As a preventive measure against graft-versus-host disease, blood components prepared for infants who have received intrauterine transfusions should be:

   a. saline-washed
   b. irradiated
   c. frozen and deglycerolized
   d. group- and Rh-compatible with the mother

31. Which of the following is used for the initial compatibility testing in exchange transfusion therapy?

   a. maternal serum
   b. eluate prepared from infant's RBCs
   c. paternal serum
   d. infant's postexchange serum

32. In addition to removing the infant's rapidly destroyed, sensitized red blood cells, the therapeutic advantages provided by an exchange transfusion include:

1. providing compatible RBCs that will not be subjected to a shortened in vivo survival
2. improving tissue oxygenation
3. removing plasma bilirubin
4. correcting anemia in the affected infant

a. only 1, 2 and 3 are correct
b. only 1 and 3 are correct
c. only 2 and 4 are correct
d. only 4 is correct
e. all are correct

33. Which of the following measures should be employed if a donor experiences perioral paresthesia during an apheresis procedure?

a. increase flow rate
b. reduce flow rate
c. elevate donor's feet
d. have donor breathe into a paper bag

34. When the main objective of the exchange transfusion is to remove the infant's antibody-sensitized red blood cells and to control hyperbilirubinemia, the blood product of choice is(are):

1. fresh whole blood
2. washed, packed RBCs
3. frozen, deglycerolized RBCs reconstituted with fresh frozen plasma compatible with the infant's RBCs
4. heparinized blood

a. only 1, 2 and 3 are correct
b. only 1 and 3 are correct
c. only 2 and 4 are correct
d. only 4 is correct
e. all are correct

35. According to AABB Standards, platelet concentrates prepared by plateletpheresis must contain:

    a. 5.5×10^{10} platelets in 75% of units tested

    b. 5.5×10^{10} platelets in all units

    c. 3×10^{11} platelets in 75% of units tested

    d. 3×10^{11} platelets in all units

36. The enzyme responsible for conferring H activity on the red cell membrane is alpha-:

    a. galactosyl transferase
    b. N-acetylgalactosaminyl transferase
    c. L-fucosyl transferase
    d. glucosyl transferase

37. What percent of group O blood would be compatible with a serum sample that contained anti-X and anti-Y if X antigen is present on red cells of 5 out of 20 donors, and Y antigen is present on red cells of 1 out of 10 donors?

    a. 2.5
    b. 6.8
    c. 25.0
    d. 68.0

38. The following results were obtained when testing a sample from a 20-year-old, first-time blood donor. What is the most likely cause of this ABO discrepancy?

Forward Group		Reverse Group	
Anti-A	Anti-B	A_1 Cells	B Cells
neg	neg	neg	3+

    a. loss of antigen due to disease
    b. acquired B
    c. phenotype O_h "Bombay"
    d. weak subgroup of A

39. A patient is group O, Rh_o(D)-negative with anti-D and anti-K in her serum. What percentage of the general Caucasian donor population would be compatible with this patient?

   a. 0.5
   b. 2.0
   c. 3.0
   d. 6.0

40. Which of the following phenotypes will react with anti-f?

   a. rr
   b. R_1R_1
   c. R_2R_2
   d. R_1R_2

41. Red cells with which of the following genotypic structures have the least amount of LW antigen?

   a. CDe/CDe
   b. Cde/cDE
   c. cDE/cde
   d. cde/cde

42. Glycophorin B is associated with which one of the following blood groups' antigenic activity?

   a. MN
   b. Ss
   c. Wr^aWr^b
   d. Lu^a/Lu^b

43. Which of the following observations suggests that a patient's blood is the McLeod phenotype?

   a. K^-k^+
   b. K^-k^-
   c. K^-k^{+w}
   d. $K^{+w}k^+$

44. In a prenatal workup, the following results were obtained:

Forward Group				Reverse Group	
Anti-A	Anti-B	Anti-D	Rh Control	A_1 Cells	B Cells
4+	2+	4+	neg	neg	3+

DAT: negative
Antibody screen: negative

The ABO discrepancy was thought to be due to an antibody directed against acriflavin. Which of the following tests would resolve this discrepancy?

a. anti-A,B
b. additional anti-B reagents; anti-B from group A donors
c. anti-A,B and extend incubation of the reverse group
d. repeat reverse group

Questions 45 and 46 refer to the following laboratory results:

Forward Group			Reverse Group		
Anti-A	Anti-B	Anti-A_1	A_1 Cells	A_2 Cells	B Cells
4+	neg	4+	neg	2+	4+

45. The ABO discrepancy seen above is most likely due to:

a. anti-A_1
b. rouleaux
c. anti-H
d. unexpected IgG antibody present

46. Which of the following antibody screen results would you expect with the ABO discrepancy seen above?

a. negative
b. positive with all screen cells at the 37°C phase
c. positive with all screen cells at the RT phase
d. positive with all screen cells and the autologous cells at the RT phase

47. The following lectin reactions were obtained on a patient's red blood cells:

Patient's cells vs:

Arachis hypogaea	+
Salvia sclarea	-
Salvia horminum	-
Glycine soja	+
Dolichos biflorus	-

The patient's cells are most likely polyagglutinable due to exposure of which antigen?

a. T
b. Tk
c. Tn
d. Cad

48. Serologic testing on a patient with no history of transfusion revealed the following results:

Direct antiglobulin testing	3+
Indirect antiglobulin testing	0

Antibody identification performed on an ether eluate and the serum showed no reactivity when tested at the AHG phase.

Which one of the following medications is most likely responsible for these observations?

a. aldomet
b. aspirin
c. insulin
d. keflex

49. Detection of anti-D in a postpartum specimen from an Rh_o-negative woman would indicate:

a. she is a candidate for Rh immune globulin
b. she is NOT a candidate for Rh immune globulin
c. a need for further investigation to determine candidacy for Rh immune globulin
d. the presence of Rh_o-positive cells in her circulation

50. In the process of identifying an antibody, the technologist observed 2+ reactions with three of the ten cells in a panel after the immediate spin phase. These reactions disappeared following incubation at 37°C and after the antihuman globulin phase of testing. The antibody most likely responsible is:

a. anti-P_1

b. anti-Le^a

c. anti-C

d. anti-Fy^a

51. The phenomenon of an Rh_o-positive person whose serum contains anti-D with a negative autocontrol is best explained by antigen:

a. deletion
b. mosaic
c. suppression
d. none of the above

52. Mixed-field agglutination is a characteristic observation for which of the following antibodies?

a. anti-K

b. anti-Sd^a

c. anti-Js^a

d. anti-e

For questions 53 to 55, refer to the following information and panel:

A 25-year-old Caucasian woman, gravida 3, para 2, required two units of blood. The antibody screen was positive and the results of the antibody panel are shown below.

Blood Group System		Rh-Hr							Kell		Duffy		Kidd		Lewis		P	MNS				Serum Reactions		
Vial No.	Rh-Hr Code	C	D	E	c	e	C^w	V	K	k	Fy^a	Fy^b	Jk^a	Jk^b	Le^a	Le^b	P_1	M	N	S	s	IS	37C	AHG
1.	r'r	+	0	0	+	+	0	0	0	+	0	+	0	+	0	+	0	+	0	0	+	0	0	1+
2.	$R_1R_1^w$	+	+	0	0	+	+	0	0	+	+	0	+	+	+	0	+	0	+	0	+	0	0	0
3.	R_1R_1	+	+	0	0	+	0	0	0	+	+	+	0	+	0	+	0	+	+	+	0	0	0	0
4.	R_2R_2	0	+	+	+	0	0	0	0	+	0	+	+	+	0	+	+	+	+	+	0	0	0	1+
5.	r"r	0	0	+	+	+	0	0	+	+	+	+	+	0	0	+	$+^w$	0	+	0	+	0	0	1+
6.	rr V	0	0	0	+	+	0	+	0	+	0	+	+	0	0	+	$+^w$	+	0	+	+	0	0	1+
7.	rr K	0	0	0	+	+	0	0	+	0	0	+	+	+	+	0	+	+	+	0	+	0	0	1+
8.	rr Js^a	0	0	0	+	+	0	0	0	+	0	0	+	+	0	0	+	+	+	0	+	0	0	1+
9.	rr	0	0	0	+	+	0	0	0	+	0	+	+	+	+	0	0	+	0	+	0	0	0	1+
10.	rr	0	0	0	+	+	0	0	0	+	+	+	+	+	+	0	+	+	0	+	+	0	0	1+
																		Autocontrol				0	0	0

53. Which of the following antibodies would be the cause of the positive antibody screen?

    a. anti-M and anti-K
    b. anti-c and anti-E
    c. anti-s and anti-c
    d. anti-Fy^b and anti-c

54. What is the most probable genotype of this patient?

    a. rr
    b. $R_o r$
    c. r'r'
    d. R_1R_1

55. Which common antibody has **NOT** been ruled out by the panel?

    a. anti-S
    b. anti-Le^a
    c. anti-Jk^a
    d. anti-K

56. Antibody identification performed on the serum of a previously transfused patient revealed two weakly positive AHG reactions when tested against 12 group O reagent red cells. Four of five type-specific donor units were negative in all phases of testing, as was the autocontrol. Which of the following antibodies could be responsible for the observed reactions?

   a. anti-Bg^a

   b. anti-JMH

   c. anti-Gy^a

   d. anti-Rg^a

57. A patient's serum results revealed weakly positive reactions ($1+^w$) in 16 of 16 group O panel cells; however, no reaction was noted in the autocontrol. Further serum testing with ficin-treated panel cells demonstrated no reactivity at the AHG phase. Which one of the following antibodies is most likely responsible for these results?

   a. anti-Ch^a
   b. anti-k
   c. anti-e
   d. anti-Js^a

58. Use of EDTA plasma prevents activation of the classical complement pathway by:

   a. causing rapid decay of complement components
   b. chelating Mg ions, which prevents the assembly of C6
   c. chelating Ca ions, which prevents assembly of C1
   d. preventing chemotaxis

59. Hemolysis of the red cell occurs when which components of complement are attached?

   a. C1
   b. C3
   c. C4-C2
   d. C8-C9

60. The observed phenotypic frequencies at the Jk locus in a particular population are:

Phenotype	Number of persons
Jk(a+b-)	122
Jk(a+b+)	194
Jk(a-b+)	84

What is the gene frequency of the Jk^a in this population?

a. 0.31
b. 0.45
c. 0.55
d. 0.60

61. How many whites in a population of 100,000 will have the following combination of phenotypes?

System	Phenotype	Phenotype Frequency (%)
ABO	O	45
Gm	Fb	48
PGM_1	2-1	37
EsD	2-1	18

a. 1
b. 14
c. 144
d. 1,438

62. In a random population, 16% of the people are Rh_o-negative (rr). What percentage of the Rh_o-positive population would be heterozygous for the Rh_o(D) antigen (Rr)?

a. 36
b. 48
c. 57
d. 66

63. After injection of RhIG, a patient's serum titer against Rh_o-positive red cells was 16. Approximately how many days would it take for the titer to become 4?

a. 5
b. 10
c. 23
d. 46

64. A 65-year-old woman with adenocarcinoma of the breast and metastases to the bone marrow, liver, and lung experienced shaking, chills, and a fever of 103°F approximately 40 minutes following the transfusion of a second unit of packed red cells. She developed a cough, shortness of breath, and nailbed cyanosis. The central venous pressure was normal; radiograph revealed bilateral perihilar and basilar infiltrates without cardiac enlargement or pulmonary vascular engorgement.

The most likely explanation for the patient's symptoms is:

a. transfusion contaminated with bacteria
b. congestive heart failure due to fluid overload
c. anaphylactic transfusion reaction
d. severe febrile transfusion reaction

65. Which of the following is the first step in hemoglobin clearance from the plasma, following an intravascular hemolytic transfusion reaction?

a. reduction in plasma haptoglobin concentration
b. increase in plasma hemoglobin
c. urinary excretion of hemosiderin
d. urinary excretion of hemoglobin

66. In testing amniotic fluid, the Liley method of predicting the severity of hemolytic disease of the newborn is based on the:

a. bilirubin concentration by standard methods
b. optical density measured at 450 nm
c. Rh_o determination
d. ratio of lecithin to sphingomyelin

67. Which of the following is <u>NOT</u> a cause for rejection of a potential blood donor?

   a. hip replacement five months previous
   b. spontaneous abortion three months previous; fetus at two months gestation
   c. resides with a known hepatitis patient
   d. received a blood transfusion 22 weeks previous

68. Each of the following genotypes is possible for an individual whose red cells react as indicated below <u>EXCEPT</u>:

Antisera	Reactions
Anti-C	+
Anti-D	+
Anti-E	+
Anti-c	+
Anti-e	+

   a. R_1R_2

   b. R_1r''

   c. R_zr

   d. R_or'

69. Inhibition testing can be used to confirm antibody specificity for each of the following antibodies <u>EXCEPT</u>:

   a. anti-Sd^a
   b. anti-I
   c. anti-K
   d. anti-P_1

70. A patient was crossmatched with nine units of blood; one unit was incompatible. She had a negative antibody screening test. If all of the pretransfusion tests were valid, which of the following explanations is <u>NOT</u> a plausible cause for the incompatibility?

   a. She had an antibody directed against a low frequency antigen.
   b. Her serum contained anti-Bg^a.
   c. The unit had a positive direct antiglobulin test.
   d. Her serum contained anti-Le^a.

71. Coughing, cyanosis, and difficulty breathing are symptoms of which of the following transfusion reactions?

    a. febrile
    b. allergic
    c. circulatory overload
    d. hemolytic

72. Hypotension, nausea, flushing, fever, and chills are symptoms of which of the following transfusion reactions?

    a. allergic
    b. circulatory overload
    c. hemolytic
    d. anaphylactic

73. Hives and itching are symptoms of which of the following transfusion reactions?

    a. febrile
    b. allergic
    c. circulatory overload
    d. anaphylactic

74. Fever and chills are symptoms of which of the following transfusion reactions?

    a. hemolytic
    b. circulatory overload
    c. allergic
    d. febrile

75. Resistance to malaria is best associated with which of the following blood groups?

    a. Rh
    b. I/i
    c. P
    d. Duffy

76. Paroxysmal cold hemoglobinuria (PCH) is best associated with which blood group?

    a. Kell
    b. Duffy
    c. P
    d. I/i

77. Cold agglutinin syndrome is best associated with which blood group?

    a. Duffy
    b. P
    c. I/i
    d. Rh

78. Warm autoimmune hemolytic anemia (AIHA) is best associated with which blood group?

    a. Rh
    b. I/i
    c. P
    d. Duffy

79. The following results were obtained:

	Anti-A	Anti-B	Anti-D	D^u	DAT	Ab. Screen
Infant	4+	0	2+	NT	0	NT
Mother	1+(mf)	0	0	$+^{vw}$(mf)	NT	0

Which of the following is the most probable explanation for these results?

    a. hemolytic disease of the newborn due to antibody against a high frequency antigen
    b. large fetomaternal hemorrhage
    c. hemolytic disease of the newborn due to anti-D
    d. mother's cells are polyagglutinable

80. If a person who has donated blood three times during the previous nine months donates a fourth unit, which of the following tests must be performed on that unit?

1. ABO typing
2. antibody screen
3. Rh typing
4. HB_sAg determination

a. only 1, 2 and 3 are correct
b. only 1 and 3 are correct
c. only 2 and 4 are correct
d. only 4 is correct
e. all are correct

81. Means of reducing the incidence of post-transfusion hepatitis include:

1. screening donors for HB_sAg
2. use of frozen blood
3. use of low-risk donor population
4. use of packed cells

a. only 1, 2 and 3 are correct
b. only 1 and 3 are correct
c. only 2 and 4 are correct
d. only 4 is correct
e. all are correct

82. Basic methods currently in clinical use for freezing red blood cells include:

1. low concentration of glycerol (10% w/v)
2. low concentration of glycerol (20% w/v)
3. high concentration of glycerol (30% w/v)
4. high concentration of glycerol (40% w/v)

a. only 1, 2 and 3 are correct
b. only 1 and 3 are correct
c. only 2 and 4 are correct
d. only 4 is correct
e. all are correct

83. True statements about separating peripheral blood lymphocytes from whole blood using Ficoll-Hypaque density gradient centrifugation include:

1. Blood must be mixed with the gradient.
2. T cells are obtained.
3. The blood must be at 4°C.
4. B cells are obtained.

a. only 1, 2 and 3 are correct
b. only 1 and 3 are correct
c. only 2 and 4 are correct
d. only 4 is correct
e. all are correct

84. The method used for deglycerolization and washing of red cells must ensure:

1. adequate removal of cryoprotective agents
2. sterility
3. minimum hemolysis
4. at least 80% recovery of the original red cells following the deglycerolization process

a. only 1, 2 and 3 are correct
b. only 1 and 3 are correct
c. only 2 and 4 are correct
d. only 4 is correct
e. all are correct

85. Rejuvenation and freezing of outdated RBCs restores intracellular ATP and 2,3-DPG by incubation with:

1. inosine
2. adenine
3. pyruvate
4. phosphate

a. only 1, 2 and 3 are correct
b. only 1 and 3 are correct
c. only 2 and 4 are correct
d. only 4 is correct
e. all are correct

86. A unit of blood that has been out of your control for ten minutes, without being refrigerated, should be:

1. cultured for bacterial contamination
2. inspected for container closure
3. stored at room temperature
4. recorded to indicate return

a. only 1, 2 and 3 are correct
b. only 1 and 3 are correct
c. only 2 and 4 are correct
d. only 4 is correct
e. all are correct

87. The quality assurance program for deglycerolized RBCs includes:

1. sterility check
2. hematocrit determination
3. pH measurement
4. observation for hemolysis in last wash solution

a. only 1, 2 and 3 are correct
b. only 1 and 3 are correct
c. only 2 and 4 are correct
d. only 4 is correct
e. all are correct

88. Characteristics of polyagglutinable red cells include:

1. They are agglutinated by cord serum.
2. They are agglutinated by most adult serum.
3. They are always an acquired condition.
4. The autocontrol is usually negative.

a. only 1, 2 and 3 are correct
b. only 1 and 3 are correct
c. only 2 and 4 are correct
d. only 4 is correct
e. all are correct

89. Which of the following situations could result in an ABO discrepancy that is due to problems with the patient's RBCs?

1. an unexpected antibody
2. rouleaux
3. agammaglobulinemia
4. Tn activation

a. only 1, 2 and 3 are correct
b. only 1 and 3 are correct
c. only 2 and 4 are correct
d. only 4 is correct
e. all are correct

90. What additional testing may be indicated from the following ABO results?

Forward Group		Reverse Group	
Anti-A	Anti-B	A Cells	B Cells
4+	neg	1+	3+

1. anti-A_1 lectin
2. antibody screen
3. A_1 cells and A_2 cells
4. anti-A,B

a. only 1, 2 and 3 are correct
b. only 1 and 3 are correct
c. only 2 and 4 are correct
d. only 4 is correct
e. all are correct

91. The ABO group of an A_1 secretor will usually differ from that of an A_3 secretor in which of the following?

1. saliva inhibition of anti-A and anti-B typing serum
2. cell typing with <u>Dolichos</u> <u>biflorus</u>
3. reverses ABO typing
4. mixed-field reactions with anti-A

a. only 1, 2 and 3 are correct
b. only 1 and 3 are correct
c. only 2 and 4 are correct
d. only 4 is correct
e. all are correct

92. True statements about the Rh_{null} phenotype include:

1. It can be produced by a regulator gene $X^{o}r$, inherited in the homozygous state.
2. It can be produced by inheritance of the amorphic gene Rh_{null} in the homozygous state.
3. It results in defective red cell membranes.
4. It is D^{u} positive.

a. only 1, 2 and 3 are correct
b. only 1 and 3 are correct
c. only 2 and 4 are correct
d. only 4 is correct
e. all are correct

93. Individuals who are group A, Le(a-b+), would have present in their saliva:

1. A
2. Le^{a}
3. H
4. Le^{b}

a. only 1, 2 and 3 are correct
b. only 1 and 3 are correct
c. only 2 and 4 are correct
d. only 4 is correct
e. all are correct

94. A blood donor is group B, le le, and is a secretor. His saliva will contain which of the following blood group substances?

1. Le^{c}
2. H
3. Le^{b}
4. B

a. only 1, 2 and 3 are correct
b. only 1 and 3 are correct
c. only 2 and 4 are correct
d. only 4 is correct
e. all are correct

95. An Xg(a+) woman can bear:

1. Xg(a-) daughters
2. Xg(a+) daughters
3. Xg(a-) sons
4. Xg(a+) sons

a. only 1, 2 and 3 are correct
b. only 1 and 3 are correct
c. only 2 and 4 are correct
d. only 4 is correct
e. all are correct

96. When the red cells of an individual fail to react with anti-U, they usually fail to react with:

1. anti-M
2. anti-s
3. anti-N
4. anti-S

a. only 1, 2 and 3 are correct
b. only 1 and 3 are correct
c. only 2 and 4 are correct
d. only 4 is correct
e. all are correct

97. True statements about polyagglutinable red cells of the Tn type include:

1. They are frequently mistaken for a subgroup of A.
2. They show strong reactions with anti-A_1 lectin.
3. They react with _Salvia_ _horminum_ lectin.
4. It is considered a transient condition.

a. only 1, 2 and 3 are correct
b. only 1 and 3 are correct
c. only 2 and 4 are correct
d. only 4 is correct
e. all are correct

98. Increased sensitization of enzyme-treated red cells could be due to:

1. exposure of latent antigenic sites
2. rearrangement of antigenic moiety
3. an increase in the association constant of the reaction
4. decrease in steric hindrance

a. only 1, 2 and 3 are correct
b. only 1 and 3 are correct
c. only 2 and 4 are correct
d. only 4 is correct
e. all are correct

99. Mixed-field agglutination encountered in ABO grouping may be due to:

1. mixed cell populations
2. Tn activation
3. A subgroup
4. fetomaternal transfer

a. only 1, 2 and 3 are correct
b. only 1 and 3 are correct
c. only 2 and 4 are correct
d. only 4 is correct
e. all are correct

100. Zeta potential is:

1. a measure of the net charge between cells
2. reduced by adding albumin to red cell suspensions
3. reduced by treating red cells with enzymes
4. may be associated with sialic acid residues

a. only 1, 2 and 3 are correct
b. only 1 and 3 are correct
c. only 2 and 4 are correct
d. only 4 is correct
e. all are correct

101. True statements about the I/i antigen system include:

1. It is pathologically significant in many cases of cold autoimmune hemolytic anemia.
2. Auto anti-i can be found in sera of patients with infectious mononucleosis.
3. If tests are performed at 10°C, many i-positive people have anti-I in their sera.
4. Anti-I occurs especially in sera of group O individuals.

a. only 1, 2 and 3 are correct
b. only 1 and 3 are correct
c. only 2 and 4 are correct
d. only 4 is correct
e. all are correct

102. The phthalate ester separation technique is useful in studying:

1. positive DAT due to methyldopa
2. multiple antibody problems in recently transfused patients
3. strong cold autoagglutinins
4. transfusion reactions

a. only 1, 2 and 3 are correct
b. only 1 and 3 are correct
c. only 2 and 4 are correct
d. only 4 is correct
e. all are correct

103. True statements about microaggregates in stored blood include:

1. They increase with storage.
2. They may be a factor in cases of pulmonary insufficiency in the massively transfused patient.
3. They are composed of leukocytes, platelets, and fibrin.
4. They can be effectively removed using filters with a pore size of 170 μm.

a. only 1, 2 and 3 are correct
b. only 1 and 3 are correct
c. only 2 and 4 are correct
d. only 4 is correct
e. all are correct

104. Partial plasma exchange has been effective in:

1. hyperviscosity syndrome
2. myasthenia gravis
3. Goodpasture's disease
4. thrombotic thrombocytopenic purpura

a. only 1, 2 and 3 are correct
b. only 1 and 3 are correct
c. only 2 and 4 are correct
d. only 4 is correct
e. all are correct

105. A patient had life-threatening anemia due to warm autoantibodies. The patient's serum was reactive 2+ in AHG with all cells on a routine panel. Techniques that would be beneficial in preparing the patient's serum for compatibility testing include:

1. autoabsorption using the patient's heat-eluted, enzyme-treated cells
2. autoabsorption using the patient's ZZAP-treated cells
3. autoabsorption using the patient's chloroquine-treated cells
4. absorption of patient's serum using keflin-treated rabbit red cells

a. only 1, 2 and 3 are correct
b. only 1 and 3 are correct
c. only 2 and 4 are correct
d. only 4 is correct
e. all are correct

106. The rationale for exchange transfusion includes:

1. correction of anemia
2. replacement of antigen-positive red cells with antigen-negative cells
3. removal of bilirubin
4. removal of antibody

a. only 1, 2 and 3 are correct
b. only 1 and 3 are correct
c. only 2 and 4 are correct
d. only 4 is correct
e. all are correct

107. Blood selected for exchange transfusion should:

1. lack the RBC antigens corresponding to the maternal antibodies
2. be less than six days old
3. be negative for Hb S
4. be ABO compatible with the father

a. only 1, 2 and 3 are correct
b. only 1 and 3 are correct
c. only 2 and 4 are correct
d. only 4 is correct
e. all are correct

108. Hazards of exchange transfusion associated with the use of citrated blood include:

1. disturbances of acid-base balance
2. hypoglycemia
3. citrate toxicity
4. decrease in body temperature

a. only 1, 2 and 3 are correct
b. only 1 and 3 are correct
c. only 2 and 4 are correct
d. only 4 is correct
e. all are correct

109. Which of the following statements about ABO-hemolytic disease of the newborn are true?

1. It usually requires an exchange transfusion.
2. It can occur in the first born.
3. It frequently results in stillbirth.
4. It is frequently seen in group O mothers.

a. only 1, 2 and 3 are correct
b. only 1 and 3 are correct
c. only 2 and 4 are correct
d. only 4 is correct
e. all are correct

110. Which of the following may be found in a classic case of autoimmune hemolytic anemia?

1. positive direct antiglobulin test
2. minor crossmatch incompatibility
3. major crossmatch incompatibility
4. false-positive Rh typing

a. only 1, 2 and 3 are correct
b. only 1 and 3 are correct
c. only 2 and 4 are correct
d. only 4 is correct
e. all are correct

111. Twenty-four or more hours after birth, major threats to the infant suffering from hemolytic disease of the newborn include:

1. glucuronyl transferase deficiency
2. failure of the hematopoietic system
3. kernicterus
4. heart failure due to bleeding

a. only 1, 2 and 3 are correct
b. only 1 and 3 are correct
c. only 2 and 4 are correct
d. only 4 is correct
e. all are correct

112. Which of the following hematologic abnormalities can be found in infants affected with ABO-hemolytic disease?

1. slight anemia
2. increased reticulocyte count
3. spherocytosis
4. jaundice developing one to three days after birth

a. only 1, 2 and 3 are correct
b. only 1 and 3 are correct
c. only 2 and 4 are correct
d. only 4 is correct
e. all are correct

113. While performing routine preadministration testing for an Rh immune globulin (RhIG) candidate, a weakly positive antibody screening test was found; anti-D was identified. This antibody may be the result of:

1. massive fetomaternal hemorrhage occurring at the time of this delivery
2. passive administration of RhIG at 28 weeks gestation
3. contamination of the blood sample with Wharton's jelly
4. previous sensitization

a. only 1, 2 and 3 are correct
b. only 1 and 3 are correct
c. only 2 and 4 are correct
d. only 4 is correct
e. all are correct

114. Which of the following is the best source of HLA-compatibile leukocytes or platelets?

a. mother
b. father
c. siblings
d. cousins

115. The purpose for implementing a low-dose irradiation of blood components is to:

a. prevent posttransfusion purpura
b. prevent graft-versus-host (GVH) disease by impeding the replication of lymphocytes
c. sterilize components, preventing the transfusion of viruses
d. prevent noncardiogenic pulmonary edema

116. The best indicator of the clinical effectiveness of granulocyte transfusions is:

a. resolution of fever or other signs of infection
b. decreased production of immunoglobulins
c. increased concentration of cytotoxic antibodies
d. decreased responsiveness in MLC testing

For questions 117 and 118, refer to the following statement and laboratory results:

The following phenotypes have been derived for the patient's family below, in order to determine the best candidate for a kidney donor.

Family Member	ABO	HLA			
Father	A	A3	A28	B18	B37
Mother	B	A2	A11	B7	B40
Patient	B	A3	A11	B7	B37
Sibling 1	AB	A3	A11	B7	B37
Sibling 2	B	A2	A3	B18	B40
Sibling 3	B	A3	A11	B	B37
Sibling 4	A	A11	A28	B7	B18

117. The haplotypes of the mother are:

   a. A2-B7/A11-B40
   b. A2-A11/B7-B40
   c. A2-B40/A11-B7
   d. A2-B18/A11-B7

118. The results obtained on sibling 2 are most probably due to which of the following?

   a. crossover of the mother's chromosomes
   b. crossover of the father's chromosomes
   c. translocation of the maternal chromosomes
   d. random segregation of the paternal chromosomes

---

119. The HLA complex shows strong associations with which blood groups?

   1. MN
   2. Bg
   3. Duffy
   4. Rodgers

   a. only 1, 2 and 3 are correct
   b. only 1 and 3 are correct
   c. only 2 and 4 are correct
   d. only 4 is correct
   e. all are correct

120. DR antigens are found on:

a. macrophages and B lymphocytes
b. platelets and B lymphocytes
c. B lymphocytes and T lymphocytes
d. T lymphocytes and macrophages

121. Antibodies to DR antigens are:

1. a cause of weak positive reactions in lymphocytotoxicity testing
2. directed against T cells
3. directed against B cells
4. not complement dependent

a. only 1, 2 and 3 are correct
b. only 1 and 3 are correct
c. only 2 and 4 are correct
d. only 4 is correct
e. all are correct

122. Conditions that cause errors in HLA typing include:

1. antigen/antibody ratio imbalance
2. cross-reacting anti-sera
3. weak complement
4. red blood cell contamination

a. only 1, 2 and 3 are correct
b. only 1 and 3 are correct
c. only 2 and 4 are correct
d. only 4 is correct
e. all are correct

123. The HLA system is a useful tool for paternity testing for which of the following reasons?

1. HLA antigens are well developed at birth.
2. The HLA system demonstrates a Mendelian pattern of inheritance.
3. The HLA system is extremely polymorphic.
4. Linkage disequilibrium is demonstrated between some HLA alleles.

a. only 1, 2 and 3 are correct
b. only 1 and 3 are correct
c. only 2 and 4 are correct
d. only 4 is correct
e. all are correct

124. Granulocyte transfusions should be:

1. administered through a microaggregate filter
2. ABO and Rh_o compatible
3. infused very rapidly (15-20 minutes/unit)
4. very closely monitored throughout procedure

a. only 1, 2 and 3 are correct
b. only 1 and 3 are correct
c. only 2 and 4 are correct
d. only 4 is correct
e. all are correct

125. Determination of HLA antigens is important in screening for:

a. ABO incompatibility
b. a kidney donor
c. Rh incompatibility
d. a blood donor

126. The optimum storage temperature for platelet concentrate is:

a. 22°C
b. 4°C
c. -12°C
d. -20°C

127. Which of the following is proper procedure for preparation of platelet concentrates?

a. light spin followed by a hard spin
b. light spin followed by two hard spins
c. two light spins
d. hard spin followed by a light spin

128. Platelet concentrates prepared in a polyolefin-type container, stored at 22-24°C in 50 mL of plasma, and gently agitated can be used for up to:

a. 24 hours
b. 72 hours
c. 3 days
d. 7 days

129. Which of the following would be the best source of platelets for transfusion in the case of alloimmune neonatal thrombocytopenia?

a. father
b. mother
c. pooled platelet-rich plasma
d. polycythemic donor

130. Which of the following blood components must be prepared within six hours after phlebotomy?

a. antihemophilic factor concentrates
b. platelet concentrate
c. Rh immune globulin
d. cryoprecipitate

131. What is the minimum pH for platelet concentrates?

a. 4
b. 5
c. 6
d. 7

132. Factors that contribute to the short shelf life of room temperature-stored platelets include:

1. pH of concentrate
2. surface area of container
3. amount of plasma in concentrate
4. number of platelets in concentrate

a. only 1, 2 and 3 are correct
b. only 1 and 3 are correct
c. only 2 and 4 are correct
d. only 4 is correct
e. all are correct

133. If an anti-A2, B12 serum is absorbed by platelets that are A2, A3, B7, B8, the serum after absorption will probably react with cells that are:

1. B7
2. A2
3. B8
4. B12

a. only 1, 2 and 3 are correct
b. only 1 and 3 are correct
c. only 2 and 4 are correct
d. only 4 is correct
e. all are correct

134. According to AABB Standards, acceptable platelet concentrates must have at least:

a. 5.5×10^{10} platelets per unit in at least 75% of the units tested

b. 6.5×11^{10} platelets per unit in 75% of the units tested

c. 7.5×10^{10} platelets per unit in 100% of the units tested

d. 8.5×10^{10} platelets per unit in 95% of the units tested

135. Each platelet concentrate should raise the patient's platelet count by:

a. 500/mm^3 per square meter of body surface
b. 1,000/mm^3 per square meter of body surface
c. 3,000/mm^3 per square meter of body surface
d. 10,000/mm^3 per square meter of body surface

136. During the preparation of platelet concentrates, the blood should be:

a. chilled to 6°C
b. kept at room temperature
c. warmed to 37°C
d. heated to 57°C

137. Each unit of whole blood will yield approximately how many units of cryoprecipitate?

a. 250
b. 130
c. 80
d. 40

138. The optimum storage temperature for cryoprecipitate is:

a. 22°C
b. 4°C
c. -12°C
d. -20°C

139. Criteria determining Rh_o immune globulin eligibility include:

a. Mother is Rh_o-positive.
b. Infant is Rh_o-negative.
c. Mother has no Rh_o antibodies.
d. Infant has a positive direct antiglobulin test.

140. Plasma exchange is recommended in the treatment of patients with macroglobulinemia in order to remove:

a. antigen
b. excess IgM
c. excess IgG
d. abnormal platelets

141. The most effective component to treat a patient with fibrinogen deficiency is:

a. fresh frozen plasma
b. platelet concentrate
c. fresh whole blood
d. cryoprecipitate

142. A patient presented with the following laboratory data: decreased levels of factor VIII antigen (determined by immunologic methods), decreased levels of factor VIII clotting activity (determined by timed clot formation), a prolonged template bleeding time, and impaired aggregation of platelets in response to ristocetin. What is the treatment of choice for this disease?

a. platelet concentrate
b. lyophilized factor VIII concentrate
c. factor IX complex
d. cryoprecipitate

143. The approximate percentage of the original plasma content of factor VIII recovered in cryoprecipitate is:

   a. 10- 20
   b. 20- 40
   c. 40- 80
   d. 80-100

144. A newborn presented with petechiae, ecchymosis, and mucosal bleeding. The preferred blood component for this infant would be:

   a. whole blood
   b. fresh frozen plasma
   c. platelet concentrate
   d. cryoprecipitate

145. An acid elution stain was made using a one-hour postdelivery maternal blood sample. Two thousand cells were counted and thirty of these cells were found to contain fetal hemoglobin. It is the policy of the medical center to add one vial of Rh immune globulin to the calculated dose when the estimated volume of the hemorrhage exceeds 20 mL of whole blood. Calculate the number of vials of Rh immune globulin that would be indicated under these circumstances.

   a. 2
   b. 3
   c. 4
   d. 5

146. A patient diagnosed as having mild hemophilia A (8% factor VIII) was transfused with factor VIII concentrates in preparation for abdominal surgery. It was calculated that he would require 1,200 units of factor VIII to raise his plasma concentration to 50%. However, after infusion his factor VIII concentration rose to 65%, and remained at 50% for approximately 30 hours without further infusion. What would be the most likely explanation for this observation?

   a. Patient really had von Willebrand's disease.
   b. Factor VIII concentrates had twice the specified factor VIII concentration.
   c. Patient had an inhibitor to the factor VIII complex.
   d. Patient had idiopathic thrombocytopenic purpura.

147. A unit of fresh frozen plasma was removed from the storage freezer and placed in a water bath to thaw. The technologist did not notice that the temperature of the water bath had dropped to 25°C. Assuming proper filtration, the unit could be effectively used to treat all coagulation deficiencies EXCEPT:

a. factor VIII and fibrinogen
b. factor VIII only
c. factors V and VIII
d. factors II, VII, IX, and X

148. Each of the following is the correct storage temperature for the component listed EXCEPT:

a. cryoprecipitate -18°C
b. fresh frozen plasma (FFP) -10°C
c. frozen RBCs -65°C
d. platelet concentrate 23°C

149. Which of the following blood components contains the most factor VIII concentration relative to volume?

a. plasma
b. cryoprecipitate
c. fresh frozen plasma
d. platelet concentrate

150. Although ABO compatibility is preferred, ABO incompatible may be administered when transfusing:

a. plasma
b. cryoprecipitate
c. fresh frozen plasma
d. granulocytes

151. Which of the following blood components is a good source of factor IX for 21 days after phlebotomy?

a. platelet concentrate
b. albumin
c. cryoprecipitate
d. plasma

152. After thawing, fresh frozen plasma must be infused within:

a. 24 hours
b. 36 hours
c. 48 hours
d. 72 hours

153. In a quality assurance program, at least 75% of the bags of cryoprecipitate must contain a minimum of how many International Units of factor VIII?

    a. 60
    b. 70
    c. 80
    d. 90

154. In the liquid state, plasma must be stored at:

    a. 56°C
    b. 37°C
    c. room temperature
    d. 1-6°C

155. After thawing, reconstituted cryoprecipitate should be stored at:

    a. room temperature
    b. 37°C
    c. 10°C
    d. 1-6°C

156. After a single-volume plasma exchange on a continuous flow cell separator, the percentage of original plasma remaining in a patient is about:

    a. 5
    b. 14
    c. 37
    d. 50

157. Individuals at risk of developing graft-versus-host disease include each of the following EXCEPT:

    a. patients with congenital immune deficiency disease
    b. patients receiving total body irradiation
    c. patients on long-term hemodialysis
    d. patients with aplastic anemia immediately after allogeneic marrow transplantation

158. Ten days after transfusion of 15 units of blood a patient had a 5 g drop in hemoglobin concentration and was jaundiced. No evidence of bleeding was found. Which of the following tests would be helpful in determining whether the patient is experiencing a delayed transfusion reaction?

1. direct antiglobulin test
2. comparison of pre- and post-haptoglobin concentrations
3. testing post-transfusion serum for alloantibodies
4. plasma free hemoglobin determination

a. only 1, 2 and 3 are correct
b. only 1 and 3 are correct
c. only 2 and 4 are correct
d. only 4 is correct
e. all are correct

159. Blood derivatives or components used in the treatment of hemophilia A include:

1. factor VIII concentrates
2. fresh frozen plasma
3. cryoprecipitate
4. whole blood

a. only 1, 2 and 3 are correct
b. only 1 and 3 are correct
c. only 2 and 4 are correct
d. only 4 is correct
e. all are correct

160. A patient with hemophilia A (less than 1% factor VIII) was being treated for intra-articular bleeding in the knee joint. He was infused with sufficient cryoprecipitate calculated to raise the plasma factor VIII level to 30%. However, immediately following infusion the patient's plasma factor VIII level was measured at 2%. Possible explanations for this observation include:

1. Factor VIII inhibitor present.
2. Patient really had von Willebrand's disease.
3. Improper preparation and/or infusion of the cryoprecipitate.
4. Patient should have been given factor VIII concentrate, not cryoprecipitate.

a. only 1, 2 and 3 are correct
b. only 1 and 3 are correct
c. only 2 and 4 are correct
d. only 4 is correct
e. all are correct

161. Which of the following blood products is appropriate to give an eight-year-old male hemophiliac who is about to undergo minor surgery?

a. whole blood (banked)
b. red cell concentrate
c. platelet concentrate
d. cryoprecipitate

162. Which of the following transfusion reactions is characterized by high fever, shock, hemoglobinuria, DIC, and renal failure?

a. bacterial contamination
b. circulatory overload
c. delayed hemolytic reaction due to anti-D
d. anaphylactic

163. Which of the following transfusion reactions occurs after infusion of only a few milliliters of blood and gives no history of fever?

a. febrile
b. circulatory overload
c. anaphylactic
d. hemolytic

164. Congestive heart failure, severe headache, and/or peripheral edema occurring soon after transfusion is indicative of which type of transfusion reaction?

  a. hemolytic
  b. febrile
  c. anaphylactic
  d. circulatory overload

165. In investigating a hemolytic transfusion reaction, the pre- and post-transfusion sample should be:

  a. tested by DAT
  b. crossmatched again
  c. tested against a panel
  d. eluted and retested

166. A granulocyte transfusion is indicated if the patient has:

  a. leukemia
  b. an absolute granulocyte count of $500/mm^3$ or less
  c. a viral infection
  d. a leukocyte count of $1,000/mm^3$

167. Transfusion of which of the following is needed to help correct hypofibrinogenemia due to DIC?

  a. whole blood
  b. fresh frozen plasma
  c. cryoprecipitate
  d. platelet concentrates

Blood Bank Answer Key

1.	d	43.	c	85.	e	127.	a
2.	c	44.	b	86.	c	128.	d
3.	b	45.	c	87.	c	129.	b
4.	b	46.	c	88.	c	130.	b
5.	a	47.	a	89.	d	131.	c
6.	a	48.	d	90.	a	132.	e
7.	c	49.	c	91.	c	133.	d
8.	d	50.	b	92.	a	134.	a
9.	c	51.	b	93.	e	135.	d
10.	d	52.	b	94.	c	136.	b
11.	a	53.	b	95.	e	137.	c
12.	d	54.	d	96.	c	138.	d
13.	a	55.	d	97.	a	139.	c
14.	a	56.	a	98.	e	140.	b
15.	d	57.	a	99.	e	141.	d
16.	d	58.	c	100.	e	142.	d
17.	d	59.	d	101.	a	143.	c
18.	d	60.	c	102.	c	144.	c
19.	d	61.	d	103.	a	145.	c
20.	c	62.	b	104.	e	146.	a
21.	a	63.	d	105.	a	147.	a
22.	a	64.	d	106.	e	148.	b
23.	c	65.	a	107.	a	149.	b
24.	c	66.	b	108.	a	150.	b
25.	b	67.	b	109.	c	151.	d
26.	c	68.	d	110.	e	152.	a
27.	d	69.	c	111.	b	153.	c
28.	d	70.	d	112.	e	154.	d
29.	c	71.	c	113.	c	155.	a
30.	b	72.	c	114.	c	156.	c
31.	a	73.	b	115.	b	157.	c
32.	e	74.	d	116.	a	158.	b
33.	b	75.	d	117.	c	159.	b
34.	b	76.	c	118.	b	160.	b
35.	c	77.	c	119.	c	161.	d
36.	c	78.	a	120.	a	162.	a
37.	d	79.	b	121.	b	163.	c
38.	d	80.	e	122.	e	164.	d
39.	d	81.	b	123.	a	165.	a
40.	a	82.	c	124.	c	166.	b
41.	d	83.	c	125.	b	167.	c
42.	b	84.	e	126.	a		

CHAPTER 14

Immunology

1. The Rose-Waaler test for rheumatoid factor utilizes:

    a. washed human erythrocytes
    b. sheep erythrocytes coated with human IgG
    c. latex particles coated with rabbit IgM
    d. sheep erythrocytes coated with rabbit IgG

2. Double precipitin rings on radial immunodiffusion (RID) plates for serum haptoglobin assays can be caused by:

    a. haptoglobin-hemoglobin complexes
    b. haptoglobin-hemopexin interactions
    c. refrigeration at 4°C of RID plates during immunodiffusion
    d. antigen excess

3. The biologic function of the C42 molecule is:

    a. cytolysis
    b. to serve as a substrate of properdin factor B
    c. cleavage and activation of the C3 molecule
    d. formation and activation of the C1s molecule

4. Which of the following is not involved in host responses to foreign antigens?

    a. C-reactive protein
    b. albumin
    c. C3, C5
    d. IgM

5. Increased susceptibility to infections is caused by each of the following deficiencies <u>EXCEPT</u>:

    a. C3 deficiency
    b. alymphocytosis
    c. agranulocytosis
    d. C-reactive protein deficiency

6. Which of the following CANNOT be detected by immunoelectrophoresis?

   a. selective IgA deficiency
   b. selective light chain deficiency
   c. IgE deficiency
   d. Bence Jones proteins

7. Which of the following abnormalities CANNOT be identified on agarose gel electrophoresis?

   a. serum hypogammaglobulinemia
   b. serum polyclonal gammopathy
   c. serum monoclonal gammopathy
   d. serum selective IgA deficiency

8. Which of the following statements about immunoglobulins is true?

   a. Immunoglobulins are produced by T lymphocytes.
   b. The IgA class is determined by the y heavy chain.
   c. The IgA class exists as a serum and secretory component.
   d. There are two subclasses of IgG.

9. Select the appropriate sensitivity limit for radial immunodiffusion.

   a. 0.1 mg/dL
   b. 0.5 mg/dL
   c. less than 1-2 mg/dL
   d. less than 1 pg/dL

10. Select the appropriate sensitivity limit for electroimmunodiffusion.

   a. 0.1 mg/dL
   b. 0.5 mg/dL
   c. less than 1-2 mg/dL
   d. less than 1 pg/dL

For questions 11 to 14, refer to the following illustration and statement:

The curve below was obtained by adding increasing amounts of a soluble antigen to fixed volumes of monospecific antiserum.

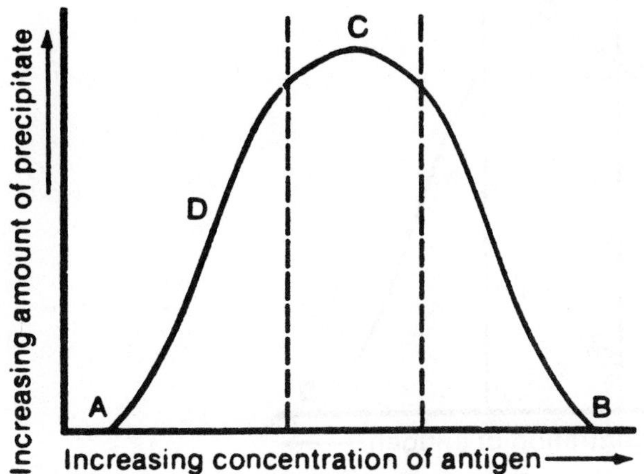

11. The area on the curve for equivalence precipitate is:

    a. A
    b. B
    c. C
    d. D

12. The area on the curve where no precipitate formed due to antigen excess is:

    a. A
    b. B
    c. C
    d. D

13. The area on the curve for prozone is:

    a. A
    b. B
    c. C
    d. D

For question 14, refer to the following illustration and statement:

The curve below was obtained by adding increasing amounts of a soluble antigen to fixed volumes of monospecific antiserum.

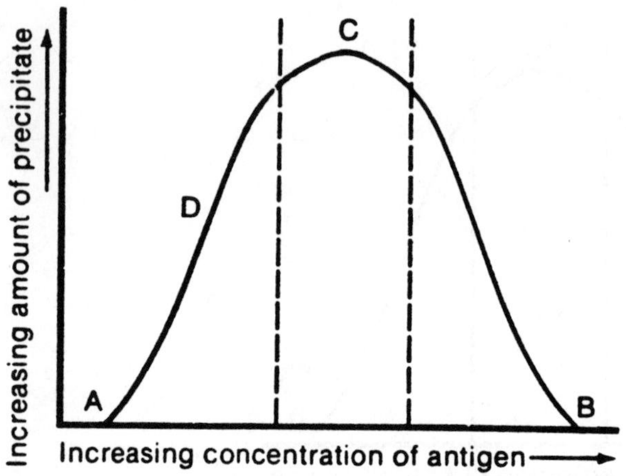

14. The area on the curve where soluble antigen-antibody complexes form is:

    a. A
    b. B
    c. C
    d. D

---

15. Select the appropriate sensitivity limit for nephelometry.

    a. 0.1 mg/dL
    b. 0.5 mg/dL
    c. less than 1-2 mg/dL
    d. less than 1 pg/dL

16. Select the appropriate sensitivity limit for radioimmunoassay (RIA).

    a. 0.1 mg/dL
    b. 0.5 mg/dL
    c. less than 1-2 mg/dL
    d. less than 1 pg/dL

17. Which of the following is a true statement about selective IgA deficiency?

   a. It is associated with a decreased incidence of allergic manifestations.
   b. There is a high concentration of secretory component in the saliva.
   c. It is associated with an increased incidence of autoimmune diseases.
   d. It is found in approximately one out of every 50 persons.

18. Which of the following is a true statement about Bruton's agammaglobulinemia?

   a. It is found only in females.
   b. There are normal numbers of circulating B cells.
   c. There are decreased to absent concentrations of immunoglobulins.
   d. The disease presents with pyogenic infections one week after birth.

19. The Epstein-Barr virus causes immunoproliferation in:

   1. infectious mononucleosis
   2. Duncan's immunoproliferative syndrome
   3. Burkitt's lymphoma
   4. nasopharyngeal carcinoma

   a. only 1, 2 and 3 are correct
   b. only 1 and 3 are correct
   c. only 2 and 4 are correct
   d. only 4 is correct
   e. all are correct

20. Which of the following could mask a monoclonal protein during immunoelectrophoresis?

   1. antigen and antibody not in proper concentration
   2. antiserum not directed against available determinants on the M component
   3. prozone effect
   4. interference of an increased concentration of albumin

   a. only 1, 2 and 3 are correct
   b. only 1 and 3 are correct
   c. only 2 and 4 are correct
   d. only 4 is correct
   e. all are correct

21. Which of the following diseases are often associated with a polyclonal hyperimmunoglobulinemia?

1. chronic infection
2. biliary cirrhosis
3. systemic lupus erythematosus
4. amyloidosis

a. only 1, 2 and 3 are correct
b. only 1 and 3 are correct
c. only 2 and 4 are correct
d. only 4 is correct
e. all are correct

22. Antigen-antibody interactions can be detected by which of the following reactions?

1. agglutination
2. flocculation
3. precipitation
4. complement fixation

a. only 1, 2 and 3 are correct
b. only 1 and 3 are correct
c. only 2 and 4 are correct
d. only 4 is correct
e. all are correct

23. The total hemolytic complement analysis:

1. detects genetic deficiencies of the complement proteins
2. can be evaluated by protein quantitation of complement components
3. is a functional measurement of the complement pathway
4. is useful in evaluating immune complex disease

a. only 1, 2 and 3 are correct
b. only 1 and 3 are correct
c. only 2 and 4 are correct
d. only 4 is correct
e. all are correct

24. The chief difference in the use of counterimmunoelectrophoresis (CIE) in the detection of antigen as opposed to the detection of antibody is the:

    a. ionic strength and pH of the veronal buffer
    b. temperature of the physiologic saline bath
    c. diameters of the reagent wells in the test plate
    d. concentration of agarose

25. Indications for the use of boronic acid buffer in a counter-immunoelectrophoresis system include:

    a. testing of a specimen from an adult
    b. testing of all urine samples
    c. inability to type pneumococcal organisms in 0.05 M barbital buffer
    d. testing of spinal fluid samples infected with type B *Neisseria meningitidis*

26. The minimum human chorionic gonadotropin (HCG) level needed for a positive rapid indirect latex slide immunoassay test is:

    a. less than 0.5 IU/mL
    b. 0.5 -1.0 IU/mL
    c. 0.75-1.5 IU/mL
    d. 1.5 -2.5 IU/mL

27. All of the following may cause false-positive indirect latex slide tests EXCEPT:

    a. significant proteinuria
    b. methadone therapy
    c. tubo-ovarian abscess
    d. a urine specific gravity of less than 1.010

28. The new radioimmunoassay procedure for serum HCG utilizes antisera against which subunit of HCG?

    a. alpha
    b. gamma
    c. chorionic
    d. beta

29. A false-positive test using the standard HCG tube immunoassay can be the result of:

    a. cross-reactivity between HCG and luteinizing hormone (LH)
    b. the binding of HCG to urine protein
    c. drug-induced increases in the zeta potential of the latex particles
    d. an HCG level of 1.0 IU/mL

30. The viral core of the hepatitis B virus (HBV) contains all of the following structures EXCEPT:

    a. viral DNA
    b. DNA polymerase
    c. HB_eAg
    d. HB_sAg

31. Patients who appear to be at high risk for the development of chronic hepatitis are those who maintain high titers of antibody to the:

    a. core antigen
    b. surface antigen
    c. e antigen
    d. delta antigen

32. The classic antibody response pattern following the contraction of hepatitis A virus (HAV) is:

    a. increase in IgM antibody; decrease in IgM antibody; increase in IgG antibody
    b. detectable presence of IgG antibody only
    c. detectable presence of IgM antibody only
    d. decrease in IgM antibody; increase in IgG antibody of the IgG3 subtype

33. The major residual split portion of C3 is which of the following?

    a. C3a
    b. C3b
    c. C4
    d. C1q

34. The component associated only with the alternative pathway of complement activation is:

    a. C4
    b. C1q
    c. properdin factor B
    d. C3a

35. The major opsonin and cell adherence factor is:

    a. C4
    b. C3b
    c. C3a
    d. properdin factor B

36. Which of the following is cleaved as a result of activation of the classical complement pathway?

    a. properdin factor B
    b. C1q
    c. C4
    d. C3b

37. Which of the following has greater than 90% accuracy only after 45 days from last normal menstrual period (LNMP)?

    a. radioreceptor assay
    b. standard HCG tube immunoassay
    c. rapid indirect latex slide immunoassay
    d. radioimmunoassay

38. Which of the following is accurate 23-32 days from last normal menstrual period?

    a. radioreceptor assay
    b. standard HCG tube immunoassay
    c. rapid indirect latex slide immunoassay
    d. radioimmunoassay

39. Which of the following shows good accuracy at 32 days or more from last normal menstrual period?

    a. radioreceptor assay
    b. standard HCG tube immunoassay
    c. rapid indirect latex slide immunoassay
    d. radioimmunoassay

40. Which of the following has greater than 90% accuracy only after 40 days from last normal menstrual period?

    a. radioreceptor assay
    b. standard HCG tube immunoassay
    c. rapid indirect latex slide immunoassay
    d. radioimmunoassay

41. Which of the following causes 90% of post-transfusion hepatitis?

    a. HAV
    b. HBV
    c. NANB
    d. HBIG

42. Which of the following is used to absorb IgG from a positive HAV antibody sample?

    a. HAV antibody, IgM type
    b. HAV antibody, IgG type
    c. staphylococcal protein A
    d. _Escherichia coli_ protein C

43. Which of the following usually indicates a remote or past infection by HAV?

    a. staphylococcal protein A
    b. HAV antibody, IgG type
    c. HAV antibody, IgM type
    d. HAV antibody, IgA type

44. Which of the following would be considered evidence of a recent hepatitis A infection?

    a. HAV antibody, IgM type
    b. HAV antibody, IgG type
    c. staphylococcal protein A
    d. _Escherichia coli_ protein C

45. The antibody initially increased in response to hepatitis A infection is:

    a. HAV antibody, IgM type
    b. HAV antibody, IgG type
    c. HAV antibody, IgA type
    d. _Escherichia coli_ protein C

46. A bacterial protein used to bind human immunoglobulins is:

a. HAV antibody, IgA type
b. *Escherichia coli* protein C
c. staphylococcal protein A
d. HAV antibody, IgG type

For questions 47 to 50, refer to the following illustration:

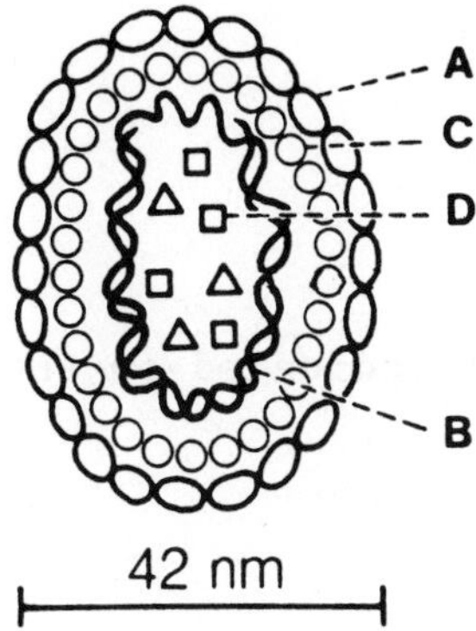

47. Select the corresponding lettered component indicated on the diagram for surface antigen.

a. A
b. B
c. C
d. D

48. Select the corresponding lettered component indicated on the diagram for e antigen.

a. A
b. B
c. C
d. D

49. Select the corresponding lettered component indicated on the diagram for core antigen.

a. A
b. B
c. C
d. D

For question 50, refer to the following illustration:

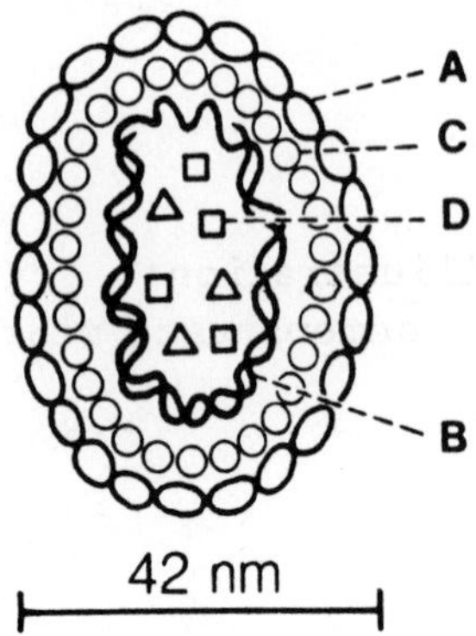

50. Select the corresponding lettered component indicated on the diagram for viral DNA.

   a. A
   b. B
   c. C
   d. D

---

51. Other hepatitis-causing viruses, such as cytomegalovirus and varicella-zoster virus, can be differentiated from HAV and HBV by:

   a. incubation period
   b. complement fixation
   c. immune electron microscopy
   d. tissue culture isolation

52. Which of the following tests have been developed to detect the presence of antibody to the hepatitis A virus?

   1. RIA
   2. immune electron microscopy
   3. complement fixation assay
   4. immune adherence test

   a. only 1, 2 and 3 are correct
   b. only 1 and 3 are correct
   c. only 2 and 4 are correct
   d. only 4 is correct
   e. all are correct

53. The 20 nm spheres and filamentous structures of the HBV are:

a. infectious
b. circulating aggregates of HB_cAg
c. circulating aggregates of HB_sAg
d. highly infectious when present in great abundance

54. Twelve weeks after onset of the disease, patients with uncomplicated acute hepatitis B usually will demonstrate which of the following in their serum?

a. HB_sAg
b. anti-HTLV
c. anti-HB_e
d. anti-HB_s

55. A medical technologist reported to her supervisor that she had accidentally stuck herself with a needle she had used in drawing blood from a person with suspected hepatitis. An incident report was filed and the tech received an ISG shot. Her test for HB_sAg was negative. An HB_sAg test was ordered on the patient's serum and was also negative. About four months later, the tech began to complain of abdominal pain, fatigue, and loss of appetite. A liver profile was ordered and results indicated only a slight rise in liver enzymes. A test for HB_sAg was negative. Which of the following could explain these findings?

1. The patient was infected with the HBV but was in the period known as the "core window."
2. The patient had hepatitis but the HB_sAg was too low to be detected by the current test method.
3. The technologist was in the period known as the "core window" when tested.
4. The technologist had contracted NANB hepatitis.

a. only 1, 2 and 3 are correct
b. only 1 and 3 are correct
c. only 2 and 4 are correct
d. only 4 is correct
e. all are correct

56. The enzyme-linked immunosorbent assay (ELISA) technique for the detection of HB_sAg:

a. requires radiolabeled C1q
b. is quantitated by degree of fluorescence
c. uses anti-HB_s linked to horseradish peroxidase
d. uses beads coated with HB_sAG

57. All of the following have been implicated as causes of infectious hepatitis EXCEPT:

a. blood transfusion
b. Epstein-Barr virus
c. contaminated water
d. mushrooms acting as hepatotoxins

58. Which of the following applies to the use of the radioreceptor assay test method in detecting HCG?

a. The Saxena test detected urine HCG levels as low as 5.0-10.0 mIU/mL.
b. The biocept G^R test could be performed in 30 minutes.
c. The radioreceptor assay test detects pregnancy with good accuracy at 23-30 days from the LNMP.
d. The test for HCG is based on the binding of HCG or LH to protein receptor plasma membranes.

59. Rheumatoid factor is:

a. an antigen found in the serum of patients with rheumatoid arthritis
b. identical to the rheumatoid arthritis precipitin
c. IgG or IgM autoantibody
d. capable of forming circulating immune complexes only when IgM-type autoantibody is present

60. The C-reactive protein assay is:

1. a sensitive measurement of the amount of tissue injury
2. a normally undetectable liver-derived serum protein
3. undetectable when inflammation clears
4. performed using immunoprecipitation, latex agglutination, "rocket electrophoresis," or immunonephelometry

a. only 1, 2 and 3 are correct
b. only 1 and 3 are correct
c. only 2 and 4 are correct
d. only 4 is correct
e. all are correct

61. The presence of immune complexes indicates:

a. polyclonal hypergammaglobulinemia
b. inflammatory tissue injury
c. protection from complement-dependent neutrophil chemotaxis
d. normal host response to antigenic exposure

62. Immune complexes:

1. form cryoglobulin precipitates when present in serum in significant amounts
2. interact with purified radiolabeled C1q
3. can activate complement pathways
4. are directly measured by the C-reactive protein assay

a. only 1, 2 and 3 are correct
b. only 1 and 3 are correct
c. only 2 and 4 are correct
d. only 4 is correct
e. all are correct

63. The complement component C3:

a. is increased (in plasma levels) when complement activation occurs
b. can be measured by immunoprecipitin assays
c. releases histamine from basophils or mast cells
d. is <u>NOT</u> involved in the alternate complement pathway

64. A chronic carrier of HBV:

   a. has chronic symptoms of hepatitis
   b. continues to carry the HBV
   c. does not transmit infection
   d. carries the HBV but is not infectious

65. Hepatitis B infection may be acquired via:

   1. blood transfusions
   2. use of illicit parenteral drugs
   3. sexual contacts with an infected person
   4. maternal-fetal infection

   a. only 1, 2 and 3 are correct
   b. only 1 and 3 are correct
   c. only 2 and 4 are correct
   d. only 4 is correct
   e. all are correct

66. Etiologic and clinical manifestations of HAV and HBV render differentiation nearly impossible because:

   1. both forms have biochemical evidence of hepatocellular damage or dysfunction
   2. histologic differentiation is not always possible during the acute phase of the disease
   3. the modes of transmission may be similar
   4. both forms of the disease are manifest by malaise, fever, abdominal pain, and anorexia

   a. only 1, 2 and 3 are correct
   b. only 1 and 3 are correct
   c. only 2 and 4 are correct
   d. only 4 is correct
   e. all are correct

67. The markers most closely associated with transmissibility of HBV infection are:

   a. HB_sAg
   b. HB_eAg
   c. HB_cAg
   d. HBVAg

68. Non-A, non-B hepatitis differs from hepatitis A and hepatitis B in that:

   a. the incubation period for NANB is highly stable
   b. NANB is associated with a high incidence of icteric hepatitis
   c. NANB is associated with a high incidence of the chronic carrier state
   d. NANB is seldom implicated in cases of post-transfusion hepatitis

69. The standard HCG tube immunoassay is:

   a. a hemagglutination-inhibition test
   b. an indirect latex test
   c. a complement fixation test
   d. less sensitive than the rapid slide test

70. The beta-HCG assays are useful in:

   1. diagnosing very early pregnancy
   2. detecting HCG in low-titer conditions
   3. detecting pregnancy in preoperative patients undergoing dilatation and curettage
   4. monitoring phases of trophoblastic disease

   a. only 1, 2 and 3 are correct
   b. only 1 and 3 are correct
   c. only 2 and 4 are correct
   d. only 4 is correct
   e. all are correct

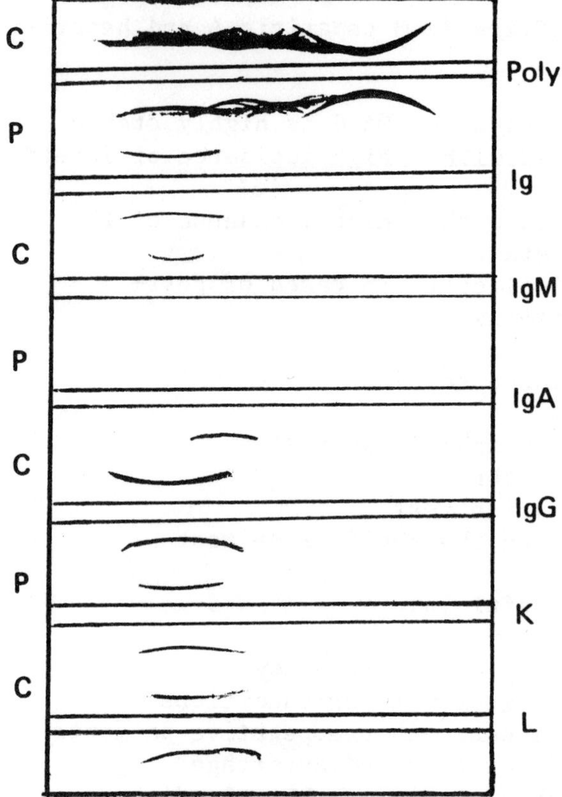

71. When the serum immunoelectrophoretic pattern has the findings depicted, appropriate studies should be performed to EXCLUDE:

   a. malignant lymphoma with monoclonal protein
   b. IgD and/or IgE myeloma
   c. heavy chain disease
   d. plasma cell leukemia

---

72. Which of the following immunologic abnormalities is associated with a high incidence of amyloidosis?

   a. alpha chain disease
   b. gamma chain disease
   c. mu chain disease
   d. IgD myeloma

73. Which of the following immunologic abnormalities is associated with malabsorption syndrome?

    a. alpha chain disease
    b. gamma chain disease
    c. IgD myeloma
    d. IgE myeloma

74. Which of the following immunologic abnormalities is associated with lymphadenopathy and fever?

    a. mu chain disease
    b. gamma chain disease
    c. alpha chain disease
    d. IgE myeloma

75. Which of the following immunologic abnormalities is most likely associated with chronic lymphocytic leukemia?

    a. IgE myeloma
    b. IgD myeloma
    c. mu chain disease
    d. gamma chain disease

76. Hereditary angioedema is characterized by:

    a. decreased activity of C3
    b. decreased activity of C1 esterase inhibitor
    c. increased activity of C1 esterase inhibitor
    d. increased activity of C2

77. A decreased ratio of synovial fluid complement to serum complement is most consistent with:

    a. pseudogout
    b. osteoarthritis
    c. rheumatoid arthritis
    d. lupus erythematosus

78. Acquired hypogammaglobulinemia is often associated with each of the following diseases <u>EXCEPT</u>:

    a. light chain variant of multiple myeloma
    b. sarcoidosis
    c. malignant lymphoma
    d. chronic lymphocytic leukemia

79. Which of the following is the most common humoral immune deficiency disease?

    a. Bruton's agammaglobulinemia
    b. IgG deficiency
    c. selective IgA deficiency
    d. Wiskott-Aldrich syndrome

80. The J-chain is associated with which of the following immunoglobulins?

    a. IgA
    b. IgG
    c. IgE
    d. IgD

81. Initiation of the activation mechanism of the alternative complement pathway differs from that of the classical pathway in that:

    a. antigen-antibody complexes containing IgM or IgG are required
    b. endotoxin alone cannot initiate activation
    c. C1 component of complement is involved
    d. antigen-antibody complexes containing IgA or IgE may initiate activation

82. The C3b component of complement:

    a. is undetectable in pathologic sera
    b. is a component of the C3 cleaving enzyme of the classical pathway
    c. is cleaved by C3 inactivator into C3c and C3d
    d. migrates farther toward the cathode than C3

83. The serum hemolytic complement level (CH50):

    a. is a measure of total complement activity
    b. provides the same information as a serum factor B level
    c. is detectable when any component of the classical system is congenitally absent
    d. can be calculated from the serum concentrations of the individual components

84. Which of the following has been associated with patients who have homozygous C3 deficiency?

a. undetectable hemolytic complement activity in the serum
b. systemic lupus erythematosus
c. no detectable disease
d. a lifelong history of life-threatening infections

85. A benign monoclonal gammopathy:

a. usually is associated with a decrease in other immunoglobulins
b. occasionally is associated with monoclonal light chains in the urine
c. occurs in approximately 10% of people over the age of 70
d. usually is of the IgM class

86. In measuring serum immunoglobulins by radial immunodiffusion, the:

a. square of the diameter of the precipitin ring in the Mancini method is inversely proportional to the amount of specific immunoglobulin present in the serum
b. precipitin line occurs in a zone of equivalence between antigen and antibody
c. diameter of the precipitin ring in the Fahey technique is directly proportional to the molecular weight of the immunoglobulin being measured
d. test as performed by the Fahey technique is insensitive to temperature variations

87. Which of the following is commonly associated with selective IgA deficiency?

a. anti-milk antibodies
b. antibodies against IgD
c. decreased occurrence of autoantibodies
d. serum IgA level between 100 and 200 mg/dL

88. Idiopathic late-onset immunoglobulin deficiency (common variable immune deficiency) is commonly associated with neoplasia of the:

1. genitourinary system
2. gastrointestinal tract
3. nerve tissue
4. lymphoid tissue

a. only 1, 2 and 3 are correct
b. only 1 and 3 are correct
c. only 2 and 4 are correct
d. only 4 is correct
e. all are correct

89. True statements about lupus nephritis include:

a. only classical components of the complement system may be deposited in the glomeruli
b. tubulointerstitial deposits of immunoglobulin and/or complement are rare
c. IgA is rarely deposited in the glomeruli
d. immunofluorescence may be positive in glomeruli that are normal by light microscopy

90. A 26-year-old nurse developed fatigue, a low-grade fever, polyarthralgia, and urticaria. Two months earlier she had cared for a patient with hepatitis. Which of the following findings is likely to be observed in this nurse?

a. a negative hepatitis B surface antigen test
b. elevated AST (SGOT) and ALT (SGPT) activities
c. an increased CH50 level
d. a positive Mono Spot test

91. A 55-year-old woman is seen by a physician because of palpable purpura, arthritis, Raynaud's phenomenon, and renal symptoms. A cryoprecipitate is present in the serum. Further studies are likely to show:

1. polyclonal IgG and monoclonal IgM in the cryoprecipitate
2. a decreased serum CH50 level
3. necrotizing arteritis on skin biopsy
4. rheumatoid factor within the glomerular deposits

a. only 1, 2 and 3 are correct
b. only 1 and 3 are correct
c. only 2 and 4 are correct
d. only 4 is correct
e. all are correct

92. A 67-year-old woman is seen by a physician because of progressive myalgia of the upper extremities and the sudden onset of blindness in the right eye. Laboratory studies would be likely to show:

a. high titer rheumatoid factor
b. giant cell arteritis on right temporal artery biopsy
c. decreased serum IgA
d. normal erythrocyte sedimentation rate

93. True statements about the antibody response to infection with group A, β hemolytic streptococci include:

a. eighty to 90% of patients with streptococcal pharyngitis who are treated will have significant rises (greater than two tubes) in their antistreptolysin O (ASO) titers
b. the anti-DNase B titer is a less sensitive index of nephritogenic skin infections than the ASO titer
c. rheumatic fever is more likely to be present in individuals who have strong antibody responses than in those who have weak responses
d. the anti-DNase B antibody titer is a more sensitive indicator than anti-group A specific carbohydrate titers for the detection of rheumatic fever

94. Anticomplementary activity in a complement fixation test can be caused by:

1. heparin
2. prolonged storage at -20°C
3. EDTA
4. serum from patients with active rheumatoid arthritis

a. only 1, 2 and 3 are correct
b. only 1 and 3 are correct
c. only 2 and 4 are correct
d. only 4 is correct
e. all are correct

95. The fluorescent treponemal antibody absorption (FTA-ABS) test for the serologic diagnosis of syphilis is:

a. less sensitive and specific than the VDRL if properly performed
b. likely to remain positive after adequate antibiotic therapy
c. currently recommended for testing cerebrospinal fluid
d. preferred over dark-field microscopy for diagnosing primary syphilis

For questions 96 to 99, refer to the following diagram:

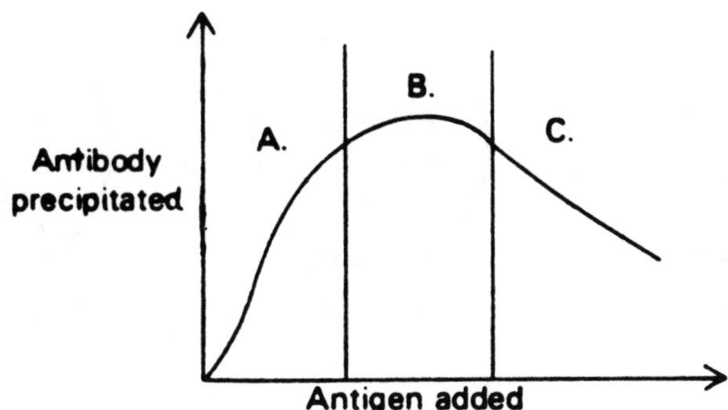

96. The zone in which the addition of more antibody would result in the formation of additional precipitate is:

a. Zone A
b. Zone B
c. Zone C

97. The zone in which the MOST extensive lattice of antigen and antibody exists is:

a. Zone A
b. Zone B
c. Zone C

98. The zone which contains the greatest amount of free antigen in the supernatant is:

a. Zone A
b. Zone B
c. Zone C

99. The antigen could be accurately quantitated in:

a. Zone A
b. Zone B
c. Zone C

For questions 100 to 103, refer to the following illustration:

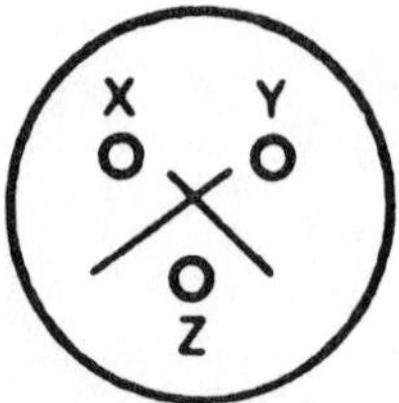

Figure #1

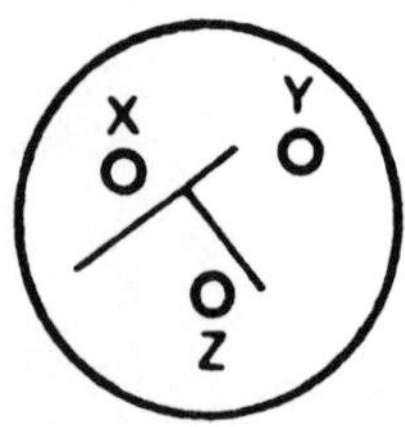

Figure #2

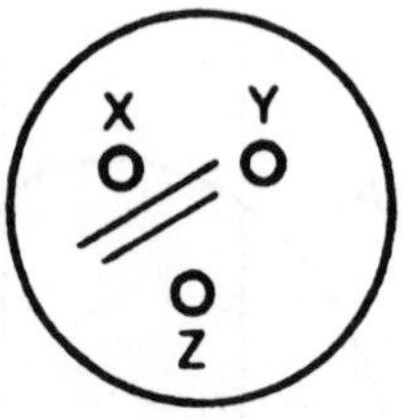

Figure #3

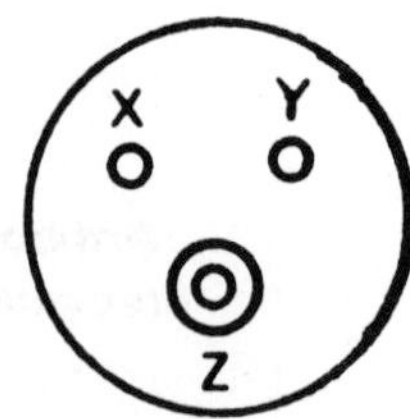

Figure #4

100. Which of the above figures demonstrates a reaction pattern of nonidentity?

  a. Figure #1
  b. Figure #2
  c. Figure #3
  d. Figure #4

101. Which of the above figures demonstrates a reaction pattern showing two different antigenic molecular species?

  a. Figure #1
  b. Figure #2
  c. Figure #3
  d. Figure #4

102. Which of the above figures demonstrates a reaction pattern of partial identity?

  a. Figure #1
  b. Figure #2
  c. Figure #3
  d. Figure #4

103. A nonspecific precipitant reaction is demonstrated in:

  a. Figure #1
  b. Figure #2
  c. Figure #3
  d. Figure #4

104. The hyperviscosity syndrome may be seen in monoclonal disease of which of the following immunoglobulin classes?

1. IgA
2. IgM
3. IgG
4. IgD

a. only 1, 2 and 3 are correct
b. only 1 and 3 are correct
c. only 2 and 4 are correct
d. only 4 is correct
e. all are correct

105. Antibody class and antibody subclass are determined by major physiochemical differences and antigenic variation found primarily in the:

a. constant region of heavy chain
b. constant region of light chain
c. variable regions of heavy and light chains
d. constant regions of heavy and light chains

106. Antibody idiotype is dictated by:

a. constant region of heavy chain
b. constant region of light chain
c. variable regions of heavy and light chains
d. constant regions of heavy and light chains

107. Antibody allotype is determined by:

a. constant region of heavy chain
b. constant region of light chain
c. variable regions of heavy and light chains
d. constant regions of heavy and light chains

108. Hereditary deficiency of early complement components C1r, C1s, C4, and C2 is associated with:

a. pneumococcal septicemia
b. small bowel obstruction
c. systemic lupus erythematosus
d. gonococcemia

109. Which of the following findings is associated with a hereditary deficiency of C3?

   a. pneumococcal septicemia
   b. small bowel obstruction
   c. systemic lupus erythematosus
   d. gonococcemia

110. Hereditary deficiency of late components of complements C5, C6, C7, or C8 can be associated with which of the following conditions?

   a. pneumococcal septicemia
   b. small bowel obstruction
   c. systemic lupus erythematosus
   d. gonococcemia

111. Edema is most likely associated with:

   a. C1
   b. C1, 4
   c. "C2 kinin"
   d. C3a

112. Weak chemotactic factor is most likely associated with:

   a. C3a
   b. C1
   c. "C2 kinin"
   d. C1, 4

113. Viral neutralization is most likely associated with:

   a. C1
   b. C1, 4
   c. "C2 kinin"
   d. C3a

114. Potent anaphylatoxin is most likely associated with:

   a. C1
   b. C1, 4
   c. "C2 kinin"
   d. C3a

115. Which of the following activities is associated with C3b?

a. opsonization
b. weak anaphylatoxin
c. vasoconstriction
d. potent chemotactic factor

116. Which of the following activities is associated with C3b?

a. vasoconstriction
b. lysis
c. bone marrow neutrophil release
d. macrophage migration inhibition factor

117. Which of the following activities is associated with C5a?

a. opsonization
b. vasoconstriction
c. potent chemotactic factor
d. bone marrow neutrophil

118. Infantile X-linked agammaglobulinemia is referred to as:

a. Bruton's agammaglobulinemia
b. DiGeorge syndrome
c. Swiss-type agammaglobulinemia
d. ataxia telangiectasia

119. Immunodeficiency with thrombocytopenia and eczema is often referred to as:

a. DiGeorge syndrome
b. Bruton's agammaglobulinemia
c. ataxia telangiectasia
d. Wiskott-Aldrich syndrome

120. Severe combined immunodeficiency disease is referred to as:

a. Bruton's agammaglobulinemia
b. Swiss-type agammaglobulinemia
c. DiGeorge syndrome
d. Wiskott-Aldrich syndrome

121. Combined immunodeficiency disease with loss of muscle coordination is referred to as:

  a. DiGeorge syndrome
  b. Bruton's agammaglobulinemia
  c. ataxia telangiectasia
  d. Wiskott-Aldrich syndrome

122. A transfusion reaction will activate which of the following immunopathologic mechanisms?

  a. reaginic sensitivity
  b. Arthus reaction
  c. delayed hypersensitivity
  d. complement-dependent antibody cytotoxicity

123. High titers of anti-mitochondrial antibodies may be found in:

  a. rheumatoid arthritis
  b. systemic lupus erythematosus
  c. biliary cirrhosis
  d. acute hepatitis

124. High titers of anti-microsomal antibodies are most often found in:

  a. rheumatoid arthritis
  b. systemic lupus erythematosus
  c. chronic hepatitis
  d. thyroid disease

125. Active systemic lupus erythematosus patients often have which of the following test results?

  a. high titers of anti-microsomal antibodies
  b. high titers of anti-smooth muscle antibodies
  c. marked decrease in serum CH50
  d. decreased serum immunoglobulin levels

126. Systemic lupus erythematosus patients often have which of the following test results?

  a. high titers of DNA antibody
  b. decreased serum immunoglobulin levels
  c. high titers of anti-smooth muscle antibodies
  d. high titers of anti-mitochondria antibody

127. High titers of anti-smooth muscle antibodies are found most often in:

a. systemic lupus erythematosus
b. rheumatoid arthritis
c. chronic active hepatitis
d. celiac disease

128. Which of the following patterns obtained by a fluorescent antinuclear antibody (ANA) test best corresponds to a low serum CH50 level and a high level of anti-nDNA?

a. speckled pattern
b. rim pattern
c. diffuse pattern
d. nucleolar pattern

129. Anti-RNA antibodies are often present in individuals having an antinuclear antibody immunofluorescent pattern which is:

a. speckled
b. rim
c. diffuse
d. nucleolar

130. Anti-extractable nuclear antigens are most likely associated with which of the following antinuclear antibody immunofluorescent patterns?

a. speckled
b. rim
c. diffuse
d. nucleolar

131. Celiac disease is often characterized by an increase in:

a. anti-reticulin antibody
b. anti-prickle cell desmosome antibody
c. anti-smooth muscle antibody
d. anti-glomerular basement antibody

132. Anti-prickle cell desmosome antibody is most often associated with:

a. celiac disease
b. pemphigus vulgaris
c. Goodpasture's syndrome
d. chronic active hepatitis

133. Anti-glomerular basement membrane antibody is most often associated with:

   a. systemic lupus erythematosus
   b. celiac disease
   c. chronic active hepatitis
   d. Goodpasture's disease

134. Bence Jones protein consists of:

   a. immunoglobulin catabolic fragments in the urine
   b. monoclonal light chains synthesized _de novo_
   c. any light chains in the urine
   d. Fab fragments of a monoclonal protein

135. Monoclonal IgD proteins are unusual in that they are:

   a. mostly lambda type and associated with Bence Jones proteinuria
   b. mostly lambda type and rarely associated with Bence Jones proteinuria
   c. mostly kappa type and associated with Bence Jones proteinuria
   d. highly resistant to enzymatic fragmentation

136. A patient's serum IgA as measured by radial immunodiffusion was 40 mg/dL. Another laboratory reported absent IgA. A possible explanation for this discrepancy is:

   a. rabbit antiserum was used in the RID plates
   b. the IgA has an Fc deletion
   c. the IgA antiserum has kappa specificity
   d. the serum has antibodies against a protein in the antiserum

137. A patient with a known hereditary deficiency of complement develops generalized urticaria each time he takes a shower. The most likely explanation is that the patient lacks:

   a. C1 esterase inhibitor and is overproducing "C2 kinin"
   b. C3b inactivator and is overproducing "C2 kinin"
   c. C3b inactivator and is overproducing C3a
   d. C4b inactivator and is overproducing C3a

138. Which of the following monoclonal proteins is most commonly associated with non-Hodgkin's lymphoma?

a. IgA
b. IgD
c. IgE
d. IgM

139. In the urine of a patient with serum monoclonal IgG lambda, the Bence Jones protein usually is:

a. nonreactive to Fab-specific antisera; has the same electrophoretic mobility as the IgG lambda
b. reactive to Fc-specific antisera; has a different electrophoretic mobility from the IgG lambda
c. reactive to lambda antisera; has a different electrophoretic mobility from the IgG lambda
d. reactive to kappa antisera; has a different electrophoretic mobility from the IgG lambda

140. Deficiency of which of the following immunoglobulins is known to have produced anaphylactic reactions following blood transfusion?

a. IgA
b. IgD
c. IgE
d. IgG

141. The pathogenesis of common variable immunodeficiency is most likely due to:

a. absence of B cells
b. decreased helper activity
c. increased suppressor cell activity
d. inappropriate antigen presentation by macrophages

142. The latex agglutination titer commonly considered as the lower limit of positivity for a diagnostic criterion of rheumatoid arthritis is:

a. 1:2
b. 1:40
c. 1:160
d. 1:640

143. A 16-year-old boy with infectious mononucleosis has a cold agglutinin titer of 1:2,000. An important consideration of this antibody's clinical relevance is the:

a. thermal range
b. titer at 4°C
c. specificity
d. light chain type

144. A serologic test for syphilis (STS) that depends upon the detection of cardiolipin-lecithin-cholesterol antigen is:

a. treponemal antibody absorption (FTA-ABS)
b. rapid plasma reagin (RPR)
c. Treponema pallidum hemagglutination assay (TPHA)
d. Treponema pallidum immobilization (TPI)

145. In the FTA-ABS test, the presence of a beaded pattern of fluorescence along the treponeme indicates:

a. positive identification of Treponema pallidum
b. presumptive diagnosis of active syphilis
c. presence of nontreponemal antibody (NTA)
d. false-positive reaction

146. The serologic test for syphilis that is easy to perform, can be interpreted objectively, and is recommended as a confirmatory test for the diagnosis of secondary or late-stage syphilis is:

a. VDRL
b. TPI
c. FTA-ABS
d. MHA-TP

147. The most important use of a nontreponemal antibody (NTA) test alone is in:

a. establishing the diagnosis of acute active syphilis
b. establishing the diagnosis of chronic syphilis
c. evaluating the success of therapy
d. determining the prevalence of disease in the general population

148. The serologic test for syphilis recommended for detecting antibody in cerebrospinal fluid is:

a. NTA
b. TPI
c. FTA-ABS
d. TPHA

149. The initial immune response following fetal infection with rubella is the production of:

a. IgG antibody
b. IgA antibody
c. IgM antibody
d. both IgG and IgA antibody

150. The serologic test for rubella that is most apt to produce a false-positive result due to the presence of nonspecific serum inhibitors is:

a. complement fixation
b. hemagglutination inhibition
c. immunofluorescence
d. hemolysis-in-gel

151. The serologic test that can be modified to selectively detect only specific IgM antibody is:

a. complement fixation
b. immunofluorescence
c. hemagglutination inhibition
d. passive hemagglutination

152. Within one week after exposure to rash illness, a maternal serum hemagglutination inhibition titer that is equal to or greater than 1:8 indicates:

a. immunity to rubella
b. evidence of acute rubella infection
c. susceptibility to rubella infection
d. absence of acute rubella

153. Which IgG subclass is most efficient at crossing the placenta?

a. IgG1
b. IgG2
c. IgG3
d. Each is equally efficient

154. Areas of the immunoglobulin molecule that are referred to as "domains" are:

   a. formed by intrachain disulfide bonds
   b. formed by interchain disulfide bonds
   c. used for classification of molecules
   d. insignificant

155. The area of the immunoglobulin molecule referred to as the "hinge" region is located between which domains?

   a. VH and VL
   b. CH1 and CH2
   c. CH2 and CH3
   d. CH3 and VL

156. Which class of immunoglobulin is thought to function as an antigenic receptor site on the surface of immature B lymphocytes?

   a. IgD
   b. IgM
   c. IgA
   d. IgG

157. Each of the following complement proteins is involved in the alternative pathway <u>EXCEPT</u>:

   a. C2
   b. C5
   c. C7
   d. C8

158. The biologic activities of complement components include each of the following <u>EXCEPT</u>:

   a. chemotaxis
   b. immune adherence
   c. placental transfer
   d. anaphylatoxin activity

159. Which of the following does <u>NOT</u> activate the classical complement pathway?

   a. IgG1
   b. IgG2
   c. IgG3
   d. IgG4

160. Characteristics of the IgG class of immunoglobulins include each of the following EXCEPT:

a. it is the most abundant immunoglobulin in the body fluids
b. it is the first immunoglobulin produced by the fetus
c. it has the ability to cross the placenta
d. it is the primary immunoglobulin involved in secondary immunization

161. Which of the following is the "recognition unit" in the classical complement pathway?

a. C1
b. C3
c. C4, C2, C3
d. C5, C6, C7, C8, C9

162. Which of the following is the "activation unit" in the classical complement pathway?

a. C1
b. C3
c. C4, C2, C3
d. C5, C6, C7, C8, C9

163. Which of the following is the "membrane attack unit" in the clinical complement pathway?

a. C1
b. C3
c. C4, C2, C3
d. C5, C6, C7, C8, C9

164. Increasing the amount of antigen in a hemagglutination reaction, while keeping the amount of antibody constant, would:

1. increase the amount of antigen-antibody complex formed
2. decrease the value of K (the equilibrium constant of the reaction) according to the law of mass action
3. decrease the number of antibody molecules attached to each cell
4. increase the sensitivity of the agglutination phase of the reaction

a. only 1, 2 and 3 are correct
b. only 1 and 3 are correct
c. only 2 and 4 are correct
d. only 4 is correct
e. all are correct

165. A functional deficiency of C1-esterase inhibitors is seen in:

a. severe rheumatoid arthritis
b. hereditary angioneurotic edema
c. systemic lupus erythematosus
d. chronic alcoholic cirrhosis

166. Patients suffering from Waldenström's macroglobulinemia demonstrate excessively increased concentrations of which of the following?

a. IgG
b. IgA
c. IgM
d. IgD

167. The presence of Hb_sAg, anti-HB_c, and often Hb_eAg is characteristic of:

a. early acute phase HBV
b. early convalescent phase HBV
c. recovery phase of acute phase HBV
d. carrier state of acute HBV

168. The disappearance of HB_sAg and HB_eAg, the persistence of anti-HB_c, the appearance of anti-HB_s, and often of anti-HB_e indicate:

a. early acute phase HBV
b. early convalescent phase HBV
c. recovery phase of acute phase HVB
d. carrier state of acute HBV

169. The immunoglobulin class typically found to be present in saliva, tears, and other secretions is:

a. IgG
b. IgA
c. IgM
d. IgD

170. The immunoglobulin class which passes easily through the placenta is:

a. IgG
b. IgA
c. IgM
d. IgD

For question 171, refer to the illustration below:

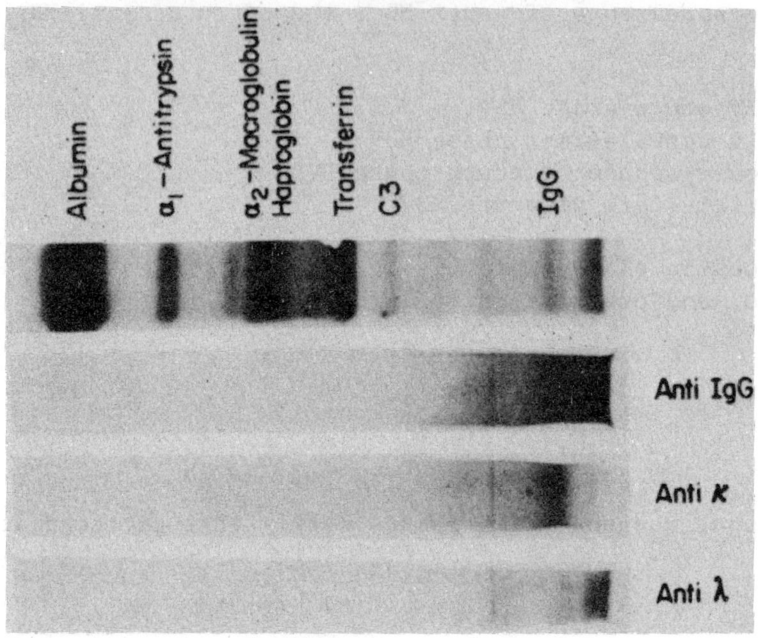

171. The immunofixation (IFE) pattern above demonstrates:

   a. monoclonal IgG kappa
   b. polyclonal IgG
   c. two monoclonal proteins, IgG kappa and IgG lambda
   d. monoclonal IgG lambda

---

172. The immunoglobulin class associated with hypersensitivity or allergenic reactions is:

   a. IgA
   b. IgM
   c. IgD
   d. IgE

173. A single and reliable screening test for detecting neonatal infection in the absence of clinical signs is:

   a. serum immunoelectrophoresis
   b. differential leukocyte count
   c. nitroblue tetrazolium (NBT) test
   d. quantitative serum IgM determination

For question 174, refer to the illustration below:

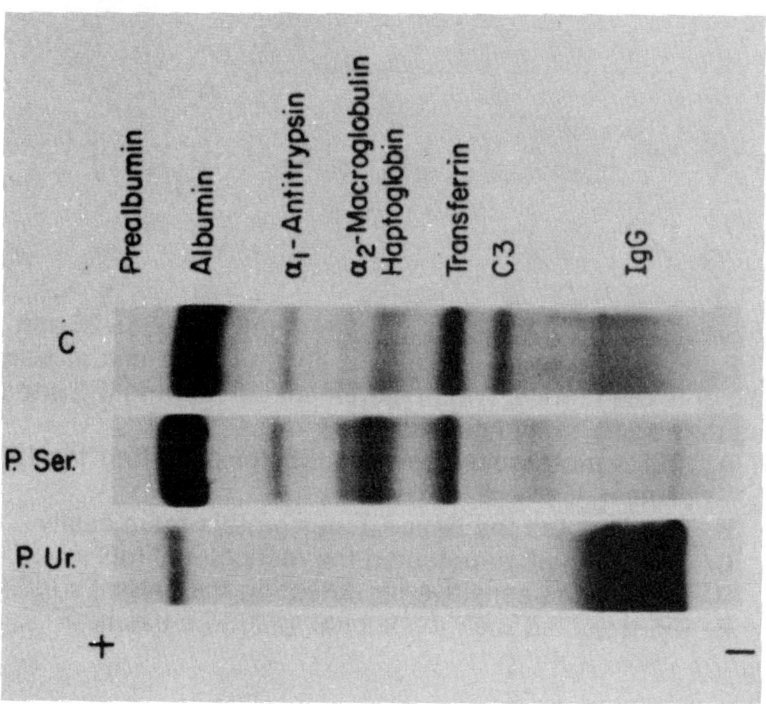

174. The large urinary protein band has a large anodal shoulder. What is the most probable reason for this observation?

a. The protein represents polyclonal light chains.

b. The protein is Bence Jones protein partially altered by enzymatic digestion.

c. The protein is Fc and Fab fragments of serum IgG.

d. The protein is Fc and pFc fragments of serum IgG.

For questions 175 and 176, refer to the illustration below:

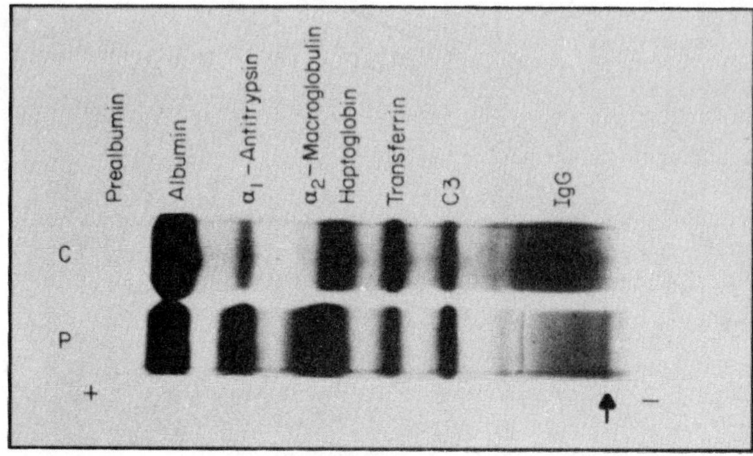

175. The patient is a 9-year-old girl with pancytopenia and an elevated sedimentation rate. The band indicated by the arrow is most likely:

   a. lysozyme
   b. monoclonal IgA
   c. C-reactive protein
   d. monoclonal light chains

176. The electrophoretic pattern above is described as:

   a. acute-phase reaction pattern
   b. iron-deficiency anemia pattern
   c. monoclonal gammopathy pattern
   d. immune deficiency pattern

For questions 177 and 178, refer to the illustration below:

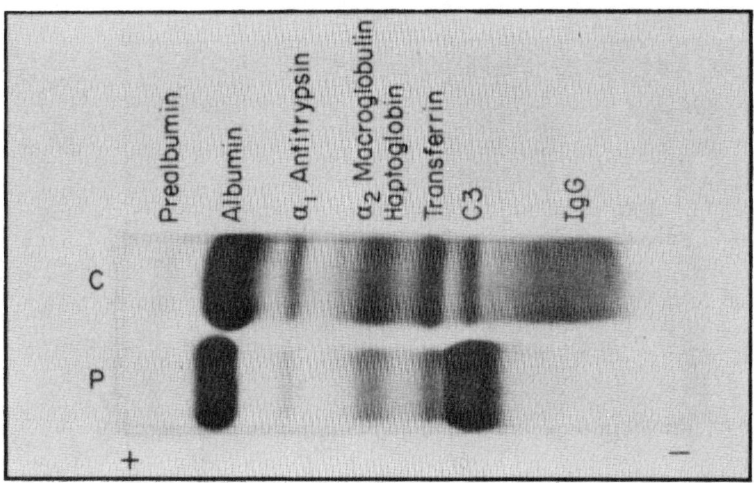

177. The pattern above is consistent with:

 a. nephrotic syndrome
 b. iron deficiency
 c. monoclonal gammopathy
 d. beta-gamma bridging

178. This pattern should be further evaluated by:

 a. serum immunofixation studies
 b. serum ultracentrifugation
 c. iron and total iron-binding capacity
 d. measurement of total cholesterol and triglyceride levels

For question 179, refer to the illustration below:

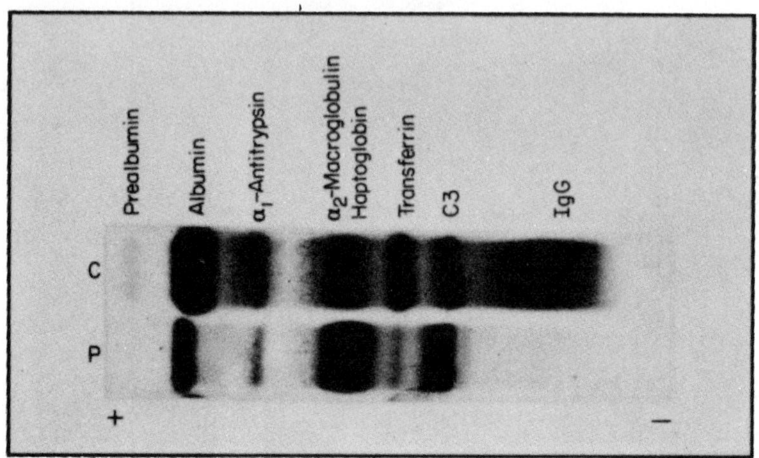

179. The serum (P) was obtained from a 4-year-old boy with proteinuria (4+). This pattern is consistent with:

   a. nephrotic syndrome
   b. tubular pattern
   c. prerenal pattern
   d. monoclonal gammopathy

For question 180, refer to the illustration below:

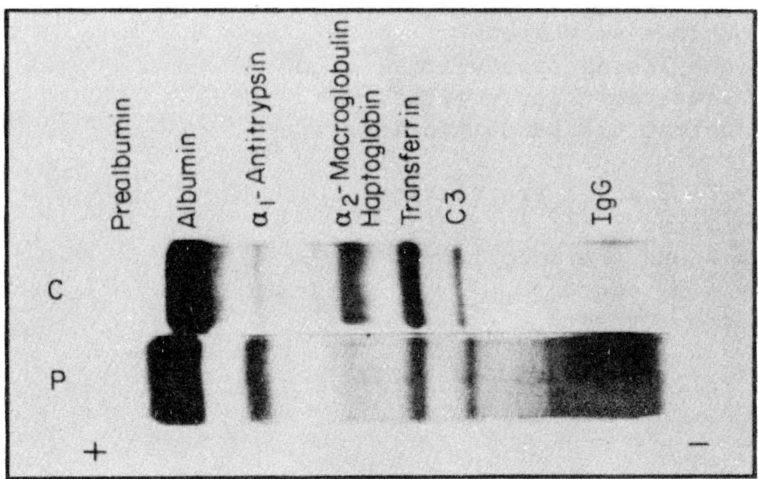

180. Based on the above pattern, what additional assay should be performed?

   a. measurement of haptoglobin level
   b. measurement of iron and iron-binding capacity
   c. phenotype alpha-1-antitrypsin
   d. measurement of total cholesterol and triglycerides

---

181. Which of the following is the major difference between a fluorescent microscope with epi-illumination and a fluorescent microscope with transmitted light?

   a. The transmitted light microscope has a barrier filter.
   b. The transmitted light microscope has an exciter filter.
   c. The transmitted light microscope uses a halogen light source.
   d. The epi-illuminated microscope has a dichroic mirror.

182. HLA-B27 antigen has been found in a high percentage of patients with:

1. Reiter's syndrome
2. ankylosing spondylitis
3. acute anterior uveitis
4. dermatitis herpetiformis

a. only 1, 2 and 3 are correct
b. only 1 and 3 are correct
c. only 2 and 4 are correct
d. only 4 is correct
e. all are correct

183. Which of the following are associated with cell mediated immunity?

1. sheep erythrocyte rosettes (E-rosettes)
2. phytohemagglutination (PHA) stimulation
3. thymic dependence
4. intrinsic surface immunoglobulins

a. only 1, 2 and 3 are correct
b. only 1 and 3 are correct
c. only 2 and 4 are correct
d. only 4 is correct
e. all are correct

184. Which of the following releases histamine and other mediators from basophils?

a. C3a
b. properdin factor B
c. C1q
d. C4

185. The Raji cell line:

a. has membrane receptors for C3b
b. is used in an assay to measure insoluble immune complexes
c. is a human T-type lymphoblastoid cell line
d. has high affinity membrane receptors for IgG-Fc

186. Charcot-Leyden crystals are usually associated with an immune response and are thought to be the breakdown products of:

   a. monocytes
   b. lymphocytes
   c. eosinophils
   d. basophils

187. Which of the following mediators is released during T cell activation?

   a. immunoglobulins
   b. thymosin
   c. serotonin
   d. lymphokines

188. Which of the following is an important marker for the presence of immature T cells in patients with leukemia and lymphomas?

   a. terminal deoxynucleotidyl transferase (TdT)
   b. adenosine deaminase
   c. glucose-6-phosphate dehydrogenase
   d. purine nucleoside phosphorylase

189. T cell lymphocytes that possess Fc receptors for aggregated IgM have been found to be specific for which of the following types of T cell functions?

   a. suppressor
   b. prosuppressor
   c. cytotoxic
   d. helper

190. Which T cell malignancy may retain "helper" activity with regard to immunoglobulin synthesis by B cells?

   a. Hodgkin's lymphoma
   b. acute lymphocytic leukemia (ALL)
   c. Sezary syndrome
   d. chronic lymphocytic leukemia (CLL)

191. Each of the following is a B lymphocyte assay technique <u>EXCEPT</u>:

   a. surface immunoglobulin determination
   b. cytoplasmic immunoglobulin determination
   c. E-rosettes
   d. EAC-rosettes

192. A patient with glomerulonephritis has a slightly decreased CH50 level, a 50% decrease in the C3 level, and normal C1, C4, and C2 levels. An immunofluorescent study of a renal biopsy from this patient may show:

1. only C3 in the deposits on the glomerular basement membrane
2. C3 and properdin in the deposits on the glomerular basement membrane
3. C3, properdin, and IgG immunoglobulin in the deposits on the glomerular basement membrane
4. C3 and IgA immunoglobulin in the deposits on the glomerular basement membrane

a. only 1, 2 and 3 are correct
b. only 1 and 3 are correct
c. only 2 and 4 are correct
d. only 4 is correct
e. all are correct

193. Immunologic surveillance of tumors is thought to be affected by:

a. B lymphocytes and T lymphocytes
b. B lymphocytes and macrophages
c. T lymphocytes and macrophages
d. macrophages and lymphokines

194. Failure to reduce nitroblue tetrazolium by polymorphonuclear leukocytes following endotoxin stimulation is found in:

a. rheumatoid arthritis
b. Staphylococcus aureus septicemia
c. DiGeorge syndrome
d. chronic granulomatous disease

195. The thymus from a patient with a severe combined T and B cell deficiency should show which of the following anatomic changes?

a. corticomedullary demarcation
b. presence of Hassall's corpuscles
c. much fatty infiltration
d. total mass greater than one gram

196. Cells from a patient with leukemic reticuloendotheliosis (hairy cell leukemia) have immunologic and functional features of:

a. mast cells and B lymphocytes
b. B lymphocytes and granulocytes
c. granulocytes and monocytes
d. B lymphocytes and monocytes

197. T cell help is required for a B cell response to:

1. purified protein derivative (PPD)
2. keyhole limpet hemocyanin
3. tetanus toxoid
4. pneumococcal polysaccharide

a. only 1, 2 and 3 are correct
b. only 1 and 3 are correct
c. only 2 and 4 are correct
d. only 4 is correct
e. all are correct

198. Which of the following cells respond best to concanavalin A?

a. T lymphocytes
b. B lymphocytes
c. macrophages
d. eosinophils

199. Sheep red blood cell rosette formation is characteristic of:

a. B lymphocytes
b. T lymphocytes
c. monocytes
d. B lymphocytes and T lymphocytes

200. C3 and Fc receptors are present on:

a. B lymphocytes
b. monocytes
c. B lymphocytes and monocytes
d. neither B lymphocytes nor monocytes

201. A 4-year-old girl has acute lymphoblastic leukemia. Her leukemia cells would most likely be:

a. B cells
b. T cells
c. null cells
d. monocytes

202. A patient demonstrating abnormal cerebriform lymphocytes, which form rosettes with sheep red blood cells, and lacks C3 receptors or surface membrane markers most likely has:

a. Hodgkin's disease
b. acute lymphocytic leukemia
c. chronic lymphocytic leukemia
d. Sezary syndrome

203. HLA-B8 antigen has been associated with which one of the following diseases?

a. ankylosing spondylitis and myasthenia gravis
b. celiac disease and ankylosing spondylitis
c. myasthenia gravis and celiac disease
d. Reiter's disease and multiple sclerosis

204. HLA-B27 antigen has been associated with which of the following diseases?

a. ankylosing spondylitis
b. myasthenia gravis
c. multiple sclerosis
d. celiac disease

205. HLA typing of a family yields the following results:

	Locus A	Locus B
Father	(8, 12)	(17, 22)
Mother	(7, 12)	(13, 27)

On the basis of these genotypes, you would predict the possibility of ankylosing spondylitis in:

a. 75% of their children
b. 50% of their children
c. 25% of their children
d. female children only

IMMUNOLOGY

206. Which of the following is an important cellular mediator of immune complex tissue injury?

    a. monocyte
    b. neutrophil
    c. basophil
    d. eosinophil

207. Rejection of transplanted organs is usually the result of:

    a. lack of immunosuppression
    b. incompatibility for minor histocompatibility antigens
    c. improper crossmatching interpretation
    d. T cell activation

208. The biologic functions of T cells include:

    1. suppression of the immune response
    2. secretion of lymphokines
    3. killer cell activity
    4. secretion of immunoglobulins

    a. only 1, 2 and 3 are correct
    b. only 1 and 3 are correct
    c. only 2 and 4 are correct
    d. only 4 is correct
    e. all are correct

209. Which of the following is a true statement about autoimmune diseases?

    a. They are associated with HLA-B and HLA-D antigens.
    b. They are B cell disorders.
    c. All autoimmune disorders are drug induced.
    d. Most autoimmune diseases are caused by viral infections.

210. Tissue injury in systemic rheumatic disorders such as systemic lupus erythematosus is thought to be caused by:

    a. selective proteinuria
    b. decreased plasma C3 levels
    c. deposition of immune complexes
    d. renal nuclear antigens

211. A homogeneous nuclear fluorescence pattern is associated with which antigen?

a. ribonucleoprotein
b. Sm antigen
c. DNA
d. deoxyribonucleoprotein

212. All of the following are true statements about the "LE cell" (lupus erythematosus cell) test EXCEPT:

a. It is a test method for detection of antinuclear antibodies (ANA).
b. LE cells are neutrophils with cytoplasmic basophilic inclusions.
c. The basophilic inclusions are nuclear fragments from disrupted cells.
d. Complement-fixing ANA disrupts certain cells by opsonization, making nuclear material available to neutrophils.

213. The indirect ANA-IFA method uses the following target substrate tissues EXCEPT:

a. human erythrocytes
b. human epithelial cells
c. rat kidney
d. mouse liver

214. Autoantibody studies to detect different antinuclear antibodies:

a. include RIA techniques to measure antibodies to single- and double-stranded DNA
b. give precise diagnostic information associated with the pattern of nuclear fluorescence
c. are always negative in patients with no evidence of disease
d. do not include the ANA-IFA test; they must be differentiated by using other special test substrates, such as the Wil_2 lymphoblastoid cell line

215. Incompatibility by which of the following procedures is an absolute contraindication to allotransplantation?

a. mixed lymphocyte culture
b. HLA typing
c. Rh typing
d. ABO typing

216. Mixed lymphocyte culture (MLC) can be used effectively for:

1. selecting donors for organ allotransplantation
2. predicting graft-vs-host reaction in bone marrow transplantation
3. diagnosing immunodeficiency syndromes affecting T lymphocytes
4. detecting tolerance after allotransplantation

a. only 1, 2 and 3 are correct
b. only 1 and 3 are correct
c. only 2 and 4 are correct
d. only 4 is correct
e. all are correct

217. Serum alpha-fetoprotein levels may be elevated in patients with which of the following disorders?

1. hepatocellular carcinoma
2. embryonal cell carcinoma
3. viral hepatitis
4. chronic active hepatitis

a. only 1, 2 and 3 are correct
b. only 1 and 3 are correct
c. only 2 and 4 are correct
d. only 4 is correct
e. all are correct

218. Carcinoembryonic antigen levels may be elevated in the serum of patients with which of the following disorders?

1. severe alcoholic cirrhosis of the liver
2. ulcerative colitis
3. adenocarcinoma of the sigmoid colon
4. embryonal carcinoma of the testes

a. only 1, 2 and 3 are correct
b. only 1 and 3 are correct
c. only 2 and 4 are correct
d. only 4 is correct
e. all are correct

219. A 28-year-old man is seen by a physician because of several months of intermittent low back pain and the acute onset of right swelling and conjunctivitis. Laboratory studies would be likely to show:

   a. a decreased synovial fluid CH50 level
   b. low serum CH50 level
   c. positive HLA-B27 antigen test
   d. rheumatoid factor in the synovial fluid

220. A true statement about antithyroid antibodies is:

   a. they may be directed against thyroglobulin or microsomal antigens
   b. their titers are reliable in children with suspected thyroiditis
   c. they are rarely present in patients with Grave's disease
   d. they are rarely present in patients with parietal cell antibodies

221. Which of the following lymphoproliferative disorders is often associated with autoimmune phenomenon and hypergamma-globulinemia?

   a. Burkitt's lymphoma
   b. immunoblastic lymphadenopathy
   c. acute lymphoblastic leukemia
   d. histiocytic lymphoma

222. For several months a 31-year-old woman has had migratory polyarthritis and a skin rash. Upon admission to the hospital, the following laboratory data were obtained:

	Patient	Normal
Leukocyte count	4.7	5.0-10.0
Differential	Normal	
Serum hemolytic complement	Less than 22U	80-150U
C3 (by RID)	117U	96-148U
C4 (by RID)	31U	24- 40U
ANA (1:10 dilution)	Positive in a homogenous pattern	
Rheumatoid factor test	Negative	
Urinalysis	Protein 1+; occasional RBC's	

This patient's test results are consistent with:

a. dermatomyositis
b. C2 deficiency
c. systemic lupus erythematosus
d. mixed connective tissue disease

223. Immunologic enhancement of tumors and renal allografts is thought to be mediated by:

a. T lymphocytes
b. antibodies and antigen-antibody complexes
c. B lymphocytes
d. C3 and C5

224. A procedure for the detection of circulating immune complexes in human sera uses Raji cells which are:

a. thymic lymphocytes
b. B cells from a patient with Burkitt's lymphoma
c. peritoneal macrophages
d. polymorphonuclear neutrophils

225. Which of the following terms describes a graft between genetically unidentical individuals?

a. autograft
b. isograft
c. allograft
d. xenograft

226. In pernicious anemia, which of the following antibodies is detected?

a. anti-mitochondrial
b. anti-smooth muscle
c. anti-DNA
d. anti-parietal cell

227. In primary biliary cirrhosis, which of the following antibodies is seen in high titers?

a. anti-mitochondrial
b. anti-smooth muscle
c. anti-DNA
d. anti-parietal cell

228. In chronic active hepatitis, titers greater than 1:100 of which of the following antibodies are seen?

a. anti-mitochondrial
b. anti-smooth muscle
c. anti-DNA
d. anti-parietal cell

229. In the indirect antinuclear antibody test, a homogeneous pattern indicates the presence of antibody to:

a. cryoglobulin
b. Sm
c. RNA
d. DNA

230. In the indirect antinuclear antibody test, a speckled pattern indicates the presence of antibody to:

a. cryoglobulin
b. Sm
c. RNA
d. DNA

231. Reaginic sensitivity is most commonly associated with:

a. transfusion reaction
b. anaphylactic reaction
c. contact sensitivity to inorganic chemicals
d. bacterial septicemia

232. Delayed hypersensitivity is related to:

a. contact sensitivity to inorganic chemicals
b. transfusion reaction
c. anaphylactic reaction
d. bacterial septicemia

233. Decreased delayed hypersensitivity measured by skin testing is seen commonly in each of the following <u>EXCEPT</u>:

a. Hodgkin's disease
b. sarcoidosis
c. Wiskott-Aldrich syndrome
d. children between one and two years of age

234. Increased concentrations of alpha-fetoprotein (AFP) in adults are most characteristically associated with:

a. hepatocellular carcinoma
b. alcoholic cirrhosis
c. chronic active hepatitis
d. multiple myeloma

235. Which of the following is used to detect anti-allergen IgE?

a. RIA
b. IEP
c. RAST
d. CRP

236. The leukocyte histamine release test is useful in detecting:

a. eosinophilic chemotactic factor
b. slow reacting substance
c. cellular cytotoxicity
d. anti-allergen IgE

237. In skin tests for allergy, a wheal and flare development is indicative of:

a. immediate sensitivity
b. delayed hypersensitivity
c. anergy
d. Arthus reaction

Immunology Answer Key

1. d
2. a
3. c
4. b
5. d
6. c
7. d
8. c
9. c
10. b
11. c
12. b
13. a
14. d
15. a
16. d
17. c
18. c
19. e
20. a
21. e
22. e
23. b
24. a
25. c
26. d
27. d
28. d
29. a
30. d
31. d
32. a
33. b
34. c
35. b
36. c
37. c
38. d
39. a
40. b
41. c
42. c
43. b
44. a
45. a
46. c
47. a
48. d
49. c
50. b
51. d
52. e
53. c
54. d
55. e
56. c
57. d
58. d
59. c
60. e
61. d
62. a
63. b
64. b
65. e
66. a
67. b
68. c
69. a
70. e
71. b
72. d
73. a
74. b
75. c
76. b
77. c
78. b
79. c
80. a
81. d
82. c
83. a
84. d
85. b
86. b
87. a
88. c
89. d
90. b
91. e
92. b
93. c
94. e
95. b
96. c
97. b
98. c
99. a
100. a
101. c
102. b
103. d
104. a
105. a
106. c
107. d
108. c
109. a
110. d
111. c
112. a
113. b
114. d
115. a
116. c
117. c
118. a
119. d
120. b
121. c
122. d
123. c
124. d
125. c
126. a
127. c
128. b
129. d
130. a
131. a
132. b
133. d
134. b
135. a
136. d
137. a
138. d
139. c
140. a
141. c
142. c
143. a
144. b
145. d
146. d
147. c
148. b
149. c
150. b
151. b
152. a
153. a
154. a
155. b
156. b
157. a
158. c
159. d
160. b
161. a
162. c
163. d
164. a
165. b
166. c
167. a
168. c
169. b
170. a
171. c
172. d
173. d
174. b
175. c
176. a
177. c
178. a
179. a
180. a
181. d
182. a
183. a
184. a
185. a
186. c
187. d
188. a

Immunology Answer Key (continued)

189. d
190. c
191. c
192. a
193. c
194. d
195. c
196. d
197. a
198. a
199. b
200. c
201. c
202. d
203. c
204. a
205. c
206. b
207. d
208. a
209. a
210. c
211. d
212. d
213. a
214. a
215. d
216. e
217. e
218. a
219. c
220. a
221. b
222. b
223. b
224. b
225. c
226. d
227. a
228. b
229. d
230. b
231. b
232. a
233. d
234. a
235. c
236. d
237. a

CHAPTER 15

Body Fluids/Urinalysis

1. On bright-light microscopic examination of a urinary sediment, round refractile globules are noted in cells encapsulated within a hyaline matrix. The technologist suspects the globules are lipid-laden renal tubular cells. Of the following types of microscopy, the one that will be MOST helpful in the definitive identification of this urinary structure is:

   a. phase-contrast
   b. immunofluorescent
   c. interference-contrast
   d. polarized-light

2. Which of the following would be affected by allowing a urine specimen to remain at room temperature for three hours before analysis?

   a. occult blood
   b. specific gravity
   c. pH
   d. protein

3. A 4-year-old girl has edema that is most obvious in her eyelids. Laboratory studies reveal:

Serum albumin	1.8 g/dL (385 µmol/L)
Serum cholesterol	450 mg/dL (11.7 mmol/L)
Serum urea nitrogen	20 mg/dL (7.1 mmol/L)
Urinalysis	Protein 4+; hyaline, granular, and fatty casts

   This is most compatible with:

   a. acute poststreptococcal glomerulonephritis
   b. minimal change glomerular disease
   c. acute pyelonephritis
   d. diabetes mellitus

4. Which of the following urinary parameters are measured during the course of concentration and dilution tests to assess renal tubular function?

   a. urea nitrogen and creatinine
   b. osmolality and specific gravity
   c. sodium and chloride
   d. sodium and osmolality

For questions 5 and 6, refer to the following illustration:

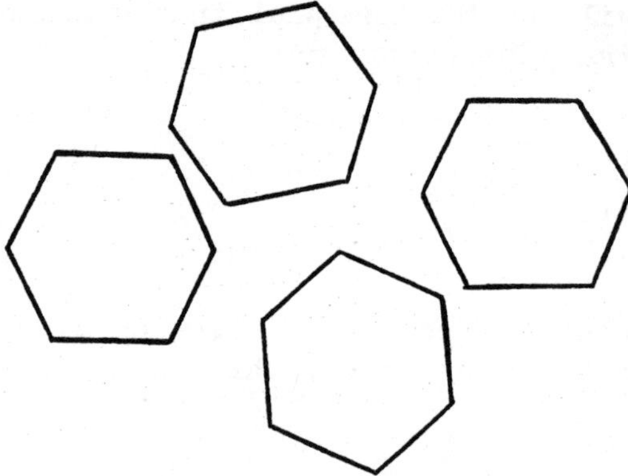

5. Colorless crystals, such as those depicted above, were seen in a urine specimen. This patient is most likely to have which of the following clinical conditions?

   a. gout
   b. renal damage
   c. bilirubinuria
   d. cystinosis

6. The colorless crystals depicted above would be found in a urine which has a(n):

   a. acid pH
   b. alkaline pH
   c. neutral pH
   d. variable pH

7. The part of the kidney in which there is selective retention and excretion of various substances and in which the concentration of urine occurs is the:

   a. glomerulus
   b. papilla
   c. tubule
   d. ureter

8. On bright-light microscopic examination of a urinary sediment, round refractile globules are noted in cells encapsulated within a hyaline matrix. A polarized-light microscopic examination of the urinary structure showed the globules to be birefringent in the shape of Maltese crosses. These urinary structures can be identified as:

   a. waxy casts associated with advanced tubular atrophy
   b. granular casts containing plasma protein aggregates
   c. crystal casts associated with obstruction due to tubular damage
   d. fatty casts containing lipid-laden renal tubular cells

9. A urinalysis performed on a 27-year-old woman yields the following results:

Reagent Strip Analysis		Microscopic	
Specific gravity	1.008	WBC/HPF	20-30
pH	5.0	RBC/HPF	30-55
Protein	2+	Casts/LPF	
Glucose	negative	Hyaline	5-7
Ketones	negative	RBC	0-2
Bilirubin	negative	Epithelial	1-3
Blood	3+	Coarse granular	2-3
Nitrite	negative	Waxy	1-3
Leukocyte	positive	Uric acid crystals	moderate
Urobilinogen	0.1 Ehrlich units/dL		

The above are MOST consistent with:

   a. yeast infections
   b. pyelonephritis
   c. bacterial cystitis
   d. glomerulonephritis

10. A urinalysis performed on a 27-year-old woman yields the following results:

Reagent Strip Analysis	
Specific Gravity	1.008
pH	5.0
Protein	2+
Glucose	negative
Ketones	negative
Bilirubin	negative
Blood	3+
Nitrite	negative
Leukocyte	positive
Urobilinogen	0.1 Ehrlich units/dL

Microscopic	
WBC/HPF	20-30
RBC/HPF	30-55
Casts/LPF	
Hyaline	5-7
RBC	0-2
Epithelial	1-3
Coarse granular	2-3
Waxy	1-3
Uric acid crystals	moderate

The above data are consistent with:

a. a vegetarian diet
b. gout
c. biliary obstruction
d. chronic renal disease

11. The following results were obtained on an unpreserved urine specimen at 8:00 a.m.:

pH	5.5
Protein	2+
Glucose	3+
Ketones	3+
Blood	negative
Bilirubin	positive
Nitrite	positive

If this specimen is reanalyzed at 3:00 p.m., which of the following results is most apt to be changed by exposure to light?

a. pH
b. protein
c. ketones
d. bilirubin

12. Urinalysis testing is performed on a urine specimen which was left at 25°C for eight hours prior to testing. If bacteria are seen in the microscopic analysis, which of the following test results will most likely be inaccurate?

    a. protein
    b. glucose
    c. blood
    d. nitrite

13. A urine specimen comes to the laboratory seven hours after it is obtained. It is acceptable for culture only if the specimen has been stored:

    a. at room temperature
    b. at 4-7°C
    c. frozen
    d. with a preservative additive

14. The following results were obtained on a urine specimen at 8:00 a.m.

pH	5.5
Protein	2+
Glucose	3+
Ketones	3+
Blood	negative
Bilirubin	positive
Nitrite	positive

    If this urine specimen was stored uncapped at 5°C without preservation and retested at 2 p.m., which of the following test results would be changed due to these storage conditions?

    a. glucose
    b. ketones
    c. protein
    d. nitrite

15. A urine specimen contaminated with bacteria is left standing unrefrigerated for seven hours. If this specimen was not preserved, which of the following tests will be most accurate?

    a. pH
    b. leukocyte esterase
    c. urobilinogen
    d. glucose

16. While performing a urinalysis, a technologist notices the urine specimen to have a fruity odor. This patient's urine most likely contains:

    a. acetone
    b. bilirubin
    c. coliform bacilli
    d. porphyrin

17. The pH of a urine specimen measures the:

    a. free sodium ions
    b. free hydrogen ions
    c. total acid excretion
    d. volatile acids

18. Some regional and public health laboratories carry out mass screening tests on the urine of newborns for a genetic disorder involving metabolism of:

    a. fructose
    b. galactose
    c. glucose
    d. lactose

19. Ketones in urine are due to:

    a. complete utilization of fatty acids
    b. faulty fat metabolism
    c. high carbohydrate diets
    d. renal tubular dysfunction

20. A test area of a urine reagent strip is impregnated with buffered sodium nitroprusside. This section will react with:

    a. acetoacetic (diacetic) acid
    b. acetone
    c. beta-hydroxybutyric acid

21. Myoglobinuria is <u>MOST</u> likely to be noted in urine specimens from patients with which of the following disorders?

    a. hemolytic anemias
    b. lower urinary tract infections
    c. myocardial infarctions
    d. paroxysmal nocturnal hemoglobinuria

22. A reagent strip area impregnated with stabilized, diazotized 2,4-dichloroaniline will yield a positive reaction with:

    a. bilirubin
    b. hemoglobin
    c. ketones
    d. urobilinogen

23. A patient with multiple myeloma collects a specimen for urinalysis immediately after having IVP radiologic studies. Which of the following is the method of choice for performing a protein screening test?

    a. reagent strip
    b. sulfosalicylic acid
    c. heat and acetic acid
    d. protein electrophoresis

24. All casts typically contain:

    a. albumin
    b. globulin
    c. immunoglobulins G and M
    d. Tamm-Horsfall glycoprotein

25. Round refractile globules noted on bright-light microscopy of a urinary sediment were birefringent with polarized light and appeared as perfect Maltese crosses. Of the following, these urinary globules are MOST likely:

    a. neutral fats
    b. starch
    c. triglycerides
    d. cholesterol

26. The presence of leukocytes in urine is known as:

    a. chyluria
    b. hematuria
    c. leukocytosis
    d. pyuria

27. Chronic progressive renal failure most likely would be associated with:

    a. an absence of urine
    b. a normal urine volume
    c. oliguria
    d. a daily excretion of approximately 3,000 mL of urine

28. The amber yellow color of urine is primarily due to:

    a. the pigment urochrome
    b. methemoglobin
    c. bilirubin
    d. homogenistic acid

29. An ammonia-like odor is characteristically associated with urines from patients who:

    a. are diabetic
    b. have hepatitis
    c. have an infection with _Proteus_ sp.
    d. have an infection with yeast

30. A urinalysis performed on a 2-week-old infant with diarrhea shows a negative reaction with the glucose oxidase reagent strip. A copper reduction tablet test should be performed to check the urine sample for the presence of:

    a. glucose
    b. galactose
    c. bilirubin
    d. ketones

31. Routine screening of urine samples for glycosuria is performed primarily to detect:

    a. glucose
    b. galactose
    c. bilirubin
    d. ketones

32. Which of the following factors will _NOT_ interfere with the reagent strip test for leukocytes?

    a. ascorbic acid
    b. formaldehyde
    c. nitrite
    d. urinary protein level of 300 mg/dL

33. While performing an analysis of a baby's urine, the technologist notices the specimen has a "mousy" odor. Of the following substances that may be excreted in urine, the one that MOST characteristically produces this odor is:

    a. phenylketone
    b. acetone
    c. coliform bacilli
    d. porphyrin

34. Hyaline casts are usually found:

    a. in the center of the coverslip
    b. under subdued light
    c. under very bright light
    d. in the supernatant

35. Which of the following can cause the kidney to be unable to concentrate and/or dilute urine?

    a. radiographic dyes
    b. exercise
    c. diabetes mellitus
    d. hormone deficiency

36. A technologist is having trouble differentiating between red blood cells, oil droplets, and yeast cells on a urine microscopy. Acetic acid should be added to the sediment to:

    a. lyse the yeast cells
    b. lyse the red blood cells
    c. dissolve the oil droplets
    d. crenate the red blood cells

37. A patient's urinalysis revealed a positive bilirubin and a decreased urobilinogen level. These results are associated with:

    a. hemolytic disease
    b. biliary obstruction
    c. hepatic disease
    d. urinary tract infection

38. Isothenuria is associated with a specific gravity which is usually:

    a. variable between 1.001 and 1.008
    b. variable between 1.015 and 1.022
    c. fixed around 1.010
    d. fixed around 1.020

39. Red-colored urine may be due to:

    a. bilirubin
    b. excess urobilin
    c. myoglobin
    d. homogenistic acid

40. A microscopic examination of a urine sediment reveals ghost cells. These red blood cells were most likely lysed due to:

    a. greater than 2% glucose concentrations
    b. specific gravity less than 1.007
    c. large amounts of ketone bodies
    d. neutral pH

41. Glycosuria testing typically is done by:

    a. yeast fermentation and glucose oxidase
    b. glucose oxidase and copper reduction
    c. chromatography and copper reduction
    d. copper reduction and yeast fermentation

42. A two-hour-old urine specimen submitted for routine urinalysis and culture yielded the following results:

pH	7.5
Specific gravity	1.008
Nitrite	negative
Culture	_Streptococcus faecalis_

Factors that may account for the negative nitrite result include:

1. pH of the urine
2. species of bacteria
3. specific gravity
4. retention time in the bladder

    a. only 1, 2 and 3 are correct
    b. only 1 and 3 are correct
    c. only 2 and 4 are correct
    d. only 4 is correct
    e. all are correct

43. Groups of people considered to be high-risk for urinary tract infections include:

    1. diabetic patients
    2. young girls
    3. pregnant women
    4. male athletes

    a. only 1, 2 and 3 are correct
    b. only 1 and 3 are correct
    c. only 2 and 4 are correct
    d. only 4 is correct
    e. all are correct

44. In which of the following conditions may ketonuria be seen?

    1. anorexia
    2. starvation
    3. cachexia
    4. diabetes mellitus

    a. only 1, 2 and 3 are correct
    b. only 1 and 3 are correct
    c. only 2 and 4 are correct
    d. only 4 is correct
    e. all are correct

45. Urinary casts can be detected using which of the following types of microscopy?

    1. polarized-light
    2. phase-contrast
    3. interference-contrast
    4. bright-light

    a. only 1, 2 and 3 are correct
    b. only 1 and 3 are correct
    c. only 2 and 4 are correct
    d. only 4 is correct
    e. all are correct

46. False results in urobilinogen testing may occur if the urine specimen is:

    1. exposed to light
    2. adjusted to a neutral pH
    3. stored at room temperature
    4. collected in a nonsterile container

    a. only 1, 2 and 3 are correct
    b. only 1 and 3 are correct
    c. only 2 and 4 are correct
    d. only 4 is correct
    e. all are correct

47. Using polarized-light microscopy, which of the following urinary elements are birefringent?

    1. cholesterol
    2. triglycerides
    3. phospholipids
    4. neutral fats

    a. only 1, 2 and 3 are correct
    b. only 1 and 3 are correct
    c. only 2 and 4 are correct
    d. only 4 is correct
    e. all are correct

48. An antidiuretic hormone deficiency is associated with a:

    a. specific gravity around 1.031
    b. low specific gravity
    c. high specific gravity
    d. variable specific gravity

49. A standard water-load dilution test is performed on a patient. A specific gravity measurement made on the urine specimen at 18.6°C using the refractometer method is 1.012. A reagent strip analysis of the specimen includes the following:

pH	8.0
Glucose	1 g/dL
Protein	1 g/dL

Correction factors that must be considered before reporting the specific gravity results include a correction for:

1. temperature
2. glucose
3. pH
4. protein

a. only 1, 2 and 3 are correct
b. only 1 and 3 are correct
c. only 2 and 4 are correct
d. only 4 is correct
e. all are correct

50. Which of the following cells may be seen in the urinary sediment as a result of vaginal contamination?

a. squamous epithelial cells
b. renal tubular cells
c. WBCs
d. RBCs

51. Which of the following findings is characteristically associated with acute pyelonephritis?

a. red cell cast
b. white cell cast
c. waxy cast
d. fatty cast

52. The type of urinary cast that is most characteristically associated with glomerular injury is a(n):

a. epithelial cell cast
b. white cell cast
c. red cell cast
d. fatty cast

53. Glitter cells are a microscopic finding of:

    a. RBCs in hypertonic urine
    b. RBCs in hypotonic urine
    c. WBCs in hypertonic urine
    d. WBCs in hypotonic urine

54. Bilirubinuria may be associated with:

    a. strenuous exercise
    b. increased destruction of red cells
    c. infectious hepatitis
    d. unconjugated bilirubinemia

55. A reagent strip test for hemoglobin has been reported positive. Microscopic examination fails to yield red blood cells. This patient's condition can be called:

    a. hematuria
    b. hemoglobinuria
    c. oliguria
    d. myoglobinuria

56. Oliguria is usually correlated with:

    a. acute glomerulonephritis
    b. diabetes mellitus
    c. hepatitis
    d. tubular damage

57. Which of the following methods are appropriate for specific gravity determination?

    1. reagent strip measurement of change in pH based on the ionic concentration
    2. hydrometers calibrated to read 1.000 in distilled water
    3. measuring refraction of light
    4. falling drop technique in organic solvent

    a. only 1, 2 and 3 are correct
    b. only 1 and 3 are correct
    c. only 2 and 4 are correct
    d. only 4 is correct
    e. all are correct

58. Glycosuria may be due to:

1. hyperglycemia
2. increased renal threshold
3. renal tubular dysfunction
4. increased glomerular filtration rate

a. only 1, 2 and 3 are correct
b. only 1 and 3 are correct
c. only 2 and 4 are correct
d. only 4 is correct
e. all are correct

59. A standard water-load dilution test is performed on a patient. A specific gravity measurement made on the urine specimen at 18.6°C using the refractometer method is 1.012. A reagent strip analysis of the specimen includes the following:

pH	8.0
Glucose	1 g/dL
Protein	1 g/dL

The corrected specific gravity to be reported is:

a. 1.012
b. 1.005
c. 1.004
d. 1.007

60. Broad waxy casts are <u>LEAST</u> likely to be associated with:

a. advanced tubular atrophy
b. end-stage renal disease
c. fatty degeneration tubular disease
d. formation in a pathologically dilated tubule

61. Which of the following fails to encourage the formation of casts in the renal tubules?

a. acid pH
b. increased protein concentration
c. diminished urine flow
d. diluted urine

62. A urine's specific gravity is directly proportional to its:

    a. turbidity
    b. dissolved solids
    c. salt content
    d. sugar content

63. Which of the following substances are excreted in the urine in the largest amount?

    a. urea and NaCl
    b. creatine and NaCl
    c. creatine and ammonia
    d. urea and glucose

64. The confirmatory test for a positive protein result by the reagent strip method uses:

    a. Ehrlich's reagent
    b. a diazo reaction
    c. sulfosalicylic acid
    d. a copper reduction tablet

65. Which of the following casts is most likely to be found in healthy people?

    a. hyaline
    b. RBC
    c. waxy
    d. WBC

66. Use of a refractometer over a urinometer is preferred due to the fact that the refractometer:

    a. uses large volume of urine and compensates for temperature
    b. uses small volume of urine and compensates for glucose
    c. uses small volume of urine and compensates for temperature
    d. uses small volume of urine and compensates for protein

67. The protein section of the urine reagent strip is MOST sensitive to:

    a. albumin
    b. mucoprotein
    c. Bence Jones protein
    d. globulin

68. Waxy casts are most easily differentiated from hyaline casts by:

a. color
b. size
c. granules
d. refractivity

69. A brown-black-colored urine would most likely contain:

a. bile pigment
b. porphyrins
c. melanin
d. blood cells

70. A milky-colored urine from a 24-year-old woman would most likely contain:

a. spermatozoa
b. many WBCs
c. RBCs
d. bilirubin

71. An abdominal fluid is submitted from surgery. The physician wants to determine if this fluid could be urine. The technologist should:

a. perform a culture
b. smell the fluid
c. test for urea, creatinine, sodium, and chloride
d. test for protein, glucose, and pH

72. When performing a routine urinalysis, the technologist notes a 2+ protein result. He should:

a. request another specimen
b. confirm with the acid precipitation test
c. test for Bence Jones protein
d. report the result obtained without further testing

73. When using the sulfosalicylic acid test, false-positive protein results may occur in the presence of:

a. ketones
b. alkaline
c. glucose
d. radiographic contrast media

74. The clarity of a urine sample should be determined:

    a. using glass tubes only, never plastic
    b. following thorough mixing of the specimen
    c. after addition of sulfosalicylic acid
    d. after the specimen cools to room temperature

75. When employing the urine reagent strip method, a false-positive protein result may occur in the presence of:

    a. large amounts of glucose
    b. x-ray contrast media
    c. Bence Jones protein
    d. highly alkaline urine

76. Microscopic analysis of a urine specimen yields a moderate amount of red blood cells in spite of a negative result for occult blood using a reagent strip. The technologist should determine if this patient has taken:

    a. vitamin C
    b. a diuretic
    c. high blood pressure medicine
    d. antibiotics

77. A patient with uncontrolled diabetes mellitus will most likely have:

    a. pale urine with a high specific gravity
    b. concentrated urine with a high specific gravity
    c. pale urine with a low specific gravity
    d. dark urine with a high specific gravity

78. Presence of which of the following cells is most commonly associated with vaginal contamination of the urine specimen?

    a. white
    b. transitional epithelial
    c. squamous epithelial
    d. glitter

79. Which of the following is the average volume of urine excreted by an adult in 24 hours?

    a. 750 mL
    b. 1,000 mL
    c. 1,500 mL
    d. 2,000 mL

80. A diet high in protein will most likely yield a urine with which of the following pH?

    a. acid
    b. neutral
    c. alkaline
    d. variable

81. The normal value for pH in a healthy adult is:

    a. 4.5
    b. 5.0
    c. 6.0
    d. 8.0

82. A 28-year-old woman is taking an antibiotic for a urinary tract infection and was told that the antibiotic would be most effective if her urine pH was acidic. This woman should be on a diet rich in:

    a. vegetables
    b. protein
    c. citrus fruits
    d. milk

83. Normal urine primarily consists of:

    a. water, protein, and sodium
    b. water, urea, and protein
    c. water, urea, and sodium chloride
    d. water, urea, and bilirubin

84. Patients with diabetes mellitus have urine with:

    a. decreased volume and decreased specific gravity
    b. decreased volume and increased specific gravity
    c. increased volume and decreased specific gravity
    d. increased volume and increased specific gravity

85. Cessation of urine flow is defined as:

    a. azotemia
    b. dysuria
    c. diuresis
    d. anuria

86. The fluid leaving the glomerulus normally has a specific gravity of:

    a. 1.001
    b. 1.010
    c. 1.020
    d. 1.030

87. Upon standing at room temperature, urine pH typically:

    a. decreases
    b. increases
    c. remains the same
    d. changes depending on bacterial concentration

88. The normal kidney does <u>NOT</u>:

    a. remove metabolic waste products from the blood
    b. regulate the acid-base balance in the body
    c. remove excess protein from the blood
    d. regulate the water content in the body

89. Antidiuretic hormone regulates the reabsorption of:

    a. water
    b. glucose
    c. potassium
    d. calcium

90. Refractive index is a comparison of:

    a. light velocity in solutions to light velocity in solids
    b. light velocity in air to light velocity in solutions
    c. light scattering by air to light scattering by solutions
    d. light scattering by particles in solution

91. Calibration of refractometers is done by measuring the specific gravity of:

    a. distilled water and protein
    b. distilled water and glucose
    c. distilled water and sodium chloride
    d. distilled water and urea

92. Oval fat bodies are defined as:

    a. squamous epithelial cells that contain lipids
    b. renal tubular epithelial cells that contain lipids
    c. free-flotating fat droplets
    d. white blood cells with phagocytized lipids

93. A 17-year-old girl decided to go on a starvation diet. After one week of starving herself, what substance would most likely be found in her urine?

    a. protein
    b. ketones
    c. glucose
    d. blood

94. Which of the following crystals is found in acidic urine?

    a. calcium carbonate
    b. calcium oxalate
    c. calcium phosphate
    d. triple phosphate

95. Which of the following reagents is used to react with ketones in the urine?

    a. sodium nitroprusside
    b. diacetic acid
    c. acetone
    d. β-hydroxybutyric acid

96. Which of the following ketone bodies is excreted in the largest amount in ketonuria?

    a. acetone
    b. diacetic acid
    c. cholesterol
    d. β-hydroxybutyric acid

97. A woman in her ninth month of pregnancy has a urine sugar which is negative with the urine reagent strip, but gives a positive reaction with the copper reduction method. The sugar most likely responsible for these results is:

    a. maltose
    b. galactose
    c. glucose
    d. lactose

98. Which of the following casts is most indicative of severe renal disease?

    a. hemoglobin
    b. granular
    c. cellular
    d. waxy

99. The following are compounds formed in the synthesis of heme.

    1. Coproporphyrinogen
    2. Porphobilinogen
    3. Uroporphyrinogen
    4. Protoporphyrinogen

    Which of the following responses list these compounds in the order in which they are formed?

    a. 4, 3, 1, 2
    b. 2, 3, 1, 4
    c. 2, 4, 3, 1
    d. 2, 1, 3, 4

100. Which of the following is the primary reagent in the copper reduction tablet?

    a. sodium carbonate
    b. copper sulfate
    c. glucose oxidase
    d. a polymerized diazonium salt

101. White blood cell casts are most likely to indicate disease of the:

    a. bladder
    b. ureter
    c. urethra
    d. kidney

102. Which of the following components are present in serum but <u>NOT</u> present in the glomerular filtrate?

    a. glucose
    b. amino acids
    c. urea
    d. large molecular weight proteins

103. A patient with renal tubular acidosis would be most likely to excrete a urine with a:

   a. low pH
   b. high pH
   c. neutral pH
   d. variable pH

104. Which of the following is an abnormal crystal described as a hexagonal plate?

   a. cystine
   b. tyrosine
   c. leucine
   d. cholesterol

105. A 21-year-old woman had glucose in her urine with a normal blood sugar. These findings are most consistent with:

   a. renal glycosuria
   b. diabetes insipidus
   c. diabetes mellitus
   d. alkaline tide

106. Which of the following crystals appears as finely scattered needles?

   a. cholesterol
   b. leucine
   c. starch
   d. tyrosine

107. Excess urine on the reagent test strip can turn a normal pH result into an acidic pH when which of the following reagents interferes?

   a. tetrabromphenol blue
   b. citrate buffer
   c. glucose oxidase
   d. alkaline copper sulfate

108. A 42-year-old man has a positive urine bilirubin and a negative urine urobilinogen test result. This is most consistent with:

   a. hepatitis
   b. normal state
   c. hemolysis
   d. biliary obstruction

109. A component seen during a microscopic urinalysis stains positively with Sudan III stain but does not polarize. This most likely is a:

a. cholesterol ester
b. neutral fat
c. lipid
d. leucine

110. Which of the following cells is the largest?

a. glitter
b. white
c. transitional epithelial
d. renal epithelial

111. What cell is MOST commonly associated with vaginal contamination?

a. white
b. transitional
c. squamous
d. glitter

112. In which of the following metabolic diseases will urine turn dark brown to black upon standing?

a. phenylketonuria
b. alkaptonuria
c. maple syrup disease
d. aminoaciduria

113. Urinary calculi most often consist of:

a. calcium
b. uric acid
c. leucine
d. cystine

114. A urine specimen which displays an elevated urobilinogen and a negative bilirubin may indicate:

a. obstruction of the biliary tract
b. hepatic damage
c. hemolytic jaundice
d. cirrhosis

115. Small round objects found in a urine sediment that dissolve after addition of dilute acetic acid and do not polarize most likely are:

a. air bubbles
b. calcium oxalate
c. RBCs
d. yeast cells

116. Tiny, colorless, dumbbell-shaped crystals were found in an alkaline urine sediment. They most likely are:

a. calcium oxalate
b. calcium carbonate
c. calcium phosphate
d. amorphous phosphate

117. A 42-year-old man is admitted to the emergency room with multiple abrasions, several broken bones, a fractured pelvis, and a crushed femur. The following urinalysis results are obtained:

Clarity	hazy	Microscopic	
Color	red-brown	Hemoglobin granular casts	3-5
Specific gravity	1.026	Amorphous	few
pH	6.0		
Protein	300 mg/dL		
Glucose	negative		
Ketones	negative		
Blood	large		
Bilirubin	negative		
Nitrite	negative		
Urobilinogen	0.1 EU/dL		

What is the MOST likely explanation for the discrepancy in the large blood, hemoglobin granular casts, and the complete absence of red cells on the microscopic analysis?

a. There is a false-positive reaction for blood on the urine reagent strip due to the large amount of protein.
b. The blood portion of the urine reagent strip is more sensitive to hemoglobin than to intact red cells.
c. RBCs have been lysed due to the pH and the specific gravity.
d. The hemoglobin granular casts which were reported may actually be myoglobin granular casts.

118. A 24-year-old obese diabetic woman had the following blood and urine test results from specimens obtained at the same time:

pH	7.5	Microscopic	
Protein	30 mg/dL	Epithelial cells	3-5
Glucose	negative	Bacteria	many
Ketone	15 mg/dL	Yeast	many
Bilirubin	negative	Amorphous	moderate
Blood	negative		
Nitrite	negative	Blood sugar	195 mg/dL
Urobilinogen	1 EU/dL		
Specific gravity	1.008		

Which of the following is the MOST likely explanation for the negative urine glucose finding?

a. There is a false-negative glucose due to oxidizing contaminants.
b. There is a false-negative glucose due to the alkaline pH.
c. The specimen is probably old and the bacteria and yeast have consumed the glucose.
d. Glucose would not be present in the urine specimen since the blood sugar was normal.

119. The following urinalysis results were obtained from an 18-year-old woman in labor:

pH	6.5	Copper reduction test	1.0 g/dL
Protein	30 gm/dL	Sulfosalicylic acid test for protein	30 mg/dL
Glucose	0.25 g/dL		
Ketone	Negative		
Bilirubin	Small (color slightly abnormal)		
Blood	Negative		
Nitrite	Negative		
Urobilinogen	0.1 EU/dL		
Specific gravity	1.025		

Which of the following is the MOST likely explanation for the positive copper reduction test?

a. Only glucose is present.
b. Only lactose is present.
c. Glucose and possibly other reducing substances/sugars are present.
d. Results are false-positive due to the presence of protein.

120. In synovial fluid, the most characteristic microscopic finding in osteoarthritis is:

a. neutrophils with 0.5-1.5 µm inclusions
b. cartilage debris
c. monosodium urate crystals
d. hemosiderin-laden macrophages

121. In synovial fluid, the most characteristic finding in rheumatoid arthritis is:

a. cartilage debris
b. monosodium urate crystals
c. hemosiderin-laden macrophages
d. neutrophils with 0.5-1.5 µm inclusions

122. In synovial fluid, the most characteristic finding in pseudogout is:

a. calcium pyrophosphate dihydrate crystals
b. cartilage debris
c. monosodium urate crystals
d. hemosiderin-laden macrophages

123. In synovial fluid, the most characteristic finding in traumatic arthritis is:

a. monosodium urate crystals
b. cartilage debris
c. calcium pyrophosphate dihydrate crystals
d. hemosiderin-laden macrophages

124. The procedure used to determine the presence of neural tube defects is:

a. lecithin/sphingomyelin ratio
b. amniotic fluid creatinine
c. measurement of absorbance at 450 nm
d. alpha-fetoprotein

125. In amniotic fluid, the procedure used to detect Rh isosensitization is:

   a. human placental lactogen (HPL)
   b. alpha-fetoprotein
   c. measurement of absorbance at 450 nm
   d. creatinine

126. Technical problems encountered during the collection of an amniotic fluid specimen caused doubt as to whether the specimen was amniotic in origin. Of the following procedures, the one that would establish that it is amniotic in origin is:

   a. measurement of absorbance at 450 nm
   b. creatinine measurement
   c. lecithin/sphingomyelin ratio
   d. HPL

127. In amniotic fluid, the procedure used to determine fetal lung maturity is:

   a. lecithin/sphingomyelin ratio
   b. creatinine
   c. measurement of absorbance at 450 nm
   d. alpha-fetoprotein

128. In amniotic fluid, the procedure most closely related to fetoplacental function is:

   a. measurement of absorbance at 450 nm
   b. creatinine
   c. lecithin/sphingomyelin ratio
   d. estriol

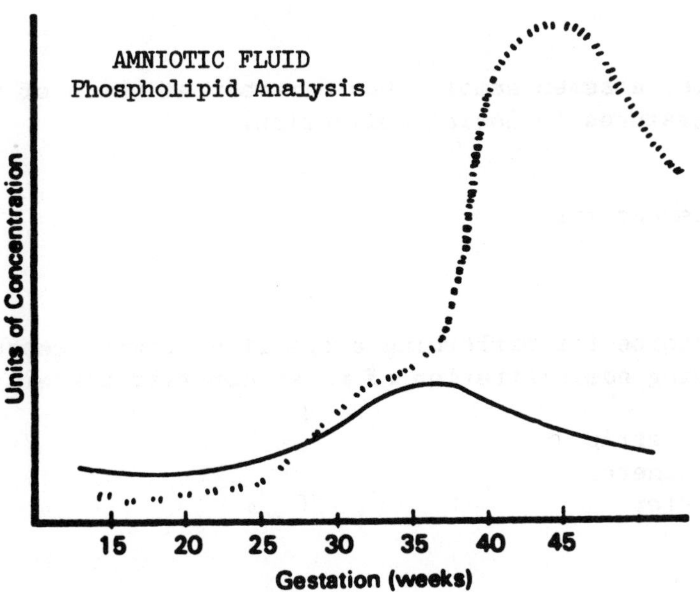

129. The class of phospholipid surfactants represented by the dotted line on the amniotic fluid analysis shown above is thought to originate in which fetal organ system?

 a. cardiovascular
 b. pulmonary
 c. hepatic
 d. placental

---

130. Which of the following determinations is useful in prenatal diagnosis of open neural tube defects?

 a. amniotic fluid alpha-fetoprotein
 b. amniotic fluid estriol
 c. maternal serum estradiol
 d. maternal serum estrone

131. Which one of the following is <u>NOT</u> a risk associated with amniocentesis?

 a. premature delivery
 b. maternal red cell immunization
 c. genetic defects
 d. fetal infection

132. For best results, a semen sample should remain at which of the following temperatures following collection?

a. 4°C
b. room temperature
c. 37°C
d. 56°C

133. The method of choice for performing a specific gravity measurement of urine following administration of x-ray contrast dyes is:

a. reagent strip
b. refractometer
c. urinometer

Body Fluids/Urinalysis Answer Key

1. d
2. c
3. b
4. b
5. d
6. d
7. c
8. d
9. d
10. d
11. d
12. b
13. b
14. b
15. b
16. a
17. b
18. b
19. b
20. a
21. c
22. a
23. c
24. d
25. d
26. d
27. d
28. a
29. c
30. b
31. b
32. c
33. a
34. b
35. d
36. b
37. b
38. c
39. c
40. b
41. b
42. b
43. a
44. e
45. e
46. b
47. b
48. b
49. c
50. a
51. b
52. c
53. d
54. c
55. b
56. a
57. e
58. b
59. b
60. c
61. d
62. b
63. a
64. c
65. a
66. c
67. a
68. d
69. c
70. b
71. c
72. b
73. d
74. b
75. d
76. a
77. a
78. c
79. c
80. a
81. c
82. b
83. c
84. d
85. d
86. b
87. b
88. c
89. a
90. b
91. c
92. b
93. b
94. b
95. a
96. d
97. d
98. d
99. b
100. b
101. d
102. d
103. b
104. a
105. a
106. d
107. b
108. d
109. b
110. c
111. c
112. b
113. a
114. c
115. c
116. b
117. b
118. c
119. c
120. b
121. d
122. a
123. b
124. d
125. c
126. b
127. a
128. d
129. b
130. a
131. c
132. c
133. a

CHAPTER 16

Laboratory Operations

1. The statistical term for the average value is the:

   a. mode
   b. median
   c. mean
   d. coefficient of variation

2. An index of precision is statistically known as the:

   a. median
   b. mean
   c. standard deviation
   d. coefficient of variation

3. The most frequent value in a collection of data is statistically known as the:

   a. mode
   b. median
   c. mean
   d. standard deviation

4. Select the most likely associated statistical term for a mathematical expression of a Gaussian curve.

   a. coefficient of variation
   b. mode
   c. median
   d. standard deviation

5. The middle value of a data set is statistically known as the:

   a. mean
   b. median
   c. mode
   d. standard deviation

6. If the correlation coefficient (r) of two variables is zero:

   a. there is complete correlation between the variables
   b. there is an absence of correlation
   c. as one variable increases, the other decreases
   d. as one variable decreases, the other increases

7. Diagnostic specificity is defined as the percentage of individuals:

   a. with a given disease who have a positive result by a given test
   b. without a given disease who have a negative result by a given test
   c. with a given disease who have a negative result by a given test
   d. without a given disease who have a positive result by a given test

8. Which of the following is a true statement about the t test?

   a. The random error of two analytical methods is compared.
   b. The difference between two variances is compared.
   c. The best linear relationship between two variables is estimated.
   d. The difference between two mean values is compared.

9. An evaluation experiment that estimates proportional error is:

   a. within-run replication
   b. interference
   c. within-day replication
   d. recovery

10. An evaluation experiment that provides the most REALISTIC estimate of random error in a routine operation is:

    a. within-run replication
    b. interference
    c. recovery
    d. day-to-day replication

11. The extent to which measurements agree with the true value of the quantity being measured is known as:

    a. reliability
    b. accuracy
    c. reproducibility
    d. precision

12. **Relative standard deviation is the preferred term for the:**

    a. **correlation coefficient**
    b. **variance**
    c. **F test**
    d. **coefficient of variation**

13. **The predictive value of a test is defined as:**

    a. $\frac{\text{true positives + true negatives}}{\text{true positives}}$

    b. $\frac{\text{true positives}}{\text{true positives + false negatives}}$

    c. $\frac{\text{true positives + true negatives}}{\text{true negatives}}$

    d. $\frac{\text{true negatives}}{\text{true negatives + false positives}}$

14. **Which of the following is NOT a source of systematic variance?**

    a. **personal bias of the analyst**
    b. **experimental error**
    c. **laboratory bias**
    d. **random error**

15. **The F test statistic is used for each of the following EXCEPT:**

    a. **random error**
    b. **accuracy**
    c. **variance**
    d. **precision**

16. **Random error is usually quantitated by calculating each of the following EXCEPT:**

    a. **mean**
    b. **F test**
    c. **standard deviation**
    d. **t test**

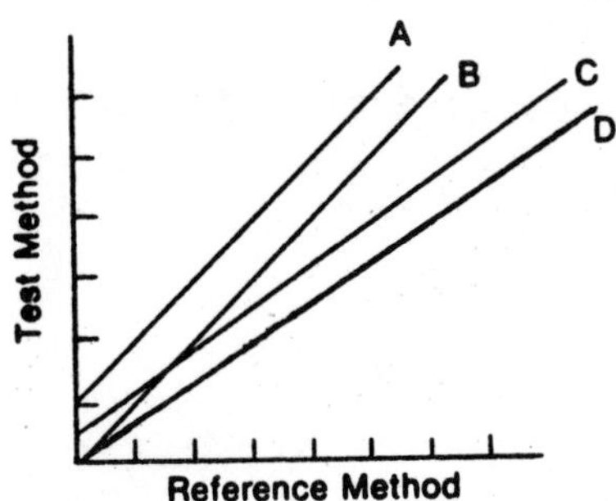

17. In the diagram above, the line which demonstrates a proportional error is:

a. line A
b. line B
c. line C
d. line D

---

18. Which of the following is the formula for standard deviation?

a. square root of the mean

b. square root of $\left(\frac{\text{sum of squared differences}}{\text{N-1}}\right)$

c. square root of the variance

d. square root of $\left(\frac{\text{mean}}{\text{sum of squared differences}}\right)$

19. Which of the following is the formula for coefficent of variation?

a. $\frac{\text{standard deviation x 100}}{\text{standard error}}$

b. $\frac{\text{mean x 100}}{\text{standard deviation}}$

c. $\frac{\text{standard deviation x 100}}{\text{mean}}$

d. $\frac{\text{variance x 100}}{\text{mean}}$

20. Given the following values:

    2.5
    3.0
    2.8
    2.2
    3.2

    What is the mean?

    a. 1.0
    b. 2.5
    c. 2.7
    d. 13.7

21. Given the following values:

    100
    120
    150
    140
    130

    What is the mean?

    a. 100
    b. 128
    c. 130
    d. 640

22. The mean for hemoglobin is 14.0 and the standard deviation is 0.20. The acceptable control range is ±2 standard deviations. What are the allowable limits for the control?

    a. 13.8-14.2
    b. 13.6-14.4
    c. 13.4-14.6
    d. 13.0-14.0

23. The mean for hemoglobin is 13.0 and the standard deviation is 0.15. The acceptable control range is ±2 standard deviations. What are the allowable limits for the control?

    a. 13.0-14.0
    b. 12.9-13.1
    c. 12.7-13.3
    d. 12.5-13.5

24. Which of the following is the formula for arithmetic mean?

a. square root of the sum of values

b. sum of values x number of values

c. $\frac{\text{number of values}}{\text{sum of values}}$

d. $\frac{\text{sum of values}}{\text{number of values}}$

25. Nonmetallic surfaces soiled with blood should be disinfected with:

a. a phenol solution
b. 5% bleach (sodium hypochlorite)
c. 70% isopropyl alcohol
d. green soap

26. Aerosol-associated laboratory infections:

a. largely occur in untrained laboratory helpers
b. usually cause clinical disease with an organism of low infectivity
c. have been associated with improper laboratory air venting
d. can occur from an accidental needle puncture wound

27. The prevention of aerosols:

a. involves the use of spray disinfectant applied on work surfaces
b. involves initial plating within a single-pass laminar airflow cabinet
c. requires the use of plastic autoclavable bags
d. can be minimized by the use of formaldehyde gas decontamination

28. A technologist on the night shift has been observed sleeping on repeated occasions by the day shift supervisor. Which of the following is the most appropriate INITIAL course of action for the day supervisor?

a. Ignore the repeated incidents.
b. Discuss the facts with the technologist's immediate supervisor.
c. Notify the personnel department of policy violations.
d. Advise the laboratory director in writing of the apparent misconduct.

29. A patient had hemoglobin and hematocrit determinations ordered at two-hour intervals. The technician who drew one of the blood samples inadvertently broke the tube enroute to the laboratory and lost the entire specimen. Rather than repeat the venipuncture, the technician reported the same result that had been obtained two hours earlier. The incident was discovered by the supervisor, who should have taken which of the following measures?

    a. Fire the technician immediately, documenting the fact that the technician had falsified a laboratory result.
    b. Suspend the technician without pay, documenting the fact that the technician had falsified a laboratory result.
    c. Counsel the technician and write a formal report documenting the fact that the technician had falsified a laboratory result.
    d. Discuss the matter with the technician informally, warning the technician never to falsify laboratory results again.

30. A major laboratory policy change is going to take place that will affect a significant portion of the laboratory employees. In order to minimize the resistance to change, the supervisor should:

    a. announce the change one day after it goes into effect
    b. discuss the change in detail with all concerned, well in advance
    c. announce only the positive aspects in advance
    d. discuss only the positive aspects with those concerned

31. Which piece of legislation guarantees employees the right to engage in self-organization and collective bargaining through representatives of their choice, or to refrain from these activities?

    a. Taft-Hartley Bill
    b. Wagner Act
    c. Clinical Laboratory Improvement Act (CLIA)
    d. National Labor Relations Act

32. According to most organizational theorists, managerial functions include:

    a. planning and organizing
    b. buying and directing
    c. organizing and appraising
    d. buying and selling

33. A workload reporting system is an important part of laboratory management because it:

1. tells exactly how much should be charged per test
2. keeps personnel busy in their free time
3. counts only tests done and specimens received in the laboratory without inflating these figures by adding in quality control and standardization efforts
4. helps in planning, developing, and maintaining efficient laboratory services with administrative and budget controls

a. only 1, 2 and 3 are correct
b. only 1 and 3 are correct
c. only 2 and 4 are correct
d. only 4 is correct
e. all are correct

34. When staffing a laboratory, fundamental consideration must be given to personnel:

1. numbers
2. distribution
3. responsibilities
4. qualifications

a. only 1, 2 and 3 are correct
b. only 1 and 3 are correct
c. only 2 and 4 are correct
d. only 4 is correct
e. all are correct

35. A blood gas sample is submitted to the laboratory from the emergency room. The slip is labeled "Jane Doe #1" with no emergency room identification numbers. The syringe is unlabeled. The emergency room is calling for the results. How should this situation be handled?

a. Run the blood gas assuming that the sample is that of Jane Doe.
b. Run the blood gas, then call the emergency room to label the syringe and provide emergency room numbers.
c. Send the syringe and slip back to the emergency room for correct identification.
d. Ask the emergency room to redraw the blood gas and provide correct identification.

36. Cost studies indicate that a new $21,000 instrument will result in a savings of $9,000 per year. What is the "pay-back period" (the time required to generate sufficient savings to pay back the initial investment)?

    a. two years and four months
    b. three years with straight line depreciation
    c. five years with straight line depreciation
    d. seven years with straight line depreciation

37. Method comparison data on the CAP Proficiency Survey cannot be biased by a single laboratory's results because:

    a. each laboratory submits only one result for each serum
    b. the constituent concentrations are always within the "normal range"
    c. the serums are always homogeneous
    d. the constituent concentrations are always within the linear range of the analytical method

38. A supervisor notices that one of her technologists continues to mouth-pipet liquids when making reagents. The supervisor's best course of action is to:

    a. allow the technologist to continue this practice as long as it is not done when dealing with specimens
    b. discuss this problem with the employee immediately
    c. order a mechanical device (bulb-pipet) for employee to use
    d. compliment the employee on his rapid pipeting technique

39. What action should be taken if insufficient information is available regarding a long-term problem?

    a. Ignore the problem.
    b. Seek more information.
    c. Base decision on available information.
    d. Refer the problem to another level of management.

40. Evaluating the performance of employees should be done:

    a. annually
    b. semiannually
    c. as needed in the judgment of management
    d. as immediate feedback at regular intervals

41. Which one of the following is <u>NOT</u> a reason for doing a performance evaluation?

    a. to give employee performance feedback
    b. to determine training needs
    c. to help the employee improve performance
    d. to criticize a problem employee

42. The clinical laboratory needs to acquire a new semiautomated chemistry instrument. Although the existing instrument is only two years old and works well, a new clinic in the area sends a very large number of additional tests to the laboratory three days a week. Which one of the following is the proper "Justification Category" for the request that this situation creates?

    a. replacement
    b. volume increase
    c. no other way to do task
    d. new service

43. Documentation of the annual review of procedure manuals is best demonstrated by:

    a. initialing and dating every page
    b. signing and dating each procedure
    c. signing and dating a covering document at the front of each manual
    d. signing and dating every page

44. Package inserts may be used:

    a. in lieu of the typed procedure
    b. as a reference
    c. at the bench but not in the procedure manual
    d. if initialed and dated by the laboratory director

45. Sample sizes for microassays can be scaled down by:

    a. using reactions that decrease the molar absorptivity of the reaction products
    b. increasing the sensitivity of the signal detection method
    c. increasing the diameters of the manifolds to the continuous flow analyzers
    d. using concentration techniques

46. Benefits of microassays include:

a. increased analytical reliability
b. reduced reagent requirements
c. increased diagnostic specificity
d. reduced numbers of repeated tests

47. Most of the automated microbiology equipment currently available has been designed to replace:

a. manual susceptibility procedures
b. manual methods that are infrequently performed but are time consuming
c. repetitive manual methods that are performed daily on a large number of specimens
d. all manual methods used in the clinical microbiology laboratory

48. Which of the following peripheral storage devices in a computer system has the highest speed?

a. magnetic tape
b. core memory
c. moving head disc
d. fixed head disc

49. Which of the following is the formula for calculating the unknown concentration based on Beer's Law? (A = absorbance, C = concentration)

a. $\frac{(\text{A unknown})}{(\text{A standard})} \times \text{C standard}$

b. C standard x A unknown

c. A standard x A unknown

d. $\frac{(\text{C standard})}{(\text{A standard})} \times 100$

50. Which of the following is the formula for Rh immune globulin dose?

a. $\frac{\text{\% of fetal cells}}{50}$

b. $\frac{\text{\% of fetal cells x 50}}{30}$

c. $\frac{\text{\% of maternal cells x 50}}{30}$

d. $\frac{\text{\% of maternal cells x 30}}{30}$

51. In spectrophotometric determination, which of the following is the formula for calculating the absorbance of a solution?

a. $\frac{\text{absorptivity x light path}}{\text{concentration}}$

b. $\frac{\text{absorptivity x concentration}}{\text{light path}}$

c. absorptivity x light path x concentration

d. $\frac{\text{light path x concentration}}{\text{absorptivity}}$

52. Which of the following is the formula for calculating absorbance given the percent transmittance (%T) of a solution?

a. 1 - log of %T

b. $\frac{\text{log of \%T}}{2}$

c. 2 x log of %T

d. 2 - log of %T

53. Which of the following is the formula for calculating the number of moles of a chemical?

a. $\frac{g}{GMW}$

b. g x GMW

c. $\frac{GMW}{g}$

d. $\frac{g \times 100}{GMW}$

54. Which of the following is the formula for calculating the gram equivalent weight of a chemical?

a. MW x oxidation number

b. $\frac{\text{MW}}{\text{oxidation number}}$

c. MW + oxidation number

d. MW - oxidation number

55. Which of the following is the formula for calculating the dilution of a solution?
(V = volume, C = concentration)

a. V1 + C1 = V2 + C2
b. V1 + C2 = V2 + C1
c. V1 x C1 = V2 x C2
d. V1 x V2 = V1 x C2

56. Which of the following is the Henderson-Hasselbalch equation?

a. $pK_a = pH + \log \frac{\text{acid}}{\text{salt}}$

b. $pK_a = pH + \log \frac{\text{salt}}{\text{acid}}$

c. $pH = pK_a + \log \frac{\text{acid}}{\text{salt}}$

d. $pH = pK_a + \log \frac{\text{salt}}{\text{acid}}$

57. Which of the following is the formula for calculating a percent (w/v) solution?

a. $\frac{\text{grams of solute}}{\text{volume of solvent}} \times 100$

b. grams of solute x volume of solvent x 100

c. $\frac{\text{volume of solvent}}{\text{grams of solute}} \times 100$

d. $\frac{\text{grams of solute} \times \text{volume of solvent}}{100}$

58. When doing a manual white cell count, which formula is used to calculate the number of white cells present?

a. $\frac{\text{number of cells counted} \times \text{dilution} \times 10}{\text{number of squares counted}}$

b. $\frac{\text{number of cells counted} \times \text{dilution}}{10 \times \text{number of squares counted}}$

c. number of cells counted x dilution

d. number of cells counted x number of squares counted

59. Which of the following is the formula for absolute cell count?

a. $\frac{\text{number of cells counted}}{\text{total count}}$

b. $\frac{\text{total count}}{\text{number of cells counted}}$

c. 10 x total count

d. % of cells counted x total count

60. Which of the following is the formula for calculating the molarity of a solution?

a. $\frac{\text{number of moles of solute}}{\text{1 L of solution}}$

b. number of moles of solute x 100

c. 1 GEW of solute x 10

d. $\frac{\text{1 GEW of solute}}{\text{1 L of solution}}$

61. Which of the following is the formula for calculating the normality of a solution?

a. $\frac{\text{number of moles of solute}}{\text{1 L of solution}}$

b. $\frac{\text{1 GEW of solute}}{\text{1 L of solution}}$

c. 1 GEW of solute x 100

d. number of moles of solute x 100

62. Which of the following is the formula for mean corpuscular volume (MCV)?

a. $\frac{\text{Hgb}}{\text{RBC}}$

b. $\frac{\text{Hgb}}{\text{Hct}}$

c. $\frac{\text{Hct} \times 10}{\text{RBC}}$

d. $\frac{\text{RBC}}{\text{Hct}}$

63. Which of the following is the formula for mean corpuscular hemoglobin (MCH)?

a. $\frac{\text{Hct}}{\text{RBC}} \times 1000$

b. $\frac{\text{Hgb}}{\text{Hct}}$

c. $\frac{\text{RBC}}{\text{Hct}}$

d. $\frac{\text{Hgb} \times 10}{\text{RBC}}$

64. Which of the following is the formula for mean corpuscular hemoglobin concentration (MCHC)?

a. $\frac{\text{Hgb} \times 100}{\text{Hct}}$

b. $\frac{\text{Hgb}}{\text{RBC}}$

c. $\frac{\text{RBC}}{\text{Hct}}$

d. $\frac{\text{Hct}}{\text{RBC}} \times 1000$

65. How many grams of sulfosalicylic acid (MW = 254) are required to prepare 1 L of a 3% (w/v) solution?

a. 3
b. 30
c. 254
d. 300

66. A 1 molal solution is equivalent to:

a. a solution containing 1 mole of solute per kg of solvent
b. 1,000 mL of solution containing 1 mole of solute
c. a solution containing 1 GEW of solute in 1 L of solution
d. a 1 L solution containing 2 moles of solute

67. A 1 molar solution is equivalent to:

a. a solution containing 1 mole of solute per kg of solvent
b. 1,000 mL of solution containing 1 mole of solute
c. a solution containing 1 GEW of solute in 1 L of solution
d. a 1 L solution containing 2 moles of solute

68. A 1 normal solution is equivalent to:

a. a solution containing 1 mole of solute per kg of solvent
b. 1,000 mL of solution containing 1 mole of solute
c. a solution containing 1 GEW of solute in 1 L of solution
d. a 1 L solution containing 2 moles of solute

69. What is the molarity of a solution that contains 18.7 g of KCl (MW = 74.5) in 500 mL?

a. 0.1
b. 0.5
c. 1.0
d. 5.0

70. A series of eight tubes is set-up with 2.3 mL of diluent in each. A serial dilution is performed by adding 1.0 mL of serum to the first tube and then transferring 1.0 mL through each remaining tube. What is the serum dilution of tube 7?

a. 1:340
b. 1:1,292
c. 1:148
d. 1:4,262

71. What is the normality of a solution which contains 148 g of HCl (MW = 37) in 1,000 mL of solution?

a. 2 N
b. 3 N
c. 4 N
d. 5 N

72. A solution contains 20 g of solute dissolved in 0.5 L of water. What is the percentage of this solution?

a. 2%
b. 4%
c. 6%
d. 8%

73. A solution contains 10 g of solute dissolved in 0.5 L of water. What is the percentage of this solution?

a. 2%
b. 4%
c. 6%
d. 8%

74. A solution contains 30 g of solute dissolved in 0.5 L of water. What is the percentage of this solution?

a. 2%
b. 4%
c. 6%
d. 8%

75. A solution contains 40 g of solute dissolved in 0.5 L of water. What is the percentage of this solution?

a. 2%
b. 4%
c. 6%
d. 8%

76. A solution contains 20 g of NaCl (MW = 58) dissolved in 0.5 L of water. What is the molarity of this solution?

a. 0.35 M
b. 0.58 M
c. 0.70 M
d. 0.85 M

77. A solution contains 7.4 g of KCl (MW = 74) dissolved in 5 L of water. What is the molarity?

    a. 0.02 M
    b. 0.01 M
    c. 0.74 M
    d. 2.00 M

78. A solution contains 18.5 g of KCl (MW = 74) dissolved in 5 L of water. What is the molarity?

    a. 0.05 M
    b. 0.25 M
    c. 4.00 M
    d. 12.50 M

79. How many grams of solute are required to make 200 mL of a 10% solution?

    a. 2.5 g
    b. 5.0 g
    c. 10.0 g
    d. 20.0 g

80. How many grams of solute are required to make 200 mL of a 2.5% solution?

    a. 2.5 g
    b. 5.0 g
    c. 10.0 g
    d. 20.0 g

81. How many grams of solute are required to make 200 mL of a 5% solution?

    a. 2.5 g
    b. 5.0 g
    c. 10.0 g
    d. 20.0 g

82. How many grams of solute are required to make 200 mL of a 25% solution?

    a. 20 g
    b. 30 g
    c. 40 g
    d. 50 g

83. How many milliliters of a 3% solution can be made if 6 g of solute are available?

a. 100 mL
b. 200 mL
c. 400 mL
d. 600 mL

84. How many milliliters of a 10% solution can be made if 5 g of solute are available?

a. 10 mL
b. 30 mL
c. 50 mL
d. 70 mL

85. How many milliliters of a 5% solution can be made if 20 g of solute are available?

a. 400 mL
b. 600 mL
c. 800 mL
d. 1,000 mL

86. How many milliliters of a 20% solution can be made if 25 g of solute are available?

a. 50 mL
b. 75 mL
c. 100 mL
d. 125 mL

87. What is the mean corpuscular volume (MCV) if the hematocrit is 20, the red cell count is 2,400,000, and the hemoglobin is 5?

a. 68
b. 83
c. 100
d. 120

88. What is the mean corpuscular hemoglobin (MCH) if the hematocrit is 20, the red cell count is 1,500,000, and the hemoglobin is 6?

a. 28
b. 30
c. 40
d. 75

89. What is the MCH if the hematocrit is 20, the red cell count is 2,400,000, and the hemoglobin is 5?

 a. 21
 b. 23
 c. 25
 d. 84

90. What is the mean corpuscular hemoglobin concentration (MCHC) if the hematocrit is 20, the red cell count is 1,500,000, and the hemoglobin is 6?

 a. 28
 b. 30
 c. 40
 d. 75

91. What is the MCHC if the hematocrit is 20, the red cell count is 2,400,000, and the hemoglobin is 5?

 a. 21
 b. 25
 c. 30
 d. 34

92. Given the following data:

WBC	8,500
Differential	
Segs	56%
Bands	2%
Lymphs	30%
Monos	6%
Eos	6%

What is the absolute lymphocyte count?

 a. 170
 b. 510
 c. 2,550
 d. 4,760

93. Given the following data:

WBC	8,500
Differential	
Segs	56%
Bands	2%
Lymphs	30%
Monos	6%
Eos	6%

What is the absolute eosinophil count?

a. 170
b. 510
c. 2,550
d. 4,760

94. If the total leukocyte count is 20,000 and 50 NRBCs are seen per 100 leukocytes on the differential, what is the corrected leukocyte count?

a. 6,666
b. 10,000
c. 13,333
d. 26,666

95. If a RBC count is performed on a 1:100 dilution and the number of cells in one-fifth of a mm^2 is 600, the total RBC count is:

a. 1,500,000
b. 2,000,000
c. 3,000,000
d. 3,500,000

96. If a RBC count is performed on a 1:200 dilution and the number of cells in one-fifth of a mm^2 is 150, the total RBC count is:

a. 1,500,000
b. 2,000,000
c. 3,000,000
d. 3,500,000

97. If a WBC count is performed on a 1:10 dilution and the number of cells counted in eight squares is 120, the total WBC count is:

a. 1,200
b. 1,500
c. 12,000
d. 15,000

98. If a WBC count is performed on a 1:100 dilution and the number of cells counted in eight squares is 50, the total WBC count is:

   a. 5,000
   b. 6,250
   c. 50,000
   d. 62,500

99. A solution is prepared by adding 25 g of NaOH (MW = 40) to 0.5 L of water. What is the molarity of this solution if an additional 0.25 L of water is added to this solution?

   a. 0.25 M
   b. 0.50 M
   c. 0.75 M
   d. 0.83 M

100. What is the final serum dilution if 4 mL of water are added to 1 mL of serum?

   a. 1:3
   b. 1:4
   c. 1:5
   d. 1:6

101. Calculate the number of gram-equivalents in 80 g of NaOH (MW = 40).

   a. 1
   b. 2
   c. 3
   d. 4

102. How many grams of H_2SO_4 (MW = 98) are in 750 mL of 3 N H_2SO_4?

   a. 36 g
   b. 72 g
   c. 110 g
   d. 146 g

103. What is the normality of a solution which contains 280 g of NaOH (MW = 40) in 2,000 mL of solution?

   a. 3.5 N
   b. 5.5 N
   c. 7.0 N
   d. 8.0 N

104. How many grams of HCl (MW = 37) are in 750 mL of 3 N HCl?

a. 83 g
b. 111 g
c. 126 g
d. 222 g

105. A serum potassium is 19.5 mg/100 mL. This value is equal to how many mEq/L?

a. 3.9 mEq/L
b. 4.2 mEq/L
c. 5.0 mEq/L
d. 8.9 mEq/L

106. Which of the following solutions has a normality of 1?

a. 1 mole of H_2SO_4

b. 2 moles of HCl

c. 2 moles of H_2CO_3

d. 1 mole of H_3PO_4

107. How many milliliters of 0.25 N NaOH are needed to make 100 mL of a 0.05 N solution of NaOH?

a. 5 mL
b. 10 mL
c. 15 mL
d. 20 mL

Laboratory Operations Answer Key

1. c
2. d
3. a
4. d
5. b
6. b
7. b
8. d
9. d
10. d
11. b
12. d
13. b
14. d
15. b
16. d
17. d
18. b
19. c
20. c
21. b
22. b
23. c
24. d
25. b
26. c
27. b
28. b
29. a
30. b
31. d
32. a
33. d
34. e
35. c
36. a
37. a
38. b
39. b
40. d
41. d
42. b
43. b
44. b
45. b
46. b
47. c
48. d
49. a
50. b
51. c
52. d
53. a
54. b
55. c
56. d
57. a
58. a
59. d
60. a
61. b
62. c
63. d
64. a
65. b
66. a
67. b
68. c
69. b
70. d
71. c
72. b
73. a
74. c
75. d
76. c
77. a
78. a
79. d
80. b
81. c
82. d
83. b
84. c
85. a
86. d
87. b
88. c
89. a
90. b
91. b
92. c
93. b
94. c
95. c
96. a
97. b
98. b
99. d
100. c
101. b
102. c
103. a
104. a
105. c
106. c
107. d

APPENDIX A

GLOSSARY OF TERMS USED IN ITEM DESCRIPTORS
MEDICAL LABORATORY TECHNICIAN EXAMINATION - FEBRUARY 1984

AB	ANTIBODY
ACCEPT	ACCEPTABILITY
ACLD	ASSOCIATE CLINICAL AND LABORATORY DATA
AFB	ACID-FAST BACILLI
AG	ANTIGEN
AGGL	AGGLUTININS
ALF	ASSOCIATE LABORATORY FINDINGS
AMM	ASSOCIATE MICROSCOPIC MORPHOLOGY
ANAL	ANALYTIC
APPEAR	APPEARANCE
ASO	ANTISTREPTOLYSIN O
ASSO	ASSOCIATE
BBNK	BLOOD BANK
BF	BODY FLUIDS
BTP	BIOCHEMICAL THEORY AND PHYSIOLOGY
CALC	CALCULATE
CCD	CORRELATE CLINICAL DATA
CCLD	CORRELATE CLINICAL AND LABORATORY DATA
CGL	CHRONIC GRANULOCYTIC LEUKEMIA
CHARACT	CHARACTERISTICS
CHEM	CHEMISTRY
CK	CREATINE KINASE
CL	CLOSTRIDIUM
CLD	CORRELATE LABORATORY DATA
CRP	C-REACTIVE PROTEIN
CSF	CEREBROSPINAL FLUID
DEFI	DEFICIENCY
DFC	DEFINE FUNDAMENTAL CHARACTERISTICS
ECC	ELECTRONIC CELL COUNTER
EMM	EVALUATE MICROSCOPIC MORPHOLOGY
ESOE	EVALUATE SOURCE OF ERROR
ETR	EVALUATE TEST RESULTS
FIX	FIXATION
GNB	GRAM-NEGATIVE BACILLI
GNC	GRAM-NEGATIVE COCCI
GPB	GRAM-POSITIVE BACILLI
GPC	GRAM-POSITIVE COCCI
HEMA	HEMATOLOGY
HEMOPATHY	HEMOGLOBINOPATHY
HI	HUMORAL IMMUNITY
IBP	IDENTIFY BASIC PRINCIPLES
IBR	IDENTIFY BIOCHEMICAL REACTION
ID	IDENTIFY
IDC	IDENTIFY DISTINGUISHING CHARACTERISTICS
IDENT	IDENTIFICATION
IMM	IDENTIFY MICROSCOPIC MORPHOLOGY
IMMU	IMMUNOLOGY
ISOE	IDENTIFY SOURCE OF ERROR
MACRO	MACROSCOPIC
METH	METHODOLOGY
MEQ	MILLIEQUIVALENTS
MICR	MICROBIOLOGY
MICRO	MICROSCOPIC
MOLEC	MOLECULAR
MORPH	MORPHOLOGY
PERF	PERFORM
PHOS	PHOSPHATASE
PREPA	PREPARATION
QC	QUALITY CONTROL
RA	RHEUMATOID ARTHRITIS
RBC	RED BLOOD CELLS
REAG	REAGENT
REQUIRE	REQUIREMENTS
RX	REACTION
SCH	SPECIMEN COLLECTION AND HANDLING
SED	SEDIMENT
SELB	SELECT BLOOD PRODUCT
SELM	SELECT METHODOLOGY
SELR	SELECT REAGENT
SG	SPECIFIC GRAVITY
SLE	SYSTEMIC LUPUS ERYTHEMATOSUS
SOE	SOURCE OF ERROR
SPEC	SPECIMEN
STS	SEROLOGICAL TESTS FOR SYPHILIS
SUSCEPT	SUSCEPTABILITY
TRANS	TRANSMISSION
WBC	WHITE BLOOD CELLS

TAXONOMIC LEVELS

TAX 1 - <u>Recall</u>: Ability to recall previously learned knowledge ranging from specific facts to complete theories, solely by recognition or memorization.

TAX 2 - <u>Interpretive skills</u>: Ability to utilize recalled knowledge to interpret or apply verbal, numeric or visual data.

TAX 3 - <u>Problem Solving</u>: Ability to utilize recalled knowledge and interpretation/application of data to resolve a problem or situation and/or make an appropriate decision.

ITEM DESCRIPTOR LIST
MEDICAL LABORATORY TECHNICIAN EXAMINATION - FEBRUARY 1984

1. CHEM/ISOE/SCH/BILIRUBIN/1
2. CHEM/DFC/BUFFER/1
3. CHEM/IBP/PROTEIN/ELECTROPHORESIS/1
4. CHEM/IBP/INSTRUMENTATION/OSMOMETER/1
5. CHEM/CALC/BEER'S LAW/2
6. CHEM/SELM/METABOLISM/GLUCOSE/1
7. CHEM/IBP/ANTICOAGULANT/1
8. CHEM/DFC/BLOOD/PH/1
9. CHEM/CCD/CK/2
10. CHEM/ALF/CREATININE/1
11. CHEM/IBP/PHYSIOLOGY/IRON/1
12. CHEM/DFC/PHYSIOLOGY/LIPIDS/1
13. CHEM/CALC/MOLEC WEIGHT/2
14. CHEM/IBP/INSTRUMENTATION/FLUOROMETER/1
15. CHEM/DFC/QC/STATISTICS/1
16. CHEM/ETR/SCH/POTASSIUM/3
17. CHEM/ISOE/GLUCOSE/2
18. CHEM/DFC/BTP/CARBON DIOXIDE/1
19. CHEM/ALF/PANCREATITIS/2
20. CHEM/IBP/REAG/PROTEIN/1
21. CHEM/DFC/PHYSIOLOGY/HEMOGLOBIN/1
22. CHEM/DFC/PHYSIOLOGY/LIPIDS/1
23. CHEM/CALC/MOLAR SOLUTION/2
24. CHEM/IBP/INSTRUMENTATION/SPECTROPHOTOMETER/1
25. CHEM/IBP/IRON/PHYSIOLOGY/1
26. CHEM/IBP/ANAL METH/CREATININE/1
27. CHEM/ALF/BEER'S LAW/2
28. CHEM/ALF/LIPASE/1
29. CHEM/ETR/BLOOD GASES/2
30. CHEM/DFC/QC/STATISTICS/1
31. CHEM/ALF/STEROIDS/1
32. CHEM/CALC/MEQ/2
33. CHEM/DFC/QC/INSTRUMENTATION/1
34. CHEM/ACLD/CHLORIDE/1
35. CHEM/DFC/QC/STATISTICS/1
36. CHEM/SELR/SCH/ACID-BASE/1
37. CHEM/ISOE/ACID PHOS/1
38. CHEM/DFC/PROTEIN/ELECTROPHORESIS/1
39. CHEM/CALC/SOLUTION/PH/2
40. CHEM/IBP/ANAL METH/BILIRUBIN/1
41. CHEM/IBP/PIPET/1
42. CHEM/DFC/PREGNANCY TESTS/1
43. CHEM/ISOE/INSTRUMENTATION/CHLORIDOMETER/2
44. CHEM/IBP/SPECIAL TEST/T-3 UPTAKE/1
45. CHEM/ALF/CALCIUM/1
46. CHEM/DFC/CREATININE/CLEARANCE TEST/1
47. CHEM/ALF/ALKALINE PHOS/1
48. CHEM/SELM/SCH/GLUCOSE/1
49. CHEM/SELM/GLASSWARE/CLEANING/1
50. HEMA/DFC/WBC/ANOMALY/1
51. HEMA/DFC/PHYSIOLOGY/RBC/1
52. HEMA/ESOE/QC/3
53. HEMA/IBP/ECC/1
54. HEMA/IBP/ANTICOAGULANT/1
55. HEMA/ALF/MYELOMA/2
56. HEMA/ALF/PLATELET COUNT/1
57. HEMA/ETR/FACTOR DEFI/2
58. HEMA/SELM/SPECIAL STAIN/WBC/1
59. HEMA/CALC/WBC/DILUTION/3
60. HEMA/IBP/CLOT/RETRACTION/1
61. HEMA/IBP/COAGULATION/PATHWAY/1
62. HEMA/DFC/WBC/DEGENERATION/1
63. HEMA/IBP/PLATELET/PHYSIOLOGY/1
64. HEMA/ALF/MICRO MORPH/ANTINUCLEAR AB/2
65. HEMA/CLD/MICRO MORPH/RBC PRODUCTION/2
66. HEMA/CLD/MICRO MORPH/HEMOPATHY/3
67. HEMA/IMM/HEMOPATHY/2
68. HEMA/CLD/MICRO MORPH/OSMOTIC FRAGILITY/2
69. HEMA/AMM/SPECIAL TEST/WBC/3
70. HEMA/ALF/MYELOMA/1
71. HEMA/CALC/INDICES/RBC/2
72. HEMA/DFC/SOURCE/PLATELETS/1
73. HEMA/IBP/ECC/1
74. HEMA/DFC/PHYSIOLOGY/FACTOR SYNTHESIS/1
75. HEMA/ISOE/CELL COUNT/RBC/1
76. HEMA/IBP/ABSOLUTE COUNT/1
77. HEMA/IBP/CELL MATURATION/1
78. HEMA/ASSO/SPECIAL STAIN/RBC INCLUSIONS/1
79. HEMA/IMM/SOE/SLIDE PREPA/2
80. HEMA/IMM/RBC/2
81. HEMA/ALF/MICRO MORPH/INFECTIOUS DISEASE/2
82. HEMA/IMM/LEUKOCYTE/2
83. HEMA/IMM/WBC INCLUSION/2
84. HEMA/CCLD/CGL/2
85. HEMA/IMM/GRANULOCYTE/2
86. HEMA/ALF/MICRO MORPH/LYMPHOCYTE/3
87. HEMA/DFC/DISEASE STATE/CHILDHOOD LEUKEMIA/1
88. HEMA/ISOE/PROTHROMBIN/2
89. HEMA/DFC/AB SYNTHESIS/1
90. BF/DFC/URINE/CAST/1
91. BF/DFC/MICROSCOPE/1
92. BF/ISOE/SCH/URINE/1
93. BF/ALF/BLOOD/GLUCOSE/1
94. BF/ISOE/URINE/REAG STRIP/1
95. BF/CALC/CSF/DILUTION/2
96. BF/DFC/COMPOSITION/URINE/1
97. BF/IBP/SPECIAL STAIN/1
98. BF/CCLD/MENINGITIS/CSF/1
99. BF/ALF/URINE SED/SITE OF ORIGIN/2
100. BF/IMM/URINE SED/2
101. BF/ALF/MICRO MORPH/URINE CRYSTALS/3
102. BF/IBP/RENAL THRESHOLD/1
103. BF/ISOE/SCH/2
104. BF/IBP/URINE/REAG STRIP/1
105. BF/DFC/COMPOSITION/URINE/1
106. BF/ISOE/PREGNANCY TEST/1
107. BF/DFC/SPEC APPEAR/CSF/1
108. BF/ISOE/SCH/1
109. BF/CALC/SG/2
110. BF/ETR/COMPOSITION/PLEURAL FLUID/3
111. BF/ALF/URINALYSIS/2
112. BF/CLD/HEMATURIA/2
113. BF/IBP/ANAL METH/URINE/UROBILINOGEN/1
114. BF/ALF/MACRO MORPH/FECES/2
115. BF/ISOE/URINE/REAG STRIP/1
116. BF/IBP/ANAL METH/OCCULT BLOOD/1
117. BF/ALF/UROBILINOGEN/1
118. MICR/CALC/COLONY COUNT/URINE/2
119. MICR/DFC/PSEUDOMONAS/1
120. MICR/DFC/TRANS/DISEASE/1
121. MICR/IBP/CANDLE JAR/1
122. MICR/DFC/BACTEROIDES/1
123. MICR/IBP/ACID-FAST STAIN/1
124. MICR/ISOE/SENSITIVITY/1
125. MICR/IDC/CESTODE/1
126. MICR/DFC/MEDIA/1
127. MICR/IBP/DISINFECTION/1
128. MICR/SELM/DISINFECTION/VIRUS/1
129. MICR/ALF/SPEC SOURCE/GNC/2
130. MICR/SELM/ANAEROBE/GPB/2

ITEM DESCRIPTOR LIST
MEDICAL LABORATORY TECHNICIAN EXAMINATION - FEBRUARY 1984

131. MICR/ALF/MICRO MORPH/GROWTH REQUIRE/2
132. MICR/ISOE/SUSCEPT TEST/2
133. MICR/IBP/STERILIZATION/MEDIA/1
134. MICR/DFC/GROWTH CHARACT/STREPTOCOCCUS/1
135. MICR/SELM/CORYNEBACTERIUM/1
136. MICR/ID/MACRO MORPH/PROTEUS/1
137. MICR/ID/MACRO MORPH/AFB/1
138. MICR/SELM/SCH/PROTOZOA/1
139. MICR/IBR/GPC/1
140. MICR/IDC/CL PERFRINGENS/1
141. MICR/IBR/PROTEUS/1
142. MICR/IBR/AFB/1
143. MICR/ALF/STREPTOCOCCUS/1
144. MICR/DFC/THIOGLYCOLLATE/1
145. MICR/IBR/GPC/1
146. MICR/ALF/ANAEROBIC GNB/2
147. MICR/IBP/SPEC PREPA/AFB/1
148. MICR/IBP/MEDIA PREPA/1
149. MICR/ID/MACRO MORPH/YEAST/2
150. MICR/ID/MACRO MORPH/YEAST/2
151. MICR/IMM/YEAST/2
152. MICR/SELM/IDENT/VIRUS/1
153. MICR/IBP/SCH/SPUTUM/1
154. MICR/SELM/EPIDEMIOLOGY/GPC/1
155. MICR/ID/MACRO MORPH/GPC/1
156. MICR/IBP/QC/AUTOCLAVE/1
157. MICR/IDC/LIFE CYCLE/NEMATODE/1
158. MICR/CLD/MORPH/MOLD/2
159. BBNK/ALF/TRANSFUSION RX/1
160. IMMU/DFC/COMPLEMENT/1
161. IMMU/ALF/FEBRILE AGGL/2
162. IMMU/DFC/AG/1
163. IMMU/DFC/WIDAL TEST/1
164. IMMU/DFC/IMMUNE RESPONSE/1
165. BBNK/DFC/DONOR ACCEPT/1
166. BBNK/IBP/COMPLEMENT FIX/1
167. BBNK/DFC/ANTICOAGULANT/1
168. BBNK/ETR/PATERNITY TEST/2
169. IMMU/DFC/AUTOANTIBODY/SLE/1
170. BBNK/PERF/ABO/2
171. IMMU/ETR/STS/2
172. BBNK/IBP/STORAGE/COMPONENTS/1
173. IMMU/DFC/IMMUNOGLOBULIN/LEVELS/1
174. BBNK/DFC/COMPLEMENT/ANTICOAGULANTS
175. IMMU/ISOE/FEBRILE AGGL/3
176. BBNK/DFC/STORAGE/BLOOD PRODUCTS/1
177. IMMU/IBP/SOE/STS/1
178. BBNK/DFC/BLOOD PRESSURE/1
179. IMMU/DFC/COLD AGGL/1
180. BBNK/DFC/QC/STORAGE/1
181. IMMU/DFC/HI/AB PRODUCTION/1
182. IMMU/DFC/ASO/1
183. BBNK/DFC/LECTIN/1
184. IMMU/DFC/AG-AB RX/1
185. BBNK/SELB/FACTOR DEFI/1
186. IMMU/ALF/CRP/1
187. BBNK/DFC/ELUTION/1
188. IMMU/DFC/IMMUNOGLOBULIN/1
189. IMMU/DFC/IMMUNITY/1
190. BBNK/DFC/RH/1
191. IMMU/ALF/SLE/1
192. BBNK/ETR/COLD AB/2
193. IMMU/DFC/PROZONE/1
194. BBNK/DFC/NATURAL AB/1
195. IMMU/DFC/STS/1
196. IMMU/SELM/STS/1
197. BBNK/ETR/INCOMPATIBILITY/ABO/2
198. IMMU/ETR/QC/RA/2

GLOSSARY OF TERMS USED IN ITEM DESCRIPTORS
MEDICAL LABORATORY TECHNICIAN EXAMINATION - AUGUST 1984

AB	ANTIBODY
ACLD	ASSOCIATE CLINICAL AND LABORATORY DATA
AFB	ACID-FAST BACILLI
AG	ANTIGEN
AGGLUT	AGGLUTININ
ALF	ASSOCIATE LABORATORY FINDING
ALK	ALKALINE
AML	ACUTE MYELOCYTIC LEUKEMIA
ANAT	ANATOMY
ANLF	ANALYZE LABORATORY FINDINGS
ANTIGLOB	ANTIGLOBULIN
ASO	ANTISTREPTOLYSIN O
AST	ASPARTATE AMINOTRANSFERASE
BBNK	BLOOD BANK
BF	BODY FLUIDS
BMD	BIOCHEMICAL MANIFESTATIONS OF DISEASE
BTP	BIOCHEMICAL THEORY AND PHYSIOLOGY
CALC	CALCULATE
CHARACT	CHARACTERISTIC(S)
CHEM	CHEMISTRY
CLEAR	CLEARANCE
CLL	CHRONIC LYMPHOCYTIC LEUKEMIA
CML	CHRONIC MYELOCYTIC LEUKEMIA
COMP	COMPOSITION
CON	CONDITION(S)
CRP	C-REACTIVE PROTEIN
CSF	CEREBROSPINAL FLUID
DAT	DIRECT ANTIGLOBULIN TEST
DEFIC	DEFICIENCY
DFC	DEFINE FUNDAMENTAL CHARACTERISTICS
DIFF	DIFFERENTIAL
DIS	DISEASE
DISORD	DISORDER
ECLD	EVALUATE CLINICAL AND LABORATORY DATA
ELECTRO	ELECTROPHORESIS
ELF	EVALUATE LABORATORY FINDINGS
EMM	EVALUATE MICROSCOPIC MORPHOLOGY
ESOE	EVALUATE SOURCE OF ERROR
ESR	ERYTHROCYTE SEDIMENTATION RATE
FRAG	FRAGILITY
GNB	GRAM-NEGATIVE BACILLI
GNC	GRAM-NEGATIVE COCCI
GPB	GRAM-POSITIVE BACILLI
GPC	GRAM-POSITIVE COCCI
GTT	GLUCOSE TOLERANCE TEST
GU	GENITOURINARY
HCG	HUMAN CHORIONIC GONADOTROPIN
HDN	HEMOLYTIC DISEASE OF THE NEWBORN
HEMA	HEMATOLOGY
HEMOSTAT	HEMOSTATIC
HEPA	HEPARIN
HGBPATHY	HEMOGLOBINOPATHY
HYPOCHRO	HYPOCHROMIC
IBP	IDENTIFY BASIC PRINCIPLE
ID	IDENTIFY
IGTP	IMMUNOLOGIC GENETIC THEORY AND PRINCIPLES
IMAM	IDENTIFY MACROSCOPIC AND MICROSCOPIC MORPHO
IMM	IDENTIFY MICROSCOPIC MORPHOLOGY
IMMU	IMMUNOLOGY
ISOE	IDENTIFY SOURCE OF ERROR
ISOP	IDENTIFY STANDARD OPERATING PROCEDURE
LAP	LEUKOCYTE ALKALINE PHOSPHATASE
LD	LACTATE DEHYDROGENASE
LO	LABORATORY OPERATIONS
MACRO	MACROCYTIC
MEGALO	MEGALOBLASTIC
MICR	MICROBIOLOGY
MICRO	MICROSCOPIC
MOLEC	MOLECULAR
MONO	MONONUCLEOSIS
MORPH	MORPHOLOGY
NEUT	NEUTROPHIL
PBS	PERIPHERAL BLOOD SMEAR
PHYSIO	PHYSIOLOGY
POS	POSITIVE
PREP	PREPARATION
PROC	PROCEDURE
QA	QUALITY ASSURANCE
QC	QUALITY CONTROL
RBC	RED BLOOD CELL
REL	RELATED
REQUIRE	REQUIREMENT
REX	REACTION
SBP	SELECT BLOOD PRODUCT
SCH	SPECIMEN COLLECTION AND HANDLING
SCOA	SELECT COURSE OF ACTION
SDU	SELECT DONOR UNIT
SELM	SELECT METHOD
SELR	SELECT REAGENT
SEME	SELECT MEDIA
SLE	SYSTEMIC LUPUS ERYTHEMATOSUS
SOL	SOLUTION
STS	SEROLOGIC TESTS FOR SYPHILIS
SUSC	SUSCEPTIBILITY
TOLER	TOLERANCE
TRAN	TRANSMISSION
TX	TRANSFUSION
WBC	WHITE BLOOD CELL
X-MATCH	CROSSMATCH

TAXONOMIC LEVELS

TAX 1 - Recall:	Ability to recall or recognize previously learned (memorized) knowledge ranging from specific facts to complete theories.
TAX 2 - Interpretive skills:	Ability to utilize recalled knowledge to interpret or apply verbal, numeric or visual data.
TAX 3 - Problem Solving:	Ability to utilize recalled knowledge and the interpretation/application of distinct criteria to resolve a problem or situation and/or make an appropriate decision.

ITEM DESCRIPTOR LIST
MEDICAL LABORATORY TECHNICIAN EXAMINATION - AUGUST 1984

1. HEMA/DFC/ANAT & PHYSIO/FACTOR VIII/1
2. HEMA/DFC/ANAT & PHYSIO/PLATELETS/1
3. HEMA/ALF/MICRO MORPH/INFECTIOUS MONO/1
4. HEMA/DFC/ANAT & PHYSIO/COAGULATION FACTOR/1
5. HEMA/DFC/ANAT & PHYSIO/COAGULATION FACTOR/1
6. HEMA/DFC/HEMOGLOBIN/QC/1
7. HEMA/CALC/ABSOLUTE COUNT/2
8. HEMA/SCOA/PROTHROMBIN/QA/3
9. HEMA/DFC/MICRO MORPH/AML/1
10. HEMA/ALF/LAP/CML/1
11. HEMA/CALC/RBC INDICES/2
12. HEMA/SELM/HEMOGLOBIN S/2
13. HEMA/DFC/DRUG EFFECT/PLATELETS/1
14. HEMA/ALF/SPECIAL TESTS/PLATELET DEFIC/2
15. HEMA/ALF/COAGULATION/FACTOR DEFIC/2
16. HEMA/DFC/WBC/ANOMALY/1
17. HEMA/DFC/ANAT & PHYSIO/WBC/1
18. HEMA/IMM/PBS/WBC/2
19. HEMA/IMM/PBS/WBC/2
20. HEMA/EMM/HGBPATHY/2
21. HEMA/IMM/HGBPATHY/2
22. HEMA/EMM/OSMOTIC FRAG/2
23. HEMA/ALF/HEMOSTAT DISORD/CLOT LYSIS/2
24. HEMA/ELF/LAP/3
25. HEMA/DFC/HEMOGLOBIN F/1
26. HEMA/ELF/HYPOCHRO ANEMIA/2
27. HEMA/DFC/RBC MORPH/1
28. HEMA/DFC/ANAT & PHYSIO/COAGULATION FACTOR/1
29. HEMA/DFC/RBC INCLUSION/1
30. HEMA/CALC/TOLER LIMITS/2
31. HEMA/ALF/MYELOMA/1
32. HEMA/SELM/SCH/PEDIATRIC/1
33. HEMA/DFC/HEMOGLOBIN COMP/1
34. HEMA/DFC/WBC/DEGENERATION/1
35. HEMA/ALF/MICRO MORPH/INFECTIOUS DISEASE/2
36. HEMA/SCOA/MICRO MORPH/MEGALO ANEMIA/3
37. HEMA/ALF/MICRO MORPH/CLL/1
38. HEMA/SCOA/DIFF DIAGNOSIS/HYPOCHRO ANEMIA/2
39. HEMA/ISOE/ESR/1
40. HEMA/IBP/WBC MATURATION/1
41. HEMA/ALF/RBC MICRO MORPH/2
42. HEMA/DFC/HEMATOCRIT/1
43. HEMA/ISOP/QA/HEMOGLOBIN/1
44. BF/ISOP/URINE SEDIMENT/CASTS/1
45. BF/ALF/URINE SEDIMENT/SOURCE OF ORIGIN/1
46. BF/DFC/RENAL PHYSIO/1
47. BF/ALF/URINE PIGMENT/1
48. BF/IBP/SPECIAL STAIN/FECES/1
49. BF/ALF/COMP/PLEURAL FLUID/2
50. BF/ALF/RENAL DIS/1
51. BF/ALF/URINE SEDIMENT/CRYSTALS/1
52. BF/DFC/ANAT & PHYSIO/URINE CASTS/1
53. BF/DFC/PHYSIO/KETONURIA/1
54. BF/ISOE/CHEMICAL TEST/URINE/1
55. BF/ANLF/MICRO MORPH/URINE CRYSTALS/3
56. BF/ELF/URINE SEDIMENT/SOURCE OF ORIGIN/2
57. BF/EMM/URINE/YEAST/2
58. BF/EMM/URINE/CRYSTAL/3
59. BF/EMM/URINE/CRYSTAL/3
60. BF/ALF/URINE SEDIMENT/CRYSTALS/1
61. BF/DFC/URINE SEDIMENT/ACID PH/1
62. BF/ALF/REL CON & DISOR/AMNIOTIC FLUID/1
63. BF/ISOE/SCH/URINE/2
64. BF/ALF/SPECIAL TESTS/URINE OSMOLALITY/1
65. BF/CALC/URINE/SPECIFIC GRAVITY/2
66. BF/ISOE/URINE/REAGENT STRIP/1
67. BF/ELF/URINE SEDIMENT/BLOOD/2
68. BF/SCOA/SCH/CELL COUNT CSF/1
69. MICR/DFC/GNB/GROWTH CHARACT/1
70. MICR/IBP/SPECIMEN PREP/PARASITE/1
71. MICR/IBP/MEDIA PREP/1
72. MICR/IMAM/GPC/GROWTH CHARACT/1
73. MICR/DFC/NEMATODE/LIFE CYCLE/1
74. MICR/ALF/GNB/URINE CULTURE/1
75. MICR/ALF/GNC/GU CULTURE/2
76. MICR/ALF/GPC/BIOCHEMICAL TEST/1
77. MICR/SELM/SCH/PROTOZOA/1
78. MICR/DFC/GPB/CLOSTRIDIUM/1
79. MICR/IMAM/CESTODE/1
80. MICR/ALF/GPC/WOUND CULTURE/2
81. MICR/ALF/GNB-ANAEROBE/WOUND CULTURE/2
82. MICR/ALF/GPC/STREPTOCOCCUS/1
83. MICR/DFC/GNB/GROWTH CHARACT/1
84. MICR/IBP/LO/STERILIZATION/1
85. MICR/ELF/GNB/BIOCHEMICAL TEST/2
86. MICR/ALF/GPB/WOUND CULTURE/2
87. MICR/IBP/GPC/INFECTIOUS DISEASE/2
88. MICR/ELF/GNB/CSF CULTURE/2
89. MICR/ALF/GNB/PSEUDOMONAS/2
90. MICR/ID/GNC/CULTURE REQUIRE/1
91. MICR/SEME/GPB/CORYNEBACTERIUM/1
92. MICR/IBP/VIRAL TITER/1
93. MICR/IBP/AFB/BIOCHEMICAL TEST/1
94. MICR/DFC/GPB/CLOSTRIDIUM/1
95. MICR/IMM/YEAST/1
96. MICR/DFC/GNB/NONFERMENTATIVE/1
97. MICR/SEME/FUNGUS CULTURE/1
98. MICR/ISOE/ANTIBIOTIC SUSC/1
99. MICR/SEME/GNC/URETHRAL CULTURE/1
100. MICR/ID/MACRO MORPH/AFB/1
101. MICR/ALF/GNB/BIOCHEMICAL TESTS/2
102. MICR/IBP/GPC/BIOCHEMICAL TEST/1
103. MICR/ALF/SPIROCHETES/GROWTH REQUIRE/2
104. MICR/IBP/QC/AUTOCLAVE/1
105. MICR/CALC/URINE/COLONY COUNT/2
106. MICR/IMM/YEAST/CSF/1
107. MICR/IBP/CO2 INCUBATION/1
108. MICR/SEME/GPB/WOUND CULTURE/2
109. MICR/DFC/DIS TRANSMIT/1
110. MICR/ALF/GNB/BIOCHEMICAL TEST/2
111. MICR/IBP/GPC/BIOCHEMICAL TEST/1
112. BBNK/DFC/CRYOPRECIPITATE/1
113. BBNK/DFC/LECTIN/1
114. BBNK/IBP/SCH/COMPONENTS/1
115. BBNK/ELF/ABO TYPING/2
116. BBNK/ECLD/HEMOTHERAPY/BLOOD COMPONENT/3
117. BBNK/ALF/RH PHENOTYPE/2
118. BBNK/IBP/ADVERSE TX REX/1
119. BBNK/IBP/ABO AB/1
120. BBNK/SBP/HEMOTHERAPY/PACKED CELLS/2
121. BBNK/DFC/RH/1
122. BBNK/DFC/IGTP/RH IMMUNE GLOBULIN/1
123. BBNK/ELF/INCOMPATIBILITY/ABO/2
124. BBNK/ECLD/HEMOTHERAPY/BLOOD COMPONENT/3
125. BBNK/IBP/DONOR REQUIRE/1
126. BBNK/ALF/AB SCREEN/1
127. BBNK/IBP/AB ID/TX REX/1
128. BBNK/IBP/ANTIGLOB TEST/2
129. BBNK/DFC/ABO AB/1
130. BBNK/ELF/RBC/AB SCREEN/2

ITEM DESCRIPTOR LIST
MEDICAL LABORATORY TECHNICIAN EXAMINATION - AUGUST 1984

131. BBNK/ELF/PATERNITY TEST/2
132. BBNK/ALF/HDN/ANTIGLOB TEST/1
133. BBNK/SDU/HEMOTHERAPY/ABO/3
134. BBNK/DFC/ELUTION/1
135. BBNK/IBP/ABO GROUP/1
136. BBNK/ELF/COLD AB/2
137. BBNK/IBP/NON-SECRETOR/1
138. BBNK/IBP/PHYSIO/HDN/1
139. BBNK/ELF/X-MATCH/AUTOCONTROL/3
140. BBNK/SELM/DU TESTING/1
141. BBNK/DFC/ANTICOAGULANT/1
142. BBNK/ELF/RH GENOTYPE/2
143. IMMU/DFC/COLD AGGLUT/1
144. IMMU/IBP/DAT/1
145. IMMU/IBP/STS/1
146. IMMU/ESOE/SEROLOGIC TEST/INFECTIOUS MONO/3
147. IMMU/DFC/ASO/1
148. IMMU/ALF/CRP/1
149. IMMU/IBP/BASIC TESTS/PRECIPITATION/1
150. IMMU/ISOE/STS/BIOLOGIC FALSE-POS/1
151. IMMU/DFC/ANAT & PHYSIO/IMMUNOGLOBULIN/1
152. IMMU/DFC/BACTERIAL AG/1
153. IMMU/DFC/ANAT & PHYSIO/HCG/1
154. IMMU/ALF/FEBRILE AGGLUT/2
155. IMMU/DFC/ANAT & PHYSIO/CELLULAR IMMUNITY/1
156. IMMU/DFC/AUTOANTIBODY/SLE/1
157. IMMU/DFC/SCREENING PROC/QC/1
158. IMMU/ALF/SLE/1
159. IMMU/ACLD/INFECTIOUS MONO/HETEROPHIL/2
160. IMMU/ESOE/SCH/SEROLOGIC TEST/3
161. IMMU/ALF/PROZONE/2
162. IMMU/DFC/STS/1
163. CHEM/CALC/BEER'S LAW/2
164. CHEM/IBP/INSTRUMENTATION/CONTINUOUS FLOW/1
165. CHEM/CALC/DILUTION/2
166. CHEM/ALF/ALK PHOSPHATASE/1
167. CHEM/ALF/CREATININE/1
168. CHEM/IBP/SCH/ANTICOAGULANT/1
169. CHEM/DFC/PHYSIO/LIPIDS/1
170. CHEM/SCOA/SCH/POTASSIUM/3
171. CHEM/ALF/BEER'S LAW/2
172. CHEM/SELM/SCH/GTT/2
173. CHEM/DFC/BTP/BILIRUBIN/1
174. CHEM/DFC/PHYSIO/LIPIDS/1
175. CHEM/DFC/BTP/BUFFER/1
176. CHEM/IBP/PRECISION/1
177. CHEM/DFC/PHYSIO/UREA/1
178. CHEM/IBP/BASIC TESTS/GLUCOSE/1
179. CHEM/ALF/STEROIDS/1
180. CHEM/IBP/BTP/ELECTROLYTES/1
181. CHEM/IBP/BTP/ALBUMIN/1
182. CHEM/ESOE/SCH/ELECTROLYTES/3
183. CHEM/ESOE/GLUCOSE/3
184. CHEM/IBP/SPECIAL TESTS/T-3 UPTAKE/1
185. CHEM/ALF/CALCIUM/1
186. CHEM/DFC/PHYSIO/HEMOGLOBIN/1
187. CHEM/IBP/SPECIAL TESTS/ELECTRO/1
188. CHEM/IBP/INSTRUMENTATION/ATOMIC ABSORPTION/1
189. CHEM/ELF/BLOOD GASES/2
190. CHEM/IBP/SPECIAL TESTS/PROTEIN ELECTRO/1
191. CHEM/ELF/BMD/AMYLASE/2
192. CHEM/IBP/ANALYTIC METHOD/LIPASE/1
193. CHEM/IBP/ANALYTIC METHOD/CREATININE/1
194. CHEM/IBP/BASIC TESTS/PROTEIN/1
195. CHEM/IBP/CARBOHYDRATE/GTT/1
196. CHEM/DFC/BTP/CARBON DIOXIDE/1
197. CHEM/ALF/BMD/CREATINE KINASE/1
198. CHEM/IBP/PHYSIO/IRON/1
199. CHEM/CALC/MILLIEQUIVALENT/2
200. CHEM/DFC/LD ISOENZYMES/1
201. CHEM/ALF/PROTEIN/MYELOMA/1
202. CHEM/CALC/STANDARD SOL/2
203. CHEM/DFC/PREGNANCY TESTS/1
204. CHEM/DFC/AST/1
205. CHEM/CALC/DILUTION/2
206. CHEM/IBP/INSTRUMENTATION/BALANCE/1
207. CHEM/IBP/INSTRUMENTATION/CHROMATOGRAPHY/1
208. CHEM/DFC/PIPET TYPE/1
209. CHEM/DFC/BLOOD PH/1
210. CHEM/SELR/SCH/ACID-BASE/1
211. CHEM/DFC/INSTRUMENTATION/QC/1
212. CHEM/IBP/INSTRUMENTATION/FLAME PHOTOMETER/1
213. CHEM/SELM/SCH/GLUCOSE/1
214. CHEM/CALC/MOLEC WEIGHT/2

GLOSSARY OF TERMS USED IN ITEM DESCRIPTORS
MEDICAL LABORATORY TECHNICIAN EXAMINATION - FEBRUARY 1985

ACCEPT	ACCEPTIBILITY
ACLD	ASSOCIATE CLINICAL AND LABORATORY DATA
ACLF	ASSOCIATE CLINICAL AND LABORATORY FINDINGS
AFB	ACID-FAST BACILLI
AGGLUT	AGGLUTININ
AIHA	AUTOIMMUNE HEMOLYTIC ANEMIA
ALF	ASSOCIATE LABORATORY FINDINGS
ALK	ALKALINE
AMM	ASSOCIATE MICROSCOPIC MORPHOLOGY
ANALY	ANALYSIS
ANAT	ANATOMY
ANLF	ANALYZE LABORATORY FINDINGS
ANTIGLO	ANTIGLOBULIN
AUTO	AUTOLOGUS
BBNK	BLOOD BANK
BF	BODY FLUIDS
BMD	BIOCHEMICAL MANIFESTATIONS OF DISEASE
BTP	BIOCHEMICAL THEORY AND PHYSIOLOGY
CALC	CALCULATE
CBC	COMPLETE BLOOD COUNT
CCLF	CORRELATE CLINICAL AND LABORATORY FINDINGS
CELLU	CELLULAR
CHARACT	CHARACTERISTIC(S)
CHEM	CHEMISTRY
CHO	CARBOHYDRATE
CLD	CORRELATE LABORATORY DATA
CML	CHRONIC MYELOCYTIC LEUKEMIA
COAG	COAGULATION
COMPO	COMPONENT
COND	CONDITIONS
CSF	CEREBROSPINAL FLUID
DAT	DIRECT ANTIGLOBULIN TEST
DBP	DEFINE BASIS PRINCIPLES
DER	DERIVATIVE
DFC	DEFINE FUNDAMENTAL CHARACTERISTIC(S)
DIC	DISSEMINATED INTRAVASCULAR COAGULATION
DIS	DISEASE
DISO	DISORDER
ECC	EVALUATE CELL COUNTER
ECLD	EVALUATE CLINICAL & LABORATORY DATA
ECLF	EVALUATE CLINICAL & LABORATORY FINDINGS
ELD	EVALUATE LABORATORY DATA
ELF	EVALUATE LABORATORY FINDINGS
EMM	EVALUATE MICROSCOPIC MORPHOLOGY
ENZYM	ENZYMES
ERYTH	ERYTHROPOIETIC
ESOE	EVALUATE SOURCE OF ERROR
FIX	FIXATION
FRAG	FRAGILITY
GEN	GENETIC
GNB	GRAM-NEGATIVE BACILLI
GNC	GRAM-NEGATIVE COCCI
GNCB	GRAM-NEGATIVE COCCOBACILLI
GPB	GRAM-POSITIVE BACILLI
GPC	GRAM-POSITIVE COCCI
HDN	HEMOLYTIC DISEASE OF THE NEWBORN
HEMA	HEMATOLOGY
HEMATOPOIET	HEMATOPOIETIC
HEMOLYTC	HEMOLYTIC
HGBPATHY	HEMOGLOBINOPATHY
HLA	HUMAN LYMPHOCYTE ANTIGENS
IBP	IDENTIFY BASIC PRINCIPLE
ID	IDENTIFY
IDENT	IDENTIFICATION
IMM	IDENTIFY MICROSCOPIC MORPHOLOGY
IMMU	IMMUNOLOGY
IMMUNOFLU	IMMUNOFLUORESCENCE
INFECT	INFECTION
INFES	INFESTATION
ISOE	IDENTIFY SOURCE OF ERROR
ISOP	IDENTIFY STANDARD OPERATING PROCEDURE
LAB	LABORATORY
LAP	LEUKOCYTE ALKALINE PHOSPHATASE
LD	LACTATE DEHYDROGENASE
MACRO	MACROCYTIC
MATURA	MATURATION
METH	METHOD
MICR	MICROBIOLOGY
MICRO	MICROSCOPIC
MONO	MONONUCLEOSIS
MORPH	MORPHOLOGY
NON-CELLU	NON-CELLULAR
NOSOCOMI	NOSOCOMIAL
OP	OPERATIONS
PBS	PERIPHERAL BLOOD SMEAR
PHYSIO	PHYSIOLOGY
PNH	PAROXYSMAL NOCTURNAL HEMOGLOBINURIA
POS	POSITIVE
PREP	PREPARATION
PRIN	PRINCIPLE
PROC	PROCEDURE
PTT	ACTIVATED PARTIAL THROMBOPLASTIN TIME
QC	QUALITY CONTROL
RA	RHEUMATOID ARTHRITIS
RAST	RADIOALLERGOSORBENT TEST
RBC	RED BLOOD CELL
RCF	RELATIVE CENTRIFUGAL FORCE
REDUC	REDUCING
REL	RELATED
REQUIRE	REQUIREMENT
RETIC	RETICULOCYTE
REX	REACTION
SBP	SELECT BLOOD PRODUCT
SCH	SPECIMEN COLLECTION AND HANDLING
SCOA	SELECT COURSE OF ACTION
SDU	SELECT DONOR UNIT
SEL	SELECT
SELM	SELECT METHOD
SELR	SELECT REAGENT
SELT	SELECT TEST
SEME	SELECT MEDIA
SLE	SYSTEMIC LUPUS ERYTHEMATOSUS
SPE	SPECIMEN
SPEC	SPECIAL
STS	SEROLOGIC TESTS FOR SYPHILIS
SUBPOP	SUBPOPULATION
SUSC	SUSCEPTIBILITY
THER	THEORY
TSI	TRIPLE SUGAR IRON AGAR
TX	TRANSFUSION
WBC	WHITE BLOOD CELL

TAXONIMIC LEVELS

TAX 1 - Recall: Ability to recall or recognize previously learned (memorized) knowledge ranging from specific facts to complete theories.

TAX 2 - Interpretive skills: Ability to utilize recalled knowledge to interpret or apply verbal, numeric or visual data.

TAX 3 - Problem Solving: Ability to utilize recalled knowledge and the interpretation/application of distinct criteria to resolve a problem or situation and/or make an appropriate decision.

ITEM DESCRIPTOR LIST
MEDICAL LABORATORY TECHNICIAN EXAMINATION - FEBRUARY 1985

1. CHEM/IBP/INSTRUMENTATION/CONTINUOUS FLOW/1
2. CHEM/SELR/SCH/ACID-BASE/1
3. CHEM/SCOA/LAB OP/SAFETY/1
4. CHEM/DFC/BTP/BUFFER/1
5. CHEM/ELF/QC/LEVY-JENNINGS/2
6. CHEM/IBP/BASIC TESTS/GLUCOSE/1
7. CHEM/ALF/STEROIDS/1
8. CHEM/DFC/ENZYM REX/1
9. CHEM/DFC/BTP/COPPER/1
10. CHEM/DFC/INSTRUMENTATION/QC/1
11. CHEM/DBP/SCH/LIPID/1
12. CHEM/ALF/ALK PHOSPHATASE/1
13. CHEM/ESOE/SCH/PROTEIN & ENZYM/3
14. CHEM/ALF/PROTEIN/MYELOMA/1
15. CHEM/DFC/QC/STATISTICS/1
16. CHEM/CALC/SPEC CHEM/RADIOACTIVE DECAY/2
17. CHEM/IBP/BASIC TESTS/PROTEIN/1
18. CHEM/CALC/INSTRUMENTATION/CENTRIFUGE-RCF/2
19. CHEM/IBP/BTP/ALBUMIN/1
20. CHEM/ALF/BMD/CREATINE KINASE/1
21. CHEM/IBP/INSTRUMENTATION/BEER'S LAW/1
22. CHEM/IBP/PHYSIO/IRON/1
23. CHEM/DFC/PHYSIO/LIPIDS/1
24. CHEM/ESOE/INSTRUMENTATION/FLAME PHOTOMETRY/3
25. CHEM/DFC/BTP/CARBON DIOXIDE/1
26. CHEM/DFC/BTP/D-XYLOSE/1
27. CHEM/ESOE/SCH/ELECTROLYTES/3
28. CHEM/IBP/SPEC TESTS/T-3 UPTAKE/1
29. CHEM/IBP/AUTOMATED METH/1
30. CHEM/DFC/LD ISOENZYMES/1
31. CHEM/DFC/SPEC CHEM/ESTRIOL/1
32. CHEM/CALC/DILUTION/2
33. CHEM/ESOE/SCH/CHO/3
34. CHEM/IBP/INSTRUMENTATION/ATOMIC ABSORPTION/1
35. CHEM/SELM/LAB OP/SAFETY/2
36. CHEM/CALC/INSTRUMENTATION/SPECTROPHOTOMETER/2
37. CHEM/IBP/BMD/ACIDOSIS/2
38. CHEM/CALC/MILLIEQUIVALENT/2
39. CHEM/ESOE/INSTRUMENTATION/SPECTROPHOTOMETRY/3
40. HEMA/DFC/DIS HEMATOPOIET/CHILDHOOD LEUKEMIA/1
41. HEMA/IBP/DIFFERENTIAL/LEFT SHIFT/1
42. HEMA/ALF/HEMOSTASIS DISO/CLOT LYSIS/2
43. HEMA/ESOE/PBS/RETIC COUNT/3
44. HEMA/ECLD/RBC/PNH/2
45. HEMA/IBP/SPEC STAIN/RBC INCLUSIONS/1
46. HEMA/ALF/COAG/FACTOR DEFICIENCY/2
47. HEMA/ELF/COAG SPEC TEST/MIXING STUDY/3
48. HEMA/IMM/PBS/WBC/2
49. HEMA/EMM/PBS/PLATELET COUNT/2
50. HEMA/IMM/WBC/PBS/2
51. HEMA/IMM/RBC/PBS/2
52. HEMA/IMM/CELL MATURA WBC/2
53. HEMA/EMM/HGBPATHY/2
54. HEMA/AMM/RBC PRODUCTION/2
55. HEMA/EMM/OSMOTIC FRAG/2
56. HEMA/AMM/WBC/SPEC TEST/3
57. HEMA/ALF/WBC/ABNORMAL PROTEIN/3
58. HEMA/ALF/LAP/CML/1
59. HEMA/ALF/PLATELET COUNT/1
60. HEMA/DFC/WBC/DEGENERATION/1
61. HEMA/ALF/ABSOLUTE VALUE/CBC/2
62. HEMA/IBP/ECC/1
63. HEMA/IBP/WBC MATURA/1
64. HEMA/ALF/PBS/MULTIPLE MYELOMA/1
65. HEMA/ELF/PBS/INDICES/3
66. HEMA/CALC/RBC/INDICES/2
67. HEMA/IBP/COAG FACTOR/PATHWAY/1
68. HEMA/CALC/RBC/CHAMBER COUNT/2
69. HEMA/ELF/ERYTH DIS/SPEC TEST/2
70. HEMA/IBP/BASIC TESTS/CYANMETHEMOGLOBIN/1
71. HEMA/DFC/SCH/LABILE FACTOR/1
72. HEMA/AMM/WBC/INFECTIOUS MONO/2
73. HEMA/EMM/WBC/INFECT/3
74. HEMA/IMM/WBC/PBS/2
75. HEMA/DFC/PHYSIO/SPLEEN/1
76. HEMA/ECLD/HEMOSTASIS/DIC/3
77. HEMA/CALC/WBC COUNT/2
78. HEMA/ESOE/WBC/EOSINOPHIL COUNT/3
79. HEMA/ELF/HEMOSTASIS/FACTOR DEFICIENCY/2
80. HEMA/IBP/PLATELET/PHYSIO/1
81. BF/ISOE/SCH/URINE/2
82. BF/ISOP/URINE SEDIMENT/CASTS/1
83. BF/ALF/REL COND & DISO/URINE/1
84. BF/ALF/SPEC TESTS/URINE OSMOLALITY/1
85. BF/ALF/TRANSUDATE/2
86. BF/ALF/REL COND & DISO/AMNIOTIC FLUID/1
87. BF/ALF/URINE/MACRO APPEARANCE/1
88. BF/ELF/BASIC TEST/CSF/2
89. BF/SELM/SCH/24-HOUR URINE/1
90. BF/DFC/COMPOSITION/URINE/1
91. BF/EMM/URINE CRYSTALS/3
92. BF/EMM/URINE/YEAST/2
93. BF/ISOE/SCH/URINE/1
94. BF/IBP/ANALYZE METH/OCCULT BLOOD/1
95. BF/ALF/SPEC APPEARANCE/URINE SEDIMENT/1
96. BF/ALF/URINALYSIS/2
97. BF/DFC/PHYSIO/RENAL FUNCTION/1
98. BF/IBP/URINE/REAGENT STRIP/1
99. BF/DFC/URINE PHYSIO/CAST FORMATION/1
100. BF/ALF/REL COND & DISO/CSF/2
101. BF/ELF/URINALYSIS/REDUC SUBSTANCES/3
102. MICR/DFC/GNB/GROWTH CHARACT/1
103. MICR/IBP/BASIC TESTS/TSI/1
104. MICR/ANLF/GNB/BASIC TEST/2
105. MICR/SELM/GPC/BIOCHEMICAL TEST/1
106. MICR/DFC/MICRO-MORPH/YEAST/1
107. MICR/IBP/GPC/INFECTIOUS DIS/1
108. MICR/IBP/GNC/BIOCHEMICAL TEST/1
109. MICR/ISOE/BASIC TEST/GNB/2
110. MICR/DFC/NOSOCOMI INFECT/1
111. MICR/DFC/SUSC TEST/1
112. MICR/AMM/AMOEBA/2
113. MICR/IBP/VIRAL TITER/1
114. MICR/IMM/AMOEBA/2
115. MICR/CCLF/PARASITIC INFES/PROTOZOA/3
116. MICR/IMM/YEAST/CSF/1
117. MICR/SELM/GPC/REAGENT QC/1
118. MICR/SEME/GNC/1
119. MICR/ESOE/AFB CULTURE/SPUTUM/3
120. MICR/ELF/GPC/BASIC TEST/2
121. MICR/CALC/COLONY COUNT/URINE CULTURE/2
122. MICR/ISOP/QC/AUTOCLAVE/1
123. MICR/ANLF/GNB/BASIC TEST/2
124. MICR/SELM/GNB/BIOCHEMICAL TEST/1
125. MICR/ISOP/INCUBATOR/1
126. MICR/ISOP/SAFETY/DISINFECTANT/1
127. MICR/ISOP/BASIC TESTS/AFB/1
128. MICR/DFC/MICRO MORPH/FUNGI/1
129. MICR/IBP/GPC/BIOCHEMICAL TEST/1
130. MICR/ACLF/GNCB IDENT/BASIC TEST/2

ITEM DESCRIPTOR LIST
MEDICAL LABORATORY TECHNICIAN EXAMINATION - FEBRUARY 1985

131. MICR/CALC/URINE/COLONY COUNT/2
132. MICR/SEL/GROWTH REQUIRE/ANAEROBES/1
133. MICR/ECLF/MICRO MORPH/ANAEROBE/2
134. MICR/DFC/SELECTIVE MEDIA/1
135. MICR/SELM/MICRO MORPH/NEMATODE/1
136. MICR/DFC/GPB/CLOSTRIDIUM/1
137. MICR/DFC/ANTIBIOTIC SUSC/TUBE DILUTION/1
138. MICR/DFC/GPC/BIOCHEMICAL TEST/1
139. MICR/ESOE/ANTIBIOTIC SUSC/2
140. MICR/SELM/IDENT/VIRUS/1
141. MICR/SEME/GPB/CORYNEBACTERIUM/2
142. MICR/DFC/LIFE CYCLE/NEMATODE/1
143. MICR/SEME/ANAEROBIC GPB/WOUND CULTURE/2
144. BBNK/IBP/RBC/COMPLEMENT FIX/1
145. BBNK/ALF/RBC/RH TYPING/2
146. BBNK/IBP/SCH/PLATELETS/1
147. BBNK/DFC/STORAGE/BLOOD PRODUCTS/1
148. BBNK/DFC/DONOR REQUIRE/1
149. BBNK/IBP/DONOR REQUIRE/PLATELETS/1
150. BBNK/ELF/CROSSMATCH/AUTOCONTROL/3
151. BBNK/DFC/GEN THER & PRIN/RH IMMUNOGLOBULIN/1
152. BBNK/DFC/HEMOTHERAPY/ADVERSE REX/1
153. BBNK/ALF/RBC/AIHA/1
154. BBNK/ISOP/SCH/DONOR PREP/1
155. BBNK/IBP/RBC/ISOAGGLUTININS/1
156. BBNK/ESOE/RBC/CELL SUSPENSION/3
157. BBNK/SBP/HEMOTHERAPY/PACKED CELLS/1
158. BBNK/ELF/RBC/DONOR ACCEPT/2
159. BBNK/DFC/CRYOPRECIPITATE/1
160. BBNK/IBP/NON-SECRETOR/1
161. BBNK/IBP/HEMOTHERAPY/TX REX/1
162. BBNK/DFC/SCH/COMPATIBILITY TEST/1
163. BBNK/DFC/RBC/ANTICOAGULANT/1
164. BBNK/ELF/RBC/RH TYPING/3
165. BBNK/ALF/ABO GROUPING/2
166. BBNK/ISOP/RBC/RH TYPING/1
167. BBNK/ISOP/DAT/HDN/1
168. BBNK/SDU/HEMOTHERAPY/ABO/3
169. BBNK/DFC/LECTIN/1
170. BBNK/ELF/RBC/COLD ANTIBODY/2
171. BBNK/ECLD/HEMOTHERAPY/BLOOD COMPO/3
172. BBNK/IBP/GEN THER & PRIN/RBC ANTIGEN/2
173. BBNK/SEL/HEMOTHERAPY/BLOOD COMPO/3
174. BBNK/ALF/HEMOLYTC TX REX/2
175. BBNK/ELF/HEMOTHERAPY/EXCHANGE TX/2
176. BBNK/IBP/RBC/ANTIGLO TEST/2
177. IMMU/DFC/ANAT & PHYSIO/CELLU IMMUNITY/1
178. IMMU/ALF/SLE/1
179. IMMU/DFC/STS/1
180. IMMU/DFC/BASIC TEST/SEROLOGIC DILUTION/2
181. IMMU/ALF/FEBRILE AGGLUT/2
182. IMMU/IBP/AUTO/INDIRECT IMMUNOFLU/1
183. IMMU/ELF/STS/2
184. IMMU/DFC/AUTOANTIBODY/SLE/1
185. IMMU/ESOE/SCH/SEROLOGIC TEST/3
186. IMMU/DFC/IMMUNOGLOBULIN/1
187. IMMU/DFC/COLD AGGLUT/1
188. IMMU/ESOE/SEROLOGIC TEST/INFECTIOUS MONO/3
189. IMMU/DFC/AUTOIMMUNITY/RA/1
190. IMMU/DFC/BASIC TEST/PROZONE/1
191. IMMU/IBP/STS/1
192. IMMU/DFC/SCREENING PROC/QC/1
193. IMMU/IBP/ALLERGY/RAST/1
194. IMMU/DFC/HUMORAL/IMMUNITY/1
195. IMMU/DFC/HUMORAL/IMMUNITY/1
196. IMMU/ISOE/STS/BIOLOLIC FALSE-POS/1

GLOSSARY OF TERMS USED IN ITEM DESCRIPTORS
MEDICAL LABORATORY TECHNICIAN EXAMINATION - AUGUST 1985

&	AND
ACLD	ASSOCIATE CLINICAL AND LABORATORY DATA
ALF	ASSOCIATE LABORATORY FINDINGS
AML	ACUTE MYELOCYTIC LEUKEMIA
BBNK	BLOOD BANK
BF	BODY FLUIDS
CALC	CALCULATE
CCLD	CORRELATE CLINICAL AND LABORATORY DATA
CHEM	CHEMISTRY
CLL	CHRONIC LYMPHOCYTIC LEUKEMIA
DFC	DEFINE FUNDAMENTAL CHARACTERISTIC(S)
ECLD	EVALUATE CLINICAL AND LABORATORY DATA
ELF	EVALUATE LABORATORY FINDINGS
EMM	EVALUATE MICROSCOPIC MORPHOLOGY
ESOE	EVALUATE SOURCE OF ERROR
GNB	GRAM-NEGATIVE BACILLI
GNC	GRAM-NEGATIVE COCCI
GPB	GRAM-POSITIVE BACILLI
GPC	GRAM-POSITIVE COCCI
HCG	HUMAN CHORIONIC GONADOTROPIN
HDN	HEMOLYTIC DISEASE OF THE NEWBORN
HEMA	HEMATOLOGY
IBP	IDENTIFY BASIC PRINCIPLE(S)
IMM	IDENTIFY MICROSCOPIC MORPHOLOGY
IMMU	IMMUNOLOGY
IMVIC	INDOL, METHYL RED, VOGES-PROSKAUER, CITRATE
ISOE	IDENTIFY SOURCE OF ERROR
ISOP	IDENTIFY STANDARD OPERATING PROCEDURE
MICR	MICROBIOLOGY
PERF	PERFORM
RBC	RED BLOOD CELL
SBP	SELECT BLOOD PRODUCT
SCH	SPECIMEN COLLECTION AND HANDLING
SCOA	SELECT COURSE OF ACTION
SELM	SELECT METHOD
SLE	SYSTEMIC LUPUS ERYTHEMATOSUS
SPE	SERUM PROTEIN ELECTROPHORESIS
WBC	WHITE BLOOD CELL
X-MATCH	CROSSMATCH

TAXONIMIC LEVELS

TAX 1 - Recall:	Ability to recall or recognize previously learned (memorized) knowledge ranging from specific facts to complete theories.
TAX 2 - Interpretive skills:	Ability to utilize recalled knowledge to interpret or apply verbal, numeric or visual data.
TAX 3 - Problem Solving:	Ability to utilize recalled knowledge and the interpretation/application of distinct criteria to resolve a problem or situation and/or make an appropriate decision.

ITEM DESCRIPTOR LIST
MEDICAL LABORATORY TECHNICIAN EXAMINATION - AUGUST, 1985

1. IMMU/DFC/COMPLEMENT/1
2. IMMU/ALF/SLE/1
3. IMMU/IBP/DIRECT ANTIGLOBULIN TEST/1
4. IMMU/CCLD/C-REACTIVE PROTEIN/2
5. IMMU/DFC/AUTOIMMUNITY/RHEUMATOID ARTHRITIS/1
6. IMMU/ELF/IMMUNE RESPONSE/2
7. IMMU/IBP/SYPHILIS SEROLOGY/2
8. IMMU/ELF/SYPHILIS SEROLOGY/2
9. IMMU/DFC/PHYSIOLOGY/HCG/1
10. IMMU/IBP/AUTOIMMUNITY/IMMUNOFLUORESCENCE/1
11. IMMU/ALF/FEBRILE AGGLUTININ/2
12. IMMU/PERF/BASIC TESTS/COLD AGGLUTININ/1
13. IMMU/SELM/BASIC TEST/ALLERGY/1
14. IMMU/DFC/PHYSIOLOGY/CELLULAR IMMUNITY/1
15. IMMU/DFC/T LYMPHOCYTES/1
16. IMMU/DFC/AUTOIMMUNITY/SLE/1
17. IMMU/IBP/AUTOIMMUNITY/IMMUNOFLUORESCENCE/1
18. IMMU/DFC/HUMORAL IMMUNITY/1
19. IMMU/ESOE/BASIC TESTS/ANTISTREPTOLYSIN O/3
20. IMMU/DFC/SCH/CRYOGLOBULINS/1
21. IMMU/CALC/PROTEIN FRACTION/SPE/2
22. IMMU/IBP/SYPHILIS SEROLOGY/1
23. CHEM/IBP/OSMOLALITY/1
24. CHEM/ELF/BLOOD GASES/2
25. CHEM/ISOE/SCH/QUALITY CONTROL/1
26. CHEM/SCOA/SCH/ACID PHOSPHATASE/1
27. CHEM/DFC/PHYSIOLOGY/LIPIDS/1
28. CHEM/DFC/SCH/ANTICOAGULANT/1
29. CHEM/SCOA/SCH/POTASSIUM/3
30. CHEM/CALC/SOLUTION PREPARATION/2
31. CHEM/IBP/ENZYME ANALYSIS/ACID PHOSPHATASE/1
32. CHEM/SCOA/SAFETY/ACID BURN/2
33. CHEM/ALF/DISEASE MANIFESTATION/ACIDOSIS/2
34. CHEM/ISOE/SCH/BILIRUBIN/1
35. CHEM/DFC/SCH/BLOOD GASES/1
36. CHEM/CALC/INSTRUMENTATION/SPECTROPHOTOMETER/2
37. CHEM/ALF/CALCIUM/1
38. CHEM/IBP/DISEASE MANIFESTATION/ACIDOSIS/2
39. CHEM/CALC/MILLIEQUIVALENT/2
40. CHEM/ACLD/ENZYMES/PERNICIOUS ANEMIA/2
41. CHEM/ALF/CARDIAC ENZYMES/2
42. CHEM/IBP/BASIC TESTS/CREATININE/1
43. CHEM/ELF/CARBOHYDRATE/MALABSORPTION/2
44. CHEM/ISOE/INSTRUMENTATION/CHLORIDOMETER/2
45. CHEM/IBP/SPECIAL TESTS/T-3 UPTAKE/1
46. CHEM/DFC/INSTRUMENTATION/BLOOD GAS ELECTRODE/1
47. CHEM/ECLD/ENZYMES/MYOCARDIAL INFARCT/2
48. CHEM/CALC/STANDARD SOLUTION/2
49. CHEM/IBP/INSTRUMENTATION/FLAME PHOTOMETER/1
50. CHEM/CALC/SPECIAL CHEMISTRY/RADIOACTIVE DECAY/2
51. CHEM/ALF/BEERS LAW/2
52. CHEM/DFC/BIOCHEMICAL THEORY/BUFFER/1
53. CHEM/IBP/ENZYME ANALYSIS/LACTATE DHYDROGENASE/1
54. CHEM/CALC/UNKNOWN CONCENTRATION/2
55. CHEM/CALC/ELECTROPHORESIS/PROTEIN/2
56. CHEM/IBP/PROTEIN ELECTROPHORESIS/1
57. CHEM/IBP/SCH/HORMONE ASSAYS/1
58. CHEM/ELF/DISEASE MANIFESTATION/AMYLASE/2
59. CHEM/ESOE/GLUCOSE/3
60. CHEM/ESOE/FLAME PHOTOMETER/3
61. CHEM/CALC/LIPOPROTEINS/LOW-DENSITY/2
62. CHEM/SELM/SAFETY/ACID SOLUTION/2
63. HEMA/DFC/PHYSIOLOGY/FACTOR VIII/1
64. HEMA/ALF/HEMOSTATIC DISORDER/CLOT LYSIS/2
65. HEMA/ALF/RBC/AUTOIMMUNE HEMOLYTIC ANEMIA/2
66. HEMA/CALC/RBC/MEAN CORPUSCULAR VOLUME/2
67. HEMA/ISOP/QUALITY ASSURANCE/HEMOGLOBIN/1
68. HEMA/DFC/MICROSCOPIC MORPHOLOGY/AML/1
69. HEMA/SELM/SCH/PLATELET FUNCTION TEST/1
70. HEMA/IBP/DIFFERENTIAL/LEFT SHIFT/1
71. HEMA/CALC/WBC/ABSOLUTE COUNT/2
72. HEMA/IBP/HEPARIN/1
73. HEMA/CALC/LEUKOCYTE ALKALINE PHOSPHATASE/2
74. HEMA/ISOP/SCH/LABILE FACTOR/1
75. HEMA/ELF/PLATELET ESTIMATE/2
76. HEMA/ACLD/HEMOSTATIC DISORDER/3
77. HEMA/ALF/HEMOSTASIS/FACTOR DEFICIENCY/3
78. HEMA/IBP/WBC MATURATION/1
79. HEMA/IBP/RETICULOCYTE STAIN/1
80. HEMA/ISOE/RBC/WRIGHT STAIN/1
81. HEMA/CALC/CORRECTED WBC/2
82. HEMA/DFC/WBC COUNT/1
83. HEMA/EMM/PERIPHERAL BLOOD SMEAR/PLATELET COUNT/2
84. HEMA/IMM/BASIC TEST/DIFFERENTIAL COUNT/2
85. HEMA/ELF/CELL MATURATION/GRANULOCYTES/2
86. HEMA/SELM/ELECTROPHORESIS/HEMOGLOBINOPATHY/2
87. HEMA/SELM/WBC/SPECIAL TEST/3
88. HEMA/ISOE/RBC/SEDIMENTATION RATE/1
89. HEMA/DFC/WBC/MONOCYTE/1
90. HEMA/ELF/RBC/OSMOTIC FRAGILITY/2
91. HEMA/SELM/SCH/PEDIATRIC/1
92. HEMA/ACLD/ANEMIA/RETICULOCYTE COUNT/1
93. HEMA/CALC/TOLERANCE LIMITS/2
94. HEMA/ALF/WBC/MYELOMA/1
95. HEMA/ALF/MICROSCOPIC MORPHOLOGY/CLL/1
96. HEMA/DFC/HEMOGLOBIN COMPOSITION/1
97. HEMA/ESOE/AUTOMATED COUNT/HEMOGLOBIN/3
98. HEMA/IBP/PHYSIOLOGY/HEMOSTATIC DISORDER/1
99. HEMA/IBP/SPECIAL STAIN/RBC INCLUSIONS/1
100. HEMA/ACLD/PLATELETS/ACUTE LEUKEMIA/1
101. HEMA/ISOP/HEMOSTASIS/BLEEDING TIME/1
102. HEMA/DFC/WBC/ANOMALY/1
103. HEMA/CALC/RBC/CHAMBER COUNT/2
104. HEMA/ALF/COAGULATION TEST/2
105. BF/IBP/RENAL THRESHOLD/1
106. BF/DFC/URINE VOLUME/1
107. BF/DFC/PHYSIOLOGY/URINE CASTS/1
108. BF/DFC/OSMOLALITY/1
109. BF/ALF/URINE/MACROSCOPIC APPEARANCE/1
110. BF/ALF/URINE SEDIMENT/CRYSTALS/1
111. BF/ELF/URINE/REDUCING SUBSTANCES/3
112. BF/ESOE/SCH/URINE/2
113. BF/CALC/URINE/SPECIFIC GRAVITY/2
114. BF/ALF/MACROSCOPIC APPEARANCE/FECES/2
115. BF/ISOE/SCH/URINE/1
116. BF/ACLD/CEREBROSPINAL FLUID/TRAUMATIC TAP/2
117. BF/ELF/URINE SEDIMENT/BLOOD/2
118. BF/SCOA/SCH/CREATININE CLEARANCE/2
119. BF/IBP/ANALYTIC METHOD/URINE UROBILINOGEN/1
120. BF/SELM/SCH/24-HOUR URINE/1
121. BF/ELF/URINE SEDIMENT/SOURCE OF ORIGIN/2
122. BF/ACLD/MICROSCOPIC MORPHOLOGY/URINE SEDIMENT/3
123. BF/ACLD/MICROSCOPIC MORPHOLOGY/URINE CRYSTALS/2
124. BF/CALC/CEREBROSPINAL FLUID/CELL COUNT/2
125. BF/IBP/PHYSIOLOGY/PERITONEAL FLUID/1
126. BF/ALF/RELATED DISORDERS/AMNIOTIC FLUID/1
127. MICR/DFC/GNB/GROWTH CHARACTERISTIC/1
128. MICR/SELM/GPC/BIOCHEMICAL TEST/1
129. MICR/SELM/GPB/CORYNEBACTERIUM/2
130. MICR/DFC/GROWTH CHARACTERISTIC/STREPTOCOCCUS/1

ITEM DESCRIPTOR LIST
MEDICAL LABORATORY TECHNICIAN EXAMINATION - AUGUST, 1985

131. MICR/SCOA/BIOCHEMICAL TEST/GPC/3
132. MICR/SELM/GNC/1
133. MICR/DFC/GPB/CLOSTRIDIUM/1
134. MICR/DFC/MICROSCOPIC MORPHOLOGY/CANDIDA/1
135. MICR/ELF/GNB/BASIC TEST/2
136. MICR/IBP/GPC/INFECTIOUS DISEASE/1
137. MICR/SELM/SCH/OVA & PARASITES/3
138. MICR/ELF/LIFECYCLE/NEMATODE/3
139. MICR/SELM/SCH/OVA & PARASITES/2
140. MICR/IBP/CARBON DIOXIDE INCUBATION/1
141. MICR/IBP/MYCOBACTERIA/BIOCHEMICAL REACTION/1
142. MICR/ELF/BASIC TESTS/IMVIC/1
143. MICR/SELM/SCH/PROTOZOA/1
144. MICR/ALF/GNB/BIOCHEMICAL TESTS/2
145. MICR/ALF/GPC/WOUND CULTURE/2
146. MICR/SCOA/SCH/URINE CULTURE/3
147. MICR/SELM/BASIC TESTS/ORGANISM IDENTIFICATION/2
148. MICR/SELM/BIOCHEMICAL TEST/STREPTOCOCCUS/1
149. MICR/ELF/VIRAL TITER/1
150. MICR/SELM/WOUND CULTURE/ANAEROBES/3
151. MICR/IBP/MEDIA/2
152. MICR/IBP/SCH/OVA & PARASITES/1
153. MICR/ELF/SUSCEPTIBILITY TEST/2
154. MICR/SELM/GROWTH REQUIREMENT/BACTEROIDES/2
155. MICR/SELM/SCH/CEREBROSPINAL FLUID/1
156. MICR/IMM/MOLD/2
157. MICR/SELM/WOUND CULTURE/ANAEROBE/2
158. MICR/ACLD/GNB/WOUND CULTURE/2
159. MICR/DFC/BIOCHEMICAL TESTS/ENTEROBACTERIACEAE/1
160. MICR/ELF/GNB/BIOCHEMICAL IDENTIFICATION/3
161. MICR/IBP/SCH/MYCOBACTERIA/1
162. MICR/DFC/BASIC TESTS/GPC/1
163. MICR/ESOE/GRAM STAIN/URINE/3
164. MICR/ELF/GRAM STAIN/SPUTUM/2
165. MICR/ALF/GNC/GENITOURINARY CULTURE/2
166. MICR/ACLD/GPB/WOUND CULTURE/2
167. MICR/ELF/GNB/BIOCHEMICAL IDENTIFICATION/3
168. MICR/ELF/GNB/CEREBROSPINAL FLUID CULTURE/2
169. MICR/ELF/BIOCHEMICAL IDENTIFICATION/GPC/2
170. MICR/SELM/SCH/VIRUS CULTURE/1
171. BBNK/SELM/DU TESTING/1
172. BBNK/DFC/THEORY/RH IMMUNE GLOBULIN/1
173. BBNK/DFC/HEMOTHERAPY/RED CELLS/1
174. BBNK/ECLD/HEMOTHERAPY/FACTOR DEFICIENCY/3
175. BBNK/ELF/X-MATCH/AUTOCONTROL/3
176. BBNK/IBP/SCH/RED CELLS/1
177. BBNK/ELF/RH GENOTYPE/2
178. BBNK/DFC/LECTIN/1
179. BBNK/DFC/SCH/CRYOPRECIPITATE/1
180. BBNK/ACLD/HEMOTHERAPY/ADVERSE REACTION/2
181. BBNK/IBP/UNIT SELECTION/ABO SUBGROUPS/2
182. BBNK/ACLD/HEMOTHERAPY/ADVERSE REACTION/2
183. BBNK/ALF/RBC/AUTOIMMUNE HEMOLYTIC ANEMIA/1
184. BBNK/IBP/HUMAN LYMPHOCYTE ANTIGEN/1
185. BBNK/DFC/SCH/COMPATIBILITY TEST/1
186. BBNK/ISOP/COMPONENT PREPARATION/PLATELETS/1
187. BBNK/DFC/DONOR ACCEPTIBILITY/1
188. BBNK/IBP/COLD AGGLUTININ/1
189. BBNK/ISOP/DIRECT ANTIGLOBULIN TEST/HDN/1
190. BBNK/IBP/NON-SECRETOR/1
191. BBNK/IBP/HEMOTHERAPY/ADVERSE REACTION/1
192. BBNK/ELF/ANTIBODY IDENTIFICATION/3
193. BBNK/ELF/ANTIBODY IDENTIFICATION/3
194. BBNK/ALF/RBC/RH TYPING/2
195. BBNK/ESOE/SCH/BLOOD TYPING/2
196. BBNK/ECLD/HEMOTHERAPY/ANEMIA/3
197. BBNK/DFC/STORAGE/BLOOD PRODUCTS/1
198. BBNK/ELF/RBC/RH TYPING/3
199. BBNK/ACLD/ANTIBODY IDENTIFICATION/2
200. BBNK/ECLD/RBC/DONOR ACCEPTIBILITY/2
201. BBNK/ELF/ABO GROUPING/2
202. BBNK/ELF/ANTIBODY IDENTIFICATION/3
203. BBNK/ELF/ANTIBODY IDENTIFICATION/3
204. BBNK/ELF/INCOMPATIBILITY/ABO/2
205. BBNK/IBP/RBC/COMPLEMENT FIXATION/1
206. BBNK/SELM/HEMOTHERAPY/ADVERSE REACTION/2
207. BBNK/SBP/HEMOTHERAPY/FACTOR DEFICIENCY/2
208. BBNK/ELF/RBC ANTIGEN/SCREENING CELLS/3
209. BBNK/ISOP/SCH/X-MATCH/2
210. BBNK/IBP/SCH/PLATELETS/1
211. BBNK/DFC/ELUTION/1

GLOSSARY OF TERMS USED IN ITEM DESCRIPTORS
MEDICAL LABORATORY TECHNICIAN EXAMINATION - FEBRUARY 1986

AB	ANTIBODY(IES)
ACLD	ASSOCIATE CLINICAL AND LABORATORY DATA
AFB	ACID-FAST BACILLI
AG	ANTIGEN
AHA	AUTOIMMUNE HEMOLYTIC ANEMIA
AHG	ANTIHUMAN GLOBULIN
ALD	ASSOCIATE LABORATORY DATA
ALF	ASSOCIATE LABORATORY FINDINGS
AML	ACUTE MYELOCYTIC LEUKEMIA
ANA	ANTINUCLEAR ANTIBODY
ANLF	ANALYZE LABORATORY FINDINGS
BBNK	BLOOD BANK
BF	BODY FLUIDS
BMD	BIOCHEMICAL MANIFESTATION OF DISEASE
BTP	BIOLOGIC THEORY AND PHYSIOLOGY
CALC	CALCULATE
CHEM	CHEMISTRY
CLL	CHRONIC LYMPHOCYTIC LEUKEMIA
CSF	CEREBROSPINAL FLUID
DFC	DEFINE FUNDAMENTAL CHARACTERISTIC(S)
DIC	DISSEMINATED INTRAVASCULAR COAGULATION
ECLF	EVALUATE CLINICAL LAND LABORATORY FINDINGS
ELD	EVALUATE LABORATORY DATA
ELF	EVALUATE LABORATORY FINDINGS
EMM	EVALUATE MICROSCOPIC MORPHOLOGY
ESOE	EVALUATE SOURCE OF ERROR
GNB	GRAM-NEGATIVE BACILLI
GNC	GRAM-NEGATIVE COCCI
GPB	GRAM-POSITIVE BACILLI
GPC	GRAM-POSITIVE COCCI
HCG	HUMAN CHORIONIC GONADOTROPIN
HDN	HEMOLYTIC DISEASE OF THE NEWBORN
HEMA	HEMATOLOGY
IBP	IDENTIFY BASIC PRINCIPLE(S)
ID	IDENTIFY/IDENTIFICATION
IGTP	IMMUNOLOGIC GENETIC THEORY & PRINCIPLES
IMM	IDENTIFY MICROSCOPIC MORPHOLOGY
IMMU	IMMUNOLOGY
ISOE	IDENTIFY SOURCE OF ERROR
ISOP	IDENTIFY STANDARD OPERATING PROCEDURE
MIC	MINIMUM INHIBITORY CONCENTRATION
MICR	MICROBIOLOGY
MICRO	MICROSCOPIC
MORPH	MORPHOLOGY
PTT	ACTIVATED PARTIAL THROMBOPLASTIN TIME
QC	QUALITY CONTROL
RBC	RED BLOOD CELL
RCD	RELATED CONDITIONS AND DISORDERS
SBP	SELECT BLOOD PRODUCT
SCH	SPECIMEN COLLECTION AND HANDLING
SCOA	SELECT COURSE OF ACTION
SELB	SELECT BLOOD COMPONENT
SELM	SELECT METHOD
SELR	SELECT REAGENT
SELT	SELECT TEST
SEME	SELECT MEDIA
SGR	SELECT GROWTH REQUIREMENTS
SLE	SYSTEMIC LUPUS ERYTHEMATOSUS
STS	SEROLOGIC TESTS FOR SYPHILIS
TIBC	TOTAL IRON BINDING CAPACITY
WBC	WHITE BLOOD CELL

TAXONOMIC LEVEL

TAX 1 - Recall: Ability to recall or recognize previously learned (memorized) knowledge ranging from specific facts to complete theories.

TAX 2 - Interpretive Skills: Ability to utilize recalled knowledge to interpret or apply verbal, numeric or visual data.

TAX 3 - Problem Solving: Ability to utilize recalled knowledge and the interpretation/application of distinct criteria to resolve a problem or situation and/or make an appropriate decision.

ITEM DESCRIPTOR LIST
MEDICAL LABORATORY TECHNICIAN EXAMINATION - FEBRUARY 1986

1. BBNK/DFC/NON-CELLULAR COMPONENTS/1
2. BBNK/IBP/DONOR REQUIREMENTS/PLATELETS/1
3. BBNK/ALF/RBC/RH TYPING/2
4. BBNK/SELB/FACTOR DEFICIENCY/1
5. BBNK/IBP/BASIC TESTS/RH TYPING/1
6. BBNK/ISOP/SPECIMEN COLLECTION/LABELING/1
7. BBNK/DFC/HDN/1
8. BBNK/ALF/TRANSFUSION REACTION/1
9. BBNK/DFC/BLOOD COMPONENT/CLOTTING FACTORS/1
10. BBNK/ELF/CROSSMATCH/AUTOCONTROL/3
11. BBNK/ELF/RBC/AB SCREEN/2
12. BBNK/SBP/HEMOTHERAPY/PACKED CELLS/1
13. BBNK/ISOP/RBC/DONOR PROCESSING/1
14. BBNK/DFC/AGGLUTININ/NON-SPECIFIC COLD/1
15. BBNK/ELF/RH GENOTYPE/2
16. BBNK/ECLF/HEMOTHERAPY/BLOOD COMPONENT/3
17. BBNK/IBP/HEMOTHERAPY/TRANSFUSION REACTION/1
18. BBNK/IBP/PHYSIOLOGY/HDN/1
19. BBNK/ELF/RBC/RH TYPING/3
20. BBNK/ESOE/ABO TESTING/3
21. BBNK/DFC/SCH/CROSSMATCH/1
22. BBNK/ISOP/DIRECT ANTIGLOBULIN TEST/HDN/1
23. BBNK/ACLD/RBC/ADVERSE REACTION/2
24. BBNK/IBP/SCH/PLATELETS/1
25. BBNK/ELF/ABO TYPING/2
26. BBNK/SCOA/TRANSFUSION REACTION/2
27. BBNK/SELM/DU TESTING/1
28. BBNK/IBP/DONOR UNIT SELECTION/SUBGROUPS/2
29. BBNK/IBP/RBC/AHG TEST/2
30. BBNK/ELD/AB ID/3
31. BBNK/ALF/ABO GROUPING/2
32. BBNK/ISOP/DONOR SELECTION/1
33. BBNK/ALF/BASIC TESTS/RH IMMUNE GLOBULIN/2
34. BBNK/SELT/COMPONENT/PLATELET POOLING/2
35. BBNK/DFC/IGTP/MNS/1
36. BBNK/IBP/DONOR REQUIREMENTS/1
37. BBNK/IBP/AB ID/1
38. IMMU/DFC/BASIC TESTS/SERIAL DILUTION/1
39. IMMU/DFC/IMMUNOGLOBULIN/1
40. IMMU/ISOE/FEBRILE AGGLUTININS/3
41. IMMU/DFC/HUMORAL/IMMUNITY/1
42. IMMU/DBP/CELL PHYSIOLOGY/1
43. IMMU/IBP/DIRECT ANTIGLOBULIN TEST/1
44. IMMU/IBP/PHYSIOLOGY/IGE/1
45. IMMU/DFC/AG-AB REACTION/1
46. IMMU/ISOP/SPECIMEN COLLECTION/COLD AGGLUTININS/1
47. IMMU/ELF/STS/2
48. IMMU/DFC/AUTOANTIBODY/SLE/1
49. IMMU/IBP/RADIAL IMMUNODIFFUSION/2
50. IMMU/ISOE/COMPLEMENT-FIXATION/2
51. IMMU/DFC/ANATOMY & PHYSIOLOGY/HCG/1
52. IMMU/ALF/C-REACTIVE PROTEIN/1
53. IMMU/DFC/ANATOMY & PHYSIOLOGY/IMMUNOGLOBULIN/1
54. IMMU/ALD/ANA/2
55. IMMU/DFC/T-LYMPHOCYTES/1
56. IMMU/ISOE/RHEUMATOID ARTHRITIS/2
57. IMMU/IBP/AUTOIMMUNITY/INDIRECT IMMUNOFLUORESCENCE/1
58. IMMU/DFC/AB/AHA/1
59. CHEM/ISOE/SCH/BILIRUBIN/1
60. CHEM/DFC/BUFFER/1
61. CHEM/IBP/INSTRUMENTATION/FLAME PHOTOMETER/1
62. CHEM/DFC/GLYCOSYLATED HEMOGLOBIN/1
63. CHEM/IBP/SPECIAL TESTS/T-3 UPTAKE/1
64. CHEM/SELM/INSTRUMENT/KINETIC ASSAY/2
65. CHEM/ALF/LIPASE/1
66. CHEM/ELF/QC/LEVEY-JENNINGS/2
67. CHEM/IBP/BMD/ACIDOSIS/2
68. CHEM/IBP/BTP/ELECTROLYTES/1
69. CHEM/IBP/SALICYLATES/1
70. CHEM/ISOE/ACID PHOSPHATASE/1
71. CHEM/DFC/FETAL HEMOGLOBIN/1
72. CHEM/IBP/INSTRUMENTATION/OSMOLALITY/1
73. CHEM/ALF/BEERS LAW/2
74. CHEM/ALF/CALCIUM/1
75. CHEM/CALC/ENZYME DILUTION/2
76. CHEM/CALC/UNKNOWN CONCENTRATION/2
77. CHEM/DFC/STANDARD SOLUTION/1
78. CHEM/ACLD/ENZYMES/PROSTATE CANCER/1
79. CHEM/IBP/BASIC TESTS/PROTEIN/1
80. CHEM/DFC/QC/STATISTICS/1
81. CHEM/DFC/INSTRUMENTATION/BLOOD GAS/1
82. CHEM/DFC/BTP/COPPER/1
83. CHEM/ALF/BMD/CREATINE KINASE/1
84. CHEM/CALC/STANDARD SOL/2
85. CHEM/DFC/BTP/LIPIDS/1
86. CHEM/ISOE/INSTRUMENTATION/CHLORIDOMETER/2
87. CHEM/SCOA/SCH/POTASSIUM/3
88. CHEM/IBP/P&E/CREATININE CLEARANCE/1
89. CHEM/IBP/INSTRUMENTATION/FLUOROMETER/1
90. CHEM/ESOE/GLUCOSE/3
91. CHEM/IBP/P&E/ALBUMIN/1
92. CHEM/DFC/BLOOD PH/1
93. CHEM/DFC/PROTEIN/ELECTROPHORESIS/1
94. CHEM/CALC/SPECIAL CHEMISTRY/RADIOACTIVE DE
95. CHEM/SELR/SCH/ACID-BASE/1
96. CHEM/CALC/INSTRUMENTATION/SPECTROPHOTOMETE
97. CHEM/CALC/QC/COEFFICIENT OF VARIATION/2
98. HEMA/ALF/HEMATOCRIT/2
99. HEMA/ALF/PLATELET COUNT/1
100. HEMA/IBP/WBC MATURATION/1
101. HEMA/ALF/HEMOSTATIC DISORDER/CLOT LYSIS/2
102. HEMA/ISOP/SCH/LABILE FACTOR/1
103. HEMA/CALC/TOLERANCE LIMITS/2
104. HEMA/ACLD/COAGULATION TESTS/ASPIRIN/2
105. HEMA/CALC/WBC/ABSOLUTE COUNT/2
106. HEMA/ALF/WBC/MYELOMA/1
107. HEMA/DFC/MATURATION/RBC/1
108. HEMA/ELD/RBC MORPH/HEMOGLOBIN ELECTROPHORE
109. HEMA/IMM/BASIC TEST/DIFFERENTIAL COUNT/2
110. HEMA/ELF/CELL MATURATION/GRANULOCYTES/2
111. HEMA/SELM/ELECTROPHORESIS/HEMOGLOBINOPATHY
112. HEMA/CALC/CORRECTED WBC/2
113. HEMA/ALF/MICRO MORPH/CLL/1
114. HEMA/ECLF/HEMOSTASIS/DIC/3
115. HEMA/ALF/BASIC TESTS/ROULEAUX/1
116. HEMA/IBP/ANALYTIC TEST/PROTHROMBIN TIME/1
117. HEMA/ALF/MICRO MORPH/ANEMIA/2
118. HEMA/ELF/HEMOSTASIS/THROMBOCYTOPENIA/3
119. HEMA/ALF/MYELOMA/1
120. HEMA/DFC/LEUKOCYTE/ARTIFACTS/1
121. HEMA/DFC/CLOTTING FACTOR/1
122. HEMA/DFC/MICRO MORPH/AML/1
123. HEMA/ALF/BASIC TESTS/HEMOLYTIC ANEMIA/1
124. HEMA/IMM/SOURCE OF ERROR/SLIDE PREPARATION
125. HEMA/ALF/MICRO MORPH/RBC/2
126. HEMA/IMM/BASIC TESTS/WBC DIFFERENTIAL/2
127. HEMA/IMM/WBC INCLUSION/2
128. HEMA/SCOA/MICRO MORPH/MEGALOBLASTIC ANEMIA
129. HEMA/DFC/WBC/NORMAL MATURATION/1
130. HEMA/IBP/SPECIAL STAIN/1

ITEM DESCRIPTOR LIST
MEDICAL LABORATORY TECHNICIAN EXAMINATION - FEBRUARY 1986

1. HEMA/CALC/RBC/CHAMBER COUNT/2
2. HEMA/CALC/RBC INDICES/2
3. HEMA/IBP/SPECIAL STAIN/RBC INCLUSIONS/1
4. HEMA/ACLD/PLATELETS/ACUTE LEUKEMIA/1
5. HEMA/IBP/PLATELET/PHYSIOLOGY/1
6. HEMA/ESOE/COAG/PTT/2
7. BF/ALF/BASIC TESTS/URINE SEDIMENT/1
8. BF/ALF/CSF/GLUCOSE/1
9. BF/ELF/MICRO MORPH/URINE CRYSTALS/3
0. BF/EMM/URINE/CRYSTAL/3
1. BF/ISOE/URINE/REAGENT STRIP/1
2. BF/ALF/PERICARDIAL FLUID/WBC/2
3. BF/IBP/URINE SEDIMENT/CRYSTALS/1
4. BF/CALC/URINE/SPECIFIC GRAVITY/2
5. BF/DFC/ANATOMY & PHYSIOLOGY/URINE CASTS/1
6. BF/IBP/URINE/REAGENT STRIP/1
7. BF/ALF/RCD/AMNIOTIC FLUID/1
8. BF/CALC/CSF/CELL COUNT/2
9. BF/ACLD/MICRO MORPH/URINE SEDIMENT/3
0. BF/ELF/URINE SEDIMENT/CAST/2
1. BF/ELF/URINE SEDIMENT/2
2. BF/ALF/URINALYSIS/SEDIMENT EXAM/2
3. BF/ALF/UROBILINOGEN/1
4. BF/DFC/ANATOMY & PHYSIOLOGY/STOOL FAT/1
5. BF/ELF/URINE SEDIMENT/BLOOD/2
6. BF/ELF/URINALYSIS/REDUCING SUBSTANCES/3
7. BF/IBP/RENAL THRESHOLD/1
8. BF/IBP/CHEMICAL TEST/URINE UROBILINOGEN/1
9. BF/ISOE/SCH/URINALYSIS/2
0. MICR/ID/MACROSCOPIC MORPH/PROTEUS/1
1. MICR/ALF/GPC/WOUND CULTURE/2
2. MICR/SELM/SCH/PROTOZOA/1
3. MICR/SELM/SAFETY DISINFECTANT/VIROLOGY/1
4. MICR/IBP/SELECTIVE MEDIA/NEISSERIA/2

165. MICR/ESOE/AFB CULTURE/SPUTUM/3
166. MICR/IBP/URINE COUNT/NORMAL/1
167. MICR/ALF/SCH/NORMAL FLORA/1
168. MICR/SELM/ANAEROBIC GPB/WOUND CULTURE/2
169. MICR/IMM/AMOEBA/1
170. MICR/ALF/GNC/GENITOURINARY CULTURE/2
171. MICR/SEME/AFB/2
172. MICR/SELM/IDENTIFICATION/DIPHTHEROIDS/2
173. MICR/ISOE/BASIC TESTS/SUSCEPTIBILITY TEST/1
174. MICR/ALF/GNB/BIOCHEMICAL TESTS/2
175. MICR/IBP/VIRAL TITER/1
176. MICR/IMM/MOLD/2
177. MICR/IBP/GPC/INFECTIOUS DISEASE/1
178. MICR/SELM/GPB/CORYNEBACTERIUM/2
179. MICR/ESOE/CAMPYLOBACTER/BLOOD CULTURE/3
180. MICR/CALC/URINE/COLONY COUNT/2
181. MICR/IBP/SEROLOGICAL TEST/STREPTOCOCCI/1
182. MICR/ANLF/GNB/BIOCHEMICAL TEST/2
183. MICR/ALF/MACROSCOPIC MORPH/STREPTOCOCCI/2
184. MICR/SELM/SUSCEPTIBILITY/HAEMOPHILUS/2
185. MICR/IBP/SCH/OVA & PARASITE/1
186. MICR/ELF/MIC/2
187. MICR/DFC/ANTIBIOTIC/CLASSIFICATION/1
188. MICR/SELM/BASIC TESTS/ORGANISM ID/2
189. MICR/IBP/DISINFECTION/1
190. MICR/DFC/BASIC TESTS/GPC/1
191. MICR/IMM/FLAGELLATE/3
192. MICR/DFC/GPB/CLOSTRIDUM/1
193. MICR/IBP/CO2 INCUBATION/1
194. MICR/ID/MICRO MORPH/GARDNERELLA/1
195. MICR/ALF/BASIC TEST/CLOSTRIDIUM PERFRINGENS/1
196. MICR/ALF/PSEUDOMONAS/BIOCHEMICAL TEST/2
197. MICR/ELF/GNB/BIOCHEMICAL ID/3
198. MICR/SCOA/BIOCHEMICAL TESTS/GPC/3

GLOSSARY OF TERMS USED IN ITEM DESCRIPTORS
MEDICAL LABORATORY TECHNICIAN EXAMINATION - AUGUST 1986

AB	ANTIBODY(IES)
ACLD	ASSOCIATE CLINICAL AND LABORATORY DATA
AFB	ACID-FAST BACILLI
ALF	ASSOCIATE LABORATORY FINDING
AMM	ASSOCIATE MICROSCOPIC MORPHOLOGY
BBNK	BLOOD BANKING
BF	BODY FLUIDS
BMD	BIOCHEMICAL MANIFESTATION OF DISEASE
BTP	BIOCHEMICAL THEORY AND PHYSIOLOGY
CALC	CALCULATE
CEA	CARCINOEMBRYONIC ANTIGHEN
CGL	CHRONIC GRANULOCYTIC LEUKEMIA
CHEM	CHEMISTRY
CLL	CHRONIC LYMPHOCYTIC LEUKEMIA
DFC	DEFINE FUNDAMENTAL CHARACTERISTIC(S)
DIC	DISSEMINATED INTRAVASCULAR COAGULATION
ECLD	EVALUATE CLINICAL AND LABORATORY DATA
EDTA	ETHYLENEDIAMINETETRAACETIC ACID
ELF	EVALUATE LABORATORY FINDINGS
EMM	EVALUATE MICROSCOPIC MORPHOLOGY
ESOE	EVALUATE SOURCE OF ERROR
GNB	GRAM-NEGATIVE BACILLI
GNC	GRAM-NEGATIVE COCCI
GPB	GRAM-POSITIVE BACILLI
GPC	GRAM-POSITIVE COCCI
HCG	HUMAN CHORIONIC GONADOTROPIN
HDN	HEMOLYTIC DISEASE OF THE NEWBORN
HEMA	HEMATOLOGY
HLA	HUMAN LYMPHOCYTE ANTIGENS
IBP	IDENTIFY BASIC PRINCIPLE(S)
ID	IDENTIFY/IDENTIFICATION
IMAM	IDENTIFY MACROSCOPIC MORPHOLOGY
IMM	IDENTIFY MICROSCOPIC MORPHOLOGY
IMMU	IMMUNOLOGY
ISOE	IDENTIFY SOURCE OF ERROR
ISOP	IDENTIFY STANDARD OPERATING PROCEDURE
MACRO	MACROSCOPIC
MICR	MICROBIOLOGY
MICRO	MICROSCOPIC
MORPH	MORPHOLOGY
O-F	OXIDATIVE-FERMENTATIVE
PERF	PERFORM
P&E	PROTEINS AND ENZYMES
QC	QUALITY CONTROL
RA	RHEUMATOID ARTHRITIS
RAST	RADIOALLERGOSORBENT TEST
RBC	RED BLOOD CELL
RID	RADIAL IMMUNODIFFUSION
SCOA	SELECT COURSE OF ACTION
SDU	SELECT DONOR UNIT
SELC	SELECT COMPONENT
SELM	SELECT METHOD
SLE	SYSTEMIC LUPUS ERYTHEMATOSUS
UV	ULTRAVIOLET
WBC	WHITE BLOOD CELL
X-MATCH	CROSSMATCH

TAXONOMIC LEVELS

TAX 1 - Recall: Ability to recall or recognize previously learned (memorized) knowledge ranging from specific facts to complete theories.

TAX 2 - Interpretive Skills: Ability to utilize recalled knowledge to interpret or apply verbal, numeric or visual data.

TAX 3 - Problem Solving: Ability to utilize recalled knowledge and the interpretation/application of distinct criteria to resolve a problem or situation and/or make an appropriat decision.

ITEM DESCRIPTOR LIST
MEDICAL LABORATORY TECHNICIAN EXAMINATION - AUGUST 1986

1. MICR/IBP/MEDIA PREPARATION/ANAEROBES/2
2. MICR/ALF/MACRO MORPH/MOLD/2
3. MICR/SELM/WOUND CULTURE/ANAEROBES/3
4. MICR/SCOA/BIOCHEMICAL TEST/GPC/3
5. MICR/DFC/NORMAL FLORA/1
6. MICR/DFC/GNB/BIOCHEMICAL ID/1
7. MICR/SELM/GPB/CORYNEBACTERIUM/2
8. MICR/ELF/BIOCHEMICAL TEST/STREPTOCOCCUS/2
9. MICR/ISOE/BASIC TESTS/SUSCEPTIBILITY/2
10. MICR/ESOE/GRAM STAIN/WOUND/3
11. MICR/ID/MACRO MORPH/AFB/1
12. MICR/DFC/PSEUDOMONAS/1
13. MICR/DFC/MEDIA/1
14. MICR/ESOE/BASIC TESTS/SUSCEPTIBILITY/2
15. MICR/ELF/BIOCHEMICAL TEST/STREPTOCOCCI/2
16. MICR/ALF/GNC/GENITAL CULTURE/2
17. MICR/DFC/SCH/AFB/1
18. MICR/DFC/MICRO MORPH/AMOEBA/1
19. MICR/ACLD/GPB/WOUND CULTURE/2
20. MICR/DFC/GNB/NONFERMENTATIVE/1
21. MICR/ELF/ANAEROBIC CULTURE/2
22. MICR/DFC/MICRO MORPH/NEMATODE/1
23. MICR/SELM/ANAEROBIC GPB/WOUND CULTURE/2
24. MICR/ALF/GNB/BIOCHEMICAL TESTS/2
25. MICR/IBP/VIRUS/TRANSPORT/1
26. MICR/DFC/GPB/CLOSTRIDUM/1
27. MICR/ALF/GPC/WOUND CULTURE/2
28. MICR/DFC/GNB/GROWTH CHARACTERISTIC/1
29. MICR/ECLD/MICRO MORPH/ANAEROBE/2
30. MICR/IBP/SAFETY/FUNGAL INFECTION/1
31. MICR/IMAM/CESTODE/1
32. MICR/ESOE/SCH/GNC/3
33. MICR/DFC/BIOCHEMICAL ID/PROTEUS/1
34. MICR/ELF/O-F REACTION/2
35. MICR/ESOE/SCH/URINE CULTURE/2
36. MICR/ISOP/QC/AUTOCLAVE/1
37. MICR/SELM/SCH/BLOOD PARASITES/1
38. MICR/SELM/SCH/VIRUS CULTURE/1
39. MICR/IBP/GPC/BIOCHEMICAL TEST/1
40. MICR/ALF/GNB/BIOCHEMICAL TEST/2
41. MICR/SELM/BASIC TESTS/ORGANISM ID/2
42. BBNK/SELC/FACTOR DEFICIENCY/1
43. BBNK/IBP/HLA TYPING/1
44. BBNK/ECLD/HEMOTHERAPY/BLOOD COMPONENT/3
45. BBNK/ELF/RBC/AB SCREEN/2
46. BBNK/ESOE/RBC/CELL SUSPENSION/3
47. BBNK/ELF/ABO GROUPING/2
48. BBNK/ELF/RH GENETICS/3
49. BBNK/IBP/HEMOTHERAPY/ADVERSE REACTION/1
50. BBNK/IBP/RBC/ANTIGLOBULIN TEST/2
51. BBNK/DFC/DONOR ACCEPTIBILITY/1
52. BBNK/SCOA/RBC/ABO TESTING/1
53. BBNK/IBP/SCH/PLATELETS/1
54. BBNK/ACLD/HEMOTHERAPY/ADVERSE REACTION/2
55. BBNK/ACLD/AB ID/2
56. BBNK/SELM/SCH/LEUKOCYTE CONCENTRATE/1
57. BBNK/ALF/AB SCREEN/1
58. BBNK/ELF/AB ID/3
59. BBNK/DFC/RBC/ANTICOAGULANT/1
60. BBNK/ELF/RH GENOTYPE/2
61. BBNK/ALF/HEMOTHERAPY/ADVERSE REACTION/2
62. BBNK/ELF/ABO TYPING/2
63. BBNK/IBP/ANTI-H LECTIN/1
64. BBNK/IBP/X-MATCH/ABO SUBGROUPS/1
65. BBNK/ISOP/DONOR REQUIREMENT/1
66. BBNK/SELM/DU TESTING/1
67. BBNK/ALF/RH PHENOTYPE/2
68. BBNK/ACLD/HEMOTHERAPY/ADVERSE REACTION/2
69. BBNK/ESOE/ANTIGLOBULIN TEST/AB ID/3
70. BBNK/DFC/ABO AB/1
71. BBNK/SELC/HEMOTHERAPY/2
72. BBNK/DFC/DONOR ACCEPTIBILITY/1
73. BBNK/ISOP/ABO SUBGROUPS/1
74. BBNK/PERF/BASIC TESTS/ANTIGLOBULIN/1
75. BBNK/ACLD/HDN/AB/1
76. BBNK/IBP/ROULEAUX/1
77. IMMU/DFC/PHYSIOLOGY/IMMUNOGLOBULIN/1
78. IMMU/DFC/IMMUNITY/1
79. IMMU/SELM/SYPHILIS TESTING/1
80. IMMU/ELF/BASIC TESTS/FEBRILE AGGLUTININ/1
81. IMMU/SCOA/RID/3
82. IMMU/DFC/ANTIGEN/BACTERIAL/1
83. IMMU/ESOE/QC/RA TEST/3
84. IMMU/IBP/BASIC TESTS/PRECIPITATION/1
85. IMMU/DFC/AUTOANTIBODY/SLE/1
86. IMMU/DFC/B LYMPHOCYTES/1
87. IMMU/DFC/SYPHILIS TESTS/1
88. IMMU/IBP/AUTOIMMUNITY/IMMUNOFLUORESCENCE/1
89. IMMU/DFC/PHYSIOLOGY/HUMORAL IMMUNITY/1
90. IMMU/SELM/SLE/1
91. IMMU/DFC/IMMUME RESPONSE/1
92. IMMU/ALF/PROZONE/2
93. IMMU/DFC/BASIC TESTS/RAST/1
94. IMMU/DFC/T LYMPHOCYTES/1
95. IMMU/DFC/ANATOMY/HCG/1
96. CHEM/SELM/SCH/GLUCOSE/1
97. CHEM/DFC/BLOOD PH/1
98. CHEM/IBP/BASIC TESTS/PROTEIN/1
99. CHEM/DFC/INSTRUMENTATION/BEERS LAW/1
100. CHEM/DFC/QC/STATISTICS/1
101. CHEM/ALF/INSTRUMENTATION/BEERS LAW/2
102. CHEM/DFC/BTP/LIPOPROTEINS/1
103. CHEM/CALC/SAMPLE DILUTION/2
104. CHEM/ELF/QC/GLUCOSE/2
105. CHEM/IBP/INSTRUMENTATION/CHROMATOGRAPHY/1
106. CHEM/IBP/SPECIAL TESTS/T-3 UPTAKE/1
107. CHEM/IBP/GLASSWARE/1
108. CHEM/ESOE/SCH/P&E/3
109. CHEM/DFC/BTP/BILIRUBIN/1
110. CHEM/ALF/PROTEIN/MYELOMA/1
111. CHEM/CALC/STANDARD SOLUTION/2
112. CHEM/ALF/STEROIDS/1
113. CHEM/IBP/SCH/HORMONE ASSAYS/1
114. CHEM/DFC/BTP/COPPER/1
115. CHEM/ELF/P&E/GLOBULIN/3
116. CHEM/DFC/NORMAL SOLUTION/1
117. CHEM/IBP/BTP/ALBUMIN/1
118. CHEM/CALC/DILUTION/2
119. CHEM/IBP/UV SPECTRUM/1
120. CHEM/IBP/BMD/ACIDOSIS/2
121. CHEM/DFC/CREATININE/CLEARANCE TEST/1
122. CHEM/IBP/P&E/LACTATE DEHYDROGENASE/1
123. CHEM/SCOA/SCH/POTASSIUM/3
124. CHEM/IBP/BTP/ELECTROLYTES/1
125. CHEM/ALF/ELECTROLYTES/CALCIUM/1
126. CHEM/DFC/BTP/LIPIDS/1
127. CHEM/IBP/INSTRUMENTATION/BLOOD GAS/1
128. CHEM/DFC/BTP/AMMONIA/1
129. CHEM/IBP/BTP/CHLORIDE/1
130. CHEM/ELF/CARBOHYDRATE/MALABSORPTION/2

ITEM DESCRIPTOR LIST
MEDICAL LABORATORY TECHNICIAN EXAMINATION - AUGUST 1986

131. CHEM/ESOE/SCH/ELECTROLYTES/3
132. CHEM/CALC/MOLECULAR WEIGHT/2
133. CHEM/IBP/BTP/IRON/1
134. CHEM/IBP/ANALYTIC METHOD/BILIRUBIN/1
135. HEMA/DFC/DRUG EFFECT/PLATELETS/1
136. HEMA/ALF/DISEASE STATE/CLOT LYSIS/2
137. HEMA/DFC/PHYSIOLOGY/RBC/1
138. HEMA/SCOA/BASIC TESTS/HYPOCHROMIC ANEMIA/2
139. HEMA/DFC/SPECIAL STAIN/RETICULOCYTES/1
140. HEMA/ELF/HEMOSTASIS/FACTOR DEFICIENCY/2
141. HEMA/CALC/WBC DILUTION/2
142. HEMA/IBP/AUTOMATED COUNTS/1
143. HEMA/IBP/WBC MATURATION/1
144. HEMA/DFC/PLATELETS/THROMBASTHENIA/1
145. HEMA/DFC/PHYSIOLOGY/COAGULATION FACTORS/1
146. HEMA/AMM/SPECIAL TESTS/RBC FRAGILITY/2
147. HEMA/ESOE/MICRO MORPH/RBC/3
148. HEMA/IMM/WBC INCLUSIONS/2
149. HEMA/SCOA/MICRO MORPH/MEGELOBLASTIC ANEMIA/3
150. HEMA/DFC/HEMATOCRIT/1
151. HEMA/DFC/DISEASE STATES/HEMOPHILIA/1
152. HEMA/ECLD/HEMOSTASIS/DIC/3
153. HEMA/SELM/HEMOSTASIS/INTRINSIC/1
154. HEMA/DFC/WBC PHYSIOLOGY/1
155. HEMA/DFC/WBC DEGENERATION/1
156. HEMA/DFC/WBC MATURATION/1
157. HEMA/ALF/SPECIAL TESTS/PLATELET DEFICIENCY/2
158. HEMA/ESOE/RBC/QC/3
159. HEMA/ALF/MICRO MORPH/CLL/1
160. HEMA/ESOE/RBC/AUTOMATED CELL COUNT/2
161. HEMA/IBP/PLATELET PHYSIOLOGY/1
162. HEMA/ESOE/WBC/EOSINOPHIL COUNT/3
163. HEMA/DFC/RBC INCLUSION/1
164. HEMA/SELM/SPECIAL STAIN/WBC/1
165. HEMA/ALF/PHYSIOLOGY/LEUKOCYTOSIS/1
166. HEMA/ESOE/QC/WBC/3
167. HEMA/ALF/COAGULATION/FACTOR DEFICIENCY/2
168. HEMA/SCOA/RBC INDICES/3
169. HEMA/IBP/SCH/EDTA/1
170. HEMA/CALC/QC/CONTROL LIMITS/2
171. HEMA/SCOA/SCH/VENIPUNCTURE/2
172. BF/DFC/COMPOSITION/URINE/1
173. BF/ISOE/SCH/URINE SEDIMENT/1
174. BF/DFC/SCH/URINE CHEM/1
175. BF/ISOP/QC/REAGENT STRIP/1
176. BF/SELM/BASIC TESTS/FECES/1
177. BF/ALF/DISORDERS/AMNIOTIC FLUID/1
178. BF/PERF/SCH/URINE PROTEIN/1
179. BF/IBP/URINE CHEM/REAGENT STRIP/1
180. BF/DFC/URINE/CELLULAR ELEMENT/1
181. BF/ALF/URINE PIGMENT/1
182. BF/ALF/MICRO MORPH/URINE SEDIMENT/2
183. BF/EMM/URINE/REAGENT STRIP/2
184. BF/ALF/MICRO MORPH/URINE SEDIMENT/2
185. BF/DFC/PHYSIOLOGY/TRANSUDATE/1
186. BF/DFC/ANATOMY/URINE CASTS/1
187. BF/ISOE/URINE CHEM/REAGENT STRIP/1
188. BF/ELF/URINE SEDIMENT/BLOOD/2
189. BF/ISOE/URINE CHEM/REAGENT STRIP/1
190. BF/DFC/PHYSIOLOGY/KIDNEY/1

GLOSSARY OF TERMS USED IN ITEM DESCRIPTORS
MEDICAL LABORATORY TECHNICIAN EXAMINATION - FEBRUARY 1987

AB	ANTIBODY
ABE	ACID BASE AND ELECTROLYTES
ACLF	ASSOCIATE CLINICAL AND LABORATORY FINDINGS
AFB	ACID-FAST BACILLI
AG	ANTIGEN
AIHA	AUTOIMMUNE HEMOLYTIC ANEMIA
ALF	ASSOCIATE LABORATORY FINDINGS
AML	ACUTE MYELOID LEUKEMIA
AMM	ASSOCIATE MICROSCOPIC MORPHOLOGY
ANA	ANTINUCLEAR ANTIBODY
ANAT & PHYSIO	ANATOMY AND PHYSIOLOGY
ASO	ANTISTREPTOLYSIN O
BBNK	BLOOD BANK
BF	BODY FLUID
BMD	BIOCHEMICAL MANIFESTATIONS OF DISEASE
BTP	BIOCHEMICAL THEORY AND PHYSIOLOGY
CALC	CALCULATE
CGL	CHRONIC GRANULOCYTIC LEUKEMIA
CHEM	CHEMISTRY
CSF	CEREBROSPINAL FLUID
DAT	DIRECT ANTIGLOBULIN TEST
DFC	DEFINE FUNDAMENTAL CHARACTERISTIC(S)
ECLF	EVALUATE CLINICAL AND LABORATORY FINDINGS
ELF	EVALUATE LABORATORY FINDINGS
ESOE	EVALUATE SOURCE OF ERROR
FSP	FIBRIN SPLIT PRODUCTS
GEN THER & PRIN	GENETIC THEORY AND PRINCIPLES
GNB	GRAM-NEGATIVE BACILLI
GNC	GRAM-NEGATIVE COCCI
GNCB	GRAM-NEGATIVE COCCOBACILLUS
GPB	GRAM-POSITIVE BACILLI
GPC	GRAM-POSITIVE COCCI
HCG	HUMAN CHORIONIC GONADOTROPIN
HDN	HEMOLYTIC DISEASE OF THE NEWBORN
HEMA	HEMATOLOGY
HGB	HEMOGLOBIN
HLA	HUMAN LYMPHOCYTE ANTIGENS
IBP	IDENTIFY BASIC PRINCIPLE(S)
IMM	IDENTIFY MICROSCOPIC MORPHOLOGY
IMMU	IMMUNOLOGY
IMMU MAN OF DIS	IMMUNOLOGIC MANIFESTATION OF DISEASE
ISOE	IDENTIFY SOURCE OF ERROR
ISOP	IDENTIFY STANDARD OPERATING PROCEDURE
LAB OP	LABORATORY OPERATIONS
LAP	LEUKOCYTE ALKALINE PHOSPHATASE
LDL	LOW DENSITY LIPOPROTEIN
MIC	MINIMUM INHIBITORY CONCENTRATION
MICR	MICROBIOLOGY
MICRO MORPH	MICROSCOPIC MORPHOLOGY
P&E	PROTEIN AND ENZYMES
QC	QUALITY CONTROL
RBC	RED BLOOD CELL
SCH	SPECIMEN COLLECTION AND HANDLING
SCOA	SELECT COURSE OF ACTION
SDU	SELECT DONOR UNIT
SEBP	SELECT BLOOD PRODUCT
SELC	SELECT COMPONENT
SELM	SELECT METHOD
SELR	SELECT REAGENT
SLE	SYSTEMIC LUPUS ERYTHEMATOSUS
WBC	WHITE BLOOD CELL

TAXONOMIC LEVELS

TAX 1 - Recall: Ability to recall or recognize previously learned (memorized) knowledge ranging from specific facts to complete theories.

TAX 2 - Interpretive Skills: Ability to utilize recalled knowledge to interpret or apply verbal, numeric or visual data.

TAX 3 - Problem Solving: Ability to utilize recalled knowledge and the interpretation/application of distinct criteria to resolve a problem or situation and/or make an appropriate decision.

ITEM DESCRIPTOR LIST
MEDICAL LABORATORY TECHNICIAN EXAMINATION - FEBRUARY 1987

1. BF/ACLF/CSF/TRAUMATIC TAP/2
2. BF/DFC/COMPOSITION/URINE/1
3. BF/ELF/URINE/REDUCING SUBSTANCES/3
4. BF/ELF/URINE SEDIMENT/BLOOD/2
5. BF/SELM/SCH/24-HOUR URINE/1
6. BF/DFC/PHYSIOLOGY/KETONURIA/1
7. BF/DFC/ANATOMY/URINE CASTS/1
8. BF/DFC/URINE PHYSIOLOGY/CAST FORMATION/1
9. BF/IBP/RENAL THRESHOLD/1
10. BF/ISOE/URINE CHEM/REAGENT STRIP/1
11. BF/ALF/URINE/CAST/2
12. BF/ELF/URINE SEDIMENT/CAST/2
13. BF/ALF/MICRO MORPH/REAGENT STRIP/2
14. BF/ALF/URINE SEDIMENT/2
15. BF/ALF/URINALYSIS/2
16. BF/ALF/MENINGITIS/CSF/1
17. BF/ISOE/SCH/URINE/2
18. BF/ALF/COMPOSITION/PLEURAL FLUID/2
19. MICR/SELM/MICRO MORPH/NEMATODE/1
20. MICR/CALC/COLONY COUNT/URINE CULTURE/2
21. MICR/SELM/WOUND CULTURE/ANAEROBES/3
22. MICR/ALF/GPB/CLOSTRIDIUM/1
23. MICR/SELM/BIOCHEMICAL TEST/STREPTOCOCCUS/1
24. MICR/ISOP/SCH/AFB/1
25. MICR/IBP/SCH/OVA & PARASITE/1
26. MICR/ALF/MICRO MORPH/AMOEBA/2
27. MICR/IBP/MEDIA PREPARATION/1
28. MICR/IBP/GPC/BIOCHEMICAL TEST/1
29. MICR/ELF/GNB/CSF CULTURE/2
30. MICR/IBP/GNC/CULTURE REQUIREMENT/1
31. MICR/SELM/GNB/BIOCHEMICAL TEST/1
32. MICR/SELM/SCH/PROTOZOA/1
33. MICR/IBP/SCH/AFB/1
34. MICR/IMM/MOLD/2
35. MICR/IMM/YEAST/2
36. MICR/ALF/GPC/BIOCHEMICAL TEST/1
37. MICR/ALF/URINE CULTURE/2
38. MICR/ELF/ENTEROBACTER/3
39. MICR/ISOE/BASIC TEST/GNB/2
40. MICR/SELM/GPC/REAGENT QC/1
41. MICR/DFC/GPC/BIOCHEMICAL TEST/1
42. MICR/IMM/GARDNERELLA/1
43. MICR/ALF/GNC/GENITAL CULTURE/2
44. MICR/ACLF/GNCB/EAR CULTURE/2
45. MICR/ECLF/MICRO MORPH/ANAEROBE/2
46. MICR/SELM/SCH/VIRUS CULTURE/1
47. MICR/ACLF/BIOCHEMICAL TEST/GNB/2
48. MICR/ISOP/QC/AUTOCLAVE/1
49. MICR/SELM/SUSCEPTIBILITY/HAEMOPHILUS/2
50. MICR/ELF/MIC/2
51. MICR/DFC/BACTEROIDES/1
52. MICR/SELM/ANAEROBIC GPB/WOUND CULTURE/2
53. MICR/SELM/GPB/CORYNEBACTERIUM/2
54. BBNK/DFC/LECTIN/1
55. BBNK/IBP/HEMOTHERAPY/ABO SUBGROUPS/1
56. BBNK/SELC/FACTOR DEFICIENCY/1
57. BBNK/IBP/HLA TYPING/1
58. BBNK/ACLF/HEMOTHERAPY/ADVERSE REACTION/2
59. BBNK/ELF/AB IDENTIFICATION/3
60. BBNK/SELM/COMPONENT/PLATELET POOLING/2
61. BBNK/ALF/ABO GROUPING/2
62. BBNK/ESOE/ABO TESTING/3
63. BBNK/IBP/RBC/ISOAGGLUTININS/1
64. BBNK/DFC/ELUTION/1
65. BBNK/ACLF/HEMOTHERAPY/ADVERSE REACTION/2
66. BBNK/ELF/RBC AG/SCREENING CELLS/3
67. BBNK/ALF/HEMOTHERAPY/ADVERSE REACTION/2
68. BBNK/ELF/CROSSMATCH/AUTOCONTROL/3
69. BBNK/DFC/ABO AB/1
70. BBNK/IBP/HEMOTHERAPY/ADVERSE REACTION/1
71. BBNK/ECLF/HEMOTHERAPY/BLOOD COMPONENT/3
72. BBNK/ISOP/DAT/HDN/1
73. BBNK/IBP/STORAGE/PLATELETS/1
74. BBNK/SCOA/ADVERSE REACTION/2
75. BBNK/SCOA/RH IMMUNE GLOBULIN/3
76. BBNK/DFC/BLOOD COMPONENT/CLOTTING FACTORS/1
77. BBNK/ACLF/RBC/ADVERSE REACTION/2
78. BBNK/IBP/RBC/ANTIGLOBULIN TEST/2
79. BBNK/ALF/DAT/1
80. BBNK/ELF/RBC/COLD AB/2
81. BBNK/IBP/ABO GROUP/1
82. BBNK/ELF/ABO TYPING/2
83. BBNK/IBP/AB IDENTIFICATION/MODE OF REACTION/1
84. BBNK/IBP/SCH/COMPONENTS/1
85. BBNK/IBP/PHYSIO/HDN/1
86. BBNK/DFC/RBC/ANTICOAGULANT/1
87. BBNK/ISOE/AB SCREEN/CROSSMATCH/1
88. BBNK/DFC/HDN/1
89. IMMU/DFC/BASIC TESTS/SERIAL DILUTION/1
90. IMMU/DFC/ASO/1
91. IMMU/ELF/IMMUNE RESPONSE/2
92. IMMU/DFC/IMMU MAN OF DIS/ALLERGY/1
93. IMMU/ALF/ANA/2
94. IMMU/ISOE/IMMUNOASSAY/HCG/2
95. IMMU/DFC/SCREENING PROCEDURE/QC/1
96. IMMU/IBP/AG-AB COMPLEX/1
97. IMMU/ELF/QC/RHEUMATOID FACTOR/2
98. IMMU/IBP/FLUORESCENT AB/1
99. IMMU/DFC/AUTOANTIBODY/SLE/1
100. IMMU/DFC/CELL PHYSIOLOGY/1
101. IMMU/ELF/SYPHILIS TEST/2
102. IMMU/IBP/SERODIAGNOSIS/INFECTIOUS DISEASE/1
103. IMMU/ISOE/BASIC TESTS/RHEUMATOID ARTHRITIS/2
104. IMMU/IBP/DAT/1
105. IMMU/ALF/C-REACTIVE PROTEIN/1
106. IMMU/DFC/ANAT & PHYSIO/IMMUNOGLOBULIN/1
107. IMMU/DFC/IMMUNOGLOBULIN/1
108. IMMU/DFC/ANATOMY/HCG/1
109. CHEM/IBP/ANALYTIC METHOD/LIPASE/1
110. CHEM/DFC/GLYCOSYLATED HGB/1
111. CHEM/DFC/BTP/BILIRUBIN/1
112. CHEM/CALC/SPECIAL CHEM/RADIOACTIVE DECAY/2
113. CHEM/CALC/LDL CHOLESTEROL/2
114. CHEM/IBP/P&E/CREATININE CLEARANCE/1
115. CHEM/IBP/DRUG MONITOR/DIGOXIN/1
116. CHEM/DFC/QC/STATISTICS/1
117. CHEM/ESOE/SCH/P&E/3
118. CHEM/IBP/COMPONENT/SPECTROPHOMETRY/1
119. CHEM/IBP/INSTRUMENTATION/CHROMATOGRAPHY/1
120. CHEM/DFC/SCH/CHELATING AGENT/1
121. CHEM/ELF/QC/LEVY-JENNINGS/2
122. CHEM/IBP/INSTRUMENTATION/BALANCE/1
123. CHEM/IBP/P&E/ALBUMIN/1
124. CHEM/IBP/INSTRUMENTATION/FLAME PHOTOMETER/1
125. CHEM/ELF/ABE/KETOACIDOSIS/2
126. CHEM/IBP/INSTRUMENTATION/ATOMIC ABSORPTION/1
127. CHEM/IBP/INSTRUMENTATION/FLUOROMETER/1
128. CHEM/ALF/BMD/ACIDOSIS/2
129. CHEM/ISOE/SCH/P&E/1
130. CHEM/DFC/STANDARD SOLUTION/1

ITEM DESCRIPTOR LIST
MEDICAL LABORATORY TECHNICIAN EXAMINATION - FEBRUARY 1987

131. CHEM/IBP/P&E/ELECTROPHORESIS/1
132. CHEM/ELF/CARBOHYDRATE/MALABSORPTION/2
133. CHEM/DFC/HEME DERIVATIVE/HGB ELECTROPHORESIS/1
134. CHEM/ALF/STEROIDS/1
135. CHEM/ALF/ELECTROLYTES/CALCIUM/1
136. CHEM/SELM/LAB OP/SAFETY/2
137. CHEM/ESOE/SCH/ELECTROLYTES/3
138. CHEM/IBP/P&E/LACTATE DEHYDROGENASE/1
139. CHEM/DFC/BTP/BUFFER/1
140. CHEM/SELR/SCH/ACID BASE/1
141. CHEM/IBP/BTP/IRON/1
142. CHEM/ALF/INSTRUMENTATION/BEERS LAW/2
143. CHEM/IBP/BMD/ACIDOSIS/2
144. CHEM/IBP/BASIC TESTS/PROTEIN/1
145. CHEM/IBP/BTP/ALBUMIN/1
146. CHEM/ALF/PROTEIN/MYELOMA/1
147. CHEM/ECLF/ENZYMES/MYOCARDIAL INFARCT/2
148. HEMA/CALC/WBC/ABSOLUTE COUNT/2
149. HEMA/DFC/DRUG EFFECT/PLATELETS/1
150. HEMA/ESOE/SCH/SLIDE PREPARATION/2
151. HEMA/IBP/BASIC TESTS/CYANMETHEMOGLOBIN/1
152. HEMA/IBP/SPECIAL STAIN/RBC INCLUSIONS/1
153. HEMA/ALF/HEMOSTASIS/FACTOR DEFICIENCY/3
154. HEMA/CALC/CORRECTED WBC/2
155. HEMA/ALF/RBC/AIHA/2
156. HEMA/DFC/MICRO MORPH/AML/1
157. HEMA/ELF/BLOOD SMEAR/INDICES/3
158. HEMA/CALC/RBC/CHAMBER COUNT/2
159. HEMA/ELF/AUTOMATED COUNT/2
160. HEMA/DFC/LEUKOCYTE COUNT/1
161. HEMA/DFC/ANAT & PHYSIO/COAGULATION FACTOR/1
162. HEMA/AMM/SEDIMENTATION RATE/3
163. HEMA/IMM/RBC/2
164. HEMA/IMM/WBC/2
165. HEMA/IBP/WBC MATURATION/1
166. HEMA/ALF/WBC MORPHOLOGY/MONONUCLEAR/2
167. HEMA/ISOP/FSP/FIBRINOLYSIS/2
168. HEMA/IBP/COAGULATION FACTOR/PATHWAY/1
169. HEMA/ALF/SPECIAL TESTS/PLATELET DEFICIENCY/2
170. HEMA/IBP/PHYSIOLOGY/PLATELET/1
171. HEMA/ALF/COAGULATION/FACTOR DEFICIENCY/2
172. HEMA/CALC/LAB OP/WBC STATISTICS/2
173. HEMA/IBP/WBC MATURATION/1
174. HEMA/DFC/WBC DEGENERATION/1
175. HEMA/ESOE/AUTOMATED COUNT/HGB/3
176. HEMA/CALC/RBC INDICES/2
177. HEMA/IBP/AUTOMATED COUNT/1
178. HEMA/ALF/WBC/ABNORMAL PROTEIN/3
179. HEMA/DFC/LEUKOCYTE/ARTIFACTS/1
180. HEMA/DFC/MATURATION/RBC/1
181. HEMA/ACLF/ANEMIA/RETICULOCYTE COUNT/1
182. HEMA/ISOP/SCH/LABILE FACTOR/1
183. HEMA/DFC/ANAT & PHYSIO/COAGULATION FACTOR/1
184. HEMA/CALC/QC/CONTROL LIMITS/2

APPENDIX B

GLOSSARY OF TERMS USED IN ITEM DESCRIPTORS
MEDICAL TECHNOLOGIST EXAMINATION - FEBRUARY 1982

AB	ANTIBODY
ABN	ABNORMAL
AFB	ACID-FAST BACILLI
AG	ANTIGEN
AGG	AGGLUTINATION
AMTS	AMOUNTS
ANA	ANTINUCLEAR ANTIBODY
ANYL	ANALYTIC
ASO	ANTISTREPTOLYSIN O
BACT	BACTERIOLOGY
BBNK	BLOOD BANK
BIOCHEM	BIOCHEMICAL
BLD	BLOOD
CALC	CALCULATE
CBC	COMPLETE BLOOD COUNT
CCD	CORRELATE CLINICAL DATA
CHAR	CHARACTERISTIC
CHEM	CHEMISTRY/CHEMICAL
CLD	CORRELATE LABORATORY DATA
CLIN	CLINICAL
COA	COURSE OF ACTION
COAG	COAGULATION
COMP	COMPONENT
CONT	CONTINUOUS
COR	CORRECT
CSF	CEREBROSPINAL FLUID
CRP	C-REACTIVE PROTEIN
DFC	DEFINE FUNDAMENTAL CHARACTERISTICS
DIFF	DIFFERENTIATION
EIA	ENZYME IMMUNOASSAY
ELECTROPHOR	ELECTROPHORESIS
ENDO	ENDOCRINE
ESR	ERYTHROCYTE SEDIMENTATION RATE
EQ	EQUIVALENT
EXAM	EXAMINATION
FIND	FINDING(S)
FUO	FEVER OF UNDETERMINED ORIGIN
GNB	GRAM-NEGATIVE BACILLI
GNC	GRAM-NEGATIVE COCCI
GPB	GRAM-POSITIVE BACILLI
GPC	GRAM- POSITIVE COCCI
GTT	GLUCOSE TOLERANCE TEST
HBSAG	HEPATITIS B SURFACE ANTIGEN
H-C	HEMATOLOGY-COAGULATION
HDN	HEMOLYTIC DISEASE OF THE NEWBORN
HGB	HEMOGLOBIN
ID	IDENTIFICATION/IDENTIFY
IG	IMMUNOGLOBULIN
IMMU	IMMUNOLOGY
INFECT	INFECTION
INST	INSTRUMENTATION
INTERP	INTERPRETATION
LAB	LABORATORY
LD	LACTATE DEHYDROGENASE
MACRO	MACROSCOPIC
MALAB	MALABSORPTION
MATH	CALCULATION(S)
METH	METHODOLOGY
MIC	MINIMUM INHIBITORY CONCENTRATION
MICRO	MICROSCOPIC
MISC	MISCELLANEOUS
MORPH	MORPHOLOGY
PA	PERNICIOUS ANEMIA
PHYSIO	PHYSIOLOGY
P-M	PARASITOLOGY-MYCOLOGY
PREP	PREPARATION
PROB	PROBLEM
QC	QUALITY CONTROL
QUAL	QUALITATIVE
RA	RHEUMATOID ARTHRITIS
RBC	RED BLOOD CELL
R&D	RESEARCH AND DEVELOPMENT
REACT	REACTION
RESP	RESPIRATORY
RID	RADIAL IMMUNODIFFUSION
SCREEN	SCREENING
SED	SEDIMENT
SIGN	SIGNIFICANCE
SOE	SOURCE OF ERROR
SPEC	SPECIMEN
STS	SEROLOGIC TESTS FOR SYPHILIS
TRANSFU	TRANSFUSION
TRBL-SHOOT	TROUBLE-SHOOTING
UCG	URINARY CHORIONIC GONADOTROPINS
URIN	URINALYSIS
VMA	VANILLYLMANDELIC ACID
X-MATCH	CROSSMATCH
WBC	WHITE BLOOD CELL
WD	WOUND

TAXONOMIC LEVELS

TAX 1. Ability to recall previously learned knowledge ranging from specific facts to complete theories, solely by recognition or memorization.

TAX 2. Ability to calculate values or interpret the general significance of verbal or visual data.

TAX 3. Ability to utilize verbal or visual data for the resolution of a problem or situation.

ITEM DESCRIPTOR LIST
MEDICAL TECHNOLOGIST EXAMINATION - FEBRUARY 1982

1. H-C/DFC/ABN MORPH/WBC/1
2. H-C/DFC/ESR/2
3. H-C/DFC/SPECIAL STAINS/WBC/1
4. H-C/DFC/COR COUNTS/PARTICLE COUNTER/1
5. H-C/DFC/SPECIAL STAINS/WBC/1
6. H-C/DFC/PHYSIO/PLATELET CONSTITUENT/1
7. H-C/CCD/MORPH/RBC/3
8. H-C/DFC/LAB FIND/MULTIPLE MYELOMA/2
9. H-C/DFC/PHYSIO/RBC DESTRUCTION/1
10. H-C/CALC/CHAMBER COUNT/RBC/2
11. H-C/SELECT METH/SPECIAL STAIN/WBC/1
12. H-C/DFC/HEMOSTASIS/EXTRINSIC PATHWAY/1
13. H-C/DFC/SOE/MANUAL HGB/2
14. H-C/DFC/SOE/HGB ID/2
15. H-C/DFC/LAB FIND/FACTOR DEFICIENCY/2
16. H-C/DFC/LAB FIND/FACTOR DEFICIENCY/2
17. H-C/CCD/MORPH/RBC/2
18. H-C/DFC/PHYSIO/PA/1
19. H-C/DFC/CLIN SIGN/CLOT RETRACTION/1
20. H-C/DFC/MORPH/WBC/1
21. H-C/CLD/COR COUNT/WBC/3
22. H-C/CLD/MORPH/RBC/3
23. H-C/CLD/MORPH/RBC/3
24. H-C/CLD/MULTIPLE MYELOMA/3
25. H-C/CALC/ABSOLUTE COUNT/WBC/2
26. H-C/CLD/COAG TEST/FACTOR DEFICIENCY/2
27. H-C/CLD/SOE/PARTICLE COUNTER/1
28. H-C/CCD/SPECIAL STAINS/WBC/3
29. H-C/DFC/REACTIVE MORPH/LYMPHOCYTES/2
30. H-C/DFC/STANDARDS/INSTRUMENT CALIBRATION/1
31. H-C/CCD/PHYSIO/RBC SURVIVAL/3
32. H-C/CLD/MORPH/RBC/2
33. H-C/CLD/INCLUSION BODIES/RBC/3
34. H-C/CLD/MORPH/WBC/3
35. H-C/DFC/CYTOGENETICS/LEUKEMIA/1
36. H-C/DFC/LAB FIND/AGRANULOCYTOSIS/1
37. H-C/DFC/LAB FIND/FACTOR DEFICIENCY/1
38. H-C/DFC/DRUG EFFECTS/COAG TESTS/1
39. H-C/DFC/PHYSIO DISTRIBUTION/WBC/1
40. URIN/DFC/CAST FORMATION/RED CELL CASTS/1
41. MISC/DFC/STANDARD DEVIATION/1
42. MATH/CALC/PERCENT SOLUTION/2
43. URIN/CCD/LAB FIND/PROTEINURIA/2
44. MATH/CALC/MOLAR SOLUTION/2
45. MISC/DFC/STANDARD SOLUTION/QC/1
46. URIN/CCD/SED EXAM/CELL ORIGIN/3
47. URIN/CCD/SED EXAM/CELL ORIGIN/3
48. URIN/CCD/LAB FIND/CASTS/3
49. URIN/CLD/SED EXAM/CYSTINE/3
50. URIN/CLD/PIGMENT/3
51. URIN/DFC/LAB FIND/UROBILINOGEN/1
52. MISC/DFC/GROSS APPEARANCE/CSF/1
53. MATH/CALC/EQ AMTS/HYDROUS ANHYDROUS/2
54. MISC/DFC/LENS SYSTEM/MICROSCOPE/2
55. URIN/DFC/QC/REFRACTOMETER/1
56. MATH/CALC/METRIC UNITS/2
57. MISC/DFC/PROPER USAGE/PIPET/1
58. URIN/CLD/SED EXAM/CRYSTAL/3
59. URIN/CCD/LAB FIND/CASTS/3
60. URIN/CLD/DEGENERATION/CASTS/3
61. URIN/DFC/PHYSIO/CLEARANCE TEST/1
62. MISC/DFC/SPEC COLL/CSF/1
63. URIN/DFC/SOE/SPECIFIC GRAVITY/1
64. MISC/DFC/EQUATION/BEERS LAW/1
65. MISC/DFC/PHYSIO/JOINT FLUID/1
66. URIN/CLD/QUAL ASSAY/REDUCING SUBSTANCES/2
67. URIN/DFC/REAGENT STRIP/KETONES/1
68. MATH/CALC/PH/2
69. MISC/DFC/STANDARD PROTOCOL/R&D/1
70. URIN/CLD/SED EXAM/CRYSTALS/3
71. URIN/CLD/SPECIAL STAIN/SEDIMENT/3
72. URIN/DFC/CONSTITUANTS/SEDIMENT/1
73. MISC/DFC/ACIDS/1
74. MISC/DFC/GAUSSIAN DISTRIBUTION/1
75. MISC/DFC/SAMPLE/QC/1
76. URIN/DFC/REAGENT STRIP/PROTEIN/1
77. MISC/DFC/ANYL METH/FECAL FAT/1
78. MISC/DFC/ISOTOPE/1
79. BACT/SELECT METH/BIOCHEM ID/GPC/3
80. BACT/DFC/MOTILITY/ENTEROBACTERIACEAE/1
81. BACT/CLD/MICRO MORPH/SPIROCHETE/2
82. BACT/SELECT METH/BIOCHEM ID/HAEMOPHILUS/3
83. BACT/CLD/QC/MEDIA/2
84. BACT/DFC/ID CHAR/MEDIA/1
85. BACT/DFC/ID CHAR/MEDIA/1
86. BACT/CLD/BIOCHEM ID/ANAEROBIC GPC/2
87. BACT/CLD/CSF/GPB/2
88. BACT/CLD/WD INFECT/GNC/2
89. P-M/CLD/MICRO MORPH/DERMATOPHYTE/3
90. BACT/DFC/MACRO MORPH/GPB/1
91. BACT/CLD/BIOCHEM ID/ENTEROBACTERIACEAE/1
92. BACT/CLD/LAB FIND/MIC/3
93. P-M/CLD/MICRO MORPH/PROTOZOA/2
94. BACT/CLD/BIOCHEM ID/NONFERMENTER/2
95. BACT/CLD/BIOCHEM ID/PROTEUS/2
96. BACT/DFC/MACRO MORPH/AFB/1
97. BACT/CLD/QC/KIRBY BAUER/3
98. MISC/DFC/SPECIFIC SOURCE/VIRUS/1
99. P-M/CLD/MICRO MORPH/DIMORPHIC FUNGI/1
100. BACT/DFC/ID/GNC/2
101. P-M/CLD/MICRO MORPH/PLASMODIUM/3
102. P-M/CLD/MICRO MORPH/CESTODE/3
103. P-M/CLD/MICRO MORPH/INTESTINAL PROTOZOA/3
104. P-M/CLD/WD INFECT/SUBCUTANEOUS MYCOSIS/2
105. BACT/SELECT METH/BIOCHEM ID/GPC/3
106. BACT/DFC/STERILIZATION/MEDIA PREPARATION/1
107. BACT/SELECT METH/GROWTH REQUIREMENT/GPB/1
108. BACT/CLD/SPEC COLL/BLD CULTURE/3
109. P-M/DFC/ARTIFACTS/STOOL EXAM/1
110. BACT/DFC/GROWTH REQUIREMENTS/MYCOPLASMA/1
111. BACT/DFC/QC/GASPACK JAR/1
112. BACT/CLD/ID CHAR/ANAEROBIC GNB/1
113. BACT/CLD/WD INFECT/GNB/2
114. IMMU/DFC/PROZONE/1
115. BBNK/DFC/X-MATCH/AUTOAGGLUTININS/1
116. IMMU/DFC/ANYL METH/HBS-AG/1
117. BBNK/CCD/COA/PROB ID/3
118. IMMU/DFC/SOE/COMPLEMENT FIXATION/1
119. BBNK/DFC/GENOTYPE/RH/1
120. IMMU/DFC/ANYL METH/RID/2
121. BBNK/DFC/QC/ANTISERA/1
122. BBNK/DFC/DONOR REQUIREMENTS/1
123. BBNK/DFC/DONOR REQUIREMENTS/1
124. IMMU/CCD/LAB FIND/STS/3
125. IMMU/DFC/ANTIBODY/1
126. IMMU/DFC/ANYL METH/UCG PREGNANCY TEST/1
127. IMMU/CCD/LAB FIND/FUO/3
128. BBNK/DFC/ANTICOAGULANT/1
129. IMMU/CCD/LAB FIND/STS/3
130. BBNK/COA/EMERGENCY TRANSFU/3

ITEM DESCRIPTOR LIST
MEDICAL TECHNOLOGIST EXAMINATION - FEBRUARY 1982

131. IMMU/CLD/SOE/ANA/3
132. BBNK/DFC/GENE FUNCTION/ABO SYSTEM/1
133. IMMU/DFC/PHYSIO FUNCTION/IG/1
134. BBNK/DFC/METH/COMP PREP/1
135. IMMU/DFC/ANYL METH/RA TEST/1
136. BBNK/DFC/BLD STORAGE/1
137. IMMU/CLD/IMMUNODIFFUSION/3
138. IMMU/CLD/IMMUNODIFFUSION/3
139. BBNK/DFC/ENZYME TREATMENT/AG/1
140. BBNK/CLD/CELL PANEL/AB ID/3
141. BBNK/DFC/ETIOLOGY/HEMOLYTIC TRANSFU REACT/2
142. IMMU/DFC/IMMUNITY/1
143. BBNK/DFC/LAB FIND/SECRETOR STATUS/2
144. IMMU/DFC/COMPLEMENT/AG-AB INTERACTION/1
145. BBNK/CCD/COA/EMERGENCY TRANSFU/3
146. IMMU/DFC/STRUCTURE/ABN IG/1
147. BBNK/CCD/LAB FIND/RH GENOTYPE/2
148. IMMU/DFC/REACT TYPES/AG-AB INTERACTION/1
149. IMMU/DFC/AUTOANTIBODY/IMMUNE DISEASE/2
150. BBNK/DFC/LAB FIND/HDN/1
151. IMMU/DFC/PHYSIO/CRP/1
152. BBNK/DFC/QC/ANTISERA/1
153. IMMU/CCD/SOE/COLD AGG/2
154. IMMU/DFC/INTERP/HETEROPHILE AGG TEST/1
155. CHEM/CALC/CONCENTRATION/BILIRUBIN/2
156. CHEM/DFC/ELECTROPHOR/PROTEIN/1
157. CHEM/DFC/PHYSIO/TRACE ELEMENTS/1
158. CHEM/DFC/METABOLISM/BILIRUBIN/1
159. CHEM/DFC/TRBL-SHOOT/CHLORIDOMETER/2
160. CHEM/DFC/SOE/CALCIUM/1
161. CHEM/CLD/GTT/2
162. CHEM/DFC/PHYSIO/ENZYME DISORDER/1
163. CHEM/DFC/CLIN SIGN/CREATININE CLEARANCE/2
164. CHEM/CLD/BLD GASES/METABOLIC DISORDERS/2
165. CHEM/CLD/BLD GASES/METABOLIC DISORDERS/2
166. CHEM/CLD/BLD GASES/METABOLIC DISORDERS/2
167. CHEM/DFC/HORMONE/1
168. CHEM/DFC/ANYL METH/EIA/1
169. CHEM/DFC/ANYL METH/GLUCOSE/1
170. CHEM/DFC/SOE/ELECTROLYTES/1
171. CHEM/DFC/ANYL METH/ENZYME REACTION/1
172. CHEM/DFC/SOE/AMNIOTIC FLUID/1
173. CHEM/SEL METH/SCREEN TEST/MALAB/1
174. CHEM/DFC/LAB FIND/LIPOPROTEINS/1
175. CHEM/CLD/CLIN SIGN/LD ISOENZYMES/1
176. CHEM/CCD/LAB FIND/DIABETIS/3
177. CHEM/DFC/ANYL METH/PROTEIN/1
178. CHEM/SELECT METH/DIAGNOSIS/ENDO TUMOR/2
179. CHEM/DFC/INST/CONT FLOW/1
180. CHEM/DFC/LAB FIND/IRON/1
181. CHEM/DFC/SOE/ELECTROLYTES/1
182. CHEM/DFC/ANYL METH/UREA/1
183. CHEM/CCD/LAB FIND/BILIRUBIN/2
184. CHEM/DFC/LAB FIND/LIPOPROTEINEMIA/1
185. CHEM/DFC/LAB FIND/FETAL MATURITY/1
186. CHEM/DFC/INST/PH METER/1
187. CHEM/DFC/SPEC COLL/GLUCOSE/1
188. CHEM/DFC/ANYL METH/PROTEIN ELECTROPHOR/1
189. CHEM/DFC/ANYL METH/UREA/1
190. CHEM/CCD/SOE/VMA
191. CHEM/CCD/LAB FIND/PANCREATITIS/2
192. CHEM/DFC/TRBL-SHOOT/CENTRIFUGE/2
193. CHEM/DFC/PHYSIO/CARBON MONOXIDE POISON/1
194. CHEM/CCD/LAB FIND/LEUKEMIA/1
195. CHEM/DFC/PHYSICAL PROPERTIES/GLOBULINS/1

GLOSSARY OF TERMS USED IN ITEM DESCRIPTORS
MEDICAL TECHNOLOGIST EXAMINATION - AUGUST 1982

	ANTIBODY
NOR	ABNORMALITY
B	ACID-FAST BACILLI
	ANTIGEN
G	AGGLUTINATION
K	ALKALINE
L	ACUTE MYELOCYTIC LEUKEMIA
PEAR	APPEARANCE
CT	BACTERIOLOGY
NK	BLOOD BANK
	BODY FLUIDS
OCHEM	BIOCHEMICAL
LC	CALCULATE
PY	CAPACITY
	CORRELATE CLINICAL DATA
D	CORRELATE CLINICAL AND LABORATORY DATA
EM	CHEMISTRY
AR	CLEARANCE
	CORRELATE LABORATORY DATA
LEC	COLLECTION
S	COLLECT SPECIMEN
	COMPETITIVE PROTEIN BINDING
	CEREBROSPINAL FLUID
	COPPER
I	DEFICIENCY
	DEFINE FUNDAMENTAL CHARACTERISTIC(S)
	DETERMINE RESULT VALIDITY
FUN	DYSFUNCTION
C	ELECTRONIC COMPLETE BLOOD COUNT
	EVALUATE MICROMORPHOLOGY
	ELECTRONIC PLATELET COUNT
	EVALUATE TEST RESULTS
R	EVALUATE RESULTS
	FETO-MATERNAL HEMORRHAGE
C	FUNCTION
	GRAM-POSITIVE BACILLI
	GRAM-POSITIVE COCCI
	HEMOLYTIC ANEMIA
	HEMOLYTIC DISEASE OF THE NEWBORN
A	HEMATOLOGY
OPATHY	HEMOGLOBINOPATHY
	INDIRECT ANTIGLOBULIN TEST
	IDENTIFY BASIC PRINCIPLE(S)
	INTERPRET BIOCHEMICAL REACTION
	IDENTIFY
	IRON DEFICIENCY ANEMIA
	IDENTIFY DISTINGUISHING CHARACTERISTICS
NT	IDENTIFICATION

IF	IMMUNOFLUORESCENCE
IMMU	IMMUNOLOGY
INFLAM	INFLAMMATORY
INTR	INTERPRET RESULTS
LE	LUPUS ERYTHEMATOSUS
METH	METHODOLOGY
MG	MILLIGRAM
MIC	MINIMUM INHIBITORY CONCENTRATION
MICR	MICROBIOLOGY
MICRO	MICROSCOPIC
ML	MILLILITER
MORPH	MORPHOLOGY
MYCO	MYCOBACTERIA
NPN	NONPROTEIN NITROGEN
PAS	PERIODIC ACID-SCHIFF
PE	PSEUDOMEMBRANOUS ENTEROCOLITIS
PRES	PREPARE SPECIMENS
PROCE	PROCEDURE
PS	PROBLEM SOLVING
QC	QUALITY CONTROL
RADIO	RADIOACTIVE
RBC	RED BLOOD CELL
R&D	RESEARCH AND DEVELOPMENT
REPR	REPORT RESULTS
REQUIRE	REQUIREMENTS
RESP	RESPIRATORY
REX	REACTION
SD	STANDARD DEVIATION
SED	SEDIMENTATION
SEL	SELECT
SELB	SELECT BLOOD
SELM	SELECT METHOD
SEME	SELECT MEDIA
SOL	SOLUTION
SOP	STANDARD OPERATING PROCEDURE
SPE	SERUM PROTEIN ELECTROPHORESIS
SPECT	SPECTROPHOTOMETER
STS	SEROLOGIC TESTS FOR SYPHILIS
SUPPRESS	SUPPRESSION
TRANS	TRANSMISSION
TRANSFU	TRANSFUSION
TREAT	TREATMENT
TS	TROUBLESHOOT
UV	ULTRAVIOLET
VAL	VALIDATE
WBC	WHITE BLOOD CELL
X-MATCH	CROSSMATCH

TAXONOMIC LEVELS

1. Ability to recall previously learned knowledge ranging from specific facts to complete theories, solely by recognition or memorization.
2. Ability to calculate values or interpret the general significance of verbal or visual dat
3. Ability to utilize verbal or visual data for the resolution of a problem or situation.

ITEM DESCRIPTOR LIST
MEDICAL TECHNOLOGIST EXAMINATION - AUGUST 1982

1. BF/CLD/CSF/MENINGITIS/2
2. CHEM/IBP/GLASSWARE//1
3. BF/ID/URINE/METABOLITE/1
4. IMMU/CALC/RBC SUSPENSION//2
5. BF/REPR/CHEM/24-HOUR URINE/3
6. CHEM/CALC/MG PER ML//2
7. BF/ID/URINE TEST/ACETONE/1
8. CHEM/CALC/RADIO DECAY//2
9. BF/SEL/TEST REQUIRE/SEMEN ANALYSIS/1
10. BF/IBP/R&D//1
11. BF/CCLD/REAGENT STRIP/PROTEIN/3
12. CHEM/CALC/PERCENT SOL//2
13. BF/CCLD/URINE CRYSTAL/METABOLIC ERROR/3
14. CHEM/CALC/NORMALITY//2
15. BF/CCLD/URINE/CELLULAR CAST/2
16. CHEM/DFC/PH//1
17. BF/CLD/SPECIMEN COLLEC/CSF/2
18. BF/CCLD/URINE SEDIMENT/CELLS AND CASTS/3
19. BF/CLD/BIOCHEM TEST/URINE CRYSTAL/3
20. BF/CCLD/URINE SEDIMENT/CELL/2
21. BF/ID/NORMAL URINE/CRYSTAL/2
22. BF/CLD/REAGENT STRIP/PIGMENT/3
23. CHEM/IBP/BUFFER//1
24. BF/REPR/URINE/REDUCING SUBSTANCE/3
25. BF/DFC/REAGENT STRIP/PROTEIN/1
26. CHEM/IBP/QC//1
27. CHEM/IBP/SD//1
28. CHEM/EVAR/QC/PRECISION/2
29. BF/CLD/SOURCE OF ERROR/URINE COLLEC/2
30. BF/ID/SPECIAL STAIN/URINE SEDIMENT/2
31. BF/ID/METHOD/MICROSCOPY/2
32. CHEM/CALC/PERCENT TRANS//2
33. CHEM/IBP/LINEARITY/BEER'S LAW/1
34. BF/DFC/SPECIMEN APPEAR/CSF/1
35. CHEM/CALC/DILUTION//2
36. BF/CALC/URINE DILUTION//2
37. CHEM/CALC/MOLALITY//2
38. BF/IBP/BILIRUBIN TEST/FECES/1
39. MICR/SEME/GPB//1
40. MICR/DFC/STERILIZATION/MEDIA/1
41. MICR/CLD/BIOCHEM IDENT/GPC/3
42. MICR/PRES/CONCENTRATION/AFB/1
43. MICR/SEME/STOOL//2
44. MICR/CCLD/STREPTOCOCCUS//2
45 MICR/CLD/GPC/3
46. MICR/DFC/SOP/INCUBATOR/1
47. MICR/CLD/PE//3
48. MICR/CLD/PHYSIOLOGY/STREPTOCOCCUS/2
49. MICR/IDC/DEMATIACEOUS/FUNGUS/2
50. MICR/IDC/DERMATOPHYTE//2
51. MICR/SEME/YEAST//2
52. MICR/CLD/IDENT/YEAST/2
53. MICR/IDC/GPB//1
54. MICR/COLS/ANAEROBIC BACT//2
55. MICR/TS/QC/MEDIA/3
56. MICR/CLD/IDENT/ACTINOMYCES/2
57. MICR/IDC/GPC/ANAEROBES/1
58. MICR/CLD/IDENT/ENTEROBACTER/2
59. MICR/CLD/IDENT/GPB/2
60. MICR/ID/MICRO MORPH/AMOEBA/2
61. MICR/ID/MICRO MORPH/MICROFILARIA/2
62. MICR/ID/MICRO MORPH/PLASMODIUM/2
63. MICR/IDC/FLAGELLATES//2
64. MICR/SELM/CULTURE/FUNGI/1
65. MICR/CCLD/GPB//2
66. MICR/SELM/DETECTION/ATYPICAL AFB/2
67. MICR/REPR/MIC//2
68. MICR/IBP/CULTURE REQUIRE/AFB/1
69. MICR/CLD/IDENT/NEMATODE/1
70. MICR/IDC/MICRO IDENT/SHIGELLA/1
71. MICR/TS/QC/KIRBY BAUER/2
72. MICR/TS/QC/MEDIA/2
73. MICR/IBR/NIACIN//2
74. MICR/CLD/IDENT/BACTEROIDES/2
75. MICR/DFC/ATYPICAL MYCO//1
76. IMMU/DFC/IMMUNOGLOBULIN//1
77. BBNK/DFC/RBC AG//1
78. IMMU/CLD/SEROLOGY/MYCOPLASMA/2
79. BBNK/SELB/HDN/EXCHANGE TRANSFU/3
80. BBNK/PS/DONOR UNIT//2
81. BBNK/INTR/AB PANEL//3
82. IMMU/DFC/COMPLEMENT/AG-AB INTERACTION/
83. IMMU/VAL/TEST RESULTS/ ANTISTREPTOLYSI
84. BBNK/DFC/ANALYTIC PROCE/COOMBS TEST/1
85. BBNK/IBP/IAT//1
86. BBNK/IBP/IAT//1
87. BBNK/DFC/IMMUNOGLOBULINS/HDN/1
88. IMMU/TS/IF//3
89. BBNK/CCD/TRANSFU REX//3
90. BBNK/DFC/HDN/ABO SYSTEM/1
91. BBNK/ETR/PROBLEM X-MATCH//2
92. BBNK/IBP/STORAGE REQUIRE//1
93. IMMU/IBP/AGG REX//1
94. IMMU/DFC/IMMUNE SUPPRESS//1
95. BBNK/CCLD/FMH//3
96. IMMU/DFC/SENSITIVITY//1
97. BBNK/DFC/RH AG//1
98. BBNK/PS/DONOR SITUATION//3
99. IMMU/DFC/COMPLEMENT//1
100. BBNK/CCLD/BLOOD SELECTION//2
101. IMMU/PS/QC/ANTISTREPTOLYSIN O/3
102. IMMU/DFC/PROZONE//1
103. BBNK/INTR/PROBLEM X-MATCH//2
104. IMMU/CCLD/STS//2
105. IMMU/CCLD/INFLAM RESPONSE//2
106. BBNK/PS/DONOR SOURCE//2
107. IMMU/INTR/IMMUNODIFFUSION//3
108. BBNK/IBP/ANTICOAGULANTS//1
109. BBNK/DFC/ABO AG//1
110. BBNK/CCLD/PATERNITY TEST//2
111. IMMU/CLD/LE//3
112. BBNK/DFC/ANTISERUM/RH TYPING/1
113. IMMU/DFC/ACTIVE IMMUNITY//1
114. IMMU/CCD/DEVELOPMENT/ACTIVE IMMUNITY/2
115. IMMU/DFC/ANALYTIC PROCE/VDRL/1
116. BBNK/IBP/AGG REX//1
117. BBNK/SELM/RH TYPING//1
118. BBNK/ETR/PROBLEM X-MATCH//3
119. IMMU/INTR/FEBRILE AGG//2
120. CHEM/IBP/ANALYTIC METH/TRIGLYCERIDES/1
121. CHEM/DFC/PHYSIOLOGY/PROTEIN/1
122. CHEM/DFC/CU METABOLISM//1
123. CHEM/IBP/ANALYTIC METH/GLUCOSE/1
124. CHEM/DFC/PRINCIPLE/PHOSPHATE/1
125. CHEM/ETR/THYROID FUNC//3
126. CHEM/ID/SOURCE OF ERROR/BLOOD GAS SAM
127. CHEM/ETR/LIPIDS//2
128. CHEM/ETR/HEME PIGMENTS//3
129. CHEM/IBP/ANALYTIC METH/UREA/1
130. CHEM/ETR/ABNOR SPE//3

ITEM DESCRIPTOR LIST
MEDICAL TECHNOLOGIST EXAMINATION - AUGUST 1982

131. CHEM/DFC/CREATINE KINASE//2
132. CHEM/DRV/CSF/GLUCOSE/1
133. CHEM/CCD/ELECTROLYTES//2
134. CHEM/DFC/ACID-BASE ABNOR//2
135. CHEM/SELM/HDN//1
136. CHEM/DFC/PHYSIOLOGY/KETOSTEROIDS/1
137. CHEM/IBP/ANALYTIC METH/UREA/1
138. CHEM/SELM/PROTEINURIA//1
139. CHEM/ID/SPECIMEN COLLEC/ENZYME/1
140. CHEM/ID/SAFETY SYMBOL//1
141. CHEM/DFC/PHYSIOLOGY/ESTRIOL LEVEL/1
142. CHEM/DFC/PRESERVATION/GLUCOSE/1
143. CHEM/IBP/ANALYTIC METH/IRON/1
144. CHEM/ETR/BEER'S LAW/2
145. CHEM/IBP/ANTICOAGULANT/BLOOD GAS/1
146. CHEM/CLD/NPN//2
147. CHEM/IBP/ANALYTIC METH/AMINO ACIDS/1
148. CHEM/IBP/ANALYTIC METH/UV SPECT/1
149. CHEM/DFC/OSMOLARITY//1
150. CHEM/CCLD/DIABETES//3
151. CHEM/DFC/PHYSIOLOGY/KETOSTEROIDS/1
152. CHEM/TS/COULOMETER//2
153. CHEM/ETR/RESP ACIDOSIS//3
154. CHEM/DFC/COMPONENT/SPECT/1
155. CHEM/ID/SOURCE OF ERROR/BILIRUBIN/1
156. CHEM/DFC/ELECTROPHORESIS//1
157. CHEM/ETR/ALK PHOSPHATASE//1
158. CHEM/DFC/CENTRIFUGE/CALIBRATION/1
159. CHEM/IBP/ANALYTIC METH/SPE/1
160. CHEM/DFC/CREATININE CLEA//2
161. CHEM/IBP/CPB//1
162. HEMA/DFC/WBC ANOMALY//1
163. HEMA/IBP/EPC//1
164. HEMA/IBP/SPECIAL STAIN/RBC INCLUSIONS/1
165. HEMA/CLD/AML//3
166. HEMA/CLD/PLATELET DYSFUN//2
167. HEMA/DFC/CYTOGENETICS/LEUKEMIA/1
168. HEMA/CALC/RBC INDICES//2
169. HEMA/CLD/FACTOR DEFI//3
170. HEMA/IBP/SPECIAL STAIN/RETICULOCYTE/1
171. HEMA/IBP/ABSORBED PLASMA//1
172. HEMA/ID/RBC INCLUSION//2
173. HEMA/ID/ABNORMAL CELL//2
174. HEMA/SELM/SPECIAL STAIN//2
175. HEMA/ID/MICRO MORPH/GRANULOCYTE/3
176. HEMA/EMM/ERYTHROCYTES//3
177. HEMA/EMM/HEMOPATHY//3
178. HEMA/CLD/BONE MARROW/SPE/3
179. HEMA/SELM/SPECIMEN COLLEC/VENIPUNCTURE/1
180. HEMA/CLD/SPECIAL STAIN/WBC/3
181. HEMA/ID/SOURCE OF ERROR/HEMOGLOBIN/2
182. HEMA/IBP/CELL MATURATION//1
183. HEMA/DFC/SYNTHESIS/COAGULATION FACTOR/1
184. HEMA/CCLD/IDA//2
185. HEMA/IBP/COAGULATION/CLOT LYSIS TEST/1
186. HEMA/CLD/FACTOR DEFI//2
187. HEMA/IBP/SPECIAL STAIN/PAS/1
188. HEMA/ETR/COAGULATION/FACTOR DEFI TEST/2
189. HEMA/IBP/ANALYTIC METH/SICKLE CELL TEST/1
190. HEMA/SELM/SPECIAL STAIN/WBC/1
191. HEMA/ETR/SED RATE//1
192. HEMA/SELM/HEMATOPOIESIS//1
193. HEMA/ID/SOURCE OF ERROR/BLEEDING TIME/1
194. HEMA/CLD/HA//3
195. HEMA/ID/RBC INCLUSIONS//3
196. HEMA/ID/MICRO MORPH/WBC/2
197. HEMA/CLD/RBC MORPH/HA/2
198. HEMA/IBP/RBC DESTRUCTION//1
199. HEMA/CCLD/FACTOR DEFI//3
200. HEMA/DFC/PHYSIOLOGY/NEUTROPHIL/1

GLOSSARY OF TERMS USED IN ITEM DESCRIPTORS
MEDICAL TECHNOLOGIST EXAMINATION - FEBRUARY 1983

AA	AMINO ACID(S)
AB	ANTIBODY
ACCEPT	ACCEPTABILITY
AFB	ACID-FAST BACILLI
AG	ANTIGEN
AGGL	AGGLUTININS
ALK	ALKALINE
ANAL	ANALYTIC
ANHYDR	ANHYDROUS
ANTICOAG	ANTICOAGULANT
ANYL	ANALYSIS
APPEAR	APPEARANCE
ASO	ANTISTREPTOLYSIN O
BBNK	BLOOD BANK
BF	BODY FLUIDS
CALC	CALCULATE
CBC	COMPLETE BLOOD COUNT
CCD	CORRELATE CLINICAL DATA
CCLD	CORRELATE CLINICAL AND LABORATORY DATA
CGL	CHRONIC GRANULOCYTIC LEUKEMIA
CHARACT	CHARACTERISTIC(S)
CHEM	CHEMISTRY
CLD	CORRELATE LABORATORY DATA
COA	COURSE OF ACTION
COLLEC	COLLECTION
CONC	CONCENTRATION
COMP	COMPONENTS
COMPUT	COMPUTER
CORR	CORRELATE
CORRE	CORRECTED
CSF	CEREBROSPINAL FLUID
DEFI	DEFICIENCY
DETECT	DETECTION
DETR	DETERMINE
DFC	DEFINE FUNDAMENTAL CHARACTERISTIC(S)
DIMORPH	DIMORPHIC
DRV	DETERMINE RESULT VALIDITY
ECC	ELECTRONIC CELL COUNT
ELECTRO	ELECTROPHORESIS
ENTEROBACT	ENTEROBACTERIACEAE
ESR	ERYTHROCYTE SEDIMENTATION RATE
ETR	EVALUATE TEST RESULTS
EVA	EVALUATION
FL	FLUORESCENT
FTA	FLUORESCENT TREPONEMAL ANTIBODY TEST
FUNC	FUNCTION
FUO	FEVER OF UNDETERMINED ORIGIN
GNB	GRAM-NEGATIVE BACILLI
GNC	GRAM-NEGATIVE COCCI
GPB	GRAM-POSITIVE BACILLI
GPC	GRAM-POSITIVE COCCI
HA	HEMOLYTIC ANEMIA
HAI	HEMAGGLUTINATION INHIBITION TEST
HBSAG	HEPATITIS B SURFACE ANTIGEN
HCG	HUMAN CHORIONIC GONADOTROPIN
HEMA	HEMATOLOGY
HEMOLY	HEMOLYSIS
HEMOPATHY	HEMOGLOBINOPATHY
IBC	IDENTIFY BASIC CONCEPT(S)
IBP	IDENTIFY BASIC PRINCIPLE(S)
IBR	IDENTIFY BIOCHEMICAL REACTION
ID	IDENTIFY
IDC	IDENTIFY DISTINGUISHING CHARACTERISTICS
IDENT	IDENTIFICATION
IEP	IMMUNOELECTROPHORESIS
IMM	IDENTIFY MICROSCOPIC MORPHOLOGY
IMMU	IMMUNOLOGY
IMMUNO	IMMUNODIFFUSION
INTERACT	INTERACTION
INTEST	INTESTINAL
LAP	LEUKOCYTE ALKALINE PHOSPHATASE
LD	LACTIC DEHYDROGENASE
MA	MEGALOBLASTIC ANEMIA
MACRO	MACROSCOPIC
MAT	MATURATION
METH	METHODOLOGY
MICR	MICROBIOLOGY
MICRO	MICROSCOPIC
MINERALOCORT	MINERALOCORTICOID
MORPH	MORPHOLOGY
OF	OXIDATION-FERMENTATION
PATH	PATHOGEN
PHOS	PHOSPHATASE
PHYSIO	PHYSIOLOGICAL
PKU	PHENYLKETONURIA
PREG	PREGNANCY
PREPA	PREPARATION
PRESERV	PRESERVATION
PROP	PROPERTY
QC	QUALITY CONTROL
QUAL	QUALITATIVE
RA	RHEUMATOID ARTHRITIS
RBC	RED BLOOD CELL
REAG	REAGENT
REF	REFERRAL
REQUIRE	REQUIREMENTS
RERE	REPORT RESULTS
REX	REACTION
RID	RADIAL IMMUNODIFFUSION
SD	STANDARD DEVIATION
SED	SEDIMENT
SEL	SELECT
SELM	SELECT METHOD
SELS	SELECT STAIN
SOE	SOURCE OF ERROR
SOL	SOLUTION
SP	SPECIFIC
SPEC	SPECIMEN
SPECT	SPECTROPHOTOMETRY
STS	SEROLOGIC TESTS FOR SYPHILIS
SUB	SUBSTANCE
SUPRAVIT	SUPRAVITAL
SUSCEPT	SUSCEPTIBILITY
TRANSFU	TRANSFUSION
TS	TROUBLESHOOT
UV	ULTRAVIOLET
VI	VIRAL
WASH	WASHING
WBC	WHITE BLOOD CELL
X-MATCH	CROSSMATCH

TAXONOMIC LEVELS

TAX 1. Ability to recall previously learned knowledge ranging from specific facts to complete theories, solely by recognition or memorization.

TAX 2. Ability to calculate values or interpret the general significance of verbal or visual data.

TAX 3. Ability to utilize verbal or visual data for the resolution of a problem or situation.

ITEM DESCRIPTOR LIST
MEDICAL TECHNOLOGIST EXAMINATION - FEBRUARY 1983

1. MICR/IBP/STERILIZATION/MEDIA/1
2. MICR/ETR/GPC//2
3. MICR/IDC/MYCOPLASMA/1
4. MICR/IMM/GNC/1
5. MICR/SELM/OC/ENTEROBACT/1
6. MICR/ID/COLONY CHARACT/YEAST/2
7. MICR/IMM/MOLD/2
8. MICR/IMM/DIMORPH FUNGUS/2
9. MICR/CCD/HEPATITIS/3
10. MICR/SELM/GPB/1
11. MICR/ID/STAINING PROP/GPB/1
12. MICR/IMM/AMOEBA/1
13. MICR/CLD/WOUND/GPC/2
14. MICR/SELM/MACRO MORPH/FUNGI/1
15. MICR/IDC/LISTERIA/1
16. MICR/SELM/CSF/1
17. MICR/IBP/SUSCEPT TEST/1
18. MICR/IBP/SPEC PREPA/AFB/1
19. MICR/CCLD/ANAEROBIC/GNB/2
20. MICR/IDC/PLASMODIUM/1
21. MICR/IMM/SPUTUM/2
22. MICR/ETR/OF REX/2
23. MICR/IBR/AFB/1
24. MICR/ID/CAUSATIVE AGENT/RICKETTSIOSIS/1
25. MICR/CLD/ACTINOMYCES/3
26. MICR/IBR/AFB/1
27. MICR/IBC/SUSCEPT/ANAEROBES/1
28. MICR/ID/SOE/SUSCEPT TEST/1
29. MICR/ID/SOE/MEDIA PREPA/3
30. MICR/IBP/GROWTH REQUIRE/GPC/1
31. MICR/IDC/ENTEROBACT/1
32. MICR/ID/MORPH/TAPE WORM/2
33. MICR/IMM/INTEST NEMATODE/2
34. MICR/SELM/SPEC COLLEC/INTEST NEMATODE/2
35. MICR/IDC/ENTEROBACT/1
36. MICR/SELM/VI ISOLATION/1
37. BBNK/IBP/DONOR REQUIRE/HEPATITIS/2
38. IMMU/DFC/BENCE JONES/1
39. BBNK/DFC/BLOOD COMP/1
40. IMMU/ID/AB SOURCE/NEWBORN/1
41. BBNK/DFC/BLOOD STORAGE/1
42. IMMU/DFC/IMMUNOGLOBULIN/FUNCTION/1
43. BBNK/CCLD/COA/EMERGENCY TRANSFU/3
44. IMMU/IBP/IMMUNITY/1
45. IMMU/ID/SOE/AG-AB REX/1
46. IMMU/DFC/AUTOANTIBODY/IMMUNE DISEASE/1
47. IMMU/IBP/RID/1
48. BBNK/SELM/AB ABSORPTION/2
49. IMMU/CORR/PHYSIO CHARACT/IMMUNE RESPONSE/3
50. IMMU/IBP/PREG TEST/1
51. BBNK/DFC/X-MATCH/AUTOAGGLUTININS/1
52. IMMU/CCLD/STS/3
53. BBNK/ETR/ABO DISCREPANCY/3
54. IMMU/DFC/SOURCE/IMMUNOGLOBULIN/1
55. IMMU/IBP/AG-AB INTERACT/1
56. BBNK/DFC/GENOTYPE/RH/1
57. IMMU/IBP/FTA/1
58. IMMU/CLD/STS/3
59. BBNK/SEL/COA/PROBLEM AB IDENT/3
60. IMMU/CCLD/FUO/3
61. BBNK/SEL/BLOOD TYPE/ABO VARIANTS/1
62. IMMU/ID/SOE/COLD AGGL/2
63. BBNK/CCLD/RH/GENETICS/2
64. IMMU/IBP/ANAL METH/RA TEST/1
65. IMMU/ETR/IEP/3
66. IMMU/ID/SOE/ASO/3
67. BBNK/ETR/PHENOTYPE/3
68. IMMU/ETR/HAI/3
69. IMMU/DFC/PHYSIOLOGY/C-REACTIVE PROTEIN/1
70. BBNK/DFC/LECTIN/1
71. IMMU/ETR/HAI/1
72. IMMU/ETR/SEROLOGIC TEST/VI HEPATITIS/2
73. BBNK/DETR/DONOR ACCEPT/1
74. BBNK/DFC/AUTOAGGLUTININS/1
75. BBNK/ETR/CELL PANEL/AB IDENT/3
76. BBNK/ETR/ELUATE/HDN/3
77. IMMU/SELM/HBSAG/1
78. CHEM/CALC/BILIRUBIN CONC/2
79. CHEM/IBP/ANAL METH/PROTEIN/1
80. CHEM/ID/SOE/GAS CHROMATOGRAPHY/2
81. CHEM/IBP/ANAL METH/GLUCOSE/1
82. CHEM/IBC/AA METABOLISM/PKU/1
83. CHEM/SELM/ACID-BASE EVA/1
84. CHEM/IBP/PROTEIN/ELECTRO/1
85. CHEM/ID/SOE/BILIRUBIN/2
86. CHEM/DFC/ADRENAL MEDULLA/PHYSIOLOGY/1
87. CHEM/ID/SOE/SPEC COLLEC/2
88. CHEM/IBP/ANAL METH/SERUM IRON/1
89. CHEM/DFC/UV SPECT/1
90. CHEM/IBP/ANAL METH/CREATININE/1
91. CHEM/IBP/ANAL METH/UREA/1
92. CHEM/IBP/INSTRUMENTATION/FLUOROMETER/1
93. CHEM/IBP/COPPER/PHYSIOLOGY/1
94. CHEM/CCLD/SOURCE/ALK PHOS/2
95. CHEM/IBP/CREATININE/CLEARANCE TEST/1
96. CHEM/DFC/BILIRUBIN/1
97. CHEM/IBP/ANAL BALANCE/1
98. CHEM/DRV/URINE/SPECIFIC GRAVITY/3
99. CHEM/ID/SOE/BLOOD GAS COLLEC/2
100. CHEM/IBP/ANAL METH/PROTEIN/1
101. CHEM/ETR/LIPOPROTEIN/ELECTRO/1
102. CHEM/IBP/NEPHELOMETRY/1
103. CHEM/IBP/COPPER/1
104. CHEM/DFC/SPEC APPEAR/1
105. CHEM/ETR/LD ISOENZYMES/2
106. CHEM/IBP/INSTRUMENTATION/CHLORIDOMETER/1
107. CHEM/IBP/CHLORIDE SHIFT/1
108. CHEM/SELM/SPEC PRESERV/GLUCOSE/1
109. CHEM/IBP/ANAL METH/PHOSPHATE/1
110. CHEM/IBP/ANAL METH/STEROIDS/1
111. CHEM/CCLD/ACID-BASE/2
112. CHEM/CCLD/LIPOPROTEIN/ELECTRO/2
113. CHEM/DFC/MINERALOCORT/1
114. CHEM/SELM/TS/CENTRIFUGE/3
115. CHEM/DRV/CSF/GLUCOSE/1
116. CHEM/CALC/ANION GAP/2
117. CHEM/DFC/BLOOD BUFFERS/1
118. CHEM/DRV/BILIRUBIN/2
119. CHEM/SELM/AA/1
120. CHEM/DFC/DIGITAL COMPUT/1

ITEM DESCRIPTOR LIST
MEDICAL TECHNOLOGIST EXAMINATION - FEBRUARY 1983

121. CHEM/CLD/SOE/ELECTROLYTES/2
122. HEMA/CCLD/SUCROSE HEMOLY/1
123. HEMA/CCLD/MICRO MORPH/SMUDGE CELLS/1
124. HEMA/IBP/ECC/1
125. HEMA/DFC/HEMOGLOBIN/1
126. HEMA/CCLD/DIRECT COOMBS/2
127. HEMA/CLD/MICRO MORPH/PROTEIN ELECTRO/3
128. HEMA/CLD/MICRO MORPH/GRANULOCYTE MAT/2
129. HEMA/EMM/GRANULOCYTE MAT/2
130. HEMA/CLD/MA/3
131. HEMA/CLD/HEMOCHROMATOSIS/2
132. HEMA/CCLD/LAP/3
133. HEMA/CCLD/FACTOR DEFI/2
134. HEMA/CALC/CHAMBER COUNT/2
135. HEMA/IBP/ECC/1
136. HEMA/CALC/CORRE WBC COUNT/2
137. HEMA/CCLD/HA/2
138. HEMA/CLD/DRUG EFFECT/BLEEDING TIME/1
139. HEMA/CALC/ABSOLUTE COUNT/2
140. HEMA/ID/SOE/BLOOD SMEAR/2
141. HEMA/CLD/CBC/ACUTE LEUKEMIA/3
142. HEMA/IBP/ESR/1
143. HEMA/SELS/WBC GRANULES/1
144. HEMA/CALC/RBC INDICES/2
145. HEMA/DFC/SYNTHESIS/COAGULATION FACTOR/1
146. HEMA/DFC/SUPRAVIT STAIN/RBC INCLUSION/1
147. HEMA/CCLD/CGL/2
148. HEMA/IBP/ECC/1
149. HEMA/CLD/FACTOR DEFI/3
150. HEMA/ID/SOE/HEMOGLOBINOMETRY/1
151. HEMA/IBP/QC/SD/1
152. HEMA/DFC/AB SYNTHESIS/1
153. HEMA/CLD/MICRO MORPH/HYPOCHROMIC RBC/3
154. HEMA/CLD/MICRO MORPH/TARGET CELLS/3
155. HEMA/IMM/RBC INCLUSIONS/2
156. HEMA/IMM/WBC/2
157. HEMA/CCLD/MICRO MORPH/SCHISTOCYTES/2
158. HEMA/CCLD/HEMOPATHY/3
159. HEMA/CCLD/MA/2
160. HEMA/CLD/FACTOR DEFI/2
161. HEMA/CCLD/LAP/3
162. BF/DFC/FORMATION/URINE CRYSTALS/1
163. BF/IBP/ANAL METH/FECAL FAT/1
164. CHEM/CALC/PERCENT SOL/2
165. BF/DFC/CAST FORMATION/1
166. BF/IMM/URINE SED/2
167. CHEM/CALC/NORMALITY/2
168. CHEM/CALC/EQUIV AMOUNTS/HYDROUS VS ANHYDR/2
169. CHEM/IBP/GRAPHIC DISPLAY/BEER'S LAW/1
170. BF/DRV/URINALYSIS/MICRO/2
171. BF/CLD/CSF/MENINGITIS/2
172. BF/ETR/UROBILINOGEN/2
173. IMMU/CALC/SERUM DILUTION/2
174. CHEM/CALC/DILUTION/2
175. CHEM/DFC/BUFFER/1
176. BF/IDC/PHYSIOLOGY/SYNOVIAL FLUID/1
177. BF/DFC/CASTS/URINE/1
178. BF/ID/URINE TEST/PROTEIN/1
179. CHEM/CALC/NORMALITY/2
180. BF/DFC/REAG STRIP/URINE KETONE/1
181. CHEM/DFC/ISOTOPE/1
182. BF/IBP/REAG STRIP/PROTEIN/1
183. CHEM/CALC/SD/2
184. BF/CCLD/URINE/SP GRAVITY/2
185. BF/DFC/URINE/SP GRAVITY/1
186. IMMU/CALC/SERIAL DILUTION/2
187. MICR/IBP/MICROSCOPE/1
188. BF/IBP/TEST COMP/SEMEN ANALYSIS/1
189. BF/CLD/URINE/SP GRAVITY/1
190. HEMA/DFC/GAUSSIAN DIST/1
191. CHEM/DFC/ACIDS/1
192. BF/DFC/SPEC ACCEPT/URINE/1
193. BF/DFC/TRANSUDATES/1
194. URIN/CLD/QUAL ASSAY/REDUCING SUB/2
195. BF/CCLD/MICRO MORPH/URINE CAST/3
196. BF/CLD/MICRO MORPH/URINE CRYSTALS/2
197. BF/CLD/MICRO MORPH/DEGENERATIVE CASTS/3
198. HEMA/DFC/SD/1
199. BF/RERE/CHEM/24-HOUR URINE/3
200. CHEM/SELM/GLASSWARE WASH/1
201. BF/ID/SOE/PREG TEST/1

GLOSSARY OF TERMS USED IN ITEM DESCRIPTORS
MEDICAL TECHNOLOGIST EXAMINATION - AUGUST 1983

AAT	ALANINE AMINO TRANSFERASE
AB	ANTIBODY
ABNOR	ABNORMALITY
ACC	AUTOMATED CELL COUNT
AG	ANTIGEN
AGGL	AGGLUTININS
AHG	ANTIHUMAN GLOBULIN
ALF	ASSOCIATE LABORATORY FINDINGS
AMM	ASSOCIATE MICROSCOPIC MORPHOLOGY
ANA	ANTINUCLEAR ANTIBODY
ANAL	ANALYZE
ANYL	ANALYTIC
APPEAR	APPEARANCE
ARF	ASSOCIATE RELATED FINDINGS
ASO	ANTISTREPTOLYSIN O
ASSO	ASSOCIATE
BBNK	BLOOD BANK
BF	BODY FLUIDS
BMD	BIOCHEMICAL MANIFESTATION OF DISEASE
BTP	BIOCHEMICAL THEORY AND PHYSIOLOGY
CALC	CALCULATE
CBC	COMPLETE BLOOD COUNT
CCLD	CORRELATE CLINICAL AND LABORATORY DATA
CGL	CHRONIC GRANULOCYTIC LEUKEMIA
CHARACT	CHARACTERISTICS
CHEM	CHEMISTRY
CK	CREATINE KINASE
CLD	CORRELATE LABORATORY DATA
CLEAR	CLEARANCE
CLL	CHRONIC LYMPHOCYTIC LEUKEMIA
COMP	COMPONENTS
CONSTIT	CONSTITUENTS
CREAT	CREATININE
CRP	C-REACTIVE PROTEIN
CSF	CEREBROSPINAL FLUID
DEFI	DEFICIENCY
DFC	DEFINE FUNDAMENTAL CHARACTERISTIC(S)
ELECTRO	ELECTROPHORESIS
EM	EMERGENCY
ESOE	EVALUATE SOURCE OF ERROR
ESR	ERYTHROCYTE SEDIMENTATION RATE
ETR	EVALUATE TEST RESULTS
EVAL	EVALUATE
EX	EXCHANGE
FIX	FIXATION
GLC	GAS-LIQUID CHROMATOGRAPHY
GTT	GLUCOSE TOLERANCE TEST
HCG	HUMAN CHORIONIC GONADOTROPIN
HEMA	HEMATOLOGY
HEMAT	HEMATOLOGIC
HEMOPATHY	HEMOGLOBINOPATHY
HHE	HENDERSON-HASSELBACH EQUATION
IBP	IDENTIFY BASIC PRINCIPLE(S)
ID	IDENTIFY
IDA	IRON DEFICIENCY ANEMIA
IDENT	IDENTIFICATION
IDS	INFECTIOUS DISEASE SEROLOGY
IG	IMMUNOGLOBULIN
IGTP	IMMUNOLOGIC GENETIC THEORY AND PRINCIPLES
IMM	IDENTIFY MICROSCOPIC MORPHOLOGY
IMMU	IMMUNOLOGY
IMMUNO	IMMUNODIFFUSION
ISOE	IDENTIFY SOURCE OF ERROR
LAP	LEUKOCYTE ALKALINE PHOSPHATASE
LE	LUPUS ERYTHEMATOSUS
LO	LABORATORY OPERATIONS
MACRO	MACROSCOPIC
METH	METHODOLOGY
MICR	MICROBIOLOGY
MICRO	MICROSCOPIC
MORPH	MORPHOLOGY
PERF	PERFORM
PREPA	PREPARATION
RBC	RED BLOOD CELL
RCD	RELATED CONDITIONS AND DISORDERS
REAG	REAGENT
REQUIRE	REQUIREMENTS
REX	REACTION
SCH	SPECIMEN COLLECTION AND HANDLING
SED	SEDIMENT
SEL	SELECT
SELM	SELECT METHOD
SOL	SOLUTION
SOO	SITE OF ORIGIN
SPEC	SPECIMEN
SPECT	SPECTROPHOTOMETER
STS	SEROLOGIC TESTS FOR SYPHILIS
SUSCEPT	SUSCEPTIBILITY
TRANS	TRANSMISSION
WBC	WHITE BLOOD CELL

TAXONOMIC LEVELS

TAX 1. Ability to recall previously learned knowledge ranging from specific facts to complete theories, solely by recognition or memorization.

TAX 2. Ability to calculate values or interpret the general significance of verbal or visual data.

TAX 3. Ability to utilize verbal or visual data for the resolution of a problem or situation.

ITEM DESCRIPTOR LIST
MEDICAL TECHNOLOGIST EXAMINATION - AUGUST 1983

1. IMMU/ALF/BASIC TESTS/CRP/2
2. BBNK/CLD/IGTP/RH/2
3. IMMU/DFC/BASIC TESTS/COMPLEMENT FIX/1
4. BBNK/DFC/IGTP/RH AG/1
5. IMMU/DFC/QUALITY CONTROL/STATISTICS/1
6. IMMU/ALF/IMMUNITY/1
7. BBNK/SEL/BLOOD COMP/EX TRANSFUSION/3
8. IMMU/CCLD/STS/2
9. IMMU/DFC/SPECIAL TESTS/IMMUNOFLUORESCENCE/1
10. BBNK/IBP/AHG/1
11. IMMU/DFC/ACTIVE IMMUNITY/1
12. BBNK/SEL/DONOR REQUIRE/1
13. IMMU/ETR/BASIC TESTS/FEBRILE AGGL/2
14. IMMU/DFC/BENCE JONES/1
15. IMMU/DFC/BASIC TESTS/WEIL-FELIX/1
16. IMMU/ETR/IMMUNO/3
17. BBNK/ETR/BASIC TESTS/AHG/2
18. IMMU/DFC/BASIC TESTS/ASO/1
19. IMMU/ID/AG SITES/IG/1
20. IMMU/ID/IG/1
21. BBNK/IBP/SCH/COMP PREPA/1
22. BBNK/ETR/BASIC TESTS/AB IDENT/3
23. BBNK/DFC/ANTISERUM/RH TYPING/1
24. IMMU/DFC/AB/1
25. BBNK/DFC/IGTP/ABO/1
26. IMMU/ETR/BASIC TESTS/COLD AGGL/2
27. IMMU/DFC/IGTP/PROZONE/1
28. BBNK/SEL/BLOOD COMP/2
29. BBNK/SEL/COMP/EM TRANSFUSION/2
30. IMMU/DFC/IGTP/IG/1
31. IMMU/CCLD/LE/3
32. BBNK/IBP/SCH/ANTICOAGULANT/1
33. IMMU/DFC/IGTP/COMPLEMENT/1
34. BBNK/CCLD/ADVERSE REX/TRANSFUSION/3
35. IMMU/PERF/BASIC TESTS/HCG/2
36. BBNK/ARF/AB/HEMOLYTIC ANEMIA/2
37. IMMU/ISOE/BASIC TESTS/ANA/2
38. BBNK/IBP/BASIC TESTS/RH IG/1
39. CHEM/IBP/BASIC TESTS/UREA/1
40. CHEM/ESOE/SPECT/2
41. CHEM/SELM/SPECIAL TESTS/PROTEIN ABNOR/1
42. CHEM/IBP/INSTRUMENTATION/ATOMIC ABSORPTION/1
43. CHEM/CCLD/BMD/LIPASE/2
44. CHEM/IBP/ANYL METH/GLUCOSE/1
45. CHEM/CCLD/BMD/ELECTROLYTES/2
46. CHEM/ISOE/SCH/BLOOD GAS/2
47. CHEM/IBP/AAT/1
48. CHEM/CLD/CARBOHYDRATES/GTT/2
49. CHEM/DFC/BTP/ALBUMIN/1
50. CHEM/CALC/BASIC TESTS/BILIRUBIN/2
51. CHEM/PERF/BASIC TESTS/CHOLESTEROL/1
52. CHEM/EVAL/SCH/2
53. CHEM/SELM/BTP/BLOOD GAS/1
54. CHEM/CCLD/BMD/ISOENZYMES/2
55. CHEM/IBP/SPECIAL TESTS/AMINO ACID/1
56. CHEM/IBP/SPECIAL TESTS/CREAT CLEAR/1
57. CHEM/IBP/BTP/BILIRUBIN/1
58. CHEM/CCLD/SPECIAL TESTS/ESTRIOL/2
59. CHEM/DFC/INSTRUMENTATION/SPECT/1
60. CHEM/IBP/CARBOHYDRATES/D-XYLOSE/1
61. CHEM/ISOE/ELECTROLYTES/1
62. CHEM/CCLD/BMD/BLOOD GAS/2
63. CHEM/CCLD/BMD/CK/2
64. CHEM/IBP/SPECIAL TESTS/CREAT CLEAR/1
65. CHEM/PERF/BASIC TESTS/BILIRUBIN/2
66. CHEM/IBP/INSTRUMENTATION/ELECTRODE/2
67. CHEM/ETR/BTP/LIPIDS/2
68. CHEM/ETR/SPEC/CARBOHYDRATES/3
69. CHEM/ASSO/BMD/ACIDOSIS/2
70. CHEM/EVAL/SCH/POTASSIUM/2
71. CHEM/IBP/PROTEIN/ELECTRO/1
72. CHEM/ESOE/SCH/BILIRUBIN/1
73. CHEM/IBP/BASIC TESTS/UREA/1
74. CHEM/DFC/BTP/CATECHOLAMINE/1
75. CHEM/IBP/INSTRUMENTATION/GLC/1
76. CHEM/DFC/BTP/LIPIDS/1
77. CHEM/PERF/IDENT/GLC/3
78. CHEM/CCLD/SPECIAL TESTS/LIPOPROTEIN/2
79. HEMA/ASSO/ANEMIA/RETICULOCYTE COUNT/2
80. HEMA/CCLD/SECONDARY IDA/2
81. HEMA/ID/INCLUSION/WBC/1
82. HEMA/ISOE/HEMOGLOBIN/SPECT/2
83. HEMA/CALC/CORRECTED COUNT/WBC/2
84. HEMA/ID/FACTOR/COAGULATION/1
85. HEMA/ALF/FACTOR DEFI/2
86. HEMA/ASSO/CYTOGENETICS/CGL/1
87. HEMA/ALF/BASIC TESTS/HEMAT DISEASE/2
88. HEMA/ESOE/NORMAL RANGE/2
89. HEMA/ANAL/RBC INDICES/MORPH/3
90. HEMA/IBP/HEMOSTASIS/PLATELET CONSTIT/1
91. HEMA/ALF/FACTOR DEFI/2
92. HEMA/ALF/SPECIAL TESTS/STAIN/2
93. HEMA/CLD/BASIC TESTS/ACUTE LEUKEMIA/3
94. HEMA/IBP/HEMOSTASIS/1
95. HEMA/ID/VITAMIN K/COAGULATION/1
96. HEMA/IMM/RBC/MACROCYTIC ANEMIA/2
97. HEMA/IMM/CLL/2
98. HEMA/AMM/RBC PHYSIOLOGY/2
99. HEMA/ETR/SPECIAL TESTS/HEMOPATHY/3
100. HEMA/IMM/WBC/ANOMALY/2
101. HEMA/IMM/RBC INCLUSIONS/2
102. HEMA/ASSO/SPECIAL TESTS/OSMOTIC FRAGILITY/2
103. HEMA/ESOE/ACC/2
104. HEMA/CALC/ABSOLUTE COUNT/WBC/2
105. HEMA/IBP/ACC/1
106. HEMA/CALC/LAP SCORE/2
107. HEMA/CCLD/SPECIAL TESTS/IDA/3
108. HEMA/CLD/FACTOR DEFI/2
109. HEMA/IMM/MATURATION/MYELOCYTIC SERIES/1
110. HEMA/CCLD/MICRO MORPH/BURNS/2
111. HEMA/CCLD/MICRO MORPH/SMUDGE CELLS/1
112. HEMA/IBP/ACC/1
113. HEMA/ETR/RBC INDICES/IDA/3
114. BF/CALC/MAGNIFICATION/2
115. BF/DFC/SCH/URINE PH/1
116. CHEM/DFC/QUALITY CONTROL/STATISTICS/1
117. BF/IBP/RCD/AMNIOTIC FLUID/1
118. BF/ISOE/SCH/URINE/1
119. BF/DFC/PHYSIOLOGY/CLEAR TEST/1
120. BF/CALC/GASTRIC PH/2
121. BF/DFC/PHYSIOLOGY/RENAL THRESHOLD/1
122. CHEM/CALC/REAG PREPA/SOL CONCENTRATION/2
123. BF/CALC/URINE/SPECIFIC GRAVITY/2
124. CHEM/DFC/LO/SAFETY/1
125. CHEM/CALC/BUFFER/SOL/2
126. BF/IBP/BASIC TESTS/FECAL BILIRUBIN/1
127. CHEM/CALC/REAG PREPA/SOL CONCENTRATION/2
128. BF/ETR/URINE/REDUCING SUBSTANCE/3
129. BF/CCLD/RCD/URINE SED/2
130. BF/ISOE/URINE/SPECIFIC GRAVITY/1

ITEM DESCRIPTOR LIST
MEDICAL TECHNOLOGIST EXAMINATION - AUGUST 1983

131. CHEM/CALC/BLOOD GAS/HHE/2
132. CHEM/CALC/REAG PREPA/SOL CONCENTRATION/2
133. BF/SELM/SCH/CSF/1
134. BBNK/CALC/RBC SUSPENSION/2
135. BF/CCLD/RCD/URINE SED/3
136. BF/IMM/URINE CRYSTAL/2
137. BF/IMM/URINE CRYSTAL/2
138. BF/ALF/URINE SED/SOO/2
139. BF/ALF/URINE SED/CHEMICAL TEST/3
140. CHEM/CALC/SPECIAL TESTS/RADIOACTIVE DECAY/2
141. BF/CCLD/URINE/PROTEIN/2
142. CHEM/CALC/CALCIUM/EQUIVALENT WEIGHT/1
143. BF/IBP/BASIC TESTS/URINE PROTEIN/1
144. CHEM/IBP/LO/GLASSWARE/1
145. BF/IBP/BASIC TESTS/URINE SED/1
146. CHEM/CALC/BASIC TESTS/PERCENT TRANS/2
147. CHEM/DFC/BTP/ACID-BASE/1
148. BF/DFC/GROSS APPEAR/CSF/1
149. BF/ESOE/SCH/URINALYSIS/2
150. CHEM/DFC/QUALITY CONTROL/SAMPLE/1
151. BF/IBP/BASIC TESTS/URINE KETONES/1
152. MICR/ALF/SPECIAL TESTS/STAPHYLOCOCCUS/2
153. MICR/SEL/BASIC TESTS/STREPTOCOCCUS/2
154. MICR/SEL/GROWTH REQUIRE/CLOSTRIDIUM/2
155. MICR/ETR/BASIC TESTS/STREPTOCOCCUS/2
156. MICR/EVAL/BASIC TESTS/SHIGELLA/2
157. MICR/IMM/DIMORPHIC FUNGI/1
158. MICR/IMM/NEMATODE/1
159. MICR/SELM/GROWTH REQUIRE/MYCOPLASMA/1
160. MICR/CCLD/MORPH/LISTERIA/2
161. MICR/ID/MACRO MORPH/CLOSTRIDIUM/1
162. MICR/CCLD/GROWTH CHARACT/BACTEROIDES/2
163. MICR/CLD/YEAST/2
164. MICR/SELM/BASIC TESTS/MYCOBACTERIA/1
165. MICR/SELM/BASIC TESTS/MYCOBACTERIA/1
166. MICR/IMM/DIPHASIC FUNGUS/2
167. MICR/IMM/YEAST/2
168. MICR/ISOE/SCH/NEMATODE/1
169. MICR/IBP/IDS/VIRAL/1
170. MICR/ESOE/SCH/BLOOD CULTURE/3
171. MICR/ASSO/INFECTION/HAEMOPHILUS/1
172. MICR/ETR/BASIC TESTS/SUSCEPT/3
173. MICR/IMM/NEMATODE/1
174. MICR/SEL/BASIC TESTS/NEISSERIA/1
175. MICR/EVAL/BASIC TESTS/PSEUDOMONAS/3
176. MICR/IBP/SELECTIVE MEDIA/1
177. MICR/DFC/MACRO MORPH/MYCOBACTERIA/1
178. MICR/ETR/BASIC TESTS/SUSCEPT/2
179. MICR/IMM/AMOEBA/2
180. MICR/IMM/PLASMODIUM/2
181. MICR/EVAL/BASIC TESTS/PROTEUS/2
182. MICR/CCLD/MICRO MORPH/SPIROCHETE/2
183. MICR/IBP/QUALITY CONTROL/1
184. MICR/IMM/DIMORPHIC FUNGI/1
185. MICR/ESOE/SCH/BLOOD CULTURE/2
186. MICR/EVAL/BASIC TESTS/ENTEROBACTER/3
187. MICR/ALF/ACTINOMYCES/2
188. MICR/IBP/LO/STERILIZATION/1
189. MICR/SELM/QUALITY CONTROL/REAG/1

GLOSSARY OF TERMS USED IN ITEM DESCRIPTORS
MEDICAL TECHNOLOGIST EXAMINATION - FEBRUARY 1984

AB	ANTIBODY
ACCEPT	ACCEPTABILITY
ACLD	ASSOCIATE CLINICAL AND LABORATORY DATA
AG	ANTIGEN
AIHA	AUTOIMMUNE HEMOLYTIC ANEMIA
ALF	ASSOCIATE LABORATORY FINDINGS
ANAL	ANALYTIC
ANHYD	ANHYDROUS
ANYL	ANALYZE
APPEAR	APPEARANCE
ASSO	ASSOCIATE
BBNK	BLOOD BANK
BF	BODY FLUIDS
BIOCHEM	BIOCHEMICAL
CALC	CALCULATE
CCD	CORRELATE CLINICAL DATA
CCLD	CORRELATE CLINICAL AND LABORATORY DATA
CHARACT	CHARACTERISTICS
CHEM	CHEMISTRY
CK	CREATINE KINASE
CLD	CORRELATE LABORATORY DATA
CLEAR	CLEARANCE
CLL	CHRONIC LYMPHOCYTIC LEUKEMIA
COA	COURSE OF ACTION
CREAT	CREATININE
CSF	CEREBROSPINAL FLUID
DEFI	DEFICIENCY
DFC	DEFINE FUNDAMENTAL CHARACTERISTICS
ECC	ELECTRONIC CELL COUNTER
EMM	EVALUATE MICROSCOPIC MORPHOLOGY
ESOE	EVALUATE SOURCE OF ERROR
ESR	ERYTHROCYTE SEDIMENTATION RATE
ETR	EVALUATE TEST RESULTS
EVAL	EVALUATE
FIX	FIXATION
FUO	FEVER OF UNDETERMINED ORIGIN
GNB	GRAM-NEGATIVE BACILLI
GNC	GRAM-NEGATIVE COCCI
GPB	GRAM-POSITIVE BACILLI
GPC	GRAM-POSITIVE COCCI
GTT	GLUCOSE TOLERANCE TEST
HAI	HEMAGGLUTINATION INHIBITION
HEMA	HEMATOLOGY
HEMOLY	HEMOLYSIS
HEMOPATHY	HEMOGLOBINOPATHY
IBP	IDENTIFY BASIC PRINCIPLES
ID	IDENTIFY
IDC	IDENTIFY DISTINGUISHING CHARACTERISTICS
IDENT	IDENTIFICATION
IEP	IMMUNOELECTROPHORESIS
IMM	IDENTIFY MICROSCOPIC MORPHOLOGY
IMMU	IMMUNOLOGY
INTERACT	INTERACTION
ISOE	IDENTIFY SOURCE OF ERROR
KOH	POTASSIUM HYDROXIDE
LAP	LEUKOCYTE ALKALINE PHOSPHATASE
LO	LABORATORY OPERATIONS
METH	METHODOLOGY
MICR	MICROBIOLOGY
MICRO	MICROSCOPIC
MORPH	MORPHOLOGY
NPN	NONPROTEIN NITROGEN
PERF	PERFORM
PREPA	PREPARATION
QC	QUALITY CONTROL
RA	RHEUMATOID ARTHRITIS
RBC	RED BLOOD CELLS
REAG	REAGENT
REQUIRE	REQUIREMENTS
RID	RADIAL IMMUNODIFFUSION
RX	REACTION
SCH	SPECIMEN COLLECTION AND HANDLING
SD	STANDARD DEVIATION
SED	SEDIMENT
SELM	SELECT METHODOLOGY
SOE	SOURCE OF ERROR
SOL	SOLUTION
SPEC	SPECIMEN
SPECT	SPECTROSCOPY
STS	SEROLOGICAL TESTS FOR SYPHILIS
TRANS	TRANSMISSION
TREAT	TREATMENT
TX	TRANSFUSION
UV	ULTRAVIOLET
VS	VERSUS
WBC	WHITE BLOOD CELLS

TAXONOMIC LEVELS

TAX 1 - Recall: Ability to recall previously learned knowledge ranging from specific facts to complete theories, solely by recognition or memorization.

TAX 2 - Interpretive skills: Ability to utilize recalled knowledge to interpret or apply verbal, numeric or visual data.

TAX 3 - Problem Solving: Ability to utilize recalled knowledge and interpretation/application of data to resolve a problem or situation and/or make an appropriate decision.

ITEM DESCRIPTOR LIST
MEDICAL TECHNOLOGIST EXAMINATION - FEBRUARY 1984

1. CHEM/IBP/INSTRUMENTATION/ELECTRODE/1
2. CHEM/ETR/CRITICAL VALUES/ACID-BASE/2
3. CHEM/IBP/OSMOLALITY/1
4. CHEM/CALC/CONCENTRATION/MILLIEQUIVALENTS/2
5. CHEM/IBP/PHYSIOLOGY/PROTEIN/1
6. CHEM/ID/SAFETY SYMBOL/1
7. CHEM/CALC/AMOUNTS/HYDROUS VS ANHYD/2
8. CHEM/CCLD/MUSCLE DISEASE/ENZYMES/2
9. CHEM/IBP/ANAL METH/UREA/1
10. CHEM/SELM/LO/SAFETY/1
11. CHEM/IBP/INSTRUMENTATION/CENTRIFUGE/1
12. CHEM/IBP/PROTEIN/ELECTROPHORESIS/1
13. CHEM/IBP/ANAL METH/GLUCOSE/1
14. CHEM/ETR/DILUTION/BEER'S LAW/3
15. CHEM/CALC/DILUTION/2
16. CHEM/CCLD/LIPOPROTEIN/ELECTROPHORESIS/2
17. CHEM/IBP/ANAL METH/SERUM IRON/1
18. CHEM/DFC/BLOOD BUFFERS/1
19. CHEM/IBP/FUNCTION/ENZYMES/1
20. CHEM/DFC/PROTEIN/ELECTROPHORESIS/1
21. CHEM/CALC/METRIC UNITS/2
22. CHEM/SELM/WASHING/GLASSWARE/1
23. CHEM/ETR/BILE PIGMENTS/3
24. CHEM/IBP/INSTRUMENTATION/CHLORIDOMETER/1
25. CHEM/IBP/GRAPHIC DISPLAY/BEER'S LAW/1
26. CHEM/ISOE/SCH/LIPIDS/1
27. CHEM/ISOE/UREA NITROGEN/2
28. CHEM/DFC/UV SPECT/1
29. CHEM/CALC/PERCENT TRANS/2
30. CHEM/IBP/PHYSIOLOGY/NPN/1
31. CHEM/IBP/SECRETION/HORMONE/1
32. CHEM/DFC/QC/PRECISION/1
33. CHEM/ISOE/SCH/BLOOD GAS/2
34. CHEM/DFC/ACIDS/1
35. CHEM/CALC/MOLAR SOL/2
36. CHEM/SELM/EVALUATION/ACID-BASE/1
37. CHEM/CALC/QC/SD/2
38. CHEM/CCLD/CATECHOLAMINES/2
39. CHEM/IBP/BUFFER/1
40. CHEM/IBP/CHROMATOGRAPHY/1
41. CHEM/ISOE/SCH/BILIRUBIN/1
42. CHEM/IBP/SPECIAL TEST/CREAT CLEAR/1
43. CHEM/CALC/ANION GAP/2
44. CHEM/DFC/CK/ISOENZYMES/1
45. CHEM/DFC/ISOTOPE/1
46. HEMA/ISOE/PLATELET COUNT/2
47. HEMA/SELM/SPECIAL STAIN/RBC INCLUSIONS/1
48. HEMA/DFC/MATURATION/BLOOD CELLS/1
49. HEMA/ETR/ECC/2
50. HEMA/CALC/ABSOLUTE COUNT/WBC/2
51. HEMA/DFC/MATURATION/CELLS/1
52. HEMA/CLD/FACTOR DEFI/2
53. HEMA/DFC/ANTICOAGULANT/1
54. HEMA/CCLD/FACTOR DEFI/2
55. HEMA/IBP/SPECIAL STAIN/WBC/1
56. HEMA/DFC/PHYSIOLOGY/RBC/1
57. HEMA/ETR/QC/PROTHROMBIN TIME/2
58. HEMA/IBP/ECC/1
59. HEMA/DFC/HEMOGLOBIN F/1
60. HEMA/CCLD/LAP/3
61. HEMA/IMM/MONOCYTE/2
62. HEMA/EMM/RBC/MACROCYTIC ANEMIA/3
63. HEMA/EMM/CLL/3
64. HEMA/IMM/RBC PHYSIOLOGY/2
65. HEMA/IMM/WBC MORPH/ANOMALY/2
66. HEMA/IMM/RBC FRAGILITY/2
67. HEMA/ESOE/ECC/3
68. HEMA/CCLD/AIHA/2
69. HEMA/CLD/DRUG EFFECT/BLEEDING TIME/1
70. HEMA/DFC/AB SYNTHESIS/1
71. HEMA/IBP/SCH/BLOOD COLLECTION/3
72. HEMA/ACLD/SUCROSE HEMOLY/1
73. HEMA/CCLD/MICRO MORPH/RBC/3
74. HEMA/CALC/CELL COUNT/2
75. HEMA/IBP/ESR/1
76. HEMA/DFC/SD/1
77. HEMA/IBP/QC/SD/1
78. HEMA/DFC/SYNTHESIS/COAGULATION FACTOR/1
79. HEMA/DFC/HEMOPATHY/SOLUBILITY TEST/1
80. HEMA/IMM/RBC/BURNS/1
81. HEMA/DFC/FACTOR DEFI/1
82. HEMA/CCLD/ANEMIA/SPHEROCYTIC/2
83. HEMA/CCLD/ANEMIA/MEGALOBLASTIC/2
84. BF/SELM/URINE TEST/PROTEIN/1
85. BF/CLD/URINE/SPECIFIC GRAVITY/1
86. BF/SELM/FETAL MATURITY/1
87. BF/DFC/TRANSUDATES/1
88. BF/ASSO/CSF/BLOOD/1
89. BF/ETR/SEMINAL FLUID/2
90. BF/ALF/URINE/1
91. BF/DFC/RED CELL CASTS/1
92. BF/ETR/URINE/SPECIFIC GRAVITY/3
93. BF/CCLD/MENINGITIS/3
94. BF/ALF/URINE/METABOLIC DISEASE/1
95. BF/CCLD/URINE/SPECIFIC GRAVITY/3
96. BF/ESOE/SPEC/24 HOUR URINE/2
97. BF/ETR/BILE PIGMENT/1
98. BF/DFC/URINE/SPECIFIC GRAVITY/1
99. BF/ESOE/URINALYSIS/MICRO/3
100. BF/IBP/ANAL METH/SEMEN ANALYSIS/1
101. BF/ALF/SED EXAMINATION/CRYSTALS/2
102. BF/ID/SPECIAL STAIN/URINE SED/2
103. BF/ID/MICRO TECHNIQUE/2
104. BF/SELM/MALABSORPTION/1
105. BF/IBP/ANAL METH/FECAL FAT/1
106. BF/ETR/URINE/REDUCING SUBSTANCE/2
107. BF/IBP/REAG STRIP/PROTEIN/1
108. BF/ETR/UROBILINOGEN/3
109. BF/CCLD/URINE/REDUCING SUBSTANCE/3
110. BF/DFC/URINE/CAST/1
111. BF/CCLD/SOE/URINE GLUCOSE/3
112. BF/ASSO/SPEC APPEAR/URINE SED/1
113. MICR/IBP/ACID-FAST STAIN/1
114. MICR/PERF/BIOCHEM IDENT/STAPHYLOCOCCUS/2
115. MICR/SELM/IDENT/CORYNEBACTERIUM/2
116. MICR/ETR/MICRO MORPH/GPB/2
117. MICR/SELM/DISINFECTION/VIRUS/1
118. MICR/IMM/MOLD/1
119. MICR/SELM/SCH/GNB/2
120. MICR/IMM/MICROFILARIA/2
121. MICR/IMM/CESTODE OVA/2
122. MICR/IMM/AMOEBA/2
123. MICR/IMM/PROTOZOA/2
124. MICR/ETR/SEROLOGY/ENTERIC PATHOGEN/3
125. MICR/ID/MORPH/GNB/1
126. MICR/IMM/ACTINOMYCES/2
127. MICR/IDC/STREPTOCOCCI/1
128. MICR/IBP/ANTIBIOTIC/SUSCEPTIBILITY/1
129. MICR/IMM/YEAST/2
130. MICR/SELM/STERILIZATION/MEDIA/1

ITEM DESCRIPTOR LIST
MEDICAL TECHNOLOGIST EXAMINATION - FEBRUARY 1984

131. MICR/IBP/QUELLUNG/1
132. MICR/DFC/MYCOBACTERIA/PIGMENT/1
133. MICR/PERF/SCH/NASOPHARYNGEAL/1
134. MICR/CCLD/COLITIS/3
135. MICR/EVAL/IDENT/GNB/3
136. MICR/SELM/EPIDEMIOLOGY/GPC/1
137. MICR/ID/CAUSITIVE AGENT/RICKETTSIOSIS/1
138. MICR/IBP/SUSCEPTIBILITY/1
139. MICR/IBP/KOH PREPA/1
140. MICR/ALF/ANAEROBES/1
141. MICR/CCLD/GNC/2
142. MICR/PERF/QC/MEDIA/1
143. MICR/ID/GROWTH CHARACT/ACINETOBACTER/1
144. MICR/SELM/IDENT/RICKETTSIA/1
145. MICR/SELM/SCH/VIRUSES/1
146. MICR/ID/GROWTH CHARACT/STREPTOCOCCUS/1
147. MICR/CCLD/MORPH/DIPHASIC FUNGI/2
148. MICR/EVAL/GRAM STAIN/SPUTUM/3
149. MICR/ISOE/QC/SUSCEPTIBILITY/3
150. MICR/SELM/SCH/ACID-FAST BACILLI/1
151. IMMU/CLD/COLD AGGLUTININ/2
152. IMMU/ETR/IEP/2
153. BBNK/IBP/STORAGE REQUIRE/1
154. IMMU/ISOE/QC/RA TEST/3
155. BBNK/DFC/ENZYME TREAT/AG/1
156. BBNK/CALC/CELL SUSPENSION/2
157. IMMU/CCLD/FUO/3
158. BBNK/ACLD/DONOR ACCEPT/1
159. IMMU/IBP/RID/1
160. BBNK/ETR/CROSSMATCH/3
161. BBNK/ISOE/STORAGE/BLOOD/2
162. IMMU/CCLD/STS/3
163. IMMU/ANYL/PHYSIOLOGY/IMMUNE RESPONSE/3
164. BBNK/ETR/DU TEST/2
165. BBNK/CCD/COA/EMERGENCY TX/3
166. IMMU/IBP/PHYSIOLOGY/HUMORAL IMMUNITY/1
167. BBNK/ETR/CROSSMATCH/AB CHARACT/2
168. IMMU/IBP/ANAL METH/RA TEST/1
169. IMMU/DFC/AB PRODUCTION/1
170. BBNK/ETR/RH/2
171. BBNK/IBP/DONOR REQUIRE/HEPATITIS/2
172. IMMU/ETR/QC/ANTISTREPTOLYSIN O/2
173. IMMU/DFC/ALLERGY/AB PRODUCTION/1
174. IMMU/IBP/STS/1
175. BBNK/DFC/ETIOLOGY/HEMOLYTIC TX RX/1
176. BBNK/ALF/AB DETECTION/COMPONENT THERAPY/1
177. IMMU/IBP/IMMUNITY/1
178. IMMU/DFC/PHYSIOLOGY/C-REACTIVE PROTEIN/1
179. IMMU/IBP/AG-AB INTERACT/1
180. BBNK/DFC/ABO/AG/1
181. IMMU/ESOE/QC/ANTISTREPTOLYSIN O/3
182. IMMU/IBP/PROZONE/1
183. BBNK/DFC/ANTICOAGULANT/AB DETECTION/1
184. IMMU/ISOE/COMPLEMENT FIX/3
185. IMMU/ETR/HAI/2
186. IMMU/ETR/HETEROPHILE/1
187. BBNK/IBP/AB RX/1
188. BBNK/ALF/POST DONATION/HEMOGLOBIN/1
189. IMMU/DFC/AUTOANTIBODY/IMMUNE DISEASE/1
190. BBNK/ETR/CROSSMATCH/2
191. IMMU/DFC/PHYSIOLOGY/IMMUNOGLOBULIN/1

GLOSSARY OF TERMS USED IN ITEM DESCRIPTORS
MEDICAL TECHNOLOGIST EXAMINATION - AUGUST 1984

AB	ANTIBODY
ACCEPT	ACCEPTIBILITY
AFB	ACID-FAST BACILLI
AGGLUT	AGGLUTININ
AGGREG	AGGREGATION
ALF	ASSOCIATE LABORATORY FINDINGS
ALK	ALKALINE
AMM	ASSOCIATE MICROSCOPIC MORPHOLOGY
ANA	ANTINUCLEAR ANTIBODY
ANLF	ANALYZE LABORATORY FINDINGS
ANTIGLOB	ANTIGLOBULIN
BBNK	BLOOD BANK
BF	BODY FLUIDS
BIOCHEM	BIOCHEMICAL
BMD	BIOCHEMICAL MANIFESTATION OF DISEASE
BTP	BIOCHEMICAL THEORY AND PHYSIOLOGY
BUN	BLOOD UREA NITROGEN
CALC	CALCULATE
CBC	COMPLETE BLOOD COUNT
CCLD	CORRELATE CLINICAL AND LABORATORY DATA
CGL	CHRONIC GRANULOCYTIC LEUKEMIA
CHEM	CHEMISTRY
CLD	CORRELATE LABORATORY DATA
CLEAR	CLEARANCE
CLL	CHRONIC LYMPHOCYTIC LEUKEMIA
COAG	COAGULATION
CONC	CONCENTRATION
CONSTIT	CONSTITUENT
CORR	CORRECTED
CSF	CEREBROSPINAL FLUID
DFC	DEFINE FUNDAMENTAL CHARACTERISTIC
DIC	DISSEMINATED INTRAVASCULAR COAGULATION
DIS	DISEASE
DNA	DEOXYRIBONUCLEIC ACID
EDTA	ETHYLENEDIAMINETETRAACETIC ACID
ELECTROPHOR	ELECTROPHORESIS
ELF	EVALUATE LABORATORY FINDINGS
EMM	EVALUATE MICROSCOPIC MORPHOLOGY
ER	EMERGENCY
ESOE	EVALUATE SOURCE OF ERROR
ESOP	EVALUATE STANDARD OPERATING PROCEDURE
FIX	FIXATION
FRAG	FRAGILITY
GLC	GAS-LIQUID CHROMATOGRAPHY
GNB	GRAM-NEGATIVE BACILLI
GNC	GRAM-NEGATIVE COCCI
GPB	GRAM-POSITIVE BACILLI
GPC	GRAM-POSITIVE COCCI
GTT	GLUCOSE TOLERANCE TEST
HASSEL	HASSELBALCH
HDN	HEMOLYTIC DISEASE OF THE NEWBORN
HEMA	HEMATOLOGY
HGBPATH	HEMOGLOBINOPATHY
HPLC	HIGH PRESSURE LIQUID CHROMATOGRAPHY
IBP	IDENTIFY BASIC PRINCIPLE
ID	IDENTIFICATION
IGC	IDENTIFY GROWTH CHARACTERISTICS
IMM	IDENTIFY MICROSCOPIC MORPHOLOGY
IMMU	IMMUNOLOGY
INF	INFECTIOUS
ISOE	IDENTIFY SOURCE OF ERROR
ISOP	IDENTIFY STANDARD OPERATING PROCEDURE
LAP	LEUKOCYTE ALKALINE PHOSPHATASE
LD	LACTATE DEHYDROGENASE
LIPO	LIPOPROTEIN
MET	METABOLISM
MICR	MICROBIOLOGY
MIC-MAC	MICROSCOPIC-MACROSCOPIC
MICRO	MICROSCOPIC
MORPH	MORPHOLOGY
OF	OXIDATION-FERMENTATION
P&E	PROTEINS AND ENZYMES
PKU	PHENYLKETONURIA
PREP	PREPARATION
QA	QUALITY ASSURANCE
QC	QUALITY CONTROL
RA	RHEUMATOID ARTHRITIS
RAST	RADIOALLERGOSORBENT TEST
RBC	RED BLOOD CELLS
RESPON	RESPONSE
REX	REACTION
SCH	SPECIMEN COLLECTION AND HANDLING
SCOA	SELECT COURSE OF ACTION
SELM	SELECT METHOD
SERO	SEROLOGIC
SPEC	SPECIMEN
STS	SEROLOGIC TESTS FOR SYPHILIS
SUSCEPT	SUSCEPTIBILITY
TREAT	TREATMENT
TX	TRANSFUSION
WBC	WHITE BLOOD CELLS
X-MATCH	CROSSMATCH

TAXONOMIC LEVELS

TAX 1 - Recall:	Ability to recall or recognize previously learned (memorized) knowledge ranging from specific facts to complete theories.
TAX 2 - Interpretive skills:	Ability to utilize recalled knowledge to interpret or apply verbal, numeric or visual data.
TAX 3 - Problem Solving:	Ability to utilize recalled knowledge and the interpretation/application of distinct criteria to resolve a problem or situation and/or make an appropriate decision.

ITEM DESCRIPTOR LIST
MEDICAL TECHNOLOGIST EXAMINATION - AUGUST 1984

1. HEMA/IBP/AUTOMATED COUNT/1
2. HEMA/ALF/MICRO MORPH/HEMOLYTIC ANEMIA/1
3. HEMA/DFC/PLATELET/PHYSIOLOGY/1
4. HEMA/SCOA/SCH/VENIPUNCTURE/3
5. HEMA/SELM/HGBPATHY/2
6. HEMA/CCLD/ANEMIA/SPHEROCYTIC/2
7. HEMA/ELF/QC/RBC INDICES/3
8. HEMA/DFC/ABSORPTION/VITAMIN B12/1
9. HEMA/IBP/AUTOMATED COUNT/1
10. HEMA/CLD/CBC/ACUTE LEUKEMIA/3
11. HEMA/DFC/SYNTHESIS/COAG FACTOR/1
12. HEMA/CALC/CORR WBC COUNT/2
13. HEMA/ALF/SPECIAL TESTS/STAIN/2
14. HEMA/SELM/HEMOSTASIS/THROMBIN TIME/1
15. HEMA/ALF/INCLUSION/WBC/1
16. HEMA/CALC/LAP SCORE/2
17. HEMA/ELF/SPECIAL TEST/HGB F/2
18. HEMA/ELF/OSMOTIC FRAG/3
19. HEMA/EMM/RBC INDICES/3
20. HEMA/CCLD/MICRO MORPH/LEUKOCYTE/3
21. HEMA/EMM/CBC/3
22. HEMA/CCLD/MICRO MORPH/CLL/3
23. HEMA/ESOE/AUTOMATED COUNT/PLATELET/3
24. HEMA/CCLD/LAP/3
25. HEMA/ESOE/COAG TEST/QC/3
26. HEMA/ALF/CYTOGENETICS/CGL/1
27. HEMA/ELF/THROMBIN TIME/SUBSTITUTION STUDY/3
28. HEMA/IBP/QC/HEMOGLOBIN/1
29. HEMA/IBP/HEMOSTASIS/PLATELET CONSTIT/1
30. HEMA/CCLD/HEMOSTASIS/DIC/3
31. HEMA/CLD/COAG/FACTOR DEFICIENCY/2
32. HEMA/SCOA/SCH/PLATELETS/3
33. HEMA/DFC/HEMOGLOBIN F/1
34. HEMA/CCLD/CBC/APLASTIC ANEMIA/2
35. HEMA/ALF/PHYSIOLOGY/PLATELET/2
36. HEMA/ALF/COAG/FACTOR DEFICIENCY/2
37. HEMA/ELF/PLATELET COUNT/PERIPHERAL SMEAR/3
38. HEMA/CCLD/COAG/FACTOR DEFICIENCY/3
39. HEMA/CCLD/ANEMIA/MEGALOBLASTIC/2
40. HEMA/CALC/ABSOLUTE COUNT/2
41. HEMA/IBP/SCH/EDTA/1
42. HEMA/ALF/FIBRINOLYSIS/SPECIAL TEST/2
43. HEMA/SCOA/QC/RBC INDICES/3
44. BF/CLD/MICRO MORPH/URINE CRYSTAL/2
45. BF/IMM/URINE CRYSTAL/2
46. BF/AMM/URINE/CRYSTAL/2
47. BF/SELM/FETAL MATURITY/1
48. BF/DFC/TRANSUDATES/1
49. BF/ELF/URINE/SPECIFIC GRAVITY/3
50. BF/ESOE/FECES/SPEC COLLECTION/3
51. BF/ESOE/URINE/PROTEIN/3
52. BF/CCLD/MICRO MORPH/URINE CAST/3
53. BF/AMM/URINE/CRYSTAL/2
54. BF/CALC/URINE/SPECIFIC GRAVITY/2
55. BF/CCLD/URINE/PROTEIN/2
56. BF/DFC/SCH/URINE PH/1
57. BF/SELM/URINE/SEDIMENT STAIN/2
58. BF/CLD/MICRO MORPH/DEGENERATIVE CASTS/3
59. BF/CCLD/URINE/SPECIFIC GRAVITY/3
60. BF/ELF/URINE/REDUCING SUBSTANCE/3
61. BF/SCOA/CELL COUNT/PLEURAL FLUID/3
62. BF/ISOE/URINE/SPEC PROCESSING/2
63. BF/ALF/URINE/METABOLIC DIS/1
64. BF/SELM/SCH/CSF/1
65. MICR/IGC/GPB/WOUND CULTURE/2
66. MICR/SELM/GNC/BASIC TEST/1
67. MICR/CCLD/GNC/WOUND CULTURE/2
68. MICR/IGC/GNB/ACINETOBACTER/1
69. MICR/SELM/GPC/REAGENT QC/1
70. MICR/SELM/GNB/SCH/1
71. MICR/CCLD/MIC-MAC MORPH/DIPHASIC FUNGI/2
72. MICR/ELF/SCH/PARASITE/3
73. MICR/ELF/GNB/STOOL CULTURE/2
74. MICR/ALF/GNB/CSF CULTURE/1
75. MICR/ISOE/SUSCEPT TEST/1
76. MICR/ELF/GNB/PROTEUS/1
77. MICR/SELM/GPC/BLOOD CULTURE/3
78. MICR/IMM/DIPHASIC FUNGUS/2
79. MICR/IMM/YEAST/2
80. MICR/ESOE/GRAM STAIN/3
81. MICR/ELF/GNB/CSF CULTURE/3
82. MICR/ESOE/AFB/PHOTOCHROMOGEN/3
83. MICR/ALF/BIOCHEM TEST/AFB/1
84. MICR/ELF/GNB/QC BIOCHEM TEST/3
85. MICR/ANLF/GPC/URINE CULTURE/3
86. MICR/IMM/AMOEBA/2
87. MICR/IMM/PLASMODIUM/2
88. MICR/IMM/AMOEBA/2
89. MICR/ELF/GNB/OF REX/2
90. MICR/IMM/GNB/SPUTUM CULTURE/2
91. MICR/IMM/GPB/STAINING PROPERTY/1
92. MICR/SELM/SPECIAL TESTS/AFB/1
93. MICR/ESOE/SCH/BLOOD CULTURE/3
94. MICR/ESOE/SCH/FUNGI/3
95. MICR/CCLD/GPB/SINUS CULTURE/2
96. MICR/SCOA/GNB/URINE CULTURE/2
97. MICR/IBP/INF DIS SERO/VIRAL/1
98. MICR/SELM/GPB/LISTERIA/1
99. MICR/ELF/GNB/2
100. MICR/CCLD/MICRO MORPH/SPIROCHETE/2
101. MICR/SELM/SCH/SPUTUM FUNGUS/2
102. MICR/ESOE/SCH/BLOOD CULTURE/2
103. MICR/SCOA/SCH/PARASITE/2
104. MICR/SELM/SPEC PREP/AFB/1
105. MICR/ELF/GPC/EAR CULTURE/2
106. BBNK/IBP/COMPONENT PREP/PLATELETS/1
107. BBNK/IBP/X-MATCH/HIGH PROTEIN/1
108. BBNK/SCOA/BLOOD COMPONENT/EXCHANGE TX/3
109. BBNK/ELF/ANTIGLOB TEST/2
110. BBNK/ISOP/RBC/REAGENT QC/1
111. BBNK/ISOE/RH TYPING/HDN/2
112. BBNK/ELF/AB PANEL/3
113. BBNK/SCOA/AB ABSORPTION/2
114. BBNK/IBP/RBC/AB ID/1
115. BBNK/CCLD/DONOR ACCEPT/PLASMAPHORESIS/2
116. BBNK/DFC/BLOOD COMPONENT/1
117. BBNK/SCOA/BLOOD COMPONENT/2
118. BBNK/DFC/RBC/ABO DISCREPANCY/1
119. BBNK/CCLD/ADVERSE REX/TX/3
120. BBNK/ELF/GENOTYPE/2
121. BBNK/DFC/ENZYME TREAT/ANTIGEN/1
122. BBNK/ALF/HEMOTHERAPY/ADVERSE REX/2
123. BBNK/SCOA/ER TX/3
124. BBNK/ALF/AB DETECTION/COMPONENT THERAPY/1
125. BBNK/SCOA/SCH/AB ID/2
126. BBNK/ISOP/PLATELETS/SPEC STORAGE/1
127. BBNK/ELF/AB ID/3
128. BBNK/ELF/AB ID/HDN/2
129. BBNK/ISOP/RBC/DONOR REQUIREMENT/1
130. BBNK/SCOA/ER TX/2

ITEM DESCRIPTOR LIST
MEDICAL TECHNOLOGIST EXAMINATION - AUGUST 1984

131. BBNK/ELF/PROBLEM X-MATCH/3
132. BBNK/SCOA/PROBLEM AB/3
133. BBNK/ELF/X-MATCH/ER SITUATION/3
134. BBNK/ISOP/REAGENT QC/1
135. IMMU/DFC/SERO REX/PROZONE/1
136. IMMU/IBP/PHYSIOLOGY/IMMUME RESPON/3
137. IMMU/DFC/AB PRODUCTION/1
138. IMMU/IBP/RA TEST/1
139. IMMU/DFC/ALLERGY/AB PRODUCTION/1
140. IMMU/DFC/AUTOANTIBODY/RA/1
141. IMMU/ELF/AUTOIMMUNITY/DNA/2
142. IMMU/ESOE/QC/ANTISTREPTOLYSIN O/3
143. IMMU/CCLD/SERO TITER/FEBRILE/3
144. IMMU/CALC/CELL IMMUNITY/T CELLS/2
145. IMMU/IBP/PHYSIOLOGY/HUMORAL IMMUNITY/1
146. IMMU/DFC/COMPLEMENT/1
147. IMMU/ESOE/COMPLEMENT FIX/3
148. IMMU/ELF/PREGNANCY TEST/2
149. IMMU/DFC/PHYSIOLOGY/HUMORAL IMMUNITY/1
150. IMMU/ELF/FEBRILE AGGLUT/2
151. IMMU/ISOE/SCH/CELL IMMUNITY/2
152. IMMU/CCLD/STS/3
153. IMMU/ESOE/SCH/COLD AGGLUT/3
154. IMMU/ESOE/CELL IMMUNITY/T LYMPHOCYTE/3
155. CHEM/CALC/MOLAR SOLUTION/2
156. CHEM/CLD/CARBOHYDRATES/GTT/2
157. CHEM/DFC/SPEC APPEARANCE/1
158. CHEM/ESOE/SPECTRAL CURVE/3
159. CHEM/IBP/CARBOHYDRATES/D-XYLOSE/1
160. CHEM/ISOE/SCH/BLOOD GAS/2
161. CHEM/ELF/LIPIDS/QA/3
162. CHEM/CALC/BLOOD GAS/HENDERSON-HASSEL/2
163. CHEM/DFC/QC/SAMPLE/1
164. CHEM/ESOE/INSTRUMENTATION/GLC/3
165. CHEM/CCLD/SPECIAL TESTS/LIPO/2
166. CHEM/ALF/BMD/CATECHOLAMINES/1
167. CHEM/DFC/PROTEIN/ELECTROPHOR/1
168. CHEM/ALF/QA/LIPO/3
169. CHEM/IBP/AMINO ACID MET/PKU/1
170. CHEM/ESOE/INSTRUMENTATION/RIA STANDARD CURVE/3
171. CHEM/IBP/COPPER/1
172. CHEM/CLD/CARBOHYDRATES/PHYSIOLOGY/2
173. CHEM/ELF/ISOENZYME/ALK PHOSPHATASE/2
174. CHEM/CCLD/BMD/BLOOD GAS/2
175. CHEM/IBP/ENZYME REX/1
176. CHEM/CALC/% TRANSMISSION/2
177. CHEM/CALC/ANION GAP/2
178. CHEM/ESOE/INSTRUMENTATION/RIA STANDARD CURVE/3
179. CHEM/CCLD/BMD/RED BLOOD CELL ENZYMES/3
180. CHEM/ELF/LIPO ELECTROPHOR/2
181. CHEM/CLD/CARBOHYDRATES/SPEC COLLECTION/2
182. CHEM/ALF/BMD/CREATINE KINASE/1
183. CHEM/CCLD/P&E/ACID PHOSPHATASE/3
184. CHEM/ELF/LD ISOENZYMES/2
185. CHEM/SELM/BTP/BLOOD GAS/1
186. CHEM/CALC/SOLUTE CONC/2
187. CHEM/ESOE/INSTRUMENTATION/SPECTROPHOTOMETER/3
188. CHEM/CALC/SOLUTION CONC/2
189. CHEM/IBP/ANALYTIC METHOD/PHOSPHATE/1
190. CHEM/IBP/INSTRUMENTATION/NEPHELOMETRY/1
191. CHEM/CCLD/BMD/ISOENZYMES/2
192. CHEM/SELM/GLUCOSE/1
193. CHEM/IBP/ENZYME REX/1
194. CHEM/ELF/HEME DERIVATIVE/JAUNDICE/3
195. CHEM/ISOP/GTT/3
196. CHEM/CALC/QC/STANDARD DEVIATION/2
197. CHEM/IBP/INSTRUMENTATION/ATOMIC ABSORPTION/1
198. CHEM/ESOE/INSTRUMENTATION/HPLC/3
199. CHEM/ALF/SPECIAL TESTS/ESTRIOL/1
200. CHEM/CALC/% SOLUTION/2
201. CHEM/ISOP/BILIRUBIN/BEER'S LAW/2
202. CHEM/IBP/INSTRUMENTATION/ELECTRODE/2
203. CHEM/CALC/SPECIAL TESTS/RADIOACTIVE DECAY/2

GLOSSARY OF TERMS USED IN ITEM DESCRIPTORS
MEDICAL TECHNOLOGIST EXAMINATION - FEBRUARY 1985

AB	ANTIBODY(IES)
ACCEPT	ACCEPTABILITY
ACLD	ASSOCIATE CLINICAL AND LABORATORY DATA
ADD	ADDITIONAL
AFB	ACID-FAST BACILLI
AG	ANTIGEN
AGGLUT	AGGLUTININS
AIHA	AUTOIMMUNE HEMOLYTIC ANEMIA
ALF	ASSOCIATE LABORATORY FINDINGS
ALLOAB	ALLOANTIBODY
AMM	ASSOCIATE MICROSCOPIC MORPHOLOGY
ANA	ANTINUCLEAR ANTIBODY
ANALY	ANALYSIS
ANLF	ANALYZE LABORATORY FINDINGS
APPEAR	APPEARANCE
AUTOAB	AUTOANTIBODY
AUTOAGGLUT	AUTOAGGLUTININ
BBNK	BLOOD BANK
BF	BODY FLUID
BIOCHEM	BIOCHEMISTRY/BIOCHEMICAL
BMD	BIOCHEMICAL MANIFESTATION OF DISEASE
BTP	BIOCHEMICAL THEORY AND PHYSIOLOGY
CALC	CALCULATION(S)
CBC	COMPLETE BLOOD COUNT
CCLD	CORRELATE CLINICAL AND LABORATORY DATA
CELLU	CELLULAR
CGL	CHRONIC GRANULOCYTIC LEUKEMIA
CHARACTERISTI	CHARACTERISTIC(S)
CHEM	CHEMISTRY
CLD	CORRELATE LABORATORY DATA
CLL	CHRONIC LYMPHOCYTIC LEUKEMIA
CMM	CORRELATE MICROSCOPIC MORPHOLOGY
COMPO	COMPONENT
CONC	CONCENTRATION
CORR	CORRECTED
CSF	CEREBROSPINAL FLUID
CT	COUNT
CULT	CULTURE
CV	COEFFICIENT OF VARIATION
DAT	DIRECT ANTIGLOBULIN TEST
DFC	DEFINE FUNDAMENTAL CHARACTERISTICS
DIFF	DIFFERENTIAL
DIS	DISEASE
DNA	DEOXYRIBONUCLEIC ACID
EDUCAT	EDUCATIONAL
EL	ELECTROLYTES
ELECT	ELECTRODE
ELECTRO	ELECTROPHORESIS
ELF	EVALUATE LABORATORY FINDINGS
EMIT	ENZYME-MULTIPLIED IMMUNOASSAY TECHNIQUES
EMM	EVALUATE MICROSCOPIC MORPHOLOGY
ENZYM	ENZYME
ER	EMERGENCY
ERR	ERROR
ESOE	EVALUTE SOURCE OF ERROR
ETR	EVALUATE TEST RESULTS
FIX	FIXATION
FUNCT	FUNCTION
GEN	GENETIC(S)
GLU	GLUCOSE
GNB	GRAM-NEGATIVE BACILLI
GNC	GRAM-NEGATIVE COCCI
GPB	GRAM-POSITIVE BACILLI
GPC	GRAM-POSITIVE COCCI
HBS	HEPATITIS B SURFACE
HDN	HEMOLYTIC DISEASE OF THE NEWBORN
HEMA	HEMATOLOGY
IBC	IDENTIFY BASIC CONCEPT
IBP	IDENTIFY BASIC PRINCIPLE
ID	IDENTIFY/IDENTIFICATION
IMM	IDENTIFY MICROSCOPIC MORPHOLOGY
IMMU	IMMUNOLOGY
INCOMPAT	INCOMPATIBLE
INFECT	INFECTION/INFECTIOUS
INSUL	INSULIN
ISOE	IDENTIFY SOURCE OF ERROR
ISOP	IDENTIFY STANDARD OPERATING PROCEDURE
LAB	LABORATORY
LAP	LEUKOCYTE ALKALINE PHOSPHATASE
LYMPH	LYMPHOCYTE(S)
MAC	MACROSCOPIC
MACRO	MACROCYTIC
MET	METABOLISM/METABOLIC
MIC	MINIMUM INHIBITORY CONCENTRATION
MICR	MICROBIOLOGY
MICRO	MICROSCOPIC
MORPH	MORPHOLOGY
NEUTRALIZA	NEUTRALIZATION
NON-CELLU	NON-CELLULAR
OBSTR	OBSTRUCTION
OF	OXIDATIVE-FERMENTATIVE
PBS	PERIPHERAL BLOOD SMEAR
PKU	PHENYLKETONURIA
PRIN	PRINCIPLE
PTT	ACTIVATED PARTIAL THROMBOPLASTIN TIME
QA	QUALITY ASSURANCE
QC	QUALITY CONTROL
RA	RHEUMATOID ARTHRITIS
RAST	RADIOALLERGOSORBENT TEST
RBC	RED BLOOD CELL
RCD	RELATED CONDITIONS AND DISORDERS
REX	REACTION
SCH	SPECIMEN COLLECTION AND HANDLING
SCOA	SELECT COURSE OF ACTION
SELC	SELECT COMPONENT
SELECT	SELECTIVE
SELM	SELECT METHOD
SELR	SELECT REAGENT
SERO	SEROLOGIC/SEROLOGY
SI	INTERNATIONAL SYSTEM OF UNITS
SPE	SPECIMEN
SPEC	SPECIAL
STS	SEROLOGIC TESTS FOR SYPHILIS
SUBPOP	SUBPOPULATION
SUBSTA	SUBSTANCES
SUSC	SUSCEPTIBILITY
THER	THEORY
TOLERANC	TOLERANCE
TST	TEST(S)
TX	TRANSFUSION
WBC	WHITE BLOOD CELL
X-MATCH	CROSSMATCH

TAXONOMIC LEVELS

TAX 1 - Recall: Ability to recall or recognize previously learned (memorized) knowledge ranging from specific facts to complete theories.

TAX 2 - Interpretive skills: Ability to utilize recalled knowledge to interpret or apply verbal, numeric or visual data.

TAX 3 - Problem Solving: Ability to utilize recalled knowledge and the interpretation/application of distinct criteria to resolve a problem or situation and/or make an appropriate decision.

ITEM DESCRIPTOR LIST
MEDICAL TECHNOLOGY EXAMINATION - FEBRUARY 1985

1. CHEM/CCLD/BMD/EL/2
2. CHEM/IBP/ENZYM REX/1
3. CHEM/ALF/SPEC TST/ESTRIOL/1
4. CHEM/IBP/INSTRUMENT/CENTRIFUGAL ANALY/1
5. CHEM/DFC/BTP/ALBUMIN/1
6. CHEM/SCOA/PROTEIN & ENZYM/QA/3
7. CHEM/CCLD/LIPOPROTEIN/ELECTRO/2
8. CHEM/ISOE/UREA NITROGEN/2
9. CHEM/SELM/BTP/BLOOD GAS/1
10. CHEM/ETR/THYROID FUNCT/3
11. CHEM/CALC/SOLUTE CONC/2
12. CHEM/ELF/PROTEIN ELECTRO/2
13. CHEM/ESOE/SCH/CALCIUM/3
14. CHEM/CALC/QC/STANDARD DEVIATION/2
15. CHEM/IBP/INSTRUMENT/ION-SELECT-ELECT/1
16. CHEM/CCLD/BMD/ISOENZYMES/2
17. CHEM/CALC/% TRANSMISSION/2
18. CHEM/CALC/DILUTION/2
19. CHEM/IBP/CARBOHYDRATES/D-XYLOSE/1
20. CHEM/IBP/AMINO ACID MET/PKU/1
21. CHEM/ANLF/STATISTICS/CARBOHYDRATES-QA/3
22. CHEM/IBP/ANALYTIC METHOD/PHOSPHATE/1
23. CHEM/ISOE/INSTRUMENTATION/PH METER/2
24. CHEM/ALF/BMD/CATECHOLAMINES/1
25. CHEM/IBP/INSTRUMENTATION/NEPHELOMETRY/1
26. CHEM/IBP/INSTRUMENT/PHOTOMETER/1
27. CHEM/CALC/SI UNITS/EL/2
28. CHEM/IBP/INSTRUMENT/EMIT/1
29. CHEM/IBP/INSTRUMENT/FLUOROMETER/1
30. CHEM/ACLD/ACID BASE & EL/HYPOPARATHYROIDISM/2
31. CHEM/CCLD/BILE DUCT OBSTR/ENZYM/2
32. CHEM/ALF/LIPIDS/PHYSIOLOGY/2
33. CHEM/IBP/CHLORIDE SHIFT/1
34. CHEM/ANLF/CARBOHYDRATES/GLU INSUL TOLERANC/2
35. CHEM/DFC/BTP/ACID BASE/1
36. CHEM/CALC/PROTEIN & ENZYM/SERUM DILUTION/2
37. CHEM/CALC/ACID BASE & EL/CV/2
38. CHEM/ISOP/BILIRUBIN/BEER'S LAW/2
39. HEMA/ALF/PBS/ROULEAUX/2
40. HEMA/ALF/FIBRINOLYSIS/SPEC TST/2
41. HEMA/ALF/PHYSIOLOGY/PLATELET/2
42. HEMA/ID/INCLUSION/WBC/1
43. HEMA/ANLF/QC/WBC CT/3
44. HEMA/SCOA/RBC INDICES/3
45. HEMA/ALF/SPEC TST/STAIN/2
46. HEMA/CCLD/COAGULATION/FACTOR DEFICIENCY/3
47. HEMA/CALC/SPEC TST/SERUM VISCOSITY/2
48. HEMA/CALC/CORR WBC CT/2
49. HEMA/CLD/HEMOSTASIS/VON WILLEBRANDS/2
50. HEMA/ALF/CYTOGENETICS/CGL/1
51. HEMA/ELF/COAGULATION/HEPARIN NEUTRALIZA/3
52. HEMA/CCLD/MICRO MORPH/LEUKOCYTE/3
53. HEMA/ELF/LEUKOCYTE/SPEC STAIN/3
54. HEMA/ELF/ERYTHROCYTES/HEMOGLOBIN ELECTRO/3
55. HEMA/EMM/RBC/MACRO ANEMIA/3
56. HEMA/CMM/CLL/3
57. HEMA/AMM/RBC PHYSIOLOGY/2
58. HEMA/ID/RBC INCLUSION/2
59. HEMA/AMM/RBC FRAGILITY/2
60. HEMA/ESOE/AUTOMATED CT/PLATELET/3
61. HEMA/SELM/MACRO ANEMIA/2
62. HEMA/DFC/HEMOGLOBIN F/1
63. HEMA/ESOE/SCH/WBC-DIFF/3
64. HEMA/ESOE/HEMOGLOBIN/2
65. HEMA/ANLF/QC/HEMOGLOBIN/3
66. HEMA/ID/VITAMIN K/COAGULATION/1
67. HEMA/SELM/SCH/WBC CT/3
68. HEMA/DFC/ANTICOAGULANT/1
69. HEMA/ISOE/PLATELET CT/2
70. HEMA/CLD/CBC/ACUTE LEUKEMIA/3
71. HEMA/CALC/QC/HEMOGLOBIN/2
72. HEMA/CCLD/ERYTHROCYTES/ENZYMOPATHIES/2
73. HEMA/CCLD/LAP/3
74. HEMA/CALC/EOSINOPHIL CT/2
75. HEMA/ANLF/LAP SCORE/3
76. HEMA/ISOE/SCH/PBS STAIN/2
77. HEMA/ELF/PTT PROTIME/FACTOR DEFICIENCY/2
78. HEMA/IMM/MATURATION/MYELOCYTIC SERIES/1
79. HEMA/CCLD/MICRO MORPH/BURNS/2
80. BF/DFC/FORMATION/URINE CRYSTALS/1
81. BF/IBP/RCD/AMNIOTIC FLUID/1
82. BF/IBP/RCD/INBORN ERR OF MET/1
83. BF/DFC/TRANSUDATES/1
84. BF/CCLD/URINE/PROTEIN/2
85. BF/ELF/SCH/CSF/2
86. BF/DFC/GROSS APPEAR/CSF/1
87. BF/CCLD/RCD/URINE SEDIMENT/2
88. BF/ALF/URINE/CAST/2
89. BF/ALF/URINE/MICRO MORPH/2
90. BF/ALF/URINE/MICRO MORPH/2
91. BF/IMM/URINE/ARTIFACT/2
92. BF/ELF/URINE/REDUCING SUBSTA/2
93. BF/CCLD/PROTEINURIA/2
94. BF/IBP/BASIC TST/URINE PROTEIN/1
95. BF/CCLD/URINE/MYOGLOBIN/2
96. BF/ESOE/SCH/24 HOUR URINE/3
97. BF/ALF/URINE/MET DIS/1
98. BF/DFC/URINE/CAST/1
99. BF/ALF/SPE APPEAR/URINE SEDIMENT/1
100. BF/CCLD/URINE/REDUCING SUBSTA/3
101. BF/ANLF/URINE/REAGENT STRIP/3
102. MICR/IBC/SELECT MEDIA/1
103. MICR/SELM/GPC/BIOCHEM ID/2
104. MICR/SELM/GNB BIOCHEM TST/URINE CULT/3
105. MICR/ELF/GNB/OF REX/2
106. MICR/ALF/GNB/BIOCHEM ID/2
107. MICR/ANLF/GPC/BASIC TST/2
108. MICR/IBP/GPB/MAC MORPH/1
109. MICR/ELF/MICRO-MAC MORPH/ACTINOMYCETES/2
110. MICR/SELM/VIRAL ISOLATION/1
111. MICR/IMM/NEMATODE/1
112. MICR/CCLD/ANAEROBIC GNB/MAC MORPH/2
113. MICR/ESOE/QC/ANTIBIOTIC SUSC/3
114. MICR/DFC/MYCOPLASMA/1
115. MICR/SELM/SCH/AFB/1
116. MICR/SELM/GNB BIOCHEM TST/SPUTUM/2
117. MICR/SELR/QC/BIOCHEM TST/1
118. MICR/ALF/BIOCHEM TST/AFB/2
119. MICR/IBP/INFECT DIS SERO/VIRAL/1
120. MICR/ANLF/GNB-BASIC TST/STOOL CULT/3
121. MICR/ANLF/GPC/CULT CHARACTERISTI/2
122. MICR/DFC/FUNGI-BASIC TST/KOH/1
123. MICR/IMM/MOLD/2
124. MICR/IMM/DIPHASIC FUNGUS/2
125. MICR/DFC/MAC MORPH/MYCOBACTERIA/1
126. MICR/ANLF/GNB-URINE CULT/COLONY CT/3
127. MICR/ANLF/ANEROBIC GNB/MICRO-MAC MORPH/2
128. MICR/ESOE/SCH/AFB/3
129. MICR/SELM/GNC/BASIC TST/1
130. MICR/ELF/GNB BIOCHEM ID/STOOL CULT/2

ITEM DESCRIPTOR LIST
MEDICAL TECHNOLOGY EXAMINATION - FEBRUARY 1985

131. MICR/ESOE/QC/BLOOD CULT/3
132. MICR/ESOE/SCH/AFB/3
133. MICR/ANLF/GPB/BASIC TST/2
134. MICR/ESOE/SCH/SPUTUM CULT FUNGI/3
135. MICR/ESOE/AFB/SMEAR EVALUATION/3
136. MICR/IMM/AMOEBA/2
137. MICR/IMM/MICROFILARIA/2
138. MICR/IMM/PLASMODIUM/2
139. MICR/ANLF/ANTIBIOTIC SUSC/MIC/3
140. MICR/ESOE/ANTIBIOTIC SUSC/DISK DIFFUSION/3
141. MICR/ANLF/ACTINOMYCES/BASIC TST/2
142. MICR/SELM/SERO GROUPING/QUELLUNG REX/2
143. MICR/SCOA/GNB SERO TYPE/STOOL CULT/3
144. MICR/SCOA/QC/BIOCHEM TST/3
145. BBNK/DFC/ABO/GEN/1
146. BBNK/ALF/PROBLEM X-MATCH/RH AB/2
147. BBNK/DFC/DAT/1
148. BBNK/SCOA/RBC/INCOMPAT X-MATCH/3
149. BBNK/SCOA/RBC/RH PHENOTYPE/2
150. BBNK/SCOA/PROBLEM AB/3
151. BBNK/CCLD/DONOR ACCEPT/PLASMAPHORESIS/2
152. BBNK/ELF/AB ID/ALLOAB/2
153. BBNK/CCLD/FETOMATERNAL HEMORRHAGE/3
154. BBNK/ISOE/RH TYPING/HDN/2
155. BBNK/CCLD/ADVERSE TX REX/3
156. BBNK/ISOP/PLATELETS/SPE STORAGE/1
157. BBNK/CALC/CELL SUSPENSION/2
158. BBNK/ISOP/LEUKOCYTE/STORAGE/1
159. BBNK/SELC/HEMOTHERAPY/RBC/2
160. BBNK/SCOA/AB ABSORPTION/2
161. BBNK/DFC/COLD AUTOAGGLUT/1
162. BBNK/CCLD/HEMOTHERAPY/BLOOD COMPO/3
163. BBNK/ELF/PROBLEM X-MATCH/3
164. BBNK/SCOA/ADD TST/ER TX/3
165. BBNK/CCLD/HEMOTHERAPY/COMPO SELECTION/3
166. BBNK/ISOP/HEMOTHERAPY/LEUKOCYTES/1
167. BBNK/ALF/GEN THER & PRIN/RH AB/2
168. BBNK/IBP/SCH/LEUKOCYTE/1
169. BBNK/ELF/PROBLEM X-MATCH/2
170. BBNK/SCOA/BLOOD COMPO/EXCHANGE TX/3
171. BBNK/CCLD/HEMOTHERAPY/BLOOD COMPO/3
172. BBNK/ALF/HEMOTHERAPY/ADVERSE TX REX/2
173. BBNK/ELF/GENOTYPE/PATERNITY TESTING/2
174. BBNK/SCOA/BLOOD COMPO/MULTIPLE AB/2
175. BBNK/ELF/RH GENOTYPE/2
176. BBNK/IBP/BASIC TST/RH IMMUNOGLOBULIN/1
177. BBNK/ALF/RBC/AIHA/1
178. BBNK/ELF/X-MATCH/ER SITUATION/3
179. BBNK/ELF/AB ID/HDN/3
180. BBNK/ISOP/HEMOTHERAPY/ADVERSE REX/1
181. BBNK/ELF/ELUATE/HDN/3
182. BBNK/CCLD/HEMOTHERAPY/BLOOD COMPO/3
183. IMMU/DFC/ALLERGY/AB PRODUCTION/1
184. IMMU/ISOE/BASIC TST/ANA/2
185. IMMU/ESOE/CELLU IMMUNITY/T LYMPH/3
186. IMMU/ESOE/SCH/COLD AGGLUT/3
187. IMMU/ANLF/IMMUNODIFFUSION/2
188. IMMU/ELF/AUTOIMMUNITY/DNA/2
189. IMMU/ETR/QC/ANTISTREPTOLYSIN O/2
190. IMMU/ELF/FEBRILE AGGLUT/2
191. IMMU/ETR/BASIC TST/STS/2
192. IMMU/ESOE/COMPLEMENT FIX/3
193. IMMU/DFC/AUTOAB/RA/1
194. IMMU/CALC/SERIAL DILUTION/2
195. IMMU/IBP/RA TST/1
196. IMMU/IBP/IMMUNITY/1
197. IMMU/ALF/AUTOIMMUNITY/ANA/1
198. IMMU/CCLD/RUBELLA/2
199. IMMU/DFC/AB/1
200. IMMU/ISOP/CELLU IMMUNITY/LYMPH SUBPOP/1
201. IMMU/CCLD/STS/3
202. IMMU/ESOE/ALLERGY/RAST/2
203. IMMU/SELM/HBS-AG/1

GLOSSARY OF TERMS USED IN ITEM DESCRIPTORS
MEDICAL TECHNOLOGIST EXAMINATION - AUGUST 1985

&	AND
ACLD	ASSOCIATE CLINICAL AND LABORATORY DATA
ALF	ASSOCIATE LABORATORY FINDINGS
ANLF	ANALYZE LABORATORY FINDINGS
AMM	ASSOCIATE MICROSCOPIC MORPHOLOGY
BBNK	BLOOD BANK
BF	BODY FLUIDS
CALC	CALCULATE
CBC	COMPLETE BLOOD COUNT
CCLD	CORRELATE CLINICAL AND LABORATORY DATA
CHEM	CHEMISTRY
CLD	CORRELATE LABORATORY DATA
CLL	CHRONIC LYMPHOCYTIC LEUKEMIA
DFC	DEFINE FUNDAMENTAL CHARACTERISTIC(S)
ELF	EVALUATE LABORATORY FINDINGS
EMIT	ENZYME-MULTIPLIED IMMUNOASSAY
EMM	EVALUATE MICROSCOPIC MORPHOLOGY
ESOE	EVALUATE SOURCE OF ERROR
GLC	GAS-LIQUID CHROMATOGRAPHY
GNB	GRAM-NEGATIVE BACILLI
GNC	GRAM-NEGATIVE COCCI
GPB	GRAM-POSITIVE BACILLI
GPC	GRAM-POSITIVE COCCI
HDN	HEMOLYTIC DISEASE OF THE NEWBORN
HEMA	HEMATOLOGY
HPLC	HIGH PRESSURE LIQUID CHROMATOGRAPHY
IBP	IDENTIFY BASIC PRINCIPLE(S)
ID	IDENTIFY/IDENTIFICATION
IMM	IDENTIFY MICROSCOPIC MORPHOLOGY
IMMU	IMMUNOLOGY
ISOE	IDENTIFY SOURCE OF ERROR
ISOP	IDENTIFY STANDARD OPERATING PROCEDURE
MIC-MAC	MICROSCOPIC-MACROSCOPIC
MICR	MICROBIOLOGY
PBS	PERIPHERAL BLOOD SMEAR
RBC	RED BLOOD CELL
SCH	SPECIMEN COLLECTION AND HANDLING
SCOA	SELECT COURSE OF ACTION
SDU	SELECT DONOR UNIT
SELM	SELECT METHOD
UV	ULTRAVIOLET
WBC	WHITE BLOOD CELL
X-MATCH	CROSSMATCH

TAXONIMIC LEVELS

TAX 1 - <u>Recall</u>:	Ability to recall or recognize previously learned (memorized) knowledge ranging from specific facts to complete theories.
TAX 2 - <u>Interpretive skills</u>:	Ability to utilize recalled knowledge to interpret or apply verbal, numeric or visual data.
TAX 3 - <u>Problem Solving</u>:	Ability to utilize recalled knowledge and the interpretation/application of distinct criteria to resolve a problem or situation and/or make an appropriate decision.

ITEM DESCRIPTOR LIST
MEDICAL TECHNOLOGIST EXAMINATION - AUGUST, 1985

1. IMMU/DFC/PHYSIOLOGY/C-REACTIVE PROTEIN/1
2. IMMU/ISOE/BASIC TESTS/ANTINUCLEAR ANTIBODY/2
3. IMMU/ESOE/COMPLEMENT FIXATION/3
4. IMMU/DFC/CELLULAR IMMUNITY/1
5. IMMU/DFC/AUTOANTIBODY/RHEUMATOID ARTHRITIS/1
6. IMMU/CALC/SERIAL DILUTION/2
7. IMMU/ESOE/QUALITY CONTROL/ANTISTREPTOLYSIN O/3
8. IMMU/DFC/ACTIVE/IMMUNITY/1
9. IMMU/CLD/HETEROPHILE/2
10. IMMU/ELF/PREGNANCY TEST/2
11. IMMU/ALF/AUTOIMMUNITY/ANTINUCLEAR ANTIBODY/1
12. IMMU/ANLF/IMMUNODIFFUSION/2
13. IMMU/IBP/PHYSIOLOGY/IMMUNE RESPONSE/3
14. IMMU/DFC/ANTIBODY/1
15. IMMU/ESOE/SCH/COLD AGGLUTININ/3
16. IMMU/DFC/COMPLEMENT/1
17. IMMU/CALC/DILUTION/2
18. IMMU/IBP/BASIC TESTS/RHEUMATOID ARTHRITIS/1
19. IMMU/DFC/BASIC TESTS/ANTISTREPTOLYSIN O/1
20. IMMU/DFC/PHYSIOLOGY/IMMUNOGLOBULIN/1
21. CHEM/DFC/CRYOGLOBULIN/1
22. CHEM/IBP/BASIC TEST/CREATININE/1
23. CHEM/DFC/CARBOHYDRATE/TOLERANCE TESTS/1
24. CHEM/ISOE/ELECTROLYTES/1
25. CHEM/IBP/INSTRUMENTATION/FLUOROMETER/1
26. CHEM/ANLF/SPECTRAL CURVE/3
27. CHEM/CALC/BLOOD GASES/HENDERSON-HASSELBALCH/2
28. CHEM/IBP/SPECIAL TESTS/CREATININE CLEARANCE/1
29. CHEM/CALC/METRIC UNITS/2
30. CHEM/ELF/PROTEIN & ENZYME/IMMUNOELECTROPHORESIS/2
31. CHEM/ANLF/CARBOHYDRATE/TOLERANCE TESTS/2
32. CHEM/ESOE/SCH/CARBOHYDRATES/3
33. CHEM/CALC/ANION GAP/2
34. CHEM/IBP/SECRETION/HORMONE/1
35. CHEM/IBP/INSTRUMENTATION/EMIT/1
36. CHEM/IBP/BIOCHEMICAL THEORY/TRACE ELEMENTS/1
37. CHEM/ESOE/INSTRUMENTATION/SPECTROPHOTOMETER/3
38. CHEM/ESOE/SCH/CALCIUM/3
39. CHEM/CALC/SPECIAL CHEM/RADIOACTIVE DECAY/2
40. CHEM/IBP/INSTRUMENTATION/GLC/1
41. CHEM/ISOE/INSTRUMENTATION/HPLC/2
42. CHEM/ELF/THYROID FUNCTION/2
43. CHEM/IBP/ANALYTIC METHOD/SERUM IRON/1
44. CHEM/CALC/CREATININE CLEARANCE/2
45. CHEM/CCLD/DISEASE MANIFESTATION/ISOENZYMES/2
46. CHEM/ELF/PROTEIN & ENZYME/ISOENZYME RESULTS/2
47. CHEM/IBP/CHLORIDE SHIFT/1
48. CHEM/CCLD/PROTEIN & ENZYME/PROTEIN ELECTROPHORESIS/3
49. CHEM/ESOE/PROTEIN & ENZYME/AMYLASE/3
50. CHEM/IBP/PHYSIOLOGY/PROTEIN/1
51. CHEM/IBP/BIOCHEMICAL THEORY/BILIRUBIN/1
52. CHEM/IBP/COFACTOR/ENZYMES/1
53. CHEM/ESOE/INSTRUMENTATION/UV SPECTROPHOMETRY/2
54. CHEM/DFC/CREATINE KINASE/ISOENZYMES/1
55. CHEM/ALF/BIOCHEMICAL THEORY/LIPID/2
56. CHEM/CALC/LABORATORY OPERATIONS/STATISTICS/2
57. CHEM/CALC/SPECIAL CHEM/THYROID FUNCTION/2
58. CHEM/ISOE/SCH/BLOOD GASES/2
59. HEMA/ISOE/PLATELET COUNT/2
60. HEMA/ALF/PHYSIOLOGY/PLATELET/2
61. HEMA/ISOE/WBC COUNT/PHYSIOLOGY/2
62. HEMA/CALC/LEUKOCYTE ALKALINE PHOSPHATASE/2
63. HEMA/CALC/QUALITY CONTROL/HEMOGLOBIN/2
64. HEMA/IMM/MATURATION/MYELOCYTIC SERIES/1
65. HEMA/ALF/FIBRINOLYSIS/CLOT LYSIS/2
66. HEMA/CLD/CBC/ACUTE LEUKEMIA/3
67. HEMA/ANLF/QUALITY CONTROL/WBC COUNT/3
68. HEMA/ESOE/HEMOGLOBIN/2
69. HEMA/ELF/THROMBIN TIME/SUBSTITUTION STUDY/3
70. HEMA/CCLD/COAGULATION/FACTOR DEFICIENCY/3
71. HEMA/SCOA/SCH/HEMOSTASIS/2
72. HEMA/DFC/ANTICOAGULANT/1
73. HEMA/CCLD/MICROSCOPIC MORPHOLOGY/LEUKOCYTE/3
74. HEMA/ELF/HEMOGLOBIN ELECTROPHORESIS/3
75. HEMA/CCLD/PBS/PLATELET COUNT/3
76. HEMA/ELF/ERYTHROCYTE/OSMOTIC FRAGILITY/3
77. HEMA/CCLD/MICROSCOPIC MORPHOLOGY/CLL/3
78. HEMA/EMM/RBC/MACROCYTIC ANEMIA/3
79. HEMA/AMM/RBC PHYSIOLOGY/2
80. HEMA/ELF/PBS/PLATELET MORPHOLOGY/2
81. HEMA/IBP/AUTOMATED COUNT/1
82. HEMA/CCLD/AUTOIMMUNE HEMOLYTIC ANEMIA/2
83. HEMA/CCLD/CBC/APLASTIC ANEMIA/2
84. HEMA/CCLD/LEUKOCYTE ALKALINE PHOSPHATASE/3
85. HEMA/CALC/ABSOLUTE COUNT/WBC/2
86. HEMA/CCLD/ANEMIA/SPHEROCYTES/2
87. HEMA/ELF/SPECIAL TESTS/MIXING STUDY/2
88. HEMA/ALF/SPECIAL TESTS/LEUKOCYTE STAIN/2
89. HEMA/ID/INCLUSION/WBC/1
90. HEMA/DFC/HEMOGLOBIN F/1
91. HEMA/CCLD/MICROSCOPIC MORPHOLOGY/SMUDGE CELLS/1
92. HEMA/ELF/SPECIAL TESTS/HEMOGLOBIN F/2
93. HEMA/CALC/CORRECTED WBC COUNT/2
94. HEMA/ANLF/RBC INDICES/MORPHOLOGY/2
95. HEMA/ISOE/SCH/PBS STAIN/2
96. HEMA/CCLD/SPECIAL TESTS/IRON DEFICIENCY ANEMIA/
97. BF/ISOE/URINE/SPECIFIC GRAVITY/1
98. BF/DFC/FORMATION/URINE CRYSTALS/1
99. BF/IBP/REAGENT STRIP/PROTEIN/1
100. BF/ESOE/URINE/GLUCOSE/3
101. BF/ID/NORMAL URINE/CRYSTAL/2
102. BF/ALF/URINE SEDIMENT/CHEMICAL TEST/3
103. BF/AMM/URINE/CRYSTAL/2
104. BF/ESOE/SCH/24-HOUR URINE/3
105. BF/DFC/TRANSUDATES/1
106. BF/CCLD/PROTEINURIA/2
107. BF/DFC/CREATININE CLEARANCE/1
108. BF/CCLD/RELATED DISORDERS/URINE SEDIMENT/2
109. BF/ESOE/SCH/URINALYSIS/2
110. BF/SELM/SCH/CEREBROSPINAL FLUID/1
111. BF/ELF/URINE GLUCOSE/PHYSIOLOGY/2
112. BF/DFC/RED CELL CASTS/1
113. BF/SELM/MALABSORBTION/1
114. MICR/SELM/GNC/BASIC TEST/1
115. MICR/ALF/BIOCHEMICAL TEST/MYCOBACTERIA/2
116. MICR/SELM/BIOCHEMICAL ID/STREPTOCOCCUS/2
117. MICR/ELF/GNB/OXIDATION-FERMENTATION REACTION/2
118. MICR/ESOE/SUSCEPTIBILITY/DISK DIFFUSION/3
119. MICR/ELF/GNB/BIOCHEMICAL REACTION/3
120. MICR/ELF/GNB/X&V FACTOR/2
121. MICR/DFC/MYCOPLASMA/1
122. MICR/CCLD/WOUND CULTURE/ANAEROBES/2
123. MICR/ELF/GNB/CEREBROSPINAL FLUID CULTURE/3
124. MICR/ELF/GNB/BIOCHEMICAL REACTION/3
125. MICR/IMM/NEMATODE/1
126. MICR/ISOE/MYCOBACTERIA/SPECIMEN PROCESSING/3
127. MICR/ELF/BASIC TESTS/STREPTOCOCCUS/2
128. MICR/ESOE/QUALITY CONTROL/GRAM STAIN/3
129. MICR/ELF/GPC/EAR CULTURE/2
130. MICR/IMM/DIPHASIC FUNGUS/2

ITEM DESCRIPTOR LIST
MEDICAL TECHNOLOGIST EXAMINATION - AUGUST, 1985

131. MICR/IMM/MOLD/2
132. MICR/IMM/DIPHASIC FUNGUS/2
133. MICR/IMM/YEAST/2
134. MICR/ELF/GNB/MIC-MAC MORPHOLOGY/1
135. MICR/ESOE/MYCOBACTERIA/PHOTOCHROMOGEN/3
136. MICR/CCLD/ANAEROBIC GNB/MACROSCOPIC MORPHOLOGY/2
137. MICR/ELF/SCH/SPUTUM/3
138. MICR/ESOE/QUALITY CONTROL/SUSCEPTIBILITY/3
139. MICR/ANLF/GPC/URINE CULTURE/3
140. MICR/CLD/HEPATITIS/3
141. MICR/IMM/MICROFILARIA/2
142. MICR/IMM/PLASMODIUM/2
143. MICR/SELM/ID/RICKETTSIA/1
144. MICR/CCLD/MIC-MAC MORPHOLOGY/LISTERIA/2
145. MICR/CCLD/GNB/SELECTIVE MEDIA/2
146. MICR/CCLD/COLITIS/3
147. MICR/ELF/GNB/BIOCHEMICAL REACTION/2
148. MICR/SELM/BASIC TESTS/STREPTOCOCCUS/2
149. MICR/ELF/MYCOBACTERIA/SPECIMEN PROCESSING/2
150. MICR/SELM/BIOCHEMICAL ID/STAPHYLOCOCCUS/2
151. MICR/CCLD/WOUND CULTURE/ACTINOMYCETES/2
152. MICR/SELM/VIRAL ISOLATION/1
153. MICR/ESOE/WOUND CULTURE/ANAEROBES/2
154. BBNK/ISOP/SCH/PLATELETS/1
155. BBNK/ALF/INCOMPATIBLE X-MATCH/RH ANTIBODY/2
156. BBNK/ISOP/GRANULOCYTE/STORAGE/1
157. BBNK/ELF/COMPONENT SELECTION/FACTOR DEFICIENCY/3
158. BBNK/SCOA/PROBLEM ANTIBODY/3
159. BBNK/SCOA/COMPONENT/EXCHANGE TRANSFUSION/3
160. BBNK/ELF/RBC/ABO DISCREPANCY/3
161. BBNK/ELF/HEMOTHERAPY/ADVERSE REACTION/3
162. BBNK/ALF/HEMOTHERAPY/ADVERSE REACTION/2
163. BBNK/ISOP/HEMOTHERAPY/ADVERSE REACTION/1
164. BBNK/ELF/ANTIBODY PANEL/3
165. BBNK/CCLD/HEMOTHERAPY/BLOOD COMPONENT/3
166. BBNK/CALC/CELL SUSPENSION/2
167. BBNK/ELF/ELUATE/HDN/3
168. BBNK/CCLD/HEMOTHERAPY/COMPONENT SELECTION/3
169. BBNK/DFC/HEMOTHERAPY/ADVERSE REACTION/1
170. BBNK/ELF/INCOMPATIBLE X-MATCH/2
171. BBNK/CCLD/DONOR ACCEPTIBILITY/PLASMAPHERESIS/2
172. BBNK/CCLD/ADVERSE REACTION/3
173. BBNK/ALF/ABO/GENOTYPES/2
174. BBNK/SCOA/BLOOD COMPONENT/MULTIPLE ANTIBODIES/2
175. BBNK/IBP/SCH/GRANULOCYTE/1
176. BBNK/ELF/INCOMPATIBLE X-MATCH/2
177. BBNK/ELF/ANTIBODY ID/HDN/2
178. BBNK/ELF/INCOMPATIBLE X-MATCH/3
179. BBNK/IBP/RBC/ANTIBODY ID/1
180. BBNK/SDU/EXCHANGE TRANSFUSION/1
181. BBNK/SCOA/SCH/ANTIBODY ID/2
182. BBNK/ELF/GENOTYPE/PATERNITY TESTING/3
183. BBNK/SCOA/IMMUNOLOGIC PRINCIPLES/RH/3
184. BBNK/IBP/COMPONENT PREPARATION/PLATELETS/1
185. BBNK/ISOE/RH/HDN/2
186. BBNK/ALF/ANTIBODY/HEMOLYTIC ANEMIA/2
187. BBNK/CCLD/BLOOD SELECTION/2
188. BBNK/ELF/ABO DISCREPANCY/3
189. BBNK/ACLD/DONOR ACCEPTIBILITY/1
190. BBNK/ISOP/RBC/REAGENT QUALITY CONTROL/1
191. BBNK/ELF/IMMUNOLOGIC PRINCIPLES/RBC/2
192. BBNK/ISOE/STORAGE/BLOOD/2
193. BBNK/IBP/SCH/ANTICOAGULANT/1

GLOSSARY OF TERMS USED IN ITEM DESCRIPTORS
MEDICAL TECHNOLOGIST EXAMINATION - FEBRUARY 1986

AB	ANTIBODY
ACLD	ASSOCIATE CLINICAL AND LABORATORY DATA
AHA	AUTOIMMUNE HEMOLYTIC ANEMIA
AHG	ANTIHUMAN GLOBULIN
ALF	ASSOCIATE LABORATORY FINDINGS
AMM	ASSOCIATE MICROSCOPIC MORPHOLOGY
ANA	ANTINUCLEAR ANTIBODY
ANLF	ANALYZE LABORATORY FINDINGS
BBNK	BLOOD BANK
BF	BODY FLUIDS
BMD	BIOCHEMICAL MANIFESTATIONS OF DISEASE
BTP	BIOCHEMICAL THEORY AND PHYSIOLOGY
CALC	CALCULATE
CBC	COMPLETE BLOOD COUNT
CLD	CORRELATE LABORATORY DATA
CCLD	CORRELATE CLINICAL AND LABORATORY DATA
CHEM	CHEMISTRY
CHO	CARBOHYDRATE
CSF	CEREBROSPINAL FLUID
DFC	DEFINE FUNDAMENTAL CHARACTERISTIC(S)
DNA	DEOXYRIBONUCLEIC ACID
ELF	EVALUATE LABORATORY FINDINGS
ESOE	EVALUATE SOURCE OF ERROR
FDP	FIBRIN DEGRADATION PRODUCTS
GNB	GRAM-NEGATIVE BACILLI
GNC	GRAM-NEGATIVE COCCI
GPB	GRAM-POSITIVE BACILLI
GPC	GRAM-POSITIVE COCCI
HDN	HEMOLYTIC DISEASE OF THE NEWBORN
HEMA	HEMATOLOGY
IBP	IDENTIFY BASIC PRINCIPLE(S)
ID	IDENTIFY/IDENTIFICATION
IGC	IDENTIFY GROWTH CHARACTERISTICS
IMM	IDENTIFY MICROSCOPIC MORPHOLOGY
IMMU	IMMUNOLOGY/IMMUNITY
ISOE	IDENTIFY SOURCE OF ERROR
ISOP	IDENTIFY STANDARD OPERATING PROCEDURE
LAP	LEUKOCYTE ALKALINE PHOSPHATASE
LO	LABORATORY OPERATIONS
LYMPH	LYMPHOCYTE
MACRO	MACROCYTIC
MIC	MINIMUM INHIBITORY CONCENTRATION
MICR	MICROBIOLOGY
MICRO	MICROSCOPIC
MORPH	MORPHOLOGY
OF	OXIDATIVE-FERMENTATIVE
P&E	PROTEIN AND ENZYMES
PKU	PHENYLKETONURIA
PREP	PREPARATION
PTT	ACTIVATED PARTIAL THROMBOPLASTIN TIME
QC	QUALITY CONTROL
RBC	RED BLOOD CELL
RCD	RELATED CONDITIONS & DISORDERS
SBP	SELECT BLOOD PRODUCT
SCH	SPECIMEN COLLECTION AND HANDLING
SCOA	SELECT COURSE OF ACTION
SELM	SELECT METHOD
SEME	SELECT MEDIA
SUSC	SUSCEPTIBILITY
TLC	THIN LAYER CHROMATOGRAPHY
WBC	WHITE BLOOD CELL

TAXONOMIC LEVEL

TAX 1 - Recall: Ability to recall or recognize previously learned (memorized) knowledge ranging from specific facts to complete theories.

TAX 2 - Interpretive Skills: Ability to utilize recalled knowledge to interpret or apply verbal, numeric or visual data.

TAX 3 - Problem Solving: Ability to utilize recalled knowledge and the interpretation/application of distinct criteria to resolve a problem or situation and/or make an appropriate decision.

ITEM DESCRIPTOR LIST
MEDICAL TECHNOLOGIST EXAMINATION - FEBRUARY 1986

1. BBNK/IBP/DIRECT AHG/1
2. BBNK/IBP/COMPONENT PREP/PLATELETS/1
3. BBNK/ALF/INDIRECT AHG/AHA/1
4. BBNK/ELF/AB PANEL/3
5. BBNK/CCLD/DONOR ACCEPTABILITY/PLASMAPHERESIS/2
6. BBNK/CCLD/HEMOTHERAPY/BLOOD COMPONENT/3
7. BBNK/DFC/TRANSFUSION REACTION/HEMOLYTIC/1
8. BBNK/DFC/LECTIN/1
9. BBNK/SBP/TRANSFUSION/EXCHANGE/3
10. BBNK/ELF/AB ID/HDN/3
11. BBNK/IBP/SCH/GRANULOCYTE/1
12. BBNK/DFC/ABO/ANTIGENS/1
13. BBNK/ELF/ABO SUBGROUP/3
14. BBNK/IBP/HEMOTHERAPY/GRANULOCYTE/1
15. BBNK/SBP/FACTOR DEFICIENCY/3
16. BBNK/ISOP/HEMOTHERAPY/ADVERSE REACTION/1
17. BBNK/IBP/ENZYME TREATMENT/AB/1
18. BBNK/CALC/RBC SUSPENSION/2
19. BBNK/ISOE/RH TYPING/2
20. BBNK/ALF/AB DETECTION/COMPONENT THERAPY/1
21. BBNK/ELF/INCOMPATIBLE CROSSMATCH/3
22. BBNK/ELF/ABO GROUPING/SALIVA/3
23. BBNK/ALF/POST DONATION/HEMOGLOBIN/1
24. BBNK/ELF/INCOMPATIBLE CROSSMATCH/2
25. BBNK/SELM/RH TYPING/1
26. BBNK/DFC/GENETICS/RH ANTIGEN/1
27. BBNK/SCOA/PROBLEM AB/3
28. BBNK/ALF/HDN/RH/2
29. BBNK/SCOA/SCH/AB ID/2
30. BBNK/CCLD/ADVERSE REACTION/3
31. BBNK/IBP/COMPONENT PREP/PLATELETS/1
32. BBNK/SBP/TRANSFUSION/EMERGENCY/2
33. IMMU/ID/ANTIGEN SITES/IMMUNOGLOBULIN/2
34. IMMU/IBP/PROZONE/1
35. IMMU/ELF/PREGNANCY TEST/2
36. IMMU/DFC/COMPLEMENT/1
37. IMMU/DFC/AB/1
38. IMMU/DFC/QC/STATISTICS/1
39. IMMU/ELF/FLUORESCENT/ANA TEST/2
40. IMMU/ALF/AUTOIMMUNITY/ANA/3
41. IMMU/ELF/IMMUNOELECTROPHORESIS/2
42. IMMU/CALC/SERUM DILUTION/2
43. IMMU/ESOE/QC/ANTISTREPTOLYSIN O/3
44. IMMU/DFC/AUTOANTIBODY/RHEUMATOID ARTHRITIS/1
45. IMMU/DFC/PHYSIOLOGY/IMMUNOGLOBULIN/1
46. IMMU/IBP/RADIAL IMMUNODIFFUSION/1
47. IMMU/ISOP/CELL IMMU/LYMPH SUBPOPULATION/1
48. IMMU/CCLD/AB RESPONSE/HEPATITIS/2
49. IMMU/ELF/AUTOIMMUNITY/DNA/2
50. CHEM/DFC/ELECTROLYTES/CYSTIC FIBROSIS/1
51. CHEM/CALC/CONCENTRATION/MILLIEQUIVALENTS/2
52. CHEM/DFC/BTP/CATECHOLAMINE/1
53. CHEM/SELM/GLUCOSE MONITOR/2
54. CHEM/CCLD/BMD/BLOOD GAS/2
55. CHEM/IBP/INSTRUMENTATION/FLUOROMETER/1
56. CHEM/CALC/ANION GAP/2
57. CHEM/ANLF/CHO/TOLERANCE TEST/2
58. CHEM/ELF/THYROID FUNCTION/2
59. CHEM/CCLD/SPECIAL CHEM/LEAD/2
60. CHEM/ISOE/INSTRUMENTATION/ANALYTICAL BALANCE/2
61. CHEM/ISOE/SCH/LIPIDS/1
62. CHEM/IBP/BTP/BILIRUBIN/1
63. CHEM/IBP/INSTRUMENTATION/CENTRIFUGE/1
64. CHEM/ESOE/P&E/BLOOD UREA NITROGEN/3
65. CHEM/CCLD/HEME DERIVATIVE/3
66. CHEM/IBP/ATOMIC ABSORPTION/1
67. CHEM/IBP/AMINO ACID METABOLISM/PKU/1
68. CHEM/SCOA/REDUCING SUBSTANCES/FECES/2
69. CHEM/IBP/P&E/ELECTROPHORESIS/1
70. CHEM/ELF/QC/LEVEY-JENNINGS/3
71. CHEM/CCLD/BMD/ISOENZYMES/2
72. CHEM/CALC/SPECIAL CHEM/TLC/2
73. CHEM/IBP/ENZYME REACTION/1
74. CHEM/ESOE/SPECTRAL CURVE/3
75. CHEM/IBP/BASIC TESTS/UREA/1
76. CHEM/IBP/ANALYTIC METHOD/PHOSPHATE/1
77. CHEM/ANLF/P&E/ELECTROPHORESIS/3
78. CHEM/CALC/BLOOD GAS/HENDERSON-HASSELBALCH/2
79. CHEM/ALF/P&E/ENZYME KINETICS/2
80. CHEM/CCLD/BTP/RBC ENZYMES/3
81. CHEM/CALC/PERCENT/SOLUTION/2
82. CHEM/DFC/BMD/ACIDOSIS/1
83. CHEM/DFC/QC/SAMPLE/1
84. CHEM/ESOE/INSTRUMENTATION/SPECTROPHOTOMETER/3
85. CHEM/IBP/INSTRUMENTATION/CHLORODOMETER/1
86. CHEM/ACLD/ELECTROLYTES/HYPOPARATHYROIDISM/2
87. HEMA/IBP/PHYSIOLOGY/HEMATOPOIESIS/1
88. HEMA/IBP/AUTOMATED COUNT/1
89. HEMA/CCLD/DIRECT ANTIGLOBULIN TEST/2
90. HEMA/ALF/FACTOR DEFICIENCY/2
91. HEMA/ELF/LAP SCORE/3
92. HEMA/CALC/RBC INDICES/2
93. HEMA/CALC/SPECIAL TEST/SERUM VISCOSITY/2
94. HEMA/CALC/WBC/MANUAL COUNT/2
95. HEMA/IBP/SEDIMENTATION RATE/1
96. HEMA/ID/INCLUSION/WBC/1
97. HEMA/ELF/LEUKOCYTES/CYTOCHEMICAL STAIN/2
98. HEMA/CLD/ANEMIA/2
99. HEMA/ISOE/COAGULATION/PTT/2
100. HEMA/CLD/CBC/ACUTE LEUKEMIA/3
101. HEMA/DFC/ANTICOAGULANT/1
102. HEMA/ELF/OSMOTIC FRAGILITY/3
103. HEMA/CCLD/MICRO MORPH/LEUKOCYTE/3
104. HEMA/ELF/LEUKOCYTE/SPECIAL STAIN/3
105. HEMA/ELF/PLATELET MORPH/2
106. HEMA/ELF/MICRO MORPH/RBC INCLUSION/2
107. HEMA/AMM/RBC PHYSIOLOGY/2
108. HEMA/IMM/WBC MORPH/ANOMALY/2
109. HEMA/ANLF/QC/WBC COUNT/3
110. HEMA/CALC/CORRECTED COUNT/WBC/2
111. HEMA/ESOE/AUTOMATED COUNT/HEMOGLOBIN/3
112. HEMA/CCLD/VON WILLEBRANDS/2
113. HEMA/CCLD/LAP/3
114. HEMA/IBP/HEMOSTASIS/FDP/1
115. HEMA/DFC/MATURATION/BLOOD CELLS/1
116. HEMA/ELF/HEMOSTASIS/SUBSTITUTION STUDIES/3
117. HEMA/CCLD/MICRO MORPH/RBC/3
118. HEMA/ALF/PHYSIOLOGY/PLATELET/2
119. HEMA/CALC/ABSOLUTE COUNT/2
120. HEMA/ESOE/HEMOGLOBIN/2
121. HEMA/IBP/HEMOSTASIS/1
122. HEMA/ALF/FACTOR DEFICIENCY/2
123. HEMA/DFC/PLATELET PHYSIOLOGY/1
124. HEMA/CCLD/PLATELET PHYSIOLOGY/ASPIRIN/2
125. BF/IBP/BASIC TESTS/URINE KETONES/1
126. BF/ELF/URINE/SPECIFIC GRAVITY/3
127. BF/IBP/BASIC TESTS/URINE SEDIMENT/1
128. BF/ALF/CSF/BLOOD/1
129. BF/IBP/MICROSCOPY/1
130. BF/ESOE/URINALYSIS/MICROSCOPIC/3

ITEM DESCRIPTOR LIST
MEDICAL TECHNOLOGIST EXAMINATION - FEBRUARY 1986

131. BF/IBP/RCD/AMNIOTIC FLUID/1
132. BF/ID/NORMAL URINE/CRYSTAL/2
133. BF/ALF/URINE SEDIMENT/CHEMICAL TEST/3
134. BF/AMM/URINE SEDIMENT/CRYSTAL/2
135. BF/ALF/URINE/1
136. BF/ALF/URINE SEDIMENT/CELLS/2
137. BF/ALF/URINE SEDIMENT/CRYSTALS/2
138. BF/ELF/URINE/REDUCING SUBSTANCE/2
139. BF/ELF/UROBILINOGEN/3
140. BF/ESOE/SCH/24 HOUR URINE/3
141. BF/IBP/SCH/CSF/1
142. MICR/CLD/GNB/WOUND CULTURE/2
143. MICR/SELM/GPB/CSF/2
144. MICR/SELM/EPIDEMIOLOGY/GPC/1
145. MICR/IBP/ACID-FAST STAIN/1
146. MICR/ELF/GNB/BIOCHEMICAL ID/2
147. MICR/DFC/SUSC TEST/BROTH DILUTION/1
148. MICR/ELF/GNB/BIOCHEMICAL REACTION/2
149. MICR/SELM/GNC/BASIC TEST/1
150. MICR/ESOE/SCH/MYCOBACTERIA/3
151. MICR/CCLD/ANAEROBIC GNB/MACRO MORPH/2
152. MICR/ESOE/SCH/MYCOBACTERIA/3
153. MICR/IMM/MOLD/2
154. MICR/IMM/DIPHASIC FUNGUS/2
155. MICR/IMM/YEAST/2
156. MICR/ELF/SEROLOGY/ENTERIC PATHOGEN/3
157. MICR/ESOE/CAMPYLOBACTER/BLOOD CULTURE/3
158. MICR/ELF/GNB/OF REACTION/2
159. MICR/CCLD/GPB/ACTINOMYCETES/2
160. MICR/ELF/GNB/CSF CULTURE/3
161. MICR/IBP/VIRAL SEROLOGY/1
162. MICR/IMM/MICROFILARIA/2
163. MICR/IMM/PLASMODIUM/2
164. MICR/IMM/AMOEBA/2
165. MICR/IGC/GNB/ACINETOBACTER/1
166. MICR/SELM/HEMOPHILUS/SUSC/3
167. MICR/CLD/AMOEBA/3
168. MICR/ANLF/ACTINOMYCES/BASIC TEST/2
169. MICR/SCOA/FILAMENTOUS MOLD/ID TECHNIQUE/3
170. MICR/SELM/VIRAL ISOLATION/1
171. MICR/SEME/GARDNERELLA/1
172. MICR/SELM/ID/CORYNEBACTERIUM/2
173. MICR/ALF/MIC/STREPTOCOCCI/1
174. MICR/SCOA/QC/MEDIA/3
175. MICR/CCLD/GNB/SELECTIVE MEDIA/2
176. MICR/SELM/STERILIZATION/1
177. MICR/SELM/ID/RICKETTSIA/1
178. MICR/IBP/BIOCHEMICAL ID/MYCOBACTERIA/1
179. MICR/CCLD/GROWTH CHARACTERISTIC/ANAEROBES/2
180. MICR/CCLD/GNC/ANAEROBES/2

GLOSSARY OF TERMS USED IN ITEM DESCRIPTORS
MEDICAL TECHNOLOGIST EXAMINATION - AUGUST 1986

AB	ANTIBODY
ACLD	ASSOCIATE CLINICAL AND LABORATORY DATA
AFB	ACID-FAST BACILLI
AG	ANTIGEN
ALF	ASSOCIATE LABORATORY FINDINGS
AMM	ASSOCIATE MICROSCOPIC MORPHOLOGY
ANA	ANTINUCLEAR ANTIBODY
ANLF	ANALYZE LABORATORY FINDINGS
BBNK	BLOOD BANK
BF	BODY FLUIDS
BMD	BIOCHEMICAL MANIFESTATIONS OF DISEASE
BTP	BIOCHEMICAL THEORY AND PHYSIOLOGY
CALC	CALCULATE
CBC	COMPLETE BLOOD COUNT
CCLD	CORRELATE CLINICAL AND LABORATORY DATA
CHARACT	CHARACTERISTIC(S)
CHEM	CHEMISTRY
CLD	CORRELATE LABORATORY DATA
CLL	CHRONIC LYMPHOCYTIC LEUKEMIA
CSF	CEREBROSPINAL FLUID
DAT	DIRECT ANTIGLOBULIN TEST
DFC	DEFINE FUNDAMENTAL CHARACTERISTIC(S)
DNA	DEOXYRIBONUCLEIC ACID
ECLD	EVALUATE CLINICAL AND LABORATORY DATA
ELF	EVALUATE LABORATORY FINDINGS
EMM	EVALUATE MICROSCOPIC MORPHOLOGY
ESOE	EVALUATE SOURCE OF ERROR
FTA	FLUORESCENT TREPONEMAL ANTIBODY
GEN THER & PRIN	GENETIC THEORY AND PRINCIPLES
GNB	GRAM-NEGATIVE BACILLI
GNC	GRAM-NEGATIVE COCCI
GPB	GRAM-POSITIVE BACILLI
GPC	GRAM-POSITIVE COCCI
HDN	HEMOLYTIC DISEASE OF THE NEWBORN
HEMA	HEMATOLOGY
HGB	HEMOGLOBIN
HGBPATHY	HEMOGLOBINOPATHY
IBP	IDENTIFY BASIC PRINCIPLE(S)
ID	IDENTIFY/IDENTIFICATION
IGC	IDENTIFY GROWTH CHARACTERISTICS
IMM	IDENTIFY MICROSCOPIC MORPHOLOGY
IMMU	IMMUNOLOGY
ISOE	IDENTIFY SOURCE OF ERROR
ISOP	IDENTIFY STANDARD OPERATING PROCEDURE
LAP	LEUKOCYTE ALKALINE PHOSPHATASE
MACRO	MACROSCOPIC
MIC	MINIMUM INHIBITORY CONCENTRATION
MIC-MAC	MICROSCOPIC-MACROSCOPIC
MICR	MICROBIOLOGY
MICRO	MICROSCOPIC
MORPH	MORPHOLOGY
P&E	PROTEIN AND ENZYMES
PERF	PERFORM
PREP	PREPARATION
PTT	ACTIVATED PARTIAL THROMBOPLASTIN TIME
QC	QUALITY CONTROL
RAST	RADIOALLERGOSORBENT TEST
RBC	RED BLOOD CELL
SBP	SELECT BLOOD PRODUCT
SCH	SPECIMEN COLLECTION AND HANDLING
SCOA	SELECT COURSE OF ACTION
SELM	SELECT METHOD
SELR	SELECT REAGENT
SOE	SOURCE OF ERROR
TRANS	TRANSFUSION
WBC	WHITE BLOOD CELLS
X-MATCH	CROSSMATCH

TAXONOMIC LEVELS

TAX 1 - Recall: Ability to recall or recognize previously learned (memorized) knowledge ranging from specific facts to complete theories.

TAX 2 - Interpretive Skills: Ability to utilize recalled knowledge to interpret or apply verbal, numeric or visual data.

TAX 3 - Problem Solving: Ability to utilize recalled knowledge and the interpretation/application of distinct criteria to resolve a problem or situation and/or make an appropriate decision.

ITEM DESCRIPTOR LIST
MEDICAL TECHNOLOGIST EXAMINATION - AUGUST 1986

1. MICR/ALF/SPECIAL TESTS/STAPHYLOCOCCUS/2
2. MICR/SELM/GNC/BASIC TEST/1
3. MICR/ESOE/GNB/ANAEROBES/2
4. MICR/PERF/QC/MEDIA/1
5. MICR/SELM/BASIC TESTS/AFB/1
6. MICR/ELF/GNB/CSF CULTURE/3
7. MICR/ESOE/QC/SUSCEPTIBILITY/3
8. MICR/ID/GROWTH CHARACT/STREPTOCOCCUS/1
9. MICR/CCLD/GNB/STOOL CULTURE/2
10. MICR/IBP/GPB/MACRO MORPH/1
11. MICR/ANLF/SUSCEPTIBILITY/MIC/3
12. MICR/ELF/GNB/X&V FACTOR/2
13. MICR/ESOE/SCH/CSF CULTURE/3
14. MICR/ISOP/SCH/AFB/1
15. MICR/SELM/VIRAL ISOLATION/1
16. MICR/ESOE/SCH/BLOOD CULTURE/2
17. MICR/ELF/GNB/BIOCHEMICAL ID/3
18. MICR/SELM/MACRO MORPH/FUNGI/1
19. MICR/IMM/ACTINOMYCES/2
20. MICR/ESOE/SCH/FUNGAL MEDIA/3
21. MICR/ELF/MICRO MORPH/GPB/2
22. MICR/CCLD/COLITIS/3
23. MICR/ID/MORPH/TAPEWORM/2
24. MICR/SELM/SCH/NEMATODE/2
25. MICR/ISOE/GRAM STAIN/URINE/2
26. MICR/IGC/GNB/ACINETOBACTER/1
27. MICR/ANLF/MIC-MAC MORPH/ANEROBIC-GNB/2
28. MICR/ALF/PLASMODIUM/1
29. MICR/ECLD/MICRO MORPH/FUNGI/2
30. MICR/CCLD/GNC/ANAEROBES/2
31. MICR/ESOE/AFB/SMEAR EVALUATION/3
32. MICR/ELF/SCH/AFB/2
33. MICR/ALF/ANAEROBES/1
34. MICR/ANLF/GPC/URINE CULTURE/3
35. MICR/ISOE/SCH/BLOOD CULTURE/2
36. MICR/CLD/DIMORPHIC FUNGUS/2
37. MICR/IBP/VIRAL SEROLOGY/1
38. MICR/CCLD/MIC-MAC MORPH/LISTERIA/2
39. MICR/CLD/HEPATITIS/3
40. BBNK/IBP/COMPONENT PREP/PLATELETS/1
41. BBNK/ISOP/HEMOTHERAPY/ADVERSE REACTION/1
42. BBNK/SELR/AB ID/1
43. BBNK/ELF/HEMOTHERAPY/FACTOR DEFICIENCY/3
44. BBNK/ALF/DAT/HDN/1
45. BBNK/ELF/DU TEST/2
46. BBNK/SCOA/AB ID/2
47. BBNK/CCLD/HEMOTHERAPY/ADVERSE REACTION/3
48. BBNK/ELF/AB ID/ALLOANTIBODY/2
49. BBNK/SCOA/BLOOD COMPONENT/EXCHANGE TRANS/3
50. BBNK/IBP/DONOR REQUIREMENT/PLATELETS/1
51. BBNK/CCLD/HEMOTHERAPY/BLOOD COMPONENTS/3
52. BBNK/ELF/AB ID/HDN/2
53. BBNK/ELF/GEN THER & PRIN/RBC/2
54. BBNK/IBP/STORAGE REQUIREMENT/1
55. BBNK/ELF/ABO DISCREPANCY/3
56. BBNK/ELF/X-MATCH/INCOMPATIBLE/2
57. BBNK/IBP/SPECIAL TESTS/ENZYME TREATMENT/1
58. BBNK/IBP/SCH/GRANULOCYTES/1
59. BBNK/CALC/CELL SUSPENSION/2
60. BBNK/ALF/ABO/GENOTYPES/2
61. BBNK/ELF/X-MATCH/INCOMPATIBLE/3
62. BBNK/SBP/HEMOTHERAPY/RBC/1
63. BBNK/SBP/EMERGENCY TRANS/2
64. BBNK/SELR/QC/RBC ANTISERA/2
65. BBNK/ELF/DAT/2
66. BBNK/CCLD/HEMOTHERAPY/BLOOD COMPONENT/3
67. BBNK/CCLD/HEMOTHERAPY/ADVERSE REACTION/3
68. BBNK/DFC/GEN THER & PRIN/BLOOD COMPONENTS/1
69. BBNK/SBP/EMERGENCY TRANS/3
70. BBNK/SBP/HEMOTHERAPY/ADVERSE REACTION/3
71. BBNK/ELF/GENOTYPE/PATERNITY TESTING/3
72. BBNK/SCOA/SCH/AB ID/2
73. BBNK/ELF/ABO DISCREPANCY/3
74. BBNK/ANLF/HEMOTHERAPY/PLATELETS/3
75. BBNK/ISOE/STORAGE/BLOOD/2
76. BBNK/ELF/X-MATCH/INCOMPATIBLE/2
77. BBNK/ELF/RBC/ABO DISCREPANCY/3
78. BBNK/ISOP/RBC/REAGENT QC/1
79. BBNK/DFC/HEMOTHERAPY/ADVERSE REACTION/1
80. IMMU/CLD/COLD AGGLUTININ/2
81. IMMU/ISOE/BASIC TESTS/ANA/2
82. IMMU/CCLD/SYPHILIS TESTING/3
83. IMMU/ALF/BASIC TESTS/C-REACTIVE PROTEIN/2
84. IMMU/DFC/AUTOIMMUNITY/DISEASE STATE/1
85. IMMU/ELF/THYROGLOBULIN/2
86. IMMU/CALC/CELLULAR IMMUNITY/B CELLS/2
87. IMMU/IBP/BASIC TESTS/RHEUMATOID FACTOR/1
88. IMMU/CCLD/RUBELLA/2
89. IMMU/ELF/AUTOIMMUNITY/DNA/2
90. IMMU/ESOE/QC/ANTISTREPTOLYSIN O/3
91. IMMU/ESOE/SCH/COLD AGGLUTININ/3
92. IMMU/IBP/PREGNANCY TESTING/1
93. IMMU/CCLD/SEROLOGIC RESPONSE/HEPATITIS/2
94. IMMU/ELF/SEROLOGIC TESTS/VIRAL HEPATITIS/2
95. IMMU/ALF/AUTOIMMUNITY/THYROIDITIS/1
96. IMMU/IBP/AG-AB INTERACTION/1
97. IMMU/DFC/SPECIAL TESTS/IMMUNOFLUORESCENCE/1
98. IMMU/DFC/CELLULAR IMMUNITY/1
99. IMMU/IBP/FTA/1
100. IMMU/ESOE/COMPLEMENT FIXATION/3
101. CHEM/CCLD/BMD/BLOOD GAS/2
102. CHEM/IBP/P&E/ALANINE AMINOTRANSFERASE/1
103. CHEM/ELF/P&E/IMMUNOELECTROPHORESIS/2
104. CHEM/CLD/BMD/CARDIAC ENZYMES/2
105. CHEM/ANLF/QC/PRECISION/3
106. CHEM/DFC/ELECTROLYTES/IRON/1
107. CHEM/ISOE/SCH/HEMOLYSIS/1
108. CHEM/IBP/INSTRUMENTATION/BEERS LAW/1
109. CHEM/SELM/GLUCOSE/1
110. CHEM/CCLD/P&E/ALKALINE PHOSPHATASE/2
111. CHEM/IBP/ANALYTIC METHOD/UREA/1
112. CHEM/IBP/CARBOHYDRATES/D-XYLOSE/1
113. CHEM/ESOE/ACID-BASE/3
114. CHEM/ECLD/SPECIAL CHEM/ESTRIOL/2
115. CHEM/ELF/THYROID FUNCTION/2
116. CHEM/CCLD/P&E/ELECTROPHORESIS/3
117. CHEM/IBP/INSTRUMENTATION/SPECTROPHOTOMETER/1
118. CHEM/IBP/BUFFER/1
119. CHEM/CLD/SCH/CARBOHYDRATES/2
120. CHEM/ELF/P&E/IMMUNOELECTROPHORESIS/2
121. CHEM/IBP/INSTRUMENTATION/CHROMATOGRAPHY/1
122. CHEM/ELF/P&E/ISOENZYME RESULTS/2
123. CHEM/CALC/MOL WT/2
124. CHEM/IBP/BTP/BILIRUBIN/1
125. CHEM/ISOE/INSTRUMENTATION/ATOMIC ABSORPTION/2
126. CHEM/ISOE/SCH/BLOOD GAS/2
127. CHEM/IBP/PHYSIOLOGY/CREATININE/1
128. CHEM/ESOE/LIPIDS/ELECTROPHORESIS/3
129. CHEM/IBP/SECRETION/HORMONE/1
130. CHEM/ISOE/ELECTROLYTES/1

ITEM DESCRIPTOR LIST
MEDICAL TECHNOLOGIST EXAMINATION - AUGUST 1986

131. CHEM/IBP/ELECTROLYTES/ANION GAP/1
132. CHEM/CCLD/HEME DERIVATIVE/JAUNDICE/3
133. CHEM/ESOE/SCH/CALCIUM/3
134. CHEM/CCLD/TOXICOLOGY/INSECTICIDES/3
135. CHEM/ACLD/PROTEINS/ELECTROPHORESIS/2
136. CHEM/ESOE/INSTRUMENTATION/SPECTROPHOTOMETER/3
137. HEMA/DFC/AB SYNTHESIS/1
138. HEMA/ELF/RBC INDICES/IRON DEFICIENCY/3
139. HEMA/ESOE/RBC/RETICULOCYTE COUNT/3
140. HEMA/IBP/HEMOSTASIS/PLATELET FACTOR/1
141. HEMA/DFC/HGB F/1
142. HEMA/CALC/EOSINOPHIL COUNT/2
143. HEMA/CLD/FACTOR DEFICIENCY/2
144. HEMA/ESOE/SCH/PLATELET COUNT/3
145. HEMA/ELF/HEMOSTASIS/PLATELET/2
146. HEMA/CALC/QC/HGB/2
147. HEMA/ELF/RBC/HEMOLYTIC ANEMIA/2
148. HEMA/CCLD/HEMOSTASIS/2
149. HEMA/ISOE/BASIC TESTS/HGB/1
150. HEMA/CCLD/LAP/3
151. HEMA/ALF/WBC/SPECIAL STAIN/2
152. HEMA/ELF/RBC/HGB ELECTROPHORESIS/3
153. HEMA/CCLD/MICRO MORPH/CLL/3
154. HEMA/CCLD/MICRO MORPH/WBC/3
155. HEMA/CLD/MICRO MORPH/HYPOCHROMIC RBC/3
156. HEMA/IMM/MONOCYTE/2
157. HEMA/EMM/RBC/MACROCYTIC ANEMIA/3
158. HEMA/AMM/RBC PHYSIOLOGY/2
159. HEMA/SELM/HGBPATHY/2
160. HEMA/SELM/RBC INCLU/2
161. HEMA/ELF/MICRO MORPH/WBC INCLUSIONS/2
162. HEMA/ESOE/AUTOMATED COUNT/PLATELET/3
163. HEMA/CALC/WBC/CORRECTED COUNT/2
164. HEMA/CCLD/BASIC TESTS/THROMBIN TIME/2
165. HEMA/CALC/SPECIAL TESTS/SERUM VISCOSITY/2
166. HEMA/DFC/MATURATION/CELLS/1
167. HEMA/DFC/HEMOSTASIS/CLOT RETRACTION/1
168. HEMA/ESOE/HGB/2
169. HEMA/DFC/PHYSIOLOGY/GRANULOCYTE/1
170. HEMA/DFC/ANTICOAGULANT/1
171. HEMA/AMM/WBC/BURNS/1
172. HEMA/ELF/PLATELET COUNT/PERIPHERAL SMEAR/3
173. HEMA/CALC/LAP SCORE/2
174. HEMA/CLD/DRUG EFFECT/BLEEDING TIME/1
175. HEMA/ANLF/THROMBOCYTES/BLEEDING TIME/3
176. HEMA/ELF/PTT MIXING STUDY/2
177. HEMA/CCLD/CBC/APLASTIC ANEMIA/2
178. HEMA/ESOE/SCH/WBC DIFFERENTIAL/3
179. BF/IBP/MICROSCOPE/BINOCULAR/1
180. BF/IBP/BASIC TESTS/FECAL BILIRUBIN/1
181. BF/CCLD/SOE/URINE GLUCOSE/3
182. BF/ELF/SYNOVIAL FLUID/2
183. BF/ELF/URINE/REDUCING SUBSTANCE/2
184. BF/IBP/SCH/CSF/1
185. BF/SELM/URINE/SEDIMENT STAIN/2
186. BF/ALF/URINE/MICRO MORPH/2
187. BF/ELF/MICRO MORPH/REAGENT STRIP/2
188. BF/ID/MICROSCOPE TECHNIQUE/2
189. BF/CCLD/PROTEINURIA/2
190. BF/CALC/GASTRIC PH/2
191. BF/ESOE/SCH/URINALYSIS/2
192. BF/IBP/REAGENT STRIP/PROTEIN/1
193. BF/CCLD/URINE/MYOGLOBIN/2
194. BF/ELF/URINE/REDUCING SUBSTANCE/3
195. BF/ESOE/SCH/24 HOUR URINE/3
196. BF/IBP/QC/ACCURACY & PERCISION/1

GLOSSARY OF TERMS USED IN ITEM DESCRIPTORS
MEDICAL TECHNOLOGIST EXAMINATION - FEBRUARY 1987

AB	ANTIBODY
ABE	ACID-BASE & ELECTROLYTES
ACLF	ASSOCIATE CLINICAL AND LABORATORY FINDINGS
AFB	ACID-FAST BACILLI
AG	ANTIGEN
AIHA	AUTOIMMUNE HEMOLYTIC ANEMIA
ALF	ASSOCIATE LABORATORY FINDINGS
AMM	ASSOCIATE MICROSCOPIC MORPHOLOGY
ANA	ANTINUCLEAR ANTIBODY
ANAT & PHYSIO	ANATOMY AND PHYSIOLOGY
ANLF	ANALYZE LABORATORY FINDINGS
BBNK	BLOOD BANK
BF	BODY FLUID
BMD	BIOCHEMICAL MANIFESTATIONS OF DISEASE
BTP	BIOCHEMICAL THEORY AND PHYSIOLOGY
CALC	CALCULATE
CBC	COMPLETE BLOOD COUNT
CCLD	CORRELATE CLINICAL AND LABORATORY DATA
CGL	CHRONIC GRANULOCYTIC LEUKEMIA
CHEM	CHEMISTRY
CHO	CARBOHYDRATE
CLD	CORRELATE LABORATORY DATA
CLL	CHRONIC LYMPHOCYTIC LEUKEMIA
CMM	CORRELATE MICROSCOPIC MORPHOLOGY
DFC	DEFINE FUNDAMENTAL CHARACTERISTIC(S)
ELF	EVALUATE LABORATORY FINDINGS
ESOE	EVALUATE SOURCE OF ERROR
FDP	FIBRIN DEGRADATION PRODUCTS
GEN THER & PRIN	GENETIC THEORY AND PRINCIPLES
GLC	GAS LIQUID CHROMATOGRAPHY
GNB	GRAM-NEGATIVE BACILLI
GNC	GRAM-NEGATIVE COCCI
GPB	GRAM-POSITIVE BACILLI
GPC	GRAM-POSITIVE COCCI
HDN	HEMOLYTIC DISEASE OF THE NEWBORN
HEMA	HEMATOLOGY
HEMOPATHY	HEMOGLOBINOPATHY
HENDERSON-HASSEL	HENDERSON-HASSELBALCH
HGB	HEMOGLOBIN
IBP	IDENTIFY BASIC PRINCIPLE(S)
ID	IDENTIFY
IEP	IMMUNOELECTROPHORESIS
IMD	IMMUNOLOGIC MANIFESTATION OF DISEASE
IMM	IDENTIFY MICROSCOPIC MORPHOLOGY
IMMM	IDENTIFY MICROSCOPIC MACROSCOPIC MORPHOLOGY
IMMU	IMMUNOLOGY
ISOE	IDENTIFY SOURCE OF ERROR
ISOP	IDENTIFY STANDARD OPERATING PROCEDURE
LAP	LEUKOCYTE ALKALINE PHOSPHATASE
LE	LUPUS ERYTHEMATOSUS
MIC	MINIMUM INHIBITORY CONCENTRATION
MIC-MAC MORPH	MICROSCOPIC-MACROSCOPIC MORPHOLOGY
MICR	MICROBIOLOGY
MICRO	MICROSCOPIC
MICRO MORPH	MICROSCOPIC MORPHOLOGY
P&E	PROTEIN AND ENZYMES
PREP	PREPARATION
PTT	ACTIVATED PARTIAL THROMBOPLASTIN TIME
QA	QUALITY ASSURANCE
QC	QUALITY CONTROL
RBC	RED BLOOD CELL
RCD	RELATED CONDITIONS & DISORDERS
SBP	SELECT BLOOD PRODUCT
SCH	SPECIMEN COLLECTION AND HANDLING
SCOA	SELECT COURSE OF ACTION
SDU	SELECT DONOR UNIT
SELC	SELECT COMPONENT
SELM	SELECT METHOD
SELECT	SELECTION
SI	STANDARD INTERNATIONAL
SOE	SOURCE OF ERROR
TLC	THIN LAYER CHROMATOGRAPHY
TOL	TOLERANCE
WBC	WHITE BLOOD CELL

TAXONOMIC LEVELS

TAX 1 - Recall: Ability to recall or recognize previously learned (memorized) knowledge ranging from specific facts to complete theories.

TAX 2 - Interpretive Skills: Ability to utilize recalled knowledge to interpret or apply verbal, numeric or visual data.

TAX 3 - Problem Solving: Ability to utilize recalled knowledge and the interpretation/application of distinct criteria to resolve a problem or situation and/or make an appropriate decision.

ITEM DESCRIPTOR LIST
MEDICAL TECHNOLOGIST EXAMINATION - FEBRUARY 1987

1. BF/IBP/RCD/AMNIOTIC FLUID/1
2. BF/DFC/RENAL CLEARANCE/CREATININE/1
3. BF/CALC/URINE/SPECIFIC GRAVITY/2
4. BF/IBP/BASIC TESTS/URINE SEDIMENT/1
5. BF/DFC/RED CELL CASTS/1
6. BF/SELM/MALABSORPTION/1
7. BF/CCLD/SOE/URINE GLUCOSE/3
8. BF/ELF/URINE/REDUCING SUBSTANCE/2
9. BF/SBP/SCH/CEREBROSPINAL FLUID/1
10. BF/IBP/BASIC TESTS/URINE KETONES/1
11. BF/ALF/MICRO MORPH/URINE CRYSTALS/2
12. BF/ID/NORMAL URINE/CRYSTAL/2
13. BF/ALF/URINE SEDIMENT/CHEMICAL TEST/3
14. BF/ESOE/SCH/URINALYSIS/2
15. BF/CCLD/URINE/PROTEIN/2
16. BF/ESOE/URINALYSIS/MICRO/3
17. BF/CCLD/URINE/REDUCING SUBSTANCE/3
18. MICR/SELM/BASIC TESTS/STREPTOCOCCUS/2
19. MICR/CCLD/ANAEROBIC GNB/MACRO MORPH/2
20. MICR/CLD/GNB/WOUND CULTURE/2
21. MICR/ESOE/SCH/AFB/3
22. MICR/CCLD/GNB/STOOL CULTURE/2
23. MICR/IBP/GPC/1
24. MICR/ELF/SCH/INFECTIOUS DISEASE/3
25. MICR/ISOE/ANAEROBIC INCUBATION/1
26. MICR/CCLD/MIC-MAC MORPH/LISTERIA/2
27. MICR/CCLD/GPB/ACTINOMYCETES/2
28. MICR/ESOE/QC/SUSCEPTIBILITY/3
29. MICR/IMM/DIPHASIC FUNGUS/2
30. MICR/ANLF/MIC-MAC MORPH/ANAEROBIC GNB/2
31. MICR/ANLF/GPC/BASIC TEST/2
32. MICR/CCLD/COLITIS/3
33. MICR/CCLD/GNC/ANAEROBES/2
34. MICR/SELM/IDENTIFICATION/RICKETTSIA/1
35. MICR/ANLF/SUSCEPTIBILITY/MIC/3
36. MICR/IMM/YEAST/2
37. MICR/ESOE/AFB/PHOTOCHROMOGEN/3
38. MICR/SELM/VIRAL ISOLATION/1
39. MICR/IMM/AMOEBA/2
40. MICR/IMM/PLASMODIUM/2
41. MICR/IMM/CESTODE OVA/2
42. MICR/SELM/SCH/PARASITE/2
43. MICR/ELF/BIOCHEMICAL TEST/STOOL CULTURE/2
44. MICR/SCOA/GNB SEROTYPE/STOOL CULTURE/3
45. MICR/ALF/BIOCHEMICAL TEST/AFB/2
46. MICR/SCOA/MANAGEMENT/DISCIPLINARY ACTION/3
47. MICR/ELF/GNB/BIOCHEMICAL REACTIONS/2
48. MICR/ESOE/SCH/BLOOD CULTURE/2
49. MICR/SCOA/MANAGEMENT/INTERDEPARTMENT RELATIONS/3
50. MICR/CLD/HEPATITIS/3
51. MICR/ANLF/GPC/CULTURE CHARACTERISTICS/2
52. MICR/ALF/SEROLOGY VS. CULTURE/QA/3
53. MICR/SCOA/QC/MEDIA/3
54. MICR/ESOE/QC/GRAM STAIN/3
55. BBNK/ISOP/HEMOTHERAPY/ADVERSE REACTION/1
56. BBNK/SCOA/RBC/RH PHENOTYPE/3
57. BBNK/DFC/ABO/GENETICS/1
58. BBNK/SELC/HEMOTHERAPY/RBC/2
59. BBNK/ELF/COMPONENT SELECT/FACTOR DEFICIENCY/3
60. BBNK/IBP/COMPONENT PREP/PLATELETS/1
61. BBNK/IBP/RBC/AB IDENTIFICATION/1
62. BBNK/ELF/RH GENOTYPE/2
63. BBNK/CCLD/HEMOTHERAPY/BLOOD COMPONENTS/3
64. BBNK/ELF/DIRECT ANTIGLOBULIN TEST/2
65. BBNK/ALF/GEN THER & PRIN/RH ANTIBODY/2
66. BBNK/SCOA/SCH/AB ID/2
67. BBNK/ELF/ABO SUBGROUP/3
68. BBNK/ELF/CROSSMATCH/INCOMPATIBLE/3
69. BBNK/DFC/AUTOAGGLUTININS/COLD/1
70. BBNK/CCLD/HEMOTHERAPY/BLOOD COMPONENT/3
71. BBNK/ELF/RBC/ABO DISCREPANCY/3
72. BBNK/SELM/RH TYPING/1
73. BBNK/IBP/COMPONENT PREP/PLATELETS/1
74. BBNK/SCOA/GEN THER & PRIN/RH/3
75. BBNK/ELF/ABO DISCREPANCY/3
76. BBNK/SELC/HEMOTHERAPY/2
77. BBNK/ALF/HEMOTHERAPY/ADVERSE REACTION/2
78. BBNK/CCLD/HEMOTHERAPY/ADVERSE REACTION/3
79. BBNK/ISOP/REAGENT QC/1
80. BBNK/SCOA/BLOOD COMPONENT/MULTIPLE ANTIBODIES/2
81. BBNK/DFC/EDUCATION/PROGRAM DEVELOPMENT/1
82. BBNK/ISOP/RBC/REAGENT QC/1
83. BBNK/SDU/HEMOTHERAPY/EXCHANGE/1
84. BBNK/ELF/ABO DISCREPANCY/2
85. BBNK/CALC/RBC SUSPENSION/2
86. BBNK/SCOA/SPECIAL TEST/ABO DISCREPANCY/3
87. BBNK/SCOA/PROBLEM AB/3
88. BBNK/ALF/TRANSFUSION REACTION/GRANULOCYTES/1
89. BBNK/ISOE/RH TYPING/HDN/2
90. IMMU/ELF/BASIC TESTS/SYPHILIS/2
91. IMMU/ELF/FEBRILE AGGLUTININS/2
92. IMMU/ALF/IMD/AFB/1
93. IMMU/ANLF/IMMUNODIFFUSION/2
94. IMMU/CALC/CELL IMMUNITY/T CELLS/2
95. IMMU/DFC/QC/STATISTICS/1
96. IMMU/IBP/BASIC TESTS/RHEUMATOID FACTOR/1
97. IMMU/CCLD/SEROLOGIC SEQUENCE/HEPATITIS/2
98. IMMU/ELF/FLUORESCENT/ANA TEST/2
99. IMMU/CALC/SERIAL DILUTION/2
100. IMMU/ESOE/SCH/COLD AGGLUTININ/3
101. IMMU/CALC/DILUTION/2
102. IMMU/DFC/ALLERGY/AB PRODUCTION/1
103. IMMU/ELF/PREGNANCY TEST/2
104. IMMU/ESOE/CELL IMMUNITY/T CELLS/3
105. IMMU/ISOE/BASIC TESTS/ANA/2
106. IMMU/CCLD/SEROLOGIC TITER/FEBRILE/3
107. CHEM/ANLF/CHO/GLUCOSE INSULIN TOL/2
108. CHEM/ISOE/SCH/BLOOD GAS/2
109. CHEM/ALF/BMD/CREATINE KINASE/1
110. CHEM/IBP/INSTRUMENTATION/FLUOROMETER/1
111. CHEM/CALC/ANION GAP/2
112. CHEM/CCLD/SPECIAL CHEM/LEAD/2
113. CHEM/CCLD/P&E/ACID PHOSPHATASE/3
114. CHEM/IBP/CHO/D-XYLOSE/1
115. CHEM/ELF/P&E/ELECTROPHORESIS/2
116. CHEM/CCLD/BMD/BLOOD GAS/2
117. CHEM/SELM/GLUCOSE/1
118. CHEM/ELF/P&E/ISOENZYME RESULTS/2
119. CHEM/ELF/THYROID FUNCTION/2
120. CHEM/IBP/BASIC TESTS/SERUM IRON/1

ITEM DESCRIPTOR LIST
MEDICAL TECHNOLOGIST EXAMINATION - FEBRUARY 1987

121. CHEM/ESOE/SCH/CALCIUM/3
122. CHEM/ISOE/ELECTROLYTES/1
123. CHEM/ISOP/BILIRUBIN/BEERS LAW/2
124. CHEM/DFC/BTP/ALBUMIN/1
125. CHEM/SELM/BTP/BLOOD GAS/1
126. CHEM/CALC/SPECIAL CHEM/TLC/2
127. CHEM/CCLD/P&E/ELECTROPHORESIS/3
128. CHEM/ESOE/P&E/UREA NITROGEN/3
129. CHEM/IBP/INSTRUMENTATION/ION ELECTRODE/1
130. CHEM/CALC/BLOOD GAS/HENDERSON-HASSEL/2
131. CHEM/DFC/DIGITAL COMPUTER/1
132. CHEM/CALC/SPECIAL TESTS/RADIOACTIVE DECAY/2
133. CHEM/ISOE/INSTRUMENTATION/ANALYTICAL BALANCE/2
134. CHEM/ECLF/ABE/METABOLIC ACIDOSIS/2
135. CHEM/IBP/ENZYME REACTION/1
136. CHEM/SCOA/P&E/ELECTROPHORESIS/3
137. CHEM/CALC/SI UNITS/ELECTROLYTES/2
138. CHEM/ESOE/INSTRUMENTATION/GLC/3
139. CHEM/ESOE/INSTRUMENTATION/ELECTROPHORESIS/3
140. CHEM/ELF/CHO/DIABETES/2
141. HEMA/IBP/HEMOSTASIS/FDP/1
142. HEMA/ALF/FIBRINOLYSIS/SPECIAL TEST/2
143. HEMA/IMM/MATURATION/MYELOCYTIC SERIES/1
144. HEMA/DFC/PHYSIOLOGY/RBC/1
145. HEMA/ISOE/LEUKOCYTE COUNT/PHYSIOLOGY/2
146. HEMA/IBP/WBC/SPECIAL STAIN/1
147. HEMA/CALC/LEUKOCYTE COUNT/MANUAL/2
148. HEMA/ELF/SPECIAL TESTS/HGB F/2
149. HEMA/ELF/HEMOSTASIS/SUBSTITUTION STUDIES/3
150. HEMA/ALF/FACTOR DEFICIENCY/2
151. HEMA/CCLD/AIHA/2
152. HEMA/IBP/SEDIMENTATION RATE/1
153. HEMA/ESOE/AUTOMATED COUNT/HGB/3
154. HEMA/ID/INCLUSION/WBC/1
155. HEMA/ELF/OSMOTIC FRAGILITY/3
156. HEMA/ALF/MICRO MORPH/CORRECTION FOR WBC/2
157. HEMA/CCLD/MICRO MORPH/WBC/3
158. HEMA/ELF/RBC/HGB ELECTROPHORESIS/3
159. HEMA/ELF/MICRO MORPH/RED CELL INCLUSION/2
160. HEMA/CALC/CORRECTED COUNT/WBC/2
161. HEMA/CCLD/MICRO MORPH/RBC/3
162. HEMA/IBP/HEMOSTASIS/INSTRUMENTATION/1
163. HEMA/ISOP/HEMATOCRIT/1
164. HEMA/ELF/PTT MIXING STUDY/2
165. HEMA/CCLD/MICRO MORPH/SMUDGE CELLS/1
166. HEMA/CLD/HEMOSTASIS/HEMOPHILIA/2
167. HEMA/ALF/WBC/SPECIAL STAIN/2
168. HEMA/ALF/CYTOGENETICS/CGL/1
169. HEMA/CLD/CBC/ACUTE LEUKEMIA/3
170. HEMA/DFC/MANAGEMENT/MOTIVATION/1
171. HEMA/CCLD/VON WILLEBRANDS/2
172. HEMA/DFC/PLATELET/PHYSIOLOGY/1
173. HEMA/DFC/HEMOPATHY/SOLUBILITY TEST/1
174. HEMA/ANLF/LAP SCORE/3

Reading Lists

General

Barnett R: Clinical Laboratory Statistics. Second edition. Boston, Little, Brown, 1975.

Bauer JD: Clinical Laboratory Methods. Ninth edition. St. Louis, CV Mosby, 1982.

Galen RS, Gambino SR: Beyond Normality: The Predictive Value and Efficiency of Medical Diagnosis. New York, John Wiley, 1975.

Inhorn SL (ed): Quality Assurance Practices for Health Laboratories. Washington, DC, American Public Health Association, 1978.

Lee LW: Elementary Principles of Laboratory Instruments. Fifth edition. St. Louis, CV Mosby, 1983.

Raphael SS: Medical Laboratory Technology. Fourth edition. Philadelphia, WB Saunders, 1983.

Sonnenwirth AC, Leonard J (eds): Grandwohl's Clinical Laboratory Methods and Diagnosis. Eighth edition. St Louis, CV Mosby, 1980.

Sutton HE: An Introduction to Human Genetics. Third edition. Philadelphia, Saunders College Publishing, 1980.

Todd-Sanford-Davidson: Clinical Diagnosis and Management by Laboratory Methods. 17th edition. Henry JB (ed). 2 vol. Philadelphia, WB Saunders, 1984.

Westgard JO: Method Evaluation. Am J Med Technol 44:6, 1978.

Blood Bank

American Association of Blood Banks and American Red Cross: Circular of Information for the Use of Human Blood and Blood Components by Physicians. Washington, DC, American Association of Blood Banks and American Red Cross, 1978.

American Association of Blood Banks: AABB Supplement to a Seminar on Laboratory Management of Hemolysis. Washington, DC, American Association of Blood Banks, 1979.

American Association of Blood Banks: Blood, Blood Components and Derivatives in Transfusion Therapy. Washington, DC, American Association of Blood Banks, 1980.

American Association of Blood Banks: Guidelines to Transfusion Practices. Washington, DC, American Association of Blood Banks, 1980.

American Association of Blood Banks: Hemolytic Disease of the Newborn. Washington, DC, American Association of Blood Banks, 1984.

American Association of Blood Banks: Hemotherapy of the Infant and Premature. Washington, DC, American Association of Blood Banks, 1983.

American Association of Blood Banks: High Titer, Low Avidity Antibodies. Washington, DC, American Association of Blood Banks, 1979.

American Association of Blood Banks: Standards for Blood Banks and Transfusion Services. 11th edition. Washington, DC, American Association of Blood Banks, 1984.

Bell CA (ed): A Seminar on Immune Mediated Cell Destruction. Washington, DC, American Association of Blood Banks, 1981.

Bell CA (ed): A Seminar on Perinatal Blood Banking. Washington, DC, American Association of Blood Banks, 1978.

Berkman EM, Umals J (eds): Therapeutic Hemapheresis. Washington, DC, American Association of Blood Banks, 1980.

Biological Corporation of America: A Handbook of Serological Techniques for use in Investigative Immunohematology. West Chester, PA, Biological Corporation of America, 1981.

Greendyke RM: Introduction to Blood Banking. Third edition. Garden City, NY, Medical Examination Publishing Co, Inc, 1980.

Huestis DW, Bove JR, Busch J: Practical Blood Transfusion. Third edition. Boston, Little, Brown, 1981.

Issit PD, Issit CH: Applied Blood Group Serology. Third edition. Rutherford, NJ, Becton, Dickinson and Co, 1985.

Kolins J, Jones J (eds): Therapeutic Apheresis. Washington, DC, American Association of Blood Banks, 1983.

Lazarus HM, Herzig RH: Reply to Murphy Scott "Letter to the Editor" re authors' article "Platelet concentrate storage at 22°C." Transfusion 23:78, 1982.

Lockwood CM: Plasma exchange: An overview. Plasma Therapy 1:1, 1979.

Marks MR, Reid ME, Ellisor SS: Absorption of unwanted cold autoagglutinins by formaldehyde treated rabbit red blood cells. Transfusion 20:629, 1980.

Marsh WL, Johnson CL, Oyen R, et al: Anti-Sd^x a new auto-agglutinin related to the Sd^a blood group. Transfusion 20:1-8, 1980.

Miller WV, Rodey G: HLA Without Tears. Chicago, American Society of Clinical Pathologists, 1981.

Mollison PL: Blood Transfusion in Clinical Medicine. Seventh edition. London, Blackwell Scientific, 1983.

Oberman HA (ed): General Principles of Blood Transfusion. Chicago, American Medical Association, 1985.

Petz LD, Swisher SN (eds): Clinical Practice of Blood Transfusion. Edinburgh, Churchill Livingstone, 1981.

Race RR, Sanger R: Blood Groups in Man. Oxford, Blackwell Scientific, 1975.

Reid ME: The Sd blood group system. In Advances in Immuno-hematology. Rutherford, NJ, Becton, Dickinson and Co, Vol 3, No 4, 1975.

Rutman RC, Miller WV: Transfusion Therapy: Principles and Procedures. Rockville, MD, Aspen Publications, 1982.

Tregellas WM, Wallas CH (eds): Prenatal and Perinatal Immuno-hematology. Washington, DC, American Association of Blood Banks, 1981.

Widman FK (ed): Technical Manual of the American Association of Blood Banks. Ninth edition. Washington, DC, American Association of Blood Banks, 1985.

Zmijewski CM: Immunohematology. Third edition. New York, Appleton-Century-Crofts, 1978.

Chemistry

Beeler MF: Interpretations in Clinical Chemistry. Chicago, American Society of Clinical Pathologists, 1978.

Bishop ML, Duben-VonLaufen J, Fody EP (eds): Clinical Chemistry: Principles, Procedures, Correlations. Philadelphia, JB Lippincott, 1985.

Campbell JM, Campbell JB: Laboratory Mathematics. St Louis, CV Mosby, 1984.

Carter T, Wilding P: Factors involved in the determination of triglycerides in serum: An international study. Clin Chim Acta 70:433-447, 1976.

Cawley LP, Minard BJ: Enlarged Liver Associated with Jaundice. Special Topics Check Sample ST-92. Chicago, American Society of Clinical Pathologists, 1976.

Galloway HE, Fisher-Ross L: Chemistry of Proteins. Ballaire, TX, American Society for Medical Technology, 1973.

Gornall AG: Applied Biochemistry of Clinical Disorders. Philadelphia, Harper & Row, 1980.

Henry RJ, Cannon DC, Winkelman JW (eds): Clinical Chemistry: Principles and Technics. Second edition. New York, Harper & Row, 1974.

International Federation of Clinical Chemistry: Provisional recommendation on quality control in clinical chemistry. Clin Chim Acta 75:F11-F20, 1977.

Johns HE, Cunningham JR: The Physics of Radiology. Fourth edition. Springfield, IL, Charles C Thomas, 1983.

Kalman SM, Clark DR: Drug Assay: The Strategy of Therapeutic Drug Monitoring. New York, Masson, 1979.

Kaplan LA, Szabo LL: Clinical Chemistry: Interpretations and Techniques. Second edition. Philadelphia, Lea & Febiger, 1983.

Kaplan LA, Pesce AJ (eds): Clinical Chemistry: Theory, Analysis and Correlation. St Louis, CV Mosby, 1984.

Labbe RF: History and background of protoporphyrin testing. Clin Chem 23:256-259, 1977.

Lehmann HP: Metrication of clinical laboratory data in SI units. Am J Clin Pathol 65:2-18, 1976.

Lehninger AL: Principles of Biochemistry. Second edition. New York, Worth Publishers, 1982.

Lewis B (ed): The Hyperlipidemias: Clinical and Laboratory Practice. Oxford, Blackwell Scientific, 1976.

Montgomery R, Dryer RL, Conway TW, et al: Biochemistry: A Case-Oriented Approach. Fourth edition. St Louis, CV Mosby, 1983.

Odell WD, Daughaday WH (eds): Principles of Competitive Protein Binding Assays. Second edition. New York, Wiley, 1982.

Orten JM, Newhaus OW: Human Biochemistry. 10th edition. St Louis, CV Mosby, 1982.

Preston JA, Troxel DB: Biochemical Profiling in Diagnostic Medicine. Tarrytown, NY, Technicon Instruments Corporation, 1971.

Ritzmann SE, Daniels JC: Serum Protein Abnormalities: Diagnostic and Clinical Aspects. Boston, Little, Brown, 1975.

Scoggins BA, Maguire KP, Norman IR, et al: Measurement of tricyclic antidepressants. I. A review of methodology. Clin Chem 26:5-17, 1980.

Stanbury JB (ed): The Metabolic Basis of Inherited Disease. Fifth edition. New York, McGraw-Hill, 1983.

Tietz NW (ed): Textbook of Clinical Chemistry. Second edition. Philadelphia, WB Saunders, 1986.

Walmsley RN, White GH: A Guide to Diagnostic Clinical Chemistry. Melbourne, Blackwell Scientific, 1983.

Werner M (ed): Microtechniques for the Clinical Laboratory: Concepts and Applications. New York, John Wiley, 1976.

Williams, RH (ed): Textbook of Endocrinology. Sixth Edition. Philadelphia, WB Saunders, 1981.

Winstead M: Instrument Check Systems. Philadelphia, Lea & Febiger, 1971.

Zilva JF, Pannall PR (eds): Clinical Chemistry in Diagnosis and Treatment. Fourth edition. Chicago, Year Book Medical, 1985.

Hematology

Bessis M: Blood Smears Reinterpreted. New York, Springer International, 1977.

Bloom AL, Thomas DP (eds): Haemostasis and Thrombosis. Edinburg, NY, Churchill Livingstone, 1981.

Brown B: Hematology: Principles and Procedures. Fourth edition. Philadelphia, Lea & Febiger, 1984.

Chung KS, Bezeaud A, Goldsmith JC, et al: Congenital deficiency of blood clotting factors II, VII, IX and X. Blood 53:776-787, 1979.

Colman RW, Hirsch J, Marder UJ, et al: Hemostasis and Thrombosis: Basic Principles and Clinical Practice. Philadelphia, JB Lippincott, 1982.

Harker L: Hemostasis Manual. Third edition. Philadelphia, Davis, 1983.

Hegde UM, White JM, Hart GH, et al: Diagnosis of alpha-thalassemia trait from Coulter Counter indices. J Clin Pathol 30:884-889, 1977.

Hoffman GC: Thalassemia minor: A common disorder. Lab Med 6:13, 1975.

Hyland DT: Hematology problem. Am J Med Technol 47:331-332, 1981.

Kapff CT, Jandl JH: Blood Atlas and Source Book of Hematology. Boston, Little, Brown, 1981.

Lenahan J, Smith K: Hemostasis. 16th edition. Morris Plains, NJ, General Diagnosis, 1982.

Maslow WC, Beutler E, Bell CA, et al: Practical Diagnosis: Hematologic Disease. Boston, Houghton Mifflin, 1980.

Miale JB: Laboratory Medicine: Hematology. Sixth edition. St. Louis, CV Mosby, 1982.

Murano G, Bick R: Basic Concepts of Hemostasis and Thrombosis. Boca Raton, FL, CRC Press, 1980.

National Committee on Clinical Laboratory Standards: NCCLS Tentative Guidelines for the Collection Transport and Preparation of Blood Specimens for Coagulation Testings. National Committee on Clinical Laboratory Standards, vol 2, no 4, 1982.

O'Connor BH: A Color Atlas and Instruction Manual of Peripheral Blood Cell Morphology. Baltimore, Williams & Wilkins, 1984.

Owen CA, Bowie EJW, Thompson JH: The Diagnosis of Bleeding Disorders. Second edition. Boston, Little, Brown, 1975.

Penn GM, Davis T: Identification of Myeloma Proteins. Chicago, American Society of Clinical Pathologists, 1975.

Platt WR: Color Atlas and Textbook of Hematology. Second edition. Philadelphia, JB Lippincott, 1979.

Poller L (ed): Recent Advances in Blood Coagulation. Third edition. London, Churchill Livingstone, 1981.

Schumacher HR, Garvin DF, Triplett DA: Introduction to Laboratory Hematology and Hematopathology. New York, Alan R Liss, 1984.

Sirridge MS, Shannon R: Laboratory Evaluation of Hemostasis and Thrombosis. Third edition. Philadelphia, Lea & Febiger, 1983.

Thompson JM (ed): Blood Coagulation and Haemostasis: A Practical Guide. Second edtion. Edinburg, NY, Churchill Livingstone, 1980.

Triplett DA, Harms CS, Newhouse P, Clark C: Platelet Function: Laboratory Evaluation and Clinical Application. Chicago, American Society of Clinical Pathologists, 1978.

Triplett DA: Laboratory Evaluation of Coagulation. Chicago, American Society of Clinical Pathologists, 1982.

Vince-Cruz MP: What to do when Coulter model S shows super high WBC. Lab Med 6:48, 1975.

Weatherall DJ, Clegg JB: The Thalassemia Syndromes. Third edition. Oxford, Blackwell Scientific, 1981.

Williams WJ, Beutler E, Erslev AJ, et al (eds): Hematology. Third edition. New York, McGraw-Hill, 1983.

Wintrobe MM: Clinical Hematology. Eighth edition. Philadelphia, Lea & Febiger, 1981.

Immunology

Agnello V: Complement deficiency states. Medicine (Baltimore) 57(1):1, 1978.

Aitcheson CT, Peebles C, Joslin F, Tan EM: Characteristics of antinuclear antibodies in rheumatoid arthritis. Arthritis Rheum 23(5):528-538, 1980.

Bearman RM, et al: Terminal deoxynucleotidyl transferase activity in neoplastic and non-neoplastic hematopoietic cells. Am J Clin Pathol 75:794-802, 1981.

Bellanti JA: Immunology III. Philadelphia, WB Saunders, 1985.

Bergsma D (ed): Immunodeficiency in Man and Animals. Sunderland, MA, Sinauer Associates Inc, 1985.

Bollum FJ: Terminal deoxynucleotidyl transferase as a hematopoietic cell marker. Blood 54:1203-1215, 1979.

Bruynzeel PLB, Berrens L: IgE and IgG4 antibodies in specific human allergies. Int Arch Allergy Appl Immunol 58:344-350, 1979.

Budd J, Penn GM: Urinary Immunoglobulins II. Clinical Immunology Check Sample CI-34. Chicago, American Society of Clinical Pathologists, 1981.

Daneo V, Migone N, Modena V, et al: Family studies and HLA typing in ankylosing spondylitis and sacroiliitis. J Rheumatol (suppl) 3:5, 1977.

Eisin HN: Immunology. Second edition. Hagerstown, MD, Harper & Row, 1980.

Fundenberg HH, Good RA, Goodman HC, et al: Primary immunodeficiencies. Report of a World Health Organization Committee. Pediatrics 48:927-946, 1971.

Fundenberg HH, Sites DP, Caldwell JL, et al: Basic and Clinical Immunology. Third edition. Los Altos, CA, Lange Medical Publications, 1980.

Goldstein G, Mackay IR: The Human Thymus. St Louis, Warren Green, Inc, 1980.

Homburger H: IgE and IgG Antibodies in the Pathogenesis of Hypersensitivity Diseases of the Respiratory Tract. Clinical Immunology Check Sample CI-22. Chicago, American Society of Clinical Pathologists, 1980.

Kelly RH, et al: Qualitative testing for circulating immune complexes by zone electrophoresis in agarose. Clin Chem 26:396-402, 1980.

Keshgegian AA, Peiffer P: Immunofixation as an adjunct to immunoelectrophoresis in characterization of serum monoclonal immunoglobulins. Clin Chim Acta 110:337-340, 1981.

Lee CL, Lebeck LK, Wong C: Estimating paternity index from HLA typing results. Amer J Clin Pathol 74:218-23, 1980.

McGraw DJ, Kurec AS, Davey FR: Mouse erythrocyte formation: A marker for testing B lymphocytes. Am J Clin Pathol 76:117-183, 1982.

Merlini G, et al: Detection and identification of monoclonal components: Immunoelectrophoresis on agarose gel and immunofixation on cellulose acetate compared. Clin Chem 27:1862-65, 1981.

Miller WV, Holland PV, Sugarbaker E, et al: Anaphylactic reactions to IgA. Am J Clin Pathol 55:618-621, 1970.

Minard BJ: Clinical Immunology. In Tech Sample GCI-1. Hawk C (ed). Chicago, American Society of Clinical Pathologists, 1979.

Nakamura RM: Immunopathology: Clinical Laboratory Concepts and Methods. Boston, Little, Brown, 1974.

Nakamura RM, Dito WR, Tucker ES: Immunoassays in the Clinical Laboratory. Vol III. New York, Alan R Liss, 1979.

Nakamura RM, Dito WR, Tucker ES: Immunoassay - Clinical Laboratory Techniques for the 1980's. Vol IV. New York, Alan R Liss, 1983.

Parker CW (ed): Clinical Immunology. 2 vols. Philadelphia, WB Saunders, 1980.

Penn GM, et al: Gamma Heavy Chain Disease. Clinical Immunology Check Sample CI-13. Chicago, American Society of Clinical Pathologists, 1977.

Penn GM, Batya JC: Interpretation of Immunoelectrophoretic Patterns. Chicago, American Society of Clinical Pathologists, 1978.

Penn GM, Batya J: Diclonal Gammopathy (IgMK-IgGK). Clinical Immunology Check Sample CI-28. Chicago, American Society of Clinical Pathologists, 1980.

Penn GM: Clinical Use and Interpretation of Agarose-gel Electrophoretic Patterns. Chicago, American Society of Clinical Pathologists, 1981.

Penn GM: Dysgammaglobulinemia Type 1: Laboratory or Clinical Diagnosis. Clinical Immunology Check Sample CI-27. Chicago, American Society of Clinical Pathologists, 1980.

Penn GM: Resolution of Monoclonal Gammopathy Problems by Electrophoresis and Associated Immunochemical Techniques. Chicago, American Society of Clinical Pathologists, 1982.

Penn GM: The monclonal gammopathies: Laboratory detection. Lab Management 19:30-40, 1981.

Penn GM: Urinary Immunoglobulins I. Clinical Immunology Check Sample CI-18. Chicago, American Society of Clinical Pathologists, 1979.

Ritchie RF, Smith R: Immunofixation I: General principles and application to agarose gel electrophoresis. Clin Chem 22:497-499, 1976.

Ritzmann SE, Killingsworth LM: Proteins in Body Fluids, Amino Acids and Tumor Markers: Diagnostic and Clinical Aspects, New York, Alan R Liss, 1983.

Ritzmann SE: Radial immunodiffusion revisited. Lab Med 9(7-8): 23-33, 1978.

Roitt I: Essential Immunology. Fourth edition. Oxford, Blackwell Scientific, 1981.

Rose NR, Friedman H (eds): Manual of Clinical Immunology. Second edition. Washington, DC, American Society of Microbiology, 1980.

Sun T, York YL, Degnan T: Study of gammopathies with immunofixation electrophoresis. Am J Clin Pathol 72:5-11, 1979.

Sun T: Laboratory diagnosis of multiple sclerosis. Special Topics Check Sample ST-113. Chicago, American Society of Clinical Pathologists, 1980.

Whiteside TL, Rowlands DT: T cell and B cell identification in the diagnosis of lymphoproliferative disease. Am J Pathol 88:754-790, 1977.

Microbiology

Antholz R: A case of unusual bacterial diarrhea. Lab Med 10:564-65, 1979.

Ash LR, Orihel TX: Atlas of Human Parasitology. Second edition. Chicago, American Society of Clinical Pathologists, 1984.

Balows A, DeHaan RM, Dowell VR, et al: Anaerobic Bacteria: Role in Disease. Springfield, IL, Charles C Thomas, 1975.

Bannatyne RM, Clausen C, McCarthy RL: Laboratory diagnosis of upper respiratory tract infections. Cumitech 10. Washington, DC, American Society for Microbiology, 1979.

Baron S (ed): Medical Microbiology: Principles and Concepts. Menlo Park, CA, Addison-Wesley, 1982.

Bartlett JG, Brewer NS, Ryan KJ: Laboratory Diagnosis of Lower Respiratory Tract Infections. Cumitech 7. Washington JA Jr (ed). Washington, DC, American Society for Microbiology, 1978.

Baude AL, Davis CE, Fierer J (eds): Microbiology. Philadelphia, WB Saunders, 1982.

Blazevic DJ, Hall CT, Wilson ME: Practical Quality Control Procedures for the Clinical Microbiology Laboratory. Cumitech 3. Washington, DC, American Society for Microbiology, 1976.

Breed RS, Murray EGD, Smith NR, et al: Bergey's Manual of Determinative Bacteriology. Eighth edition. Baltimore, Williams & Wilkins, 1974.

Brown HW, Neva FA: Basic Clinical Parasitology. Fifth edition. New York, Appleton-Century-Crofts, 1983.

Chapman JS: The Atypical Mycobacteria and Human Mycobacteriosis. New York, Plenum, 1977.

Conant NF, Smith DT, Baker RD, Calloway JL: Manual of Clinical Mycology. Third edition. Philadelphia, WB Saunders, 1971.

Dolan CT, Koneman EW, Funkhouser JW, et al (eds): Atlases of Clinical Mycology. Chicago, American Society of Clinical Pathologists, 1975.

Duquid JP, et al: Medical Microbiology, Vol I. 13th edition. London, Churchill Livingstone, 1979.

Edberg SC, Atkinson B, Chambers C, et al: Clinical evaluation of the MICRO-ID, API 20E, and conventional media systems for identification of Enterobacteriaceae. J Clin Microbiol 10:161-7, 1979.

Finegold SM, Martin WJ, Scott EG: Bailey and Scott's Diagnostic Microbiology. Sixth edition. St Louis, CV Mosby, 1982.

Garcia LS, Ash LR: Diagnostic Parasitology: Clinical Laboratory Manual. Second edition. St Louis, CV Mosby, 1979.

Gavan TL: Agar Diffusion Susceptibility Tests. Syracuse, NY, Bristol Laboratories, 1980.

Gilardi GL: Glucose Nonfermenting Gram-Negative Bacteria in Clinical Microbiology. West Palm Beach, FL, CRC Press, Inc, 1980.

Grange JM: Mycobacterial Diseases. New York, Elsevier, 1981.

Haley LN, et al: Laboratory Methods in Medical Mycology. Fourth edition. US Department of Health, Education, and Welfare, Public Health Service. Atlanta, Centers for Disease Control, DHEW Pub No. 78-8361, 1979.

Hoeprich PD (ed): Infectious Diseases: A Modern Treatise of Infectious Processes. Third edition. New York, Harper & Row, 1983.

Isenberg HD, Schoenknecht FD, von Graevenitz A: Collection and Processing of Bacteriological Specimens. Cumitech 9. Rubin SJ (ed). Washington, DC, American Society for Microbiology, 1979.

Jawetz E, Melnick JL, Adelberg EA: A Review of Medical Microbiology. 16th edition. Los Altos, CA, Lange Medical Publications, 1984.

Jones GL, Gaither JG: Isolation and Identification of Salmonella and Shigella. US Department of Health and Human Services, Public Health Service. Atlanta, Centers for Disease Control, 1984.

Jones GL, Herbert GA (eds): Legionnaires, the Disease, the Bacterium, and Methodology. US Department of Health, Education, and Welfare, Public Health Service. Atlanta, Centers for Disease Control, 1979.

Kagan BM (ed): Antimicrobial Therapy. Third edition. Philadelphia, WB Saunders, 1980.

Kellogg DS Jr, Holmes KK, Hill GA: Laboratory diagnosis of gonorrhea. Cumitech 4. Washington, DC, American Society of Microbiology, 1976.

Kloss WE: Natural populations of the genus Staphylococcus. Ann Rev Microbiol 34:559-592, 1980.

Koneman EW, Allen SD, Dowell VR Jr, Sommers HM: Color Atlas and Textbook of Diagnostic Microbiology. Second edition. Philadelphia, JB Lippincott, 1983.

Kunin CM: Detection, Prevention and Management of Urinary Tract Infections. Third edition. Philadelphia, Lea & Febiger, 1979.

Leighton I: Prospects of automation in microbiology. Med Lab Sci 35:213-214, 1978.

Lennette EH, Balows A, Hausler WJ Jr, et al(eds): Manual of Clinical Microbiology. Fourth edition. Washington, DC, American Society for Microbiology, 1985.

Lennette EH, Schmidt NJ (eds): Diagnostic Procedures for Viral, Rickettsial and Chlamydial Infections. Fifth edition. Washington, DC, American Public Health Association, 1979.

MacFaddin JF: Biochemical Tests for Identification of Medical Bacteria. Second edition. Baltimore, Williams & Wilkins, 1980.

Mandell GL, Douglas RG Jr, Bennett JE (eds): Principles and Practice of Infectious Diseases. Second edition. New York, John Wiley, 1985.

Markell EK, Voge M: Medical Parasitology. Fifth edition. Philadelphia, WB Saunders, 1981.

McCarthy LR, Sherris JC, Anhalt JP: Collaborative Evaluation of the MS-2 Antibiotic Susceptibility Testing Instrument (Abstr). Washington, DC, American Society of Microbiology, 1978.

McGinnis MR: Laboratory Handbook of Medical Mycology. New York, Academic Press, 1980.

McLean DM: Virology in Health Care. Baltimore, Williams & Wilkins, 1980.

Miller JM, Wenthworth BB: Methods for Quality Control in Diagnostic Microbiology. Washington, DC, American Public Health Association, 1985.

Miller JM: Handbook of Specimen Collection and Handling. US Department of Health and Human Services. Public Health Service. Atlanta, Centers for Disease Control, 1984.

Morello JA, Graves MH: Automation in Clinical Microbiology. Clin Microbiol News 1:1-5, 1979.

Newsom B: A review of automation and rapid methods in microbiology. Med Lab Sci 35(3):215-222, 1978.

Nicholson DP, Koepke JA: Automicrobic system for urine. J Clin Microbiol 10(6):823-833, 1979.

Palmer DE, et al: Serodiagnosis of Mycotic Diseases. American Lecture Series. Springfield, IL, Charles C Thomas, 1977.

Rebell G, Taplin D: Dermatophytes: Their Recognition and Identification. Second revised edition. Coral Gables, FL, University of Miami Press, 1974.

Rippon JW: Medical Mycology: The Pathogenic Fungi and the Pathogenic Actinomycetes. Second edition. Philadelphia, WB Saunders, 1982.

Shea JM: Bilateral tuberculous osteomyelitis of medial humeral condyles: Infection secondary to cutaneous inoculation. JAMA 247: 821-822, 1982.

Sheth NK, Daigeneault JW: Mycobacteria on routine sputum culture plates: A potential for laboratory acquired infection. Lab Med 11: 602-623, 1980.

Somers HM, Russell JP: Clinically Significant Mycobacteria: Their Recognition and Identification. Chicago, American Society of Clinical Pathologists, 1967.

Strong BE, Kubica G: Isolation and Identification of Mycobacterium tuberculosis. US Department of Health, Education, and Welfare, Public Health Service. Atlanta, Centers for Disease Control, HEW Pub No. 81-8390, 1981.

Sutter VL, Citron DM, Finegold SM: Wadsworth Anaerobic Bacteriology Manual. Third edition. St Louis, CV Mosby, 1980.

US Department of Health, Education, and Welfare: Fluorescent Antibody Techniques and Bacterial Applications. Atlanta, DHEW Publication No. (CDC) 78-8364, 1978.

US Department of Health, Education, and Welfare, Public Health Service. Media for Isolation, Characterization and Identification of Obligately Anaerobic Bacteria. Atlanta, Centers for Disease Control, 1977.

Washington JA, Jr (ed): Laboratory Procedures in Clinical Microbiology. Second edition. New York, Springer-Verlag, Inc, 1981.

Willis TA: Anaerobic Bacteriology: Clinical and Laboratory Practice. Third edition. Boston, Butterworth, 1977.

Youmans G (ed): Tuberculosis. Philadelphia, WB Saunders, 1979.

Youmans GP, Paterson PY, Sommers HM: The Biologic and Clinical Basis of Infectious Diseases. Second edition. Philadelphia, WB Saunders, 1980.

Urinalysis and Body Fluids

Ames Division, Miles Laboratories: Modern Urine Chemistry. Elkhart, IN, Ames Division, Miles Laboratory, 1982.

Ames Division, Miles Laboratories: Factors Affecting Urine Chemistry Tests. Elkhart, IN, Ames Division, Miles Laboratories, 1982.

Graff L: A Handbook of Routine Urinalysis, Philadelphia, JB Lippincott, 1983.

Haber MH: Urinary Sediment: A Textbook Atlas. Chicago, American Society of Clinical Pathologists, 1981.

Kjeldsberg CR, Knight JA: Body Fluids: Laboratory Examination of Amniotic, Cerebrospinal, Seminal, Serous, & Synovial Fluids: A Textbook Atlas. Second edition. Chicago, Amercian Society of Clinical Pathologists, 1986.

Race GT, White MG: Basic Urinalysis. Baltimore, Harper & Row, 1979.

Ross DL, Neely AE: A Textbook of Urinalysis. New York, Appleton-Century-Crofts, 1983.

Stamey TA, Kindrachuk RW: Urinary Sediment and Urinalysis. Philadelphia, WB Saunders, 1985.

Strasinger SK: Urinalysis and Body Fluids. Philadelphia, FA Davis, 1985.

Education and Laboratory Operations

Anastasi A: Psychological Testing. Fourth edition. New York, Macmillan, 1976.

Bennington JL, et al (eds): Management and Cost Control Techniques for the Clinical Laboratory. Baltimore, University Park Press, 1977.

Becan-McBride K (ed): Textbook of Clinical Laboratory Supervision. New York, Appleton-Century-Crofts, 1982.

Berk RA (ed): Criterion-Referenced Measurement: State of the Art. Baltimore, John Hopkins University Press, 1980.

Berk RA (ed): A Guide to Criterion-Referenced Test Construction. Baltimore, John Hopkins University Press. 1984.

Bunda MA, Sanders JR (eds): Practices and Problems in Competency-Based Measurement. Washington, DC, National Council on Measurement in Education, 1979.

Elbing AO: Behavioral Decisions in Organization. Glenview, IL, Scott, Foresman, 1979.

Glass GV: Standards and criteria. J Educ Meas 15:277-290, 1978.

Gronlund NE: Individualizing Classroom Instruction. New York, Macmillan, 1974.

Hersey P, Blanchard KH: Management of Organizational Behavior: Utilizing Human Resources. Third edition. Englewood Cliffs, NJ, Prentice-Hall, 1977.

Hicks R, et al: Laboratory Instrumentation. Hagerstown, MD, Harper & Row, 1980.

Johnson JL: Clinical Laboratory Computer Systems: A Comprehensive Review. Northbrook, IL, J Lloyd Johnson Associates, 1971.

Livingston SA, Wingersky MS: Assessing the reliability of tests used to make pass/fail decisions. J Educ Meas 16:247-260, 1979.

Lundberg GD: Managing the Patient-Focused Laboratory. Oradell, NJ, Medical Economics Co, 1975.

Nedelsky L: Absolute grading standards for objective tests. Educ Psychol Meas 14:3-19, 1954.

Newell JE: Laboratory Management. Boston, Little, Brown, 1972.

Nunnally JC: Psychometric Theory. New York, McGraw-Hill, 1978.

Popham WJ (ed): Evaluation in Education: Current Applications. Berkley, CA, McCutchan Publishing Co, 1974.

Popham WJ, Lindheim E: The practical side of criterion-referenced test development. Meas Educ 9:(1), 1980.

Popham WJ: An approaching peril: Cloud-referenced tests. Phi Delta Kappan 56:614-615, 1974.

Popham WJ: Criterion-Referenced Measurement. Englewood Cliffs, NJ, Prentice-Hall, 1978.

Popham WJ: Well-crafted criterion-referenced tests. Educ Lead, November 1978:91-95.

Reynolds CR, Gutkin TB (eds): A Handbook for the Practice of School Psychology. New York, John Wiley, 1980.

Shepard L: Norm-referenced vs. criterion-referenced tests. Educ Horiz 58(1):26-32, 1979.

Shuffstall RM, Hemmaplardh B: The Hospital Laboratory: Modern Concepts of Management, Operations, and Finance. St Louis, CV Mosby, 1979.

Subkoviak MJ: Estimating reliability from a single administration of a criterion-referenced test. J Educ Meas 13:265-275, 1976.

Thorndike RL (ed): Educational Measurement. Second edition. Washington, DC, American Council on Education, 1971.

Traub R (ed): New Directions for Testing and Measurement: Methodological Developments. San Francisco, Jossey-Bass Inc, 1979.

Weisbrot JM: Statistics for the Clinical Laboratory. Philadelphia, JB Lippincott, 1985.

Wilcox RR: An approach to measuring the achievement or proficiency of an examinee. Appl Psychol Meas 4:241-251, 1980.

Williams F: Reasoning with Statistics. Second edition. New York, Holt, Rinehart & Winston. 1979.

IDENTIFICATION NUMBER | EXAM TYPE

0	0	0	0	0	0	0	0	0	0	0
1	1	1	1	1	1	1	1	1	1	1
2	2	2	2	2	2	2	2	2	2	2
3	3	3	3	3	3	3	3	3	3	3
4	4	4	4	4	4	4	4	4	4	4
5	5	5	5	5	5	5	5	5	5	5
6	6	6	6	6	6	6	6	6	6	6
7	7	7	7	7	7	7	7	7	7	7
8	8	8	8	8	8	8	8	8	8	8
9	9	9	9	9	9	9	9	9	9	9

TEST BOOKLET NUMBER

IMPORTANT DIRECTIONS FOR MARKING ANSWERS

- Use black lead pencil only (No. 2½ or softer).
- Do NOT use ink, felt tip or ballpoint pens.
- Erase cleanly any answer you wish to change.
- Make no stray marks on the answer sheet.
- Make heavy black marks that fill the circle completely.

EXAMPLES

WRONG: Fill in the circle completely.
1 (A) (B) (C) (D) (E)
2 (A) (B) (C) (D) (E)
3 (A) (B) (C) (D) (E)

WRONG: Make heavy black marks.
4 (A) (B) (C) (D) (E)

RIGHT: Make heavy black marks that fill in the circle completely.
5 (A) (B) (C) (D) (E)

NAME: ______

EXAM TYPE: ______ DATE: ______

BOARD OF REGISTRY

1 (A) (B) (C) (D) (E)
2 (A) (B) (C) (D) (E)
3 (A) (B) (C) (D) (E)
4 (A) (B) (C) (D) (E)
5 (A) (B) (C) (D) (E)
6 (A) (B) (C) (D) (E)
7 (A) (B) (C) (D) (E)
8 (A) (B) (C) (D) (E)
9 (A) (B) (C) (D) (E)
10 (A) (B) (C) (D) (E)
11 (A) (B) (C) (D) (E)
12 (A) (B) (C) (D) (E)
13 (A) (B) (C) (D) (E)
14 (A) (B) (C) (D) (E)
15 (A) (B) (C) (D) (E)
16 (A) (B) (C) (D) (E)
17 (A) (B) (C) (D) (E)
18 (A) (B) (C) (D) (E)
19 (A) (B) (C) (D) (E)
20 (A) (B) (C) (D) (E)
21 (A) (B) (C) (D) (E)
22 (A) (B) (C) (D) (E)
23 (A) (B) (C) (D) (E)
24 (A) (B) (C) (D) (E)
25 (A) (B) (C) (D) (E)
26 (A) (B) (C) (D) (E)
27 (A) (B) (C) (D) (E)
28 (A) (B) (C) (D) (E)
29 (A) (B) (C) (D) (E)
30 (A) (B) (C) (D) (E)
31 (A) (B) (C) (D) (E)
32 (A) (B) (C) (D) (E)
33 (A) (B) (C) (D) (E)
34 (A) (B) (C) (D) (E)
35 (A) (B) (C) (D) (E)
36 (A) (B) (C) (D) (E)
37 (A) (B) (C) (D) (E)
38 (A) (B) (C) (D) (E)
39 (A) (B) (C) (D) (E)
40 (A) (B) (C) (D) (E)
41 (A) (B) (C) (D) (E)
42 (A) (B) (C) (D) (E)
43 (A) (B) (C) (D) (E)
44 (A) (B) (C) (D) (E)
45 (A) (B) (C) (D) (E)
46 (A) (B) (C) (D) (E)
47 (A) (B) (C) (D) (E)
48 (A) (B) (C) (D) (E)
49 (A) (B) (C) (D) (E)
50 (A) (B) (C) (D) (E)
51 (A) (B) (C) (D) (E)
52 (A) (B) (C) (D) (E)
53 (A) (B) (C) (D) (E)
54 (A) (B) (C) (D) (E)
55 (A) (B) (C) (D) (E)
56 (A) (B) (C) (D) (E)
57 (A) (B) (C) (D) (E)
58 (A) (B) (C) (D) (E)
59 (A) (B) (C) (D) (E)
60 (A) (B) (C) (D) (E)
61 (A) (B) (C) (D) (E)
62 (A) (B) (C) (D) (E)
63 (A) (B) (C) (D) (E)
64 (A) (B) (C) (D) (E)
65 (A) (B) (C) (D) (E)
66 (A) (B) (C) (D) (E)
67 (A) (B) (C) (D) (E)
68 (A) (B) (C) (D) (E)
69 (A) (B) (C) (D) (E)
70 (A) (B) (C) (D) (E)
71 (A) (B) (C) (D) (E)
72 (A) (B) (C) (D) (E)
73 (A) (B) (C) (D) (E)
74 (A) (B) (C) (D) (E)
75 (A) (B) (C) (D) (E)
76 (A) (B) (C) (D) (E)
77 (A) (B) (C) (D) (E)
78 (A) (B) (C) (D) (E)
79 (A) (B) (C) (D) (E)
80 (A) (B) (C) (D) (E)
81 (A) (B) (C) (D) (E)
82 (A) (B) (C) (D) (E)
83 (A) (B) (C) (D) (E)
84 (A) (B) (C) (D) (E)
85 (A) (B) (C) (D) (E)
86 (A) (B) (C) (D) (E)
87 (A) (B) (C) (D) (E)
88 (A) (B) (C) (D) (E)
89 (A) (B) (C) (D) (E)
90 (A) (B) (C) (D) (E)
91 (A) (B) (C) (D) (E)
92 (A) (B) (C) (D) (E)
93 (A) (B) (C) (D) (E)
94 (A) (B) (C) (D) (E)
95 (A) (B) (C) (D) (E)
96 (A) (B) (C) (D) (E)
97 (A) (B) (C) (D) (E)
98 (A) (B) (C) (D) (E)
99 (A) (B) (C) (D) (E)
100 (A) (B) (C) (D) (E)
101 (A) (B) (C) (D) (E)
102 (A) (B) (C) (D) (E)
103 (A) (B) (C) (D) (E)
104 (A) (B) (C) (D) (E)
105 (A) (B) (C) (D) (E)
106 (A) (B) (C) (D) (E)
107 (A) (B) (C) (D) (E)
108 (A) (B) (C) (D) (E)
109 (A) (B) (C) (D) (E)
110 (A) (B) (C) (D) (E)
111 (A) (B) (C) (D) (E)
112 (A) (B) (C) (D) (E)
113 (A) (B) (C) (D) (E)
114 (A) (B) (C) (D) (E)
115 (A) (B) (C) (D) (E)
116 (A) (B) (C) (D) (E)
117 (A) (B) (C) (D) (E)
118 (A) (B) (C) (D) (E)
119 (A) (B) (C) (D) (E)
120 (A) (B) (C) (D) (E)

NCS Trans-Optic F6292-54321

SIDE ONE

BOARD OF REGISTRY

founded in 1928 by the American Society of Clinical Pathologists

Representatives from:

American Society of Clinical Pathologists
- Medical Technologists/Technicians
- Pathologists

American Academy of Microbiology
American Association of Blood Banks
American Society of Cytology
National Registry in Clinical Chemistry
American Society of Hematology
National Society for Histotechnology

IMPORTANT DIRECTIONS FOR MARKING ANSWERS

- Use black lead pencil only (No. 2½ or softer).
- Do NOT use ink, felt tip or ballpoint pens.
- Erase cleanly any answer you wish to change.
- Make no stray marks on the answer sheet.
- Make <u>heavy</u> black marks that fill the circle <u>completely</u>.

EXAMPLES

1 Ⓐ Ⓑ Ⓒ Ⓓ Ⓔ	WRONG: Fill in the circle <u>completely</u>.
2 Ⓐ Ⓑ Ⓒ Ⓓ Ⓔ	
3 Ⓐ Ⓑ Ⓒ Ⓓ Ⓔ	
4 Ⓐ Ⓑ Ⓒ Ⓓ Ⓔ	WRONG: Make <u>heavy</u> black marks.
5 Ⓐ Ⓑ Ⓒ Ⓓ ●	RIGHT: Make <u>heavy</u> black marks that fill in the circle <u>completely</u>.

121 Ⓐ Ⓑ Ⓒ Ⓓ Ⓔ	141 Ⓐ Ⓑ Ⓒ Ⓓ Ⓔ	161 Ⓐ Ⓑ Ⓒ Ⓓ Ⓔ	181 Ⓐ Ⓑ Ⓒ Ⓓ Ⓔ	201 Ⓐ Ⓑ Ⓒ Ⓓ Ⓔ	221 Ⓐ Ⓑ Ⓒ Ⓓ Ⓔ
122 Ⓐ Ⓑ Ⓒ Ⓓ Ⓔ	142 Ⓐ Ⓑ Ⓒ Ⓓ Ⓔ	162 Ⓐ Ⓑ Ⓒ Ⓓ Ⓔ	182 Ⓐ Ⓑ Ⓒ Ⓓ Ⓔ	202 Ⓐ Ⓑ Ⓒ Ⓓ Ⓔ	222 Ⓐ Ⓑ Ⓒ Ⓓ Ⓔ
123 Ⓐ Ⓑ Ⓒ Ⓓ Ⓔ	143 Ⓐ Ⓑ Ⓒ Ⓓ Ⓔ	163 Ⓐ Ⓑ Ⓒ Ⓓ Ⓔ	183 Ⓐ Ⓑ Ⓒ Ⓓ Ⓔ	203 Ⓐ Ⓑ Ⓒ Ⓓ Ⓔ	223 Ⓐ Ⓑ Ⓒ Ⓓ Ⓔ
124 Ⓐ Ⓑ Ⓒ Ⓓ Ⓔ	144 Ⓐ Ⓑ Ⓒ Ⓓ Ⓔ	164 Ⓐ Ⓑ Ⓒ Ⓓ Ⓔ	184 Ⓐ Ⓑ Ⓒ Ⓓ Ⓔ	204 Ⓐ Ⓑ Ⓒ Ⓓ Ⓔ	224 Ⓐ Ⓑ Ⓒ Ⓓ Ⓔ
125 Ⓐ Ⓑ Ⓒ Ⓓ Ⓔ	145 Ⓐ Ⓑ Ⓒ Ⓓ Ⓔ	165 Ⓐ Ⓑ Ⓒ Ⓓ Ⓔ	185 Ⓐ Ⓑ Ⓒ Ⓓ Ⓔ	205 Ⓐ Ⓑ Ⓒ Ⓓ Ⓔ	225 Ⓐ Ⓑ Ⓒ Ⓓ Ⓔ
126 Ⓐ Ⓑ Ⓒ Ⓓ Ⓔ	146 Ⓐ Ⓑ Ⓒ Ⓓ Ⓔ	166 Ⓐ Ⓑ Ⓒ Ⓓ Ⓔ	186 Ⓐ Ⓑ Ⓒ Ⓓ Ⓔ	206 Ⓐ Ⓑ Ⓒ Ⓓ Ⓔ	226 Ⓐ Ⓑ Ⓒ Ⓓ Ⓔ
127 Ⓐ Ⓑ Ⓒ Ⓓ Ⓔ	147 Ⓐ Ⓑ Ⓒ Ⓓ Ⓔ	167 Ⓐ Ⓑ Ⓒ Ⓓ Ⓔ	187 Ⓐ Ⓑ Ⓒ Ⓓ Ⓔ	207 Ⓐ Ⓑ Ⓒ Ⓓ Ⓔ	227 Ⓐ Ⓑ Ⓒ Ⓓ Ⓔ
128 Ⓐ Ⓑ Ⓒ Ⓓ Ⓔ	148 Ⓐ Ⓑ Ⓒ Ⓓ Ⓔ	168 Ⓐ Ⓑ Ⓒ Ⓓ Ⓔ	188 Ⓐ Ⓑ Ⓒ Ⓓ Ⓔ	208 Ⓐ Ⓑ Ⓒ Ⓓ Ⓔ	228 Ⓐ Ⓑ Ⓒ Ⓓ Ⓔ
129 Ⓐ Ⓑ Ⓒ Ⓓ Ⓔ	149 Ⓐ Ⓑ Ⓒ Ⓓ Ⓔ	169 Ⓐ Ⓑ Ⓒ Ⓓ Ⓔ	189 Ⓐ Ⓑ Ⓒ Ⓓ Ⓔ	209 Ⓐ Ⓑ Ⓒ Ⓓ Ⓔ	229 Ⓐ Ⓑ Ⓒ Ⓓ Ⓔ
130 Ⓐ Ⓑ Ⓒ Ⓓ Ⓔ	150 Ⓐ Ⓑ Ⓒ Ⓓ Ⓔ	170 Ⓐ Ⓑ Ⓒ Ⓓ Ⓔ	190 Ⓐ Ⓑ Ⓒ Ⓓ Ⓔ	210 Ⓐ Ⓑ Ⓒ Ⓓ Ⓔ	230 Ⓐ Ⓑ Ⓒ Ⓓ Ⓔ
131 Ⓐ Ⓑ Ⓒ Ⓓ Ⓔ	151 Ⓐ Ⓑ Ⓒ Ⓓ Ⓔ	171 Ⓐ Ⓑ Ⓒ Ⓓ Ⓔ	191 Ⓐ Ⓑ Ⓒ Ⓓ Ⓔ	211 Ⓐ Ⓑ Ⓒ Ⓓ Ⓔ	231 Ⓐ Ⓑ Ⓒ Ⓓ Ⓔ
132 Ⓐ Ⓑ Ⓒ Ⓓ Ⓔ	152 Ⓐ Ⓑ Ⓒ Ⓓ Ⓔ	172 Ⓐ Ⓑ Ⓒ Ⓓ Ⓔ	192 Ⓐ Ⓑ Ⓒ Ⓓ Ⓔ	212 Ⓐ Ⓑ Ⓒ Ⓓ Ⓔ	232 Ⓐ Ⓑ Ⓒ Ⓓ Ⓔ
133 Ⓐ Ⓑ Ⓒ Ⓓ Ⓔ	153 Ⓐ Ⓑ Ⓒ Ⓓ Ⓔ	173 Ⓐ Ⓑ Ⓒ Ⓓ Ⓔ	193 Ⓐ Ⓑ Ⓒ Ⓓ Ⓔ	213 Ⓐ Ⓑ Ⓒ Ⓓ Ⓔ	233 Ⓐ Ⓑ Ⓒ Ⓓ Ⓔ
134 Ⓐ Ⓑ Ⓒ Ⓓ Ⓔ	154 Ⓐ Ⓑ Ⓒ Ⓓ Ⓔ	174 Ⓐ Ⓑ Ⓒ Ⓓ Ⓔ	194 Ⓐ Ⓑ Ⓒ Ⓓ Ⓔ	214 Ⓐ Ⓑ Ⓒ Ⓓ Ⓔ	234 Ⓐ Ⓑ Ⓒ Ⓓ Ⓔ
135 Ⓐ Ⓑ Ⓒ Ⓓ Ⓔ	155 Ⓐ Ⓑ Ⓒ Ⓓ Ⓔ	175 Ⓐ Ⓑ Ⓒ Ⓓ Ⓔ	195 Ⓐ Ⓑ Ⓒ Ⓓ Ⓔ	215 Ⓐ Ⓑ Ⓒ Ⓓ Ⓔ	235 Ⓐ Ⓑ Ⓒ Ⓓ Ⓔ
136 Ⓐ Ⓑ Ⓒ Ⓓ Ⓔ	156 Ⓐ Ⓑ Ⓒ Ⓓ Ⓔ	176 Ⓐ Ⓑ Ⓒ Ⓓ Ⓔ	196 Ⓐ Ⓑ Ⓒ Ⓓ Ⓔ	216 Ⓐ Ⓑ Ⓒ Ⓓ Ⓔ	236 Ⓐ Ⓑ Ⓒ Ⓓ Ⓔ
137 Ⓐ Ⓑ Ⓒ Ⓓ Ⓔ	157 Ⓐ Ⓑ Ⓒ Ⓓ Ⓔ	177 Ⓐ Ⓑ Ⓒ Ⓓ Ⓔ	197 Ⓐ Ⓑ Ⓒ Ⓓ Ⓔ	217 Ⓐ Ⓑ Ⓒ Ⓓ Ⓔ	237 Ⓐ Ⓑ Ⓒ Ⓓ Ⓔ
138 Ⓐ Ⓑ Ⓒ Ⓓ Ⓔ	158 Ⓐ Ⓑ Ⓒ Ⓓ Ⓔ	178 Ⓐ Ⓑ Ⓒ Ⓓ Ⓔ	198 Ⓐ Ⓑ Ⓒ Ⓓ Ⓔ	218 Ⓐ Ⓑ Ⓒ Ⓓ Ⓔ	238 Ⓐ Ⓑ Ⓒ Ⓓ Ⓔ
139 Ⓐ Ⓑ Ⓒ Ⓓ Ⓔ	159 Ⓐ Ⓑ Ⓒ Ⓓ Ⓔ	179 Ⓐ Ⓑ Ⓒ Ⓓ Ⓔ	199 Ⓐ Ⓑ Ⓒ Ⓓ Ⓔ	219 Ⓐ Ⓑ Ⓒ Ⓓ Ⓔ	239 Ⓐ Ⓑ Ⓒ Ⓓ Ⓔ
140 Ⓐ Ⓑ Ⓒ Ⓓ Ⓔ	160 Ⓐ Ⓑ Ⓒ Ⓓ Ⓔ	180 Ⓐ Ⓑ Ⓒ Ⓓ Ⓔ	200 Ⓐ Ⓑ Ⓒ Ⓓ Ⓔ	220 Ⓐ Ⓑ Ⓒ Ⓓ Ⓔ	240 Ⓐ Ⓑ Ⓒ Ⓓ Ⓔ

IDENTIFICATION NUMBER									EXAM TYPE	
0	0	0	0	0	0	0	0	0	0	0
1	1	1	1	1	1	1	1	1	1	1
2	2	2	2	2	2	2	2	2	2	2
3	3	3	3	3	3	3	3	3	3	3
4	4	4	4	4	4	4	4	4	4	4
5	5	5	5	5	5	5	5	5	5	5
6	6	6	6	6	6	6	6	6	6	6
7	7	7	7	7	7	7	7	7	7	7
8	8	8	8	8	8	8	8	8	8	8
9	9	9	9	9	9	9	9	9	9	9

TEST BOOKLET NUMBER				

IMPORTANT DIRECTIONS FOR MARKING ANSWERS

- Use black lead pencil only (No. 2½ or softer).
- Do NOT use ink, felt tip or ballpoint pens.
- Erase cleanly any answer you wish to change.
- Make no stray marks on the answer sheet.
- Make heavy black marks that fill the circle completely.

EXAMPLES

WRONG: Fill in the circle completely.

1 Ⓧ Ⓑ Ⓒ Ⓓ Ⓔ

2 Ⓐ ✓ Ⓒ Ⓓ Ⓔ

3 Ⓐ Ⓑ Ⓒ Ⓓ Ⓔ

WRONG: Make heavy black marks.

4 Ⓐ Ⓑ Ⓒ Ⓓ Ⓔ

RIGHT: Make heavy black marks that fill in the circle completely.

5 Ⓐ Ⓑ Ⓒ Ⓓ ●

NAME: ______

EXAM TYPE: ______ DATE: ______

BOARD OF REGISTRY

1 Ⓐ Ⓑ Ⓒ Ⓓ Ⓔ	21 Ⓐ Ⓑ Ⓒ Ⓓ Ⓔ	41 Ⓐ Ⓑ Ⓒ Ⓓ Ⓔ	61 Ⓐ Ⓑ Ⓒ Ⓓ Ⓔ	81 Ⓐ Ⓑ Ⓒ Ⓓ Ⓔ	101 Ⓐ Ⓑ Ⓒ Ⓓ Ⓔ
2 Ⓐ Ⓑ Ⓒ Ⓓ Ⓔ	22 Ⓐ Ⓑ Ⓒ Ⓓ Ⓔ	42 Ⓐ Ⓑ Ⓒ Ⓓ Ⓔ	62 Ⓐ Ⓑ Ⓒ Ⓓ Ⓔ	82 Ⓐ Ⓑ Ⓒ Ⓓ Ⓔ	102 Ⓐ Ⓑ Ⓒ Ⓓ Ⓔ
3 Ⓐ Ⓑ Ⓒ Ⓓ Ⓔ	23 Ⓐ Ⓑ Ⓒ Ⓓ Ⓔ	43 Ⓐ Ⓑ Ⓒ Ⓓ Ⓔ	63 Ⓐ Ⓑ Ⓒ Ⓓ Ⓔ	83 Ⓐ Ⓑ Ⓒ Ⓓ Ⓔ	103 Ⓐ Ⓑ Ⓒ Ⓓ Ⓔ
4 Ⓐ Ⓑ Ⓒ Ⓓ Ⓔ	24 Ⓐ Ⓑ Ⓒ Ⓓ Ⓔ	44 Ⓐ Ⓑ Ⓒ Ⓓ Ⓔ	64 Ⓐ Ⓑ Ⓒ Ⓓ Ⓔ	84 Ⓐ Ⓑ Ⓒ Ⓓ Ⓔ	104 Ⓐ Ⓑ Ⓒ Ⓓ Ⓔ
5 Ⓐ Ⓑ Ⓒ Ⓓ Ⓔ	25 Ⓐ Ⓑ Ⓒ Ⓓ Ⓔ	45 Ⓐ Ⓑ Ⓒ Ⓓ Ⓔ	65 Ⓐ Ⓑ Ⓒ Ⓓ Ⓔ	85 Ⓐ Ⓑ Ⓒ Ⓓ Ⓔ	105 Ⓐ Ⓑ Ⓒ Ⓓ Ⓔ
6 Ⓐ Ⓑ Ⓒ Ⓓ Ⓔ	26 Ⓐ Ⓑ Ⓒ Ⓓ Ⓔ	46 Ⓐ Ⓑ Ⓒ Ⓓ Ⓔ	66 Ⓐ Ⓑ Ⓒ Ⓓ Ⓔ	86 Ⓐ Ⓑ Ⓒ Ⓓ Ⓔ	106 Ⓐ Ⓑ Ⓒ Ⓓ Ⓔ
7 Ⓐ Ⓑ Ⓒ Ⓓ Ⓔ	27 Ⓐ Ⓑ Ⓒ Ⓓ Ⓔ	47 Ⓐ Ⓑ Ⓒ Ⓓ Ⓔ	67 Ⓐ Ⓑ Ⓒ Ⓓ Ⓔ	87 Ⓐ Ⓑ Ⓒ Ⓓ Ⓔ	107 Ⓐ Ⓑ Ⓒ Ⓓ Ⓔ
8 Ⓐ Ⓑ Ⓒ Ⓓ Ⓔ	28 Ⓐ Ⓑ Ⓒ Ⓓ Ⓔ	48 Ⓐ Ⓑ Ⓒ Ⓓ Ⓔ	68 Ⓐ Ⓑ Ⓒ Ⓓ Ⓔ	88 Ⓐ Ⓑ Ⓒ Ⓓ Ⓔ	108 Ⓐ Ⓑ Ⓒ Ⓓ Ⓔ
9 Ⓐ Ⓑ Ⓒ Ⓓ Ⓔ	29 Ⓐ Ⓑ Ⓒ Ⓓ Ⓔ	49 Ⓐ Ⓑ Ⓒ Ⓓ Ⓔ	69 Ⓐ Ⓑ Ⓒ Ⓓ Ⓔ	89 Ⓐ Ⓑ Ⓒ Ⓓ Ⓔ	109 Ⓐ Ⓑ Ⓒ Ⓓ Ⓔ
10 Ⓐ Ⓑ Ⓒ Ⓓ Ⓔ	30 Ⓐ Ⓑ Ⓒ Ⓓ Ⓔ	50 Ⓐ Ⓑ Ⓒ Ⓓ Ⓔ	70 Ⓐ Ⓑ Ⓒ Ⓓ Ⓔ	90 Ⓐ Ⓑ Ⓒ Ⓓ Ⓔ	110 Ⓐ Ⓑ Ⓒ Ⓓ Ⓔ
11 Ⓐ Ⓑ Ⓒ Ⓓ Ⓔ	31 Ⓐ Ⓑ Ⓒ Ⓓ Ⓔ	51 Ⓐ Ⓑ Ⓒ Ⓓ Ⓔ	71 Ⓐ Ⓑ Ⓒ Ⓓ Ⓔ	91 Ⓐ Ⓑ Ⓒ Ⓓ Ⓔ	111 Ⓐ Ⓑ Ⓒ Ⓓ Ⓔ
12 Ⓐ Ⓑ Ⓒ Ⓓ Ⓔ	32 Ⓐ Ⓑ Ⓒ Ⓓ Ⓔ	52 Ⓐ Ⓑ Ⓒ Ⓓ Ⓔ	72 Ⓐ Ⓑ Ⓒ Ⓓ Ⓔ	92 Ⓐ Ⓑ Ⓒ Ⓓ Ⓔ	112 Ⓐ Ⓑ Ⓒ Ⓓ Ⓔ
13 Ⓐ Ⓑ Ⓒ Ⓓ Ⓔ	33 Ⓐ Ⓑ Ⓒ Ⓓ Ⓔ	53 Ⓐ Ⓑ Ⓒ Ⓓ Ⓔ	73 Ⓐ Ⓑ Ⓒ Ⓓ Ⓔ	93 Ⓐ Ⓑ Ⓒ Ⓓ Ⓔ	113 Ⓐ Ⓑ Ⓒ Ⓓ Ⓔ
14 Ⓐ Ⓑ Ⓒ Ⓓ Ⓔ	34 Ⓐ Ⓑ Ⓒ Ⓓ Ⓔ	54 Ⓐ Ⓑ Ⓒ Ⓓ Ⓔ	74 Ⓐ Ⓑ Ⓒ Ⓓ Ⓔ	94 Ⓐ Ⓑ Ⓒ Ⓓ Ⓔ	114 Ⓐ Ⓑ Ⓒ Ⓓ Ⓔ
15 Ⓐ Ⓑ Ⓒ Ⓓ Ⓔ	35 Ⓐ Ⓑ Ⓒ Ⓓ Ⓔ	55 Ⓐ Ⓑ Ⓒ Ⓓ Ⓔ	75 Ⓐ Ⓑ Ⓒ Ⓓ Ⓔ	95 Ⓐ Ⓑ Ⓒ Ⓓ Ⓔ	115 Ⓐ Ⓑ Ⓒ Ⓓ Ⓔ
16 Ⓐ Ⓑ Ⓒ Ⓓ Ⓔ	36 Ⓐ Ⓑ Ⓒ Ⓓ Ⓔ	56 Ⓐ Ⓑ Ⓒ Ⓓ Ⓔ	76 Ⓐ Ⓑ Ⓒ Ⓓ Ⓔ	96 Ⓐ Ⓑ Ⓒ Ⓓ Ⓔ	116 Ⓐ Ⓑ Ⓒ Ⓓ Ⓔ
17 Ⓐ Ⓑ Ⓒ Ⓓ Ⓔ	37 Ⓐ Ⓑ Ⓒ Ⓓ Ⓔ	57 Ⓐ Ⓑ Ⓒ Ⓓ Ⓔ	77 Ⓐ Ⓑ Ⓒ Ⓓ Ⓔ	97 Ⓐ Ⓑ Ⓒ Ⓓ Ⓔ	117 Ⓐ Ⓑ Ⓒ Ⓓ Ⓔ
18 Ⓐ Ⓑ Ⓒ Ⓓ Ⓔ	38 Ⓐ Ⓑ Ⓒ Ⓓ Ⓔ	58 Ⓐ Ⓑ Ⓒ Ⓓ Ⓔ	78 Ⓐ Ⓑ Ⓒ Ⓓ Ⓔ	98 Ⓐ Ⓑ Ⓒ Ⓓ Ⓔ	118 Ⓐ Ⓑ Ⓒ Ⓓ Ⓔ
19 Ⓐ Ⓑ Ⓒ Ⓓ Ⓔ	39 Ⓐ Ⓑ Ⓒ Ⓓ Ⓔ	59 Ⓐ Ⓑ Ⓒ Ⓓ Ⓔ	79 Ⓐ Ⓑ Ⓒ Ⓓ Ⓔ	99 Ⓐ Ⓑ Ⓒ Ⓓ Ⓔ	119 Ⓐ Ⓑ Ⓒ Ⓓ Ⓔ
20 Ⓐ Ⓑ Ⓒ Ⓓ Ⓔ	40 Ⓐ Ⓑ Ⓒ Ⓓ Ⓔ	60 Ⓐ Ⓑ Ⓒ Ⓓ Ⓔ	80 Ⓐ Ⓑ Ⓒ Ⓓ Ⓔ	100 Ⓐ Ⓑ Ⓒ Ⓓ Ⓔ	120 Ⓐ Ⓑ Ⓒ Ⓓ Ⓔ

NCS Trans-Optic F6292-54321

SIDE ONE

TM

BOARD OF REGISTRY

founded in 1928 by the
American Society of Clinical Pathologists

Representatives from:

American Society of Clinical Pathologists
Medical Technologists/Technicians
Pathologists
American Academy of Microbiology
American Association of Blood Banks
American Society of Cytology
National Registry in Clinical Chemistry
American Society of Hematology
National Society for Histotechnology

IMPORTANT DIRECTIONS FOR MARKING ANSWERS

- Use black lead pencil only (No. 2½ or softer).
- Do NOT use ink, felt tip or ballpoint pens.
- Erase cleanly any answer you wish to change.
- Make no stray marks on the answer sheet.
- Make heavy black marks that fill the circle completely.

EXAMPLES

WRONG: Fill in the circle completely.
1 (A) (B) (C) (D) (E)
2 (A) (B) (C) (D) (E)
3 (A) (B) (C) (D) (E)

WRONG: Make heavy black marks.
4 (A) (B) (C) (D) (E)

RIGHT: Make heavy black marks that fill in the circle completely.
5 (A) (B) (C) (D) (E)

121 (A) (B) (C) (D) (E)
122 (A) (B) (C) (D) (E)
123 (A) (B) (C) (D) (E)
124 (A) (B) (C) (D) (E)
125 (A) (B) (C) (D) (E)
126 (A) (B) (C) (D) (E)
127 (A) (B) (C) (D) (E)
128 (A) (B) (C) (D) (E)
129 (A) (B) (C) (D) (E)
130 (A) (B) (C) (D) (E)
131 (A) (B) (C) (D) (E)
132 (A) (B) (C) (D) (E)
133 (A) (B) (C) (D) (E)
134 (A) (B) (C) (D) (E)
135 (A) (B) (C) (D) (E)
136 (A) (B) (C) (D) (E)
137 (A) (B) (C) (D) (E)
138 (A) (B) (C) (D) (E)
139 (A) (B) (C) (D) (E)
140 (A) (B) (C) (D) (E)

141 (A) (B) (C) (D) (E)
142 (A) (B) (C) (D) (E)
143 (A) (B) (C) (D) (E)
144 (A) (B) (C) (D) (E)
145 (A) (B) (C) (D) (E)
146 (A) (B) (C) (D) (E)
147 (A) (B) (C) (D) (E)
148 (A) (B) (C) (D) (E)
149 (A) (B) (C) (D) (E)
150 (A) (B) (C) (D) (E)
151 (A) (B) (C) (D) (E)
152 (A) (B) (C) (D) (E)
153 (A) (B) (C) (D) (E)
154 (A) (B) (C) (D) (E)
155 (A) (B) (C) (D) (E)
156 (A) (B) (C) (D) (E)
157 (A) (B) (C) (D) (E)
158 (A) (B) (C) (D) (E)
159 (A) (B) (C) (D) (E)
160 (A) (B) (C) (D) (E)

161 (A) (B) (C) (D) (E)
162 (A) (B) (C) (D) (E)
163 (A) (B) (C) (D) (E)
164 (A) (B) (C) (D) (E)
165 (A) (B) (C) (D) (E)
166 (A) (B) (C) (D) (E)
167 (A) (B) (C) (D) (E)
168 (A) (B) (C) (D) (E)
169 (A) (B) (C) (D) (E)
170 (A) (B) (C) (D) (E)
171 (A) (B) (C) (D) (E)
172 (A) (B) (C) (D) (E)
173 (A) (B) (C) (D) (E)
174 (A) (B) (C) (D) (E)
175 (A) (B) (C) (D) (E)
176 (A) (B) (C) (D) (E)
177 (A) (B) (C) (D) (E)
178 (A) (B) (C) (D) (E)
179 (A) (B) (C) (D) (E)
180 (A) (B) (C) (D) (E)

181 (A) (B) (C) (D) (E)
182 (A) (B) (C) (D) (E)
183 (A) (B) (C) (D) (E)
184 (A) (B) (C) (D) (E)
185 (A) (B) (C) (D) (E)
186 (A) (B) (C) (D) (E)
187 (A) (B) (C) (D) (E)
188 (A) (B) (C) (D) (E)
189 (A) (B) (C) (D) (E)
190 (A) (B) (C) (D) (E)
191 (A) (B) (C) (D) (E)
192 (A) (B) (C) (D) (E)
193 (A) (B) (C) (D) (E)
194 (A) (B) (C) (D) (E)
195 (A) (B) (C) (D) (E)
196 (A) (B) (C) (D) (E)
197 (A) (B) (C) (D) (E)
198 (A) (B) (C) (D) (E)
199 (A) (B) (C) (D) (E)
200 (A) (B) (C) (D) (E)

201 (A) (B) (C) (D) (E)
202 (A) (B) (C) (D) (E)
203 (A) (B) (C) (D) (E)
204 (A) (B) (C) (D) (E)
205 (A) (B) (C) (D) (E)
206 (A) (B) (C) (D) (E)
207 (A) (B) (C) (D) (E)
208 (A) (B) (C) (D) (E)
209 (A) (B) (C) (D) (E)
210 (A) (B) (C) (D) (E)
211 (A) (B) (C) (D) (E)
212 (A) (B) (C) (D) (E)
213 (A) (B) (C) (D) (E)
214 (A) (B) (C) (D) (E)
215 (A) (B) (C) (D) (E)
216 (A) (B) (C) (D) (E)
217 (A) (B) (C) (D) (E)
218 (A) (B) (C) (D) (E)
219 (A) (B) (C) (D) (E)
220 (A) (B) (C) (D) (E)

221 (A) (B) (C) (D) (E)
222 (A) (B) (C) (D) (E)
223 (A) (B) (C) (D) (E)
224 (A) (B) (C) (D) (E)
225 (A) (B) (C) (D) (E)
226 (A) (B) (C) (D) (E)
227 (A) (B) (C) (D) (E)
228 (A) (B) (C) (D) (E)
229 (A) (B) (C) (D) (E)
230 (A) (B) (C) (D) (E)
231 (A) (B) (C) (D) (E)
232 (A) (B) (C) (D) (E)
233 (A) (B) (C) (D) (E)
234 (A) (B) (C) (D) (E)
235 (A) (B) (C) (D) (E)
236 (A) (B) (C) (D) (E)
237 (A) (B) (C) (D) (E)
238 (A) (B) (C) (D) (E)
239 (A) (B) (C) (D) (E)
240 (A) (B) (C) (D) (E)

BOARD OF REGISTRY

NAME: ____________________

EXAM TYPE: ____________________ DATE: ____________________

IDENTIFICATION NUMBER									EXAM TYPE	
⓪	⓪	⓪	⓪	⓪	⓪	⓪	⓪	⓪	⓪	⓪
①	①	①	①	①	①	①	①	①	①	①
②	②	②	②	②	②	②	②	②	②	②
③	③	③	③	③	③	③	③	③	③	③
④	④	④	④	④	④	④	④	④	④	④
⑤	⑤	⑤	⑤	⑤	⑤	⑤	⑤	⑤	⑤	⑤
⑥	⑥	⑥	⑥	⑥	⑥	⑥	⑥	⑥	⑥	⑥
⑦	⑦	⑦	⑦	⑦	⑦	⑦	⑦	⑦	⑦	⑦
⑧	⑧	⑧	⑧	⑧	⑧	⑧	⑧	⑧	⑧	⑧
⑨	⑨	⑨	⑨	⑨	⑨	⑨	⑨	⑨	⑨	⑨

TEST BOOKLET NUMBER				

IMPORTANT DIRECTIONS FOR MARKING ANSWERS

- Use black lead pencil only (No. 2½ or softer).
- Do NOT use ink, felt tip or ballpoint pens.
- Erase cleanly any answer you wish to change.
- Make no stray marks on the answer sheet.
- Make heavy black marks that fill the circle completely.

EXAMPLES

WRONG: Fill in the circle completely.

1 Ⓧ Ⓑ Ⓒ Ⓓ Ⓔ

2 Ⓐ ✓ Ⓒ Ⓓ Ⓔ

3 Ⓐ Ⓑ Ⓒ Ⓓ Ⓔ

WRONG: Make heavy black marks.

4 Ⓐ Ⓑ Ⓒ Ⓓ Ⓔ

RIGHT: Make heavy black marks that fill in the circle completely.

5 Ⓐ Ⓑ Ⓒ Ⓓ ●

1 Ⓐ Ⓑ Ⓒ Ⓓ Ⓔ	21 Ⓐ Ⓑ Ⓒ Ⓓ Ⓔ	41 Ⓐ Ⓑ Ⓒ Ⓓ Ⓔ	61 Ⓐ Ⓑ Ⓒ Ⓓ Ⓔ	81 Ⓐ Ⓑ Ⓒ Ⓓ Ⓔ	101 Ⓐ Ⓑ Ⓒ Ⓓ Ⓔ
2 Ⓐ Ⓑ Ⓒ Ⓓ Ⓔ	22 Ⓐ Ⓑ Ⓒ Ⓓ Ⓔ	42 Ⓐ Ⓑ Ⓒ Ⓓ Ⓔ	62 Ⓐ Ⓑ Ⓒ Ⓓ Ⓔ	82 Ⓐ Ⓑ Ⓒ Ⓓ Ⓔ	102 Ⓐ Ⓑ Ⓒ Ⓓ Ⓔ
3 Ⓐ Ⓑ Ⓒ Ⓓ Ⓔ	23 Ⓐ Ⓑ Ⓒ Ⓓ Ⓔ	43 Ⓐ Ⓑ Ⓒ Ⓓ Ⓔ	63 Ⓐ Ⓑ Ⓒ Ⓓ Ⓔ	83 Ⓐ Ⓑ Ⓒ Ⓓ Ⓔ	103 Ⓐ Ⓑ Ⓒ Ⓓ Ⓔ
4 Ⓐ Ⓑ Ⓒ Ⓓ Ⓔ	24 Ⓐ Ⓑ Ⓒ Ⓓ Ⓔ	44 Ⓐ Ⓑ Ⓒ Ⓓ Ⓔ	64 Ⓐ Ⓑ Ⓒ Ⓓ Ⓔ	84 Ⓐ Ⓑ Ⓒ Ⓓ Ⓔ	104 Ⓐ Ⓑ Ⓒ Ⓓ Ⓔ
5 Ⓐ Ⓑ Ⓒ Ⓓ Ⓔ	25 Ⓐ Ⓑ Ⓒ Ⓓ Ⓔ	45 Ⓐ Ⓑ Ⓒ Ⓓ Ⓔ	65 Ⓐ Ⓑ Ⓒ Ⓓ Ⓔ	85 Ⓐ Ⓑ Ⓒ Ⓓ Ⓔ	105 Ⓐ Ⓑ Ⓒ Ⓓ Ⓔ
6 Ⓐ Ⓑ Ⓒ Ⓓ Ⓔ	26 Ⓐ Ⓑ Ⓒ Ⓓ Ⓔ	46 Ⓐ Ⓑ Ⓒ Ⓓ Ⓔ	66 Ⓐ Ⓑ Ⓒ Ⓓ Ⓔ	86 Ⓐ Ⓑ Ⓒ Ⓓ Ⓔ	106 Ⓐ Ⓑ Ⓒ Ⓓ Ⓔ
7 Ⓐ Ⓑ Ⓒ Ⓓ Ⓔ	27 Ⓐ Ⓑ Ⓒ Ⓓ Ⓔ	47 Ⓐ Ⓑ Ⓒ Ⓓ Ⓔ	67 Ⓐ Ⓑ Ⓒ Ⓓ Ⓔ	87 Ⓐ Ⓑ Ⓒ Ⓓ Ⓔ	107 Ⓐ Ⓑ Ⓒ Ⓓ Ⓔ
8 Ⓐ Ⓑ Ⓒ Ⓓ Ⓔ	28 Ⓐ Ⓑ Ⓒ Ⓓ Ⓔ	48 Ⓐ Ⓑ Ⓒ Ⓓ Ⓔ	68 Ⓐ Ⓑ Ⓒ Ⓓ Ⓔ	88 Ⓐ Ⓑ Ⓒ Ⓓ Ⓔ	108 Ⓐ Ⓑ Ⓒ Ⓓ Ⓔ
9 Ⓐ Ⓑ Ⓒ Ⓓ Ⓔ	29 Ⓐ Ⓑ Ⓒ Ⓓ Ⓔ	49 Ⓐ Ⓑ Ⓒ Ⓓ Ⓔ	69 Ⓐ Ⓑ Ⓒ Ⓓ Ⓔ	89 Ⓐ Ⓑ Ⓒ Ⓓ Ⓔ	109 Ⓐ Ⓑ Ⓒ Ⓓ Ⓔ
10 Ⓐ Ⓑ Ⓒ Ⓓ Ⓔ	30 Ⓐ Ⓑ Ⓒ Ⓓ Ⓔ	50 Ⓐ Ⓑ Ⓒ Ⓓ Ⓔ	70 Ⓐ Ⓑ Ⓒ Ⓓ Ⓔ	90 Ⓐ Ⓑ Ⓒ Ⓓ Ⓔ	110 Ⓐ Ⓑ Ⓒ Ⓓ Ⓔ
11 Ⓐ Ⓑ Ⓒ Ⓓ Ⓔ	31 Ⓐ Ⓑ Ⓒ Ⓓ Ⓔ	51 Ⓐ Ⓑ Ⓒ Ⓓ Ⓔ	71 Ⓐ Ⓑ Ⓒ Ⓓ Ⓔ	91 Ⓐ Ⓑ Ⓒ Ⓓ Ⓔ	111 Ⓐ Ⓑ Ⓒ Ⓓ Ⓔ
12 Ⓐ Ⓑ Ⓒ Ⓓ Ⓔ	32 Ⓐ Ⓑ Ⓒ Ⓓ Ⓔ	52 Ⓐ Ⓑ Ⓒ Ⓓ Ⓔ	72 Ⓐ Ⓑ Ⓒ Ⓓ Ⓔ	92 Ⓐ Ⓑ Ⓒ Ⓓ Ⓔ	112 Ⓐ Ⓑ Ⓒ Ⓓ Ⓔ
13 Ⓐ Ⓑ Ⓒ Ⓓ Ⓔ	33 Ⓐ Ⓑ Ⓒ Ⓓ Ⓔ	53 Ⓐ Ⓑ Ⓒ Ⓓ Ⓔ	73 Ⓐ Ⓑ Ⓒ Ⓓ Ⓔ	93 Ⓐ Ⓑ Ⓒ Ⓓ Ⓔ	113 Ⓐ Ⓑ Ⓒ Ⓓ Ⓔ
14 Ⓐ Ⓑ Ⓒ Ⓓ Ⓔ	34 Ⓐ Ⓑ Ⓒ Ⓓ Ⓔ	54 Ⓐ Ⓑ Ⓒ Ⓓ Ⓔ	74 Ⓐ Ⓑ Ⓒ Ⓓ Ⓔ	94 Ⓐ Ⓑ Ⓒ Ⓓ Ⓔ	114 Ⓐ Ⓑ Ⓒ Ⓓ Ⓔ
15 Ⓐ Ⓑ Ⓒ Ⓓ Ⓔ	35 Ⓐ Ⓑ Ⓒ Ⓓ Ⓔ	55 Ⓐ Ⓑ Ⓒ Ⓓ Ⓔ	75 Ⓐ Ⓑ Ⓒ Ⓓ Ⓔ	95 Ⓐ Ⓑ Ⓒ Ⓓ Ⓔ	115 Ⓐ Ⓑ Ⓒ Ⓓ Ⓔ
16 Ⓐ Ⓑ Ⓒ Ⓓ Ⓔ	36 Ⓐ Ⓑ Ⓒ Ⓓ Ⓔ	56 Ⓐ Ⓑ Ⓒ Ⓓ Ⓔ	76 Ⓐ Ⓑ Ⓒ Ⓓ Ⓔ	96 Ⓐ Ⓑ Ⓒ Ⓓ Ⓔ	116 Ⓐ Ⓑ Ⓒ Ⓓ Ⓔ
17 Ⓐ Ⓑ Ⓒ Ⓓ Ⓔ	37 Ⓐ Ⓑ Ⓒ Ⓓ Ⓔ	57 Ⓐ Ⓑ Ⓒ Ⓓ Ⓔ	77 Ⓐ Ⓑ Ⓒ Ⓓ Ⓔ	97 Ⓐ Ⓑ Ⓒ Ⓓ Ⓔ	117 Ⓐ Ⓑ Ⓒ Ⓓ Ⓔ
18 Ⓐ Ⓑ Ⓒ Ⓓ Ⓔ	38 Ⓐ Ⓑ Ⓒ Ⓓ Ⓔ	58 Ⓐ Ⓑ Ⓒ Ⓓ Ⓔ	78 Ⓐ Ⓑ Ⓒ Ⓓ Ⓔ	98 Ⓐ Ⓑ Ⓒ Ⓓ Ⓔ	118 Ⓐ Ⓑ Ⓒ Ⓓ Ⓔ
19 Ⓐ Ⓑ Ⓒ Ⓓ Ⓔ	39 Ⓐ Ⓑ Ⓒ Ⓓ Ⓔ	59 Ⓐ Ⓑ Ⓒ Ⓓ Ⓔ	79 Ⓐ Ⓑ Ⓒ Ⓓ Ⓔ	99 Ⓐ Ⓑ Ⓒ Ⓓ Ⓔ	119 Ⓐ Ⓑ Ⓒ Ⓓ Ⓔ
20 Ⓐ Ⓑ Ⓒ Ⓓ Ⓔ	40 Ⓐ Ⓑ Ⓒ Ⓓ Ⓔ	60 Ⓐ Ⓑ Ⓒ Ⓓ Ⓔ	80 Ⓐ Ⓑ Ⓒ Ⓓ Ⓔ	100 Ⓐ Ⓑ Ⓒ Ⓓ Ⓔ	120 Ⓐ Ⓑ Ⓒ Ⓓ Ⓔ

NCS Trans-Optic F6292-54321

SIDE ONE

TM

BOARD OF REGISTRY

founded in 1928 by the
American Society of Clinical Pathologists

Representatives from:

American Society of Clinical Pathologists
Medical Technologists/Technicians
Pathologists
American Academy of Microbiology
American Association of Blood Banks
American Society of Cytology
National Registry in Clinical Chemistry
American Society of Hematology
National Society for Histotechnology

IMPORTANT DIRECTIONS FOR MARKING ANSWERS

- Use black lead pencil only (No. 2½ or softer).
- Do NOT use ink, felt tip or ballpoint pens.
- Erase cleanly any answer you wish to change.
- Make no stray marks on the answer sheet.
- Make heavy black marks that fill the circle completely.

EXAMPLES

1 Ⓐ Ⓑ Ⓒ Ⓓ Ⓔ — WRONG: Fill in the circle completely.
2 Ⓐ Ⓑ Ⓒ Ⓓ Ⓔ
3 Ⓐ Ⓑ Ⓒ Ⓓ Ⓔ
4 Ⓐ Ⓑ Ⓒ Ⓓ Ⓔ — WRONG: Make heavy black marks.
5 Ⓐ Ⓑ Ⓒ Ⓓ ● — RIGHT: Make heavy black marks that fill in the circle completely.

121 Ⓐ Ⓑ Ⓒ Ⓓ Ⓔ	141 Ⓐ Ⓑ Ⓒ Ⓓ Ⓔ	161 Ⓐ Ⓑ Ⓒ Ⓓ Ⓔ	181 Ⓐ Ⓑ Ⓒ Ⓓ Ⓔ	201 Ⓐ Ⓑ Ⓒ Ⓓ Ⓔ	221 Ⓐ Ⓑ Ⓒ Ⓓ Ⓔ
122 Ⓐ Ⓑ Ⓒ Ⓓ Ⓔ	142 Ⓐ Ⓑ Ⓒ Ⓓ Ⓔ	162 Ⓐ Ⓑ Ⓒ Ⓓ Ⓔ	182 Ⓐ Ⓑ Ⓒ Ⓓ Ⓔ	202 Ⓐ Ⓑ Ⓒ Ⓓ Ⓔ	222 Ⓐ Ⓑ Ⓒ Ⓓ Ⓔ
123 Ⓐ Ⓑ Ⓒ Ⓓ Ⓔ	143 Ⓐ Ⓑ Ⓒ Ⓓ Ⓔ	163 Ⓐ Ⓑ Ⓒ Ⓓ Ⓔ	183 Ⓐ Ⓑ Ⓒ Ⓓ Ⓔ	203 Ⓐ Ⓑ Ⓒ Ⓓ Ⓔ	223 Ⓐ Ⓑ Ⓒ Ⓓ Ⓔ
124 Ⓐ Ⓑ Ⓒ Ⓓ Ⓔ	144 Ⓐ Ⓑ Ⓒ Ⓓ Ⓔ	164 Ⓐ Ⓑ Ⓒ Ⓓ Ⓔ	184 Ⓐ Ⓑ Ⓒ Ⓓ Ⓔ	204 Ⓐ Ⓑ Ⓒ Ⓓ Ⓔ	224 Ⓐ Ⓑ Ⓒ Ⓓ Ⓔ
125 Ⓐ Ⓑ Ⓒ Ⓓ Ⓔ	145 Ⓐ Ⓑ Ⓒ Ⓓ Ⓔ	165 Ⓐ Ⓑ Ⓒ Ⓓ Ⓔ	185 Ⓐ Ⓑ Ⓒ Ⓓ Ⓔ	205 Ⓐ Ⓑ Ⓒ Ⓓ Ⓔ	225 Ⓐ Ⓑ Ⓒ Ⓓ Ⓔ
126 Ⓐ Ⓑ Ⓒ Ⓓ Ⓔ	146 Ⓐ Ⓑ Ⓒ Ⓓ Ⓔ	166 Ⓐ Ⓑ Ⓒ Ⓓ Ⓔ	186 Ⓐ Ⓑ Ⓒ Ⓓ Ⓔ	206 Ⓐ Ⓑ Ⓒ Ⓓ Ⓔ	226 Ⓐ Ⓑ Ⓒ Ⓓ Ⓔ
127 Ⓐ Ⓑ Ⓒ Ⓓ Ⓔ	147 Ⓐ Ⓑ Ⓒ Ⓓ Ⓔ	167 Ⓐ Ⓑ Ⓒ Ⓓ Ⓔ	187 Ⓐ Ⓑ Ⓒ Ⓓ Ⓔ	207 Ⓐ Ⓑ Ⓒ Ⓓ Ⓔ	227 Ⓐ Ⓑ Ⓒ Ⓓ Ⓔ
128 Ⓐ Ⓑ Ⓒ Ⓓ Ⓔ	148 Ⓐ Ⓑ Ⓒ Ⓓ Ⓔ	168 Ⓐ Ⓑ Ⓒ Ⓓ Ⓔ	188 Ⓐ Ⓑ Ⓒ Ⓓ Ⓔ	208 Ⓐ Ⓑ Ⓒ Ⓓ Ⓔ	228 Ⓐ Ⓑ Ⓒ Ⓓ Ⓔ
129 Ⓐ Ⓑ Ⓒ Ⓓ Ⓔ	149 Ⓐ Ⓑ Ⓒ Ⓓ Ⓔ	169 Ⓐ Ⓑ Ⓒ Ⓓ Ⓔ	189 Ⓐ Ⓑ Ⓒ Ⓓ Ⓔ	209 Ⓐ Ⓑ Ⓒ Ⓓ Ⓔ	229 Ⓐ Ⓑ Ⓒ Ⓓ Ⓔ
130 Ⓐ Ⓑ Ⓒ Ⓓ Ⓔ	150 Ⓐ Ⓑ Ⓒ Ⓓ Ⓔ	170 Ⓐ Ⓑ Ⓒ Ⓓ Ⓔ	190 Ⓐ Ⓑ Ⓒ Ⓓ Ⓔ	210 Ⓐ Ⓑ Ⓒ Ⓓ Ⓔ	230 Ⓐ Ⓑ Ⓒ Ⓓ Ⓔ
131 Ⓐ Ⓑ Ⓒ Ⓓ Ⓔ	151 Ⓐ Ⓑ Ⓒ Ⓓ Ⓔ	171 Ⓐ Ⓑ Ⓒ Ⓓ Ⓔ	191 Ⓐ Ⓑ Ⓒ Ⓓ Ⓔ	211 Ⓐ Ⓑ Ⓒ Ⓓ Ⓔ	231 Ⓐ Ⓑ Ⓒ Ⓓ Ⓔ
132 Ⓐ Ⓑ Ⓒ Ⓓ Ⓔ	152 Ⓐ Ⓑ Ⓒ Ⓓ Ⓔ	172 Ⓐ Ⓑ Ⓒ Ⓓ Ⓔ	192 Ⓐ Ⓑ Ⓒ Ⓓ Ⓔ	212 Ⓐ Ⓑ Ⓒ Ⓓ Ⓔ	232 Ⓐ Ⓑ Ⓒ Ⓓ Ⓔ
133 Ⓐ Ⓑ Ⓒ Ⓓ Ⓔ	153 Ⓐ Ⓑ Ⓒ Ⓓ Ⓔ	173 Ⓐ Ⓑ Ⓒ Ⓓ Ⓔ	193 Ⓐ Ⓑ Ⓒ Ⓓ Ⓔ	213 Ⓐ Ⓑ Ⓒ Ⓓ Ⓔ	233 Ⓐ Ⓑ Ⓒ Ⓓ Ⓔ
134 Ⓐ Ⓑ Ⓒ Ⓓ Ⓔ	154 Ⓐ Ⓑ Ⓒ Ⓓ Ⓔ	174 Ⓐ Ⓑ Ⓒ Ⓓ Ⓔ	194 Ⓐ Ⓑ Ⓒ Ⓓ Ⓔ	214 Ⓐ Ⓑ Ⓒ Ⓓ Ⓔ	234 Ⓐ Ⓑ Ⓒ Ⓓ Ⓔ
135 Ⓐ Ⓑ Ⓒ Ⓓ Ⓔ	155 Ⓐ Ⓑ Ⓒ Ⓓ Ⓔ	175 Ⓐ Ⓑ Ⓒ Ⓓ Ⓔ	195 Ⓐ Ⓑ Ⓒ Ⓓ Ⓔ	215 Ⓐ Ⓑ Ⓒ Ⓓ Ⓔ	235 Ⓐ Ⓑ Ⓒ Ⓓ Ⓔ
136 Ⓐ Ⓑ Ⓒ Ⓓ Ⓔ	156 Ⓐ Ⓑ Ⓒ Ⓓ Ⓔ	176 Ⓐ Ⓑ Ⓒ Ⓓ Ⓔ	196 Ⓐ Ⓑ Ⓒ Ⓓ Ⓔ	216 Ⓐ Ⓑ Ⓒ Ⓓ Ⓔ	236 Ⓐ Ⓑ Ⓒ Ⓓ Ⓔ
137 Ⓐ Ⓑ Ⓒ Ⓓ Ⓔ	157 Ⓐ Ⓑ Ⓒ Ⓓ Ⓔ	177 Ⓐ Ⓑ Ⓒ Ⓓ Ⓔ	197 Ⓐ Ⓑ Ⓒ Ⓓ Ⓔ	217 Ⓐ Ⓑ Ⓒ Ⓓ Ⓔ	237 Ⓐ Ⓑ Ⓒ Ⓓ Ⓔ
138 Ⓐ Ⓑ Ⓒ Ⓓ Ⓔ	158 Ⓐ Ⓑ Ⓒ Ⓓ Ⓔ	178 Ⓐ Ⓑ Ⓒ Ⓓ Ⓔ	198 Ⓐ Ⓑ Ⓒ Ⓓ Ⓔ	218 Ⓐ Ⓑ Ⓒ Ⓓ Ⓔ	238 Ⓐ Ⓑ Ⓒ Ⓓ Ⓔ
139 Ⓐ Ⓑ Ⓒ Ⓓ Ⓔ	159 Ⓐ Ⓑ Ⓒ Ⓓ Ⓔ	179 Ⓐ Ⓑ Ⓒ Ⓓ Ⓔ	199 Ⓐ Ⓑ Ⓒ Ⓓ Ⓔ	219 Ⓐ Ⓑ Ⓒ Ⓓ Ⓔ	239 Ⓐ Ⓑ Ⓒ Ⓓ Ⓔ
140 Ⓐ Ⓑ Ⓒ Ⓓ Ⓔ	160 Ⓐ Ⓑ Ⓒ Ⓓ Ⓔ	180 Ⓐ Ⓑ Ⓒ Ⓓ Ⓔ	200 Ⓐ Ⓑ Ⓒ Ⓓ Ⓔ	220 Ⓐ Ⓑ Ⓒ Ⓓ Ⓔ	240 Ⓐ Ⓑ Ⓒ Ⓓ Ⓔ

IDENTIFICATION NUMBER | EXAM TYPE

0	0	0	0	0	0	0	0	0	0	0
1	1	1	1	1	1	1	1	1	1	1
2	2	2	2	2	2	2	2	2	2	2
3	3	3	3	3	3	3	3	3	3	3
4	4	4	4	4	4	4	4	4	4	4
5	5	5	5	5	5	5	5	5	5	5
6	6	6	6	6	6	6	6	6	6	6
7	7	7	7	7	7	7	7	7	7	7
8	8	8	8	8	8	8	8	8	8	8
9	9	9	9	9	9	9	9	9	9	9

TEST BOOKLET NUMBER

IMPORTANT DIRECTIONS FOR MARKING ANSWERS

- Use black lead pencil only (No. 2½ or softer).
- Do NOT use ink, felt tip or ballpoint pens.
- Erase cleanly any answer you wish to change.
- Make no stray marks on the answer sheet.
- Make heavy black marks that fill the circle completely.

EXAMPLES

WRONG: Fill in the circle completely.
1 (A) (B) (C) (D) (E)
2 (A) (B) (C) (D) (E)
3 (A) (B) (C) (D) (E)

WRONG: Make heavy black marks.
4 (A) (B) (C) (D) (E)

RIGHT: Make heavy black marks that fill in the circle completely.
5 (A) (B) (C) (D) ●

NAME: ______

EXAM TYPE: ______ DATE: ______

BOARD OF REGISTRY

1 (A) (B) (C) (D) (E)
2 (A) (B) (C) (D) (E)
3 (A) (B) (C) (D) (E)
4 (A) (B) (C) (D) (E)
5 (A) (B) (C) (D) (E)
6 (A) (B) (C) (D) (E)
7 (A) (B) (C) (D) (E)
8 (A) (B) (C) (D) (E)
9 (A) (B) (C) (D) (E)
10 (A) (B) (C) (D) (E)
11 (A) (B) (C) (D) (E)
12 (A) (B) (C) (D) (E)
13 (A) (B) (C) (D) (E)
14 (A) (B) (C) (D) (E)
15 (A) (B) (C) (D) (E)
16 (A) (B) (C) (D) (E)
17 (A) (B) (C) (D) (E)
18 (A) (B) (C) (D) (E)
19 (A) (B) (C) (D) (E)
20 (A) (B) (C) (D) (E)
21 (A) (B) (C) (D) (E)
22 (A) (B) (C) (D) (E)
23 (A) (B) (C) (D) (E)
24 (A) (B) (C) (D) (E)
25 (A) (B) (C) (D) (E)
26 (A) (B) (C) (D) (E)
27 (A) (B) (C) (D) (E)
28 (A) (B) (C) (D) (E)
29 (A) (B) (C) (D) (E)
30 (A) (B) (C) (D) (E)
31 (A) (B) (C) (D) (E)
32 (A) (B) (C) (D) (E)
33 (A) (B) (C) (D) (E)
34 (A) (B) (C) (D) (E)
35 (A) (B) (C) (D) (E)
36 (A) (B) (C) (D) (E)
37 (A) (B) (C) (D) (E)
38 (A) (B) (C) (D) (E)
39 (A) (B) (C) (D) (E)
40 (A) (B) (C) (D) (E)
41 (A) (B) (C) (D) (E)
42 (A) (B) (C) (D) (E)
43 (A) (B) (C) (D) (E)
44 (A) (B) (C) (D) (E)
45 (A) (B) (C) (D) (E)
46 (A) (B) (C) (D) (E)
47 (A) (B) (C) (D) (E)
48 (A) (B) (C) (D) (E)
49 (A) (B) (C) (D) (E)
50 (A) (B) (C) (D) (E)
51 (A) (B) (C) (D) (E)
52 (A) (B) (C) (D) (E)
53 (A) (B) (C) (D) (E)
54 (A) (B) (C) (D) (E)
55 (A) (B) (C) (D) (E)
56 (A) (B) (C) (D) (E)
57 (A) (B) (C) (D) (E)
58 (A) (B) (C) (D) (E)
59 (A) (B) (C) (D) (E)
60 (A) (B) (C) (D) (E)
61 (A) (B) (C) (D) (E)
62 (A) (B) (C) (D) (E)
63 (A) (B) (C) (D) (E)
64 (A) (B) (C) (D) (E)
65 (A) (B) (C) (D) (E)
66 (A) (B) (C) (D) (E)
67 (A) (B) (C) (D) (E)
68 (A) (B) (C) (D) (E)
69 (A) (B) (C) (D) (E)
70 (A) (B) (C) (D) (E)
71 (A) (B) (C) (D) (E)
72 (A) (B) (C) (D) (E)
73 (A) (B) (C) (D) (E)
74 (A) (B) (C) (D) (E)
75 (A) (B) (C) (D) (E)
76 (A) (B) (C) (D) (E)
77 (A) (B) (C) (D) (E)
78 (A) (B) (C) (D) (E)
79 (A) (B) (C) (D) (E)
80 (A) (B) (C) (D) (E)
81 (A) (B) (C) (D) (E)
82 (A) (B) (C) (D) (E)
83 (A) (B) (C) (D) (E)
84 (A) (B) (C) (D) (E)
85 (A) (B) (C) (D) (E)
86 (A) (B) (C) (D) (E)
87 (A) (B) (C) (D) (E)
88 (A) (B) (C) (D) (E)
89 (A) (B) (C) (D) (E)
90 (A) (B) (C) (D) (E)
91 (A) (B) (C) (D) (E)
92 (A) (B) (C) (D) (E)
93 (A) (B) (C) (D) (E)
94 (A) (B) (C) (D) (E)
95 (A) (B) (C) (D) (E)
96 (A) (B) (C) (D) (E)
97 (A) (B) (C) (D) (E)
98 (A) (B) (C) (D) (E)
99 (A) (B) (C) (D) (E)
100 (A) (B) (C) (D) (E)
101 (A) (B) (C) (D) (E)
102 (A) (B) (C) (D) (E)
103 (A) (B) (C) (D) (E)
104 (A) (B) (C) (D) (E)
105 (A) (B) (C) (D) (E)
106 (A) (B) (C) (D) (E)
107 (A) (B) (C) (D) (E)
108 (A) (B) (C) (D) (E)
109 (A) (B) (C) (D) (E)
110 (A) (B) (C) (D) (E)
111 (A) (B) (C) (D) (E)
112 (A) (B) (C) (D) (E)
113 (A) (B) (C) (D) (E)
114 (A) (B) (C) (D) (E)
115 (A) (B) (C) (D) (E)
116 (A) (B) (C) (D) (E)
117 (A) (B) (C) (D) (E)
118 (A) (B) (C) (D) (E)
119 (A) (B) (C) (D) (E)
120 (A) (B) (C) (D) (E)

BOARD OF REGISTRY

founded in 1928 by the
American Society of Clinical Pathologists

Representatives from:

American Society of Clinical Pathologists
Medical Technologists/Technicians
Pathologists
American Academy of Microbiology
American Association of Blood Banks
American Society of Cytology
National Registry in Clinical Chemistry
American Society of Hematology
National Society for Histotechnology

IMPORTANT DIRECTIONS FOR MARKING ANSWERS

- Use black lead pencil only (No. 2½ or softer).
- Do NOT use ink, felt tip or ballpoint pens.
- Erase cleanly any answer you wish to change.
- Make no stray marks on the answer sheet.
- Make heavy black marks that fill the circle completely.

EXAMPLES

1 A B C D E — WRONG: Fill in the circle completely.
2 A B C D E
3 A B C D E
4 A B C D E — WRONG: Make heavy black marks.
5 A B C D E — RIGHT: Make heavy black marks that fill in the circle completely.

121 A B C D E	141 A B C D E	161 A B C D E	181 A B C D E	201 A B C D E	221 A B C D E
122 A B C D E	142 A B C D E	162 A B C D E	182 A B C D E	202 A B C D E	222 A B C D E
123 A B C D E	143 A B C D E	163 A B C D E	183 A B C D E	203 A B C D E	223 A B C D E
124 A B C D E	144 A B C D E	164 A B C D E	184 A B C D E	204 A B C D E	224 A B C D E
125 A B C D E	145 A B C D E	165 A B C D E	185 A B C D E	205 A B C D E	225 A B C D E
126 A B C D E	146 A B C D E	166 A B C D E	186 A B C D E	206 A B C D E	226 A B C D E
127 A B C D E	147 A B C D E	167 A B C D E	187 A B C D E	207 A B C D E	227 A B C D E
128 A B C D E	148 A B C D E	168 A B C D E	188 A B C D E	208 A B C D E	228 A B C D E
129 A B C D E	149 A B C D E	169 A B C D E	189 A B C D E	209 A B C D E	229 A B C D E
130 A B C D E	150 A B C D E	170 A B C D E	190 A B C D E	210 A B C D E	230 A B C D E
131 A B C D E	151 A B C D E	171 A B C D E	191 A B C D E	211 A B C D E	231 A B C D E
132 A B C D E	152 A B C D E	172 A B C D E	192 A B C D E	212 A B C D E	232 A B C D E
133 A B C D E	153 A B C D E	173 A B C D E	193 A B C D E	213 A B C D E	233 A B C D E
134 A B C D E	154 A B C D E	174 A B C D E	194 A B C D E	214 A B C D E	234 A B C D E
135 A B C D E	155 A B C D E	175 A B C D E	195 A B C D E	215 A B C D E	235 A B C D E
136 A B C D E	156 A B C D E	176 A B C D E	196 A B C D E	216 A B C D E	236 A B C D E
137 A B C D E	157 A B C D E	177 A B C D E	197 A B C D E	217 A B C D E	237 A B C D E
138 A B C D E	158 A B C D E	178 A B C D E	198 A B C D E	218 A B C D E	238 A B C D E
139 A B C D E	159 A B C D E	179 A B C D E	199 A B C D E	219 A B C D E	239 A B C D E
140 A B C D E	160 A B C D E	180 A B C D E	200 A B C D E	220 A B C D E	240 A B C D E

BOARD OF REGISTRY

NAME: ______________________

EXAM TYPE: ______________ DATE: ______________

IDENTIFICATION NUMBER									EXAM TYPE	
(0)	(0)	(0)	(0)	(0)	(0)	(0)	(0)	(0)	(0)	(0)
(1)	(1)	(1)	(1)	(1)	(1)	(1)	(1)	(1)	(1)	(1)
(2)	(2)	(2)	(2)	(2)	(2)	(2)	(2)	(2)	(2)	(2)
(3)	(3)	(3)	(3)	(3)	(3)	(3)	(3)	(3)	(3)	(3)
(4)	(4)	(4)	(4)	(4)	(4)	(4)	(4)	(4)	(4)	(4)
(5)	(5)	(5)	(5)	(5)	(5)	(5)	(5)	(5)	(5)	(5)
(6)	(6)	(6)	(6)	(6)	(6)	(6)	(6)	(6)	(6)	(6)
(7)	(7)	(7)	(7)	(7)	(7)	(7)	(7)	(7)	(7)	(7)
(8)	(8)	(8)	(8)	(8)	(8)	(8)	(8)	(8)	(8)	(8)
(9)	(9)	(9)	(9)	(9)	(9)	(9)	(9)	(9)	(9)	(9)

TEST BOOKLET NUMBER				

IMPORTANT DIRECTIONS FOR MARKING ANSWERS

- Use black lead pencil only (No. 2½ or softer).
- Do NOT use ink, felt tip or ballpoint pens.
- Erase cleanly any answer you wish to change.
- Make no stray marks on the answer sheet.
- Make heavy black marks that fill the circle completely.

EXAMPLES

WRONG: Fill in the circle completely.

1 (X) (B) (C) (D) (E)

2 (A) (✓) (C) (D) (E)

3 (A) (B) (●) (D) (E)

WRONG: Make heavy black marks.

4 (A) (B) (C) (D) (E)

RIGHT: Make heavy black marks that fill in the circle completely.

5 (A) (B) (C) (D) ●

1 (A) (B) (C) (D) (E)	21 (A) (B) (C) (D) (E)	41 (A) (B) (C) (D) (E)	61 (A) (B) (C) (D) (E)	81 (A) (B) (C) (D) (E)	101 (A) (B) (C) (D) (E)
2 (A) (B) (C) (D) (E)	22 (A) (B) (C) (D) (E)	42 (A) (B) (C) (D) (E)	62 (A) (B) (C) (D) (E)	82 (A) (B) (C) (D) (E)	102 (A) (B) (C) (D) (E)
3 (A) (B) (C) (D) (E)	23 (A) (B) (C) (D) (E)	43 (A) (B) (C) (D) (E)	63 (A) (B) (C) (D) (E)	83 (A) (B) (C) (D) (E)	103 (A) (B) (C) (D) (E)
4 (A) (B) (C) (D) (E)	24 (A) (B) (C) (D) (E)	44 (A) (B) (C) (D) (E)	64 (A) (B) (C) (D) (E)	84 (A) (B) (C) (D) (E)	104 (A) (B) (C) (D) (E)
5 (A) (B) (C) (D) (E)	25 (A) (B) (C) (D) (E)	45 (A) (B) (C) (D) (E)	65 (A) (B) (C) (D) (E)	85 (A) (B) (C) (D) (E)	105 (A) (B) (C) (D) (E)
6 (A) (B) (C) (D) (E)	26 (A) (B) (C) (D) (E)	46 (A) (B) (C) (D) (E)	66 (A) (B) (C) (D) (E)	86 (A) (B) (C) (D) (E)	106 (A) (B) (C) (D) (E)
7 (A) (B) (C) (D) (E)	27 (A) (B) (C) (D) (E)	47 (A) (B) (C) (D) (E)	67 (A) (B) (C) (D) (E)	87 (A) (B) (C) (D) (E)	107 (A) (B) (C) (D) (E)
8 (A) (B) (C) (D) (E)	28 (A) (B) (C) (D) (E)	48 (A) (B) (C) (D) (E)	68 (A) (B) (C) (D) (E)	88 (A) (B) (C) (D) (E)	108 (A) (B) (C) (D) (E)
9 (A) (B) (C) (D) (E)	29 (A) (B) (C) (D) (E)	49 (A) (B) (C) (D) (E)	69 (A) (B) (C) (D) (E)	89 (A) (B) (C) (D) (E)	109 (A) (B) (C) (D) (E)
10 (A) (B) (C) (D) (E)	30 (A) (B) (C) (D) (E)	50 (A) (B) (C) (D) (E)	70 (A) (B) (C) (D) (E)	90 (A) (B) (C) (D) (E)	110 (A) (B) (C) (D) (E)
11 (A) (B) (C) (D) (E)	31 (A) (B) (C) (D) (E)	51 (A) (B) (C) (D) (E)	71 (A) (B) (C) (D) (E)	91 (A) (B) (C) (D) (E)	111 (A) (B) (C) (D) (E)
12 (A) (B) (C) (D) (E)	32 (A) (B) (C) (D) (E)	52 (A) (B) (C) (D) (E)	72 (A) (B) (C) (D) (E)	92 (A) (B) (C) (D) (E)	112 (A) (B) (C) (D) (E)
13 (A) (B) (C) (D) (E)	33 (A) (B) (C) (D) (E)	53 (A) (B) (C) (D) (E)	73 (A) (B) (C) (D) (E)	93 (A) (B) (C) (D) (E)	113 (A) (B) (C) (D) (E)
14 (A) (B) (C) (D) (E)	34 (A) (B) (C) (D) (E)	54 (A) (B) (C) (D) (E)	74 (A) (B) (C) (D) (E)	94 (A) (B) (C) (D) (E)	114 (A) (B) (C) (D) (E)
15 (A) (B) (C) (D) (E)	35 (A) (B) (C) (D) (E)	55 (A) (B) (C) (D) (E)	75 (A) (B) (C) (D) (E)	95 (A) (B) (C) (D) (E)	115 (A) (B) (C) (D) (E)
16 (A) (B) (C) (D) (E)	36 (A) (B) (C) (D) (E)	56 (A) (B) (C) (D) (E)	76 (A) (B) (C) (D) (E)	96 (A) (B) (C) (D) (E)	116 (A) (B) (C) (D) (E)
17 (A) (B) (C) (D) (E)	37 (A) (B) (C) (D) (E)	57 (A) (B) (C) (D) (E)	77 (A) (B) (C) (D) (E)	97 (A) (B) (C) (D) (E)	117 (A) (B) (C) (D) (E)
18 (A) (B) (C) (D) (E)	38 (A) (B) (C) (D) (E)	58 (A) (B) (C) (D) (E)	78 (A) (B) (C) (D) (E)	98 (A) (B) (C) (D) (E)	118 (A) (B) (C) (D) (E)
19 (A) (B) (C) (D) (E)	39 (A) (B) (C) (D) (E)	59 (A) (B) (C) (D) (E)	79 (A) (B) (C) (D) (E)	99 (A) (B) (C) (D) (E)	119 (A) (B) (C) (D) (E)
20 (A) (B) (C) (D) (E)	40 (A) (B) (C) (D) (E)	60 (A) (B) (C) (D) (E)	80 (A) (B) (C) (D) (E)	100 (A) (B) (C) (D) (E)	120 (A) (B) (C) (D) (E)

NCS Trans-Optic F6292-54321

SIDE ONE

TM

BOARD OF REGISTRY

founded in 1928 by the
American Society of Clinical Pathologists

Representatives from:

American Society of Clinical Pathologists
Medical Technologists/Technicians
Pathologists
American Academy of Microbiology
American Association of Blood Banks
American Society of Cytology
National Registry in Clinical Chemistry
American Society of Hematology
National Society for Histotechnology

IMPORTANT DIRECTIONS FOR MARKING ANSWERS

- Use black lead pencil only (No. 2½ or softer).
- Do NOT use ink, felt tip or ballpoint pens.
- Erase cleanly any answer you wish to change.
- Make no stray marks on the answer sheet.
- Make heavy black marks that fill the circle completely.

EXAMPLES

1 Ⓐ Ⓑ Ⓒ Ⓓ Ⓔ WRONG: Fill in the circle completely.
2 Ⓐ Ⓑ Ⓒ Ⓓ Ⓔ
3 Ⓐ Ⓑ Ⓒ Ⓓ Ⓔ
4 Ⓐ Ⓑ Ⓒ Ⓓ Ⓔ WRONG: Make heavy black marks.
5 Ⓐ Ⓑ Ⓒ Ⓓ ● RIGHT: Make heavy black marks that fill in the circle completely.

121 Ⓐ Ⓑ Ⓒ Ⓓ Ⓔ
122 Ⓐ Ⓑ Ⓒ Ⓓ Ⓔ
123 Ⓐ Ⓑ Ⓒ Ⓓ Ⓔ
124 Ⓐ Ⓑ Ⓒ Ⓓ Ⓔ
125 Ⓐ Ⓑ Ⓒ Ⓓ Ⓔ
126 Ⓐ Ⓑ Ⓒ Ⓓ Ⓔ
127 Ⓐ Ⓑ Ⓒ Ⓓ Ⓔ
128 Ⓐ Ⓑ Ⓒ Ⓓ Ⓔ
129 Ⓐ Ⓑ Ⓒ Ⓓ Ⓔ
130 Ⓐ Ⓑ Ⓒ Ⓓ Ⓔ
131 Ⓐ Ⓑ Ⓒ Ⓓ Ⓔ
132 Ⓐ Ⓑ Ⓒ Ⓓ Ⓔ
133 Ⓐ Ⓑ Ⓒ Ⓓ Ⓔ
134 Ⓐ Ⓑ Ⓒ Ⓓ Ⓔ
135 Ⓐ Ⓑ Ⓒ Ⓓ Ⓔ
136 Ⓐ Ⓑ Ⓒ Ⓓ Ⓔ
137 Ⓐ Ⓑ Ⓒ Ⓓ Ⓔ
138 Ⓐ Ⓑ Ⓒ Ⓓ Ⓔ
139 Ⓐ Ⓑ Ⓒ Ⓓ Ⓔ
140 Ⓐ Ⓑ Ⓒ Ⓓ Ⓔ

141 Ⓐ Ⓑ Ⓒ Ⓓ Ⓔ
142 Ⓐ Ⓑ Ⓒ Ⓓ Ⓔ
143 Ⓐ Ⓑ Ⓒ Ⓓ Ⓔ
144 Ⓐ Ⓑ Ⓒ Ⓓ Ⓔ
145 Ⓐ Ⓑ Ⓒ Ⓓ Ⓔ
146 Ⓐ Ⓑ Ⓒ Ⓓ Ⓔ
147 Ⓐ Ⓑ Ⓒ Ⓓ Ⓔ
148 Ⓐ Ⓑ Ⓒ Ⓓ Ⓔ
149 Ⓐ Ⓑ Ⓒ Ⓓ Ⓔ
150 Ⓐ Ⓑ Ⓒ Ⓓ Ⓔ
151 Ⓐ Ⓑ Ⓒ Ⓓ Ⓔ
152 Ⓐ Ⓑ Ⓒ Ⓓ Ⓔ
153 Ⓐ Ⓑ Ⓒ Ⓓ Ⓔ
154 Ⓐ Ⓑ Ⓒ Ⓓ Ⓔ
155 Ⓐ Ⓑ Ⓒ Ⓓ Ⓔ
156 Ⓐ Ⓑ Ⓒ Ⓓ Ⓔ
157 Ⓐ Ⓑ Ⓒ Ⓓ Ⓔ
158 Ⓐ Ⓑ Ⓒ Ⓓ Ⓔ
159 Ⓐ Ⓑ Ⓒ Ⓓ Ⓔ
160 Ⓐ Ⓑ Ⓒ Ⓓ Ⓔ

161 Ⓐ Ⓑ Ⓒ Ⓓ Ⓔ
162 Ⓐ Ⓑ Ⓒ Ⓓ Ⓔ
163 Ⓐ Ⓑ Ⓒ Ⓓ Ⓔ
164 Ⓐ Ⓑ Ⓒ Ⓓ Ⓔ
165 Ⓐ Ⓑ Ⓒ Ⓓ Ⓔ
166 Ⓐ Ⓑ Ⓒ Ⓓ Ⓔ
167 Ⓐ Ⓑ Ⓒ Ⓓ Ⓔ
168 Ⓐ Ⓑ Ⓒ Ⓓ Ⓔ
169 Ⓐ Ⓑ Ⓒ Ⓓ Ⓔ
170 Ⓐ Ⓑ Ⓒ Ⓓ Ⓔ
171 Ⓐ Ⓑ Ⓒ Ⓓ Ⓔ
172 Ⓐ Ⓑ Ⓒ Ⓓ Ⓔ
173 Ⓐ Ⓑ Ⓒ Ⓓ Ⓔ
174 Ⓐ Ⓑ Ⓒ Ⓓ Ⓔ
175 Ⓐ Ⓑ Ⓒ Ⓓ Ⓔ
176 Ⓐ Ⓑ Ⓒ Ⓓ Ⓔ
177 Ⓐ Ⓑ Ⓒ Ⓓ Ⓔ
178 Ⓐ Ⓑ Ⓒ Ⓓ Ⓔ
179 Ⓐ Ⓑ Ⓒ Ⓓ Ⓔ
180 Ⓐ Ⓑ Ⓒ Ⓓ Ⓔ

181 Ⓐ Ⓑ Ⓒ Ⓓ Ⓔ
182 Ⓐ Ⓑ Ⓒ Ⓓ Ⓔ
183 Ⓐ Ⓑ Ⓒ Ⓓ Ⓔ
184 Ⓐ Ⓑ Ⓒ Ⓓ Ⓔ
185 Ⓐ Ⓑ Ⓒ Ⓓ Ⓔ
186 Ⓐ Ⓑ Ⓒ Ⓓ Ⓔ
187 Ⓐ Ⓑ Ⓒ Ⓓ Ⓔ
188 Ⓐ Ⓑ Ⓒ Ⓓ Ⓔ
189 Ⓐ Ⓑ Ⓒ Ⓓ Ⓔ
190 Ⓐ Ⓑ Ⓒ Ⓓ Ⓔ
191 Ⓐ Ⓑ Ⓒ Ⓓ Ⓔ
192 Ⓐ Ⓑ Ⓒ Ⓓ Ⓔ
193 Ⓐ Ⓑ Ⓒ Ⓓ Ⓔ
194 Ⓐ Ⓑ Ⓒ Ⓓ Ⓔ
195 Ⓐ Ⓑ Ⓒ Ⓓ Ⓔ
196 Ⓐ Ⓑ Ⓒ Ⓓ Ⓔ
197 Ⓐ Ⓑ Ⓒ Ⓓ Ⓔ
198 Ⓐ Ⓑ Ⓒ Ⓓ Ⓔ
199 Ⓐ Ⓑ Ⓒ Ⓓ Ⓔ
200 Ⓐ Ⓑ Ⓒ Ⓓ Ⓔ

201 Ⓐ Ⓑ Ⓒ Ⓓ Ⓔ
202 Ⓐ Ⓑ Ⓒ Ⓓ Ⓔ
203 Ⓐ Ⓑ Ⓒ Ⓓ Ⓔ
204 Ⓐ Ⓑ Ⓒ Ⓓ Ⓔ
205 Ⓐ Ⓑ Ⓒ Ⓓ Ⓔ
206 Ⓐ Ⓑ Ⓒ Ⓓ Ⓔ
207 Ⓐ Ⓑ Ⓒ Ⓓ Ⓔ
208 Ⓐ Ⓑ Ⓒ Ⓓ Ⓔ
209 Ⓐ Ⓑ Ⓒ Ⓓ Ⓔ
210 Ⓐ Ⓑ Ⓒ Ⓓ Ⓔ
211 Ⓐ Ⓑ Ⓒ Ⓓ Ⓔ
212 Ⓐ Ⓑ Ⓒ Ⓓ Ⓔ
213 Ⓐ Ⓑ Ⓒ Ⓓ Ⓔ
214 Ⓐ Ⓑ Ⓒ Ⓓ Ⓔ
215 Ⓐ Ⓑ Ⓒ Ⓓ Ⓔ
216 Ⓐ Ⓑ Ⓒ Ⓓ Ⓔ
217 Ⓐ Ⓑ Ⓒ Ⓓ Ⓔ
218 Ⓐ Ⓑ Ⓒ Ⓓ Ⓔ
219 Ⓐ Ⓑ Ⓒ Ⓓ Ⓔ
220 Ⓐ Ⓑ Ⓒ Ⓓ Ⓔ

221 Ⓐ Ⓑ Ⓒ Ⓓ Ⓔ
222 Ⓐ Ⓑ Ⓒ Ⓓ Ⓔ
223 Ⓐ Ⓑ Ⓒ Ⓓ Ⓔ
224 Ⓐ Ⓑ Ⓒ Ⓓ Ⓔ
225 Ⓐ Ⓑ Ⓒ Ⓓ Ⓔ
226 Ⓐ Ⓑ Ⓒ Ⓓ Ⓔ
227 Ⓐ Ⓑ Ⓒ Ⓓ Ⓔ
228 Ⓐ Ⓑ Ⓒ Ⓓ Ⓔ
229 Ⓐ Ⓑ Ⓒ Ⓓ Ⓔ
230 Ⓐ Ⓑ Ⓒ Ⓓ Ⓔ
231 Ⓐ Ⓑ Ⓒ Ⓓ Ⓔ
232 Ⓐ Ⓑ Ⓒ Ⓓ Ⓔ
233 Ⓐ Ⓑ Ⓒ Ⓓ Ⓔ
234 Ⓐ Ⓑ Ⓒ Ⓓ Ⓔ
235 Ⓐ Ⓑ Ⓒ Ⓓ Ⓔ
236 Ⓐ Ⓑ Ⓒ Ⓓ Ⓔ
237 Ⓐ Ⓑ Ⓒ Ⓓ Ⓔ
238 Ⓐ Ⓑ Ⓒ Ⓓ Ⓔ
239 Ⓐ Ⓑ Ⓒ Ⓓ Ⓔ
240 Ⓐ Ⓑ Ⓒ Ⓓ Ⓔ

BOARD OF REGISTRY

EXAM TYPE: ______________ DATE: ______________

IDENTIFICATION NUMBER									EXAM TYPE	
0	0	0	0	0	0	0	0	0	0	0
1	1	1	1	1	1	1	1	1	1	1
2	2	2	2	2	2	2	2	2	2	2
3	3	3	3	3	3	3	3	3	3	3
4	4	4	4	4	4	4	4	4	4	4
5	5	5	5	5	5	5	5	5	5	5
6	6	6	6	6	6	6	6	6	6	6
7	7	7	7	7	7	7	7	7	7	7
8	8	8	8	8	8	8	8	8	8	8
9	9	9	9	9	9	9	9	9	9	9

TEST BOOKLET NUMBER				

IMPORTANT DIRECTIONS FOR MARKING ANSWERS

- Use black lead pencil only (No. 2½ or softer).
- Do NOT use ink, felt tip or ballpoint pens.
- Erase cleanly any answer you wish to change.
- Make no stray marks on the answer sheet.
- Make heavy black marks that fill the circle completely.

EXAMPLES

1 Ⓐ Ⓑ Ⓒ Ⓓ Ⓔ WRONG: Fill in the circle completely.

2 Ⓐ Ⓑ Ⓒ Ⓓ Ⓔ

3 Ⓐ Ⓑ Ⓒ Ⓓ Ⓔ

4 Ⓐ Ⓑ Ⓒ Ⓓ Ⓔ WRONG: Make heavy black marks.

5 Ⓐ Ⓑ Ⓒ Ⓓ ● RIGHT: Make heavy black marks that fill in the circle completely.

1 Ⓐ Ⓑ Ⓒ Ⓓ Ⓔ	21 Ⓐ Ⓑ Ⓒ Ⓓ Ⓔ	41 Ⓐ Ⓑ Ⓒ Ⓓ Ⓔ	61 Ⓐ Ⓑ Ⓒ Ⓓ Ⓔ	81 Ⓐ Ⓑ Ⓒ Ⓓ Ⓔ	101 Ⓐ Ⓑ Ⓒ Ⓓ Ⓔ
2 Ⓐ Ⓑ Ⓒ Ⓓ Ⓔ	22 Ⓐ Ⓑ Ⓒ Ⓓ Ⓔ	42 Ⓐ Ⓑ Ⓒ Ⓓ Ⓔ	62 Ⓐ Ⓑ Ⓒ Ⓓ Ⓔ	82 Ⓐ Ⓑ Ⓒ Ⓓ Ⓔ	102 Ⓐ Ⓑ Ⓒ Ⓓ Ⓔ
3 Ⓐ Ⓑ Ⓒ Ⓓ Ⓔ	23 Ⓐ Ⓑ Ⓒ Ⓓ Ⓔ	43 Ⓐ Ⓑ Ⓒ Ⓓ Ⓔ	63 Ⓐ Ⓑ Ⓒ Ⓓ Ⓔ	83 Ⓐ Ⓑ Ⓒ Ⓓ Ⓔ	103 Ⓐ Ⓑ Ⓒ Ⓓ Ⓔ
4 Ⓐ Ⓑ Ⓒ Ⓓ Ⓔ	24 Ⓐ Ⓑ Ⓒ Ⓓ Ⓔ	44 Ⓐ Ⓑ Ⓒ Ⓓ Ⓔ	64 Ⓐ Ⓑ Ⓒ Ⓓ Ⓔ	84 Ⓐ Ⓑ Ⓒ Ⓓ Ⓔ	104 Ⓐ Ⓑ Ⓒ Ⓓ Ⓔ
5 Ⓐ Ⓑ Ⓒ Ⓓ Ⓔ	25 Ⓐ Ⓑ Ⓒ Ⓓ Ⓔ	45 Ⓐ Ⓑ Ⓒ Ⓓ Ⓔ	65 Ⓐ Ⓑ Ⓒ Ⓓ Ⓔ	85 Ⓐ Ⓑ Ⓒ Ⓓ Ⓔ	105 Ⓐ Ⓑ Ⓒ Ⓓ Ⓔ
6 Ⓐ Ⓑ Ⓒ Ⓓ Ⓔ	26 Ⓐ Ⓑ Ⓒ Ⓓ Ⓔ	46 Ⓐ Ⓑ Ⓒ Ⓓ Ⓔ	66 Ⓐ Ⓑ Ⓒ Ⓓ Ⓔ	86 Ⓐ Ⓑ Ⓒ Ⓓ Ⓔ	106 Ⓐ Ⓑ Ⓒ Ⓓ Ⓔ
7 Ⓐ Ⓑ Ⓒ Ⓓ Ⓔ	27 Ⓐ Ⓑ Ⓒ Ⓓ Ⓔ	47 Ⓐ Ⓑ Ⓒ Ⓓ Ⓔ	67 Ⓐ Ⓑ Ⓒ Ⓓ Ⓔ	87 Ⓐ Ⓑ Ⓒ Ⓓ Ⓔ	107 Ⓐ Ⓑ Ⓒ Ⓓ Ⓔ
8 Ⓐ Ⓑ Ⓒ Ⓓ Ⓔ	28 Ⓐ Ⓑ Ⓒ Ⓓ Ⓔ	48 Ⓐ Ⓑ Ⓒ Ⓓ Ⓔ	68 Ⓐ Ⓑ Ⓒ Ⓓ Ⓔ	88 Ⓐ Ⓑ Ⓒ Ⓓ Ⓔ	108 Ⓐ Ⓑ Ⓒ Ⓓ Ⓔ
9 Ⓐ Ⓑ Ⓒ Ⓓ Ⓔ	29 Ⓐ Ⓑ Ⓒ Ⓓ Ⓔ	49 Ⓐ Ⓑ Ⓒ Ⓓ Ⓔ	69 Ⓐ Ⓑ Ⓒ Ⓓ Ⓔ	89 Ⓐ Ⓑ Ⓒ Ⓓ Ⓔ	109 Ⓐ Ⓑ Ⓒ Ⓓ Ⓔ
10 Ⓐ Ⓑ Ⓒ Ⓓ Ⓔ	30 Ⓐ Ⓑ Ⓒ Ⓓ Ⓔ	50 Ⓐ Ⓑ Ⓒ Ⓓ Ⓔ	70 Ⓐ Ⓑ Ⓒ Ⓓ Ⓔ	90 Ⓐ Ⓑ Ⓒ Ⓓ Ⓔ	110 Ⓐ Ⓑ Ⓒ Ⓓ Ⓔ
11 Ⓐ Ⓑ Ⓒ Ⓓ Ⓔ	31 Ⓐ Ⓑ Ⓒ Ⓓ Ⓔ	51 Ⓐ Ⓑ Ⓒ Ⓓ Ⓔ	71 Ⓐ Ⓑ Ⓒ Ⓓ Ⓔ	91 Ⓐ Ⓑ Ⓒ Ⓓ Ⓔ	111 Ⓐ Ⓑ Ⓒ Ⓓ Ⓔ
12 Ⓐ Ⓑ Ⓒ Ⓓ Ⓔ	32 Ⓐ Ⓑ Ⓒ Ⓓ Ⓔ	52 Ⓐ Ⓑ Ⓒ Ⓓ Ⓔ	72 Ⓐ Ⓑ Ⓒ Ⓓ Ⓔ	92 Ⓐ Ⓑ Ⓒ Ⓓ Ⓔ	112 Ⓐ Ⓑ Ⓒ Ⓓ Ⓔ
13 Ⓐ Ⓑ Ⓒ Ⓓ Ⓔ	33 Ⓐ Ⓑ Ⓒ Ⓓ Ⓔ	53 Ⓐ Ⓑ Ⓒ Ⓓ Ⓔ	73 Ⓐ Ⓑ Ⓒ Ⓓ Ⓔ	93 Ⓐ Ⓑ Ⓒ Ⓓ Ⓔ	113 Ⓐ Ⓑ Ⓒ Ⓓ Ⓔ
14 Ⓐ Ⓑ Ⓒ Ⓓ Ⓔ	34 Ⓐ Ⓑ Ⓒ Ⓓ Ⓔ	54 Ⓐ Ⓑ Ⓒ Ⓓ Ⓔ	74 Ⓐ Ⓑ Ⓒ Ⓓ Ⓔ	94 Ⓐ Ⓑ Ⓒ Ⓓ Ⓔ	114 Ⓐ Ⓑ Ⓒ Ⓓ Ⓔ
15 Ⓐ Ⓑ Ⓒ Ⓓ Ⓔ	35 Ⓐ Ⓑ Ⓒ Ⓓ Ⓔ	55 Ⓐ Ⓑ Ⓒ Ⓓ Ⓔ	75 Ⓐ Ⓑ Ⓒ Ⓓ Ⓔ	95 Ⓐ Ⓑ Ⓒ Ⓓ Ⓔ	115 Ⓐ Ⓑ Ⓒ Ⓓ Ⓔ
16 Ⓐ Ⓑ Ⓒ Ⓓ Ⓔ	36 Ⓐ Ⓑ Ⓒ Ⓓ Ⓔ	56 Ⓐ Ⓑ Ⓒ Ⓓ Ⓔ	76 Ⓐ Ⓑ Ⓒ Ⓓ Ⓔ	96 Ⓐ Ⓑ Ⓒ Ⓓ Ⓔ	116 Ⓐ Ⓑ Ⓒ Ⓓ Ⓔ
17 Ⓐ Ⓑ Ⓒ Ⓓ Ⓔ	37 Ⓐ Ⓑ Ⓒ Ⓓ Ⓔ	57 Ⓐ Ⓑ Ⓒ Ⓓ Ⓔ	77 Ⓐ Ⓑ Ⓒ Ⓓ Ⓔ	97 Ⓐ Ⓑ Ⓒ Ⓓ Ⓔ	117 Ⓐ Ⓑ Ⓒ Ⓓ Ⓔ
18 Ⓐ Ⓑ Ⓒ Ⓓ Ⓔ	38 Ⓐ Ⓑ Ⓒ Ⓓ Ⓔ	58 Ⓐ Ⓑ Ⓒ Ⓓ Ⓔ	78 Ⓐ Ⓑ Ⓒ Ⓓ Ⓔ	98 Ⓐ Ⓑ Ⓒ Ⓓ Ⓔ	118 Ⓐ Ⓑ Ⓒ Ⓓ Ⓔ
19 Ⓐ Ⓑ Ⓒ Ⓓ Ⓔ	39 Ⓐ Ⓑ Ⓒ Ⓓ Ⓔ	59 Ⓐ Ⓑ Ⓒ Ⓓ Ⓔ	79 Ⓐ Ⓑ Ⓒ Ⓓ Ⓔ	99 Ⓐ Ⓑ Ⓒ Ⓓ Ⓔ	119 Ⓐ Ⓑ Ⓒ Ⓓ Ⓔ
20 Ⓐ Ⓑ Ⓒ Ⓓ Ⓔ	40 Ⓐ Ⓑ Ⓒ Ⓓ Ⓔ	60 Ⓐ Ⓑ Ⓒ Ⓓ Ⓔ	80 Ⓐ Ⓑ Ⓒ Ⓓ Ⓔ	100 Ⓐ Ⓑ Ⓒ Ⓓ Ⓔ	120 Ⓐ Ⓑ Ⓒ Ⓓ Ⓔ

NCS Trans-Optic F6292-54321

SIDE ONE

BOARD OF REGISTRY

founded in 1928 by the
American Society of Clinical Pathologists

Representatives from:

American Society of Clinical Pathologists
Medical Technologists/Technicians
Pathologists
American Academy of Microbiology
American Association of Blood Banks
American Society of Cytology
National Registry in Clinical Chemistry
American Society of Hematology
National Society for Histotechnology

IMPORTANT DIRECTIONS FOR MARKING ANSWERS

- Use black lead pencil only (No. 2½ or softer).
- Do NOT use ink, felt tip or ballpoint pens.
- Erase cleanly any answer you wish to change.
- Make no stray marks on the answer sheet.
- Make heavy black marks that fill the circle completely.

EXAMPLES

WRONG: Fill in the circle completely.
1 (A) (B) (C) (D) (E)
2 (A) (B) (C) (D) (E)
3 (A) (B) (C) (D) (E)

WRONG: Make heavy black marks.
4 (A) (B) (C) (D) (E)

RIGHT: Make heavy black marks that fill in the circle completely.
5 (A) (B) (C) (D) (E)

121 (A) (B) (C) (D) (E)	141 (A) (B) (C) (D) (E)	161 (A) (B) (C) (D) (E)	181 (A) (B) (C) (D) (E)	201 (A) (B) (C) (D) (E)	221 (A) (B) (C) (D) (E)
122 (A) (B) (C) (D) (E)	142 (A) (B) (C) (D) (E)	162 (A) (B) (C) (D) (E)	182 (A) (B) (C) (D) (E)	202 (A) (B) (C) (D) (E)	222 (A) (B) (C) (D) (E)
123 (A) (B) (C) (D) (E)	143 (A) (B) (C) (D) (E)	163 (A) (B) (C) (D) (E)	183 (A) (B) (C) (D) (E)	203 (A) (B) (C) (D) (E)	223 (A) (B) (C) (D) (E)
124 (A) (B) (C) (D) (E)	144 (A) (B) (C) (D) (E)	164 (A) (B) (C) (D) (E)	184 (A) (B) (C) (D) (E)	204 (A) (B) (C) (D) (E)	224 (A) (B) (C) (D) (E)
125 (A) (B) (C) (D) (E)	145 (A) (B) (C) (D) (E)	165 (A) (B) (C) (D) (E)	185 (A) (B) (C) (D) (E)	205 (A) (B) (C) (D) (E)	225 (A) (B) (C) (D) (E)
126 (A) (B) (C) (D) (E)	146 (A) (B) (C) (D) (E)	166 (A) (B) (C) (D) (E)	186 (A) (B) (C) (D) (E)	206 (A) (B) (C) (D) (E)	226 (A) (B) (C) (D) (E)
127 (A) (B) (C) (D) (E)	147 (A) (B) (C) (D) (E)	167 (A) (B) (C) (D) (E)	187 (A) (B) (C) (D) (E)	207 (A) (B) (C) (D) (E)	227 (A) (B) (C) (D) (E)
128 (A) (B) (C) (D) (E)	148 (A) (B) (C) (D) (E)	168 (A) (B) (C) (D) (E)	188 (A) (B) (C) (D) (E)	208 (A) (B) (C) (D) (E)	228 (A) (B) (C) (D) (E)
129 (A) (B) (C) (D) (E)	149 (A) (B) (C) (D) (E)	169 (A) (B) (C) (D) (E)	189 (A) (B) (C) (D) (E)	209 (A) (B) (C) (D) (E)	229 (A) (B) (C) (D) (E)
130 (A) (B) (C) (D) (E)	150 (A) (B) (C) (D) (E)	170 (A) (B) (C) (D) (E)	190 (A) (B) (C) (D) (E)	210 (A) (B) (C) (D) (E)	230 (A) (B) (C) (D) (E)
131 (A) (B) (C) (D) (E)	151 (A) (B) (C) (D) (E)	171 (A) (B) (C) (D) (E)	191 (A) (B) (C) (D) (E)	211 (A) (B) (C) (D) (E)	231 (A) (B) (C) (D) (E)
132 (A) (B) (C) (D) (E)	152 (A) (B) (C) (D) (E)	172 (A) (B) (C) (D) (E)	192 (A) (B) (C) (D) (E)	212 (A) (B) (C) (D) (E)	232 (A) (B) (C) (D) (E)
133 (A) (B) (C) (D) (E)	153 (A) (B) (C) (D) (E)	173 (A) (B) (C) (D) (E)	193 (A) (B) (C) (D) (E)	213 (A) (B) (C) (D) (E)	233 (A) (B) (C) (D) (E)
134 (A) (B) (C) (D) (E)	154 (A) (B) (C) (D) (E)	174 (A) (B) (C) (D) (E)	194 (A) (B) (C) (D) (E)	214 (A) (B) (C) (D) (E)	234 (A) (B) (C) (D) (E)
135 (A) (B) (C) (D) (E)	155 (A) (B) (C) (D) (E)	175 (A) (B) (C) (D) (E)	195 (A) (B) (C) (D) (E)	215 (A) (B) (C) (D) (E)	235 (A) (B) (C) (D) (E)
136 (A) (B) (C) (D) (E)	156 (A) (B) (C) (D) (E)	176 (A) (B) (C) (D) (E)	196 (A) (B) (C) (D) (E)	216 (A) (B) (C) (D) (E)	236 (A) (B) (C) (D) (E)
137 (A) (B) (C) (D) (E)	157 (A) (B) (C) (D) (E)	177 (A) (B) (C) (D) (E)	197 (A) (B) (C) (D) (E)	217 (A) (B) (C) (D) (E)	237 (A) (B) (C) (D) (E)
138 (A) (B) (C) (D) (E)	158 (A) (B) (C) (D) (E)	178 (A) (B) (C) (D) (E)	198 (A) (B) (C) (D) (E)	218 (A) (B) (C) (D) (E)	238 (A) (B) (C) (D) (E)
139 (A) (B) (C) (D) (E)	159 (A) (B) (C) (D) (E)	179 (A) (B) (C) (D) (E)	199 (A) (B) (C) (D) (E)	219 (A) (B) (C) (D) (E)	239 (A) (B) (C) (D) (E)
140 (A) (B) (C) (D) (E)	160 (A) (B) (C) (D) (E)	180 (A) (B) (C) (D) (E)	200 (A) (B) (C) (D) (E)	220 (A) (B) (C) (D) (E)	240 (A) (B) (C) (D) (E)

BOARD OF REGISTRY

NAME: ______________________

EXAM TYPE: ______________ DATE: ______________

IDENTIFICATION NUMBER									EXAM TYPE	
0	0	0	0	0	0	0	0	0	0	0
1	1	1	1	1	1	1	1	1	1	1
2	2	2	2	2	2	2	2	2	2	2
3	3	3	3	3	3	3	3	3	3	3
4	4	4	4	4	4	4	4	4	4	4
5	5	5	5	5	5	5	5	5	5	5
6	6	6	6	6	6	6	6	6	6	6
7	7	7	7	7	7	7	7	7	7	7
8	8	8	8	8	8	8	8	8	8	8
9	9	9	9	9	9	9	9	9	9	9

TEST BOOKLET NUMBER

IMPORTANT DIRECTIONS FOR MARKING ANSWERS

- Use black lead pencil only (No. 2½ or softer).
- Do NOT use ink, felt tip or ballpoint pens.
- Erase cleanly any answer you wish to change.
- Make no stray marks on the answer sheet.
- Make heavy black marks that fill the circle completely.

EXAMPLES

WRONG: Fill in the circle completely.

1 Ⓧ Ⓑ Ⓒ Ⓓ Ⓔ

2 Ⓐ ✓ Ⓒ Ⓓ Ⓔ

3 Ⓐ Ⓑ ◉ Ⓓ Ⓔ

WRONG: Make heavy black marks.

4 Ⓐ Ⓑ Ⓒ Ⓓ Ⓔ

RIGHT: Make heavy black marks that fill the circle completely.

5 Ⓐ Ⓑ Ⓒ Ⓓ ●

1 Ⓐ Ⓑ Ⓒ Ⓓ Ⓔ	21 Ⓐ Ⓑ Ⓒ Ⓓ Ⓔ	41 Ⓐ Ⓑ Ⓒ Ⓓ Ⓔ	61 Ⓐ Ⓑ Ⓒ Ⓓ Ⓔ	81 Ⓐ Ⓑ Ⓒ Ⓓ Ⓔ	101 Ⓐ Ⓑ Ⓒ Ⓓ Ⓔ
2 Ⓐ Ⓑ Ⓒ Ⓓ Ⓔ	22 Ⓐ Ⓑ Ⓒ Ⓓ Ⓔ	42 Ⓐ Ⓑ Ⓒ Ⓓ Ⓔ	62 Ⓐ Ⓑ Ⓒ Ⓓ Ⓔ	82 Ⓐ Ⓑ Ⓒ Ⓓ Ⓔ	102 Ⓐ Ⓑ Ⓒ Ⓓ Ⓔ
3 Ⓐ Ⓑ Ⓒ Ⓓ Ⓔ	23 Ⓐ Ⓑ Ⓒ Ⓓ Ⓔ	43 Ⓐ Ⓑ Ⓒ Ⓓ Ⓔ	63 Ⓐ Ⓑ Ⓒ Ⓓ Ⓔ	83 Ⓐ Ⓑ Ⓒ Ⓓ Ⓔ	103 Ⓐ Ⓑ Ⓒ Ⓓ Ⓔ
4 Ⓐ Ⓑ Ⓒ Ⓓ Ⓔ	24 Ⓐ Ⓑ Ⓒ Ⓓ Ⓔ	44 Ⓐ Ⓑ Ⓒ Ⓓ Ⓔ	64 Ⓐ Ⓑ Ⓒ Ⓓ Ⓔ	84 Ⓐ Ⓑ Ⓒ Ⓓ Ⓔ	104 Ⓐ Ⓑ Ⓒ Ⓓ Ⓔ
5 Ⓐ Ⓑ Ⓒ Ⓓ Ⓔ	25 Ⓐ Ⓑ Ⓒ Ⓓ Ⓔ	45 Ⓐ Ⓑ Ⓒ Ⓓ Ⓔ	65 Ⓐ Ⓑ Ⓒ Ⓓ Ⓔ	85 Ⓐ Ⓑ Ⓒ Ⓓ Ⓔ	105 Ⓐ Ⓑ Ⓒ Ⓓ Ⓔ
6 Ⓐ Ⓑ Ⓒ Ⓓ Ⓔ	26 Ⓐ Ⓑ Ⓒ Ⓓ Ⓔ	46 Ⓐ Ⓑ Ⓒ Ⓓ Ⓔ	66 Ⓐ Ⓑ Ⓒ Ⓓ Ⓔ	86 Ⓐ Ⓑ Ⓒ Ⓓ Ⓔ	106 Ⓐ Ⓑ Ⓒ Ⓓ Ⓔ
7 Ⓐ Ⓑ Ⓒ Ⓓ Ⓔ	27 Ⓐ Ⓑ Ⓒ Ⓓ Ⓔ	47 Ⓐ Ⓑ Ⓒ Ⓓ Ⓔ	67 Ⓐ Ⓑ Ⓒ Ⓓ Ⓔ	87 Ⓐ Ⓑ Ⓒ Ⓓ Ⓔ	107 Ⓐ Ⓑ Ⓒ Ⓓ Ⓔ
8 Ⓐ Ⓑ Ⓒ Ⓓ Ⓔ	28 Ⓐ Ⓑ Ⓒ Ⓓ Ⓔ	48 Ⓐ Ⓑ Ⓒ Ⓓ Ⓔ	68 Ⓐ Ⓑ Ⓒ Ⓓ Ⓔ	88 Ⓐ Ⓑ Ⓒ Ⓓ Ⓔ	108 Ⓐ Ⓑ Ⓒ Ⓓ Ⓔ
9 Ⓐ Ⓑ Ⓒ Ⓓ Ⓔ	29 Ⓐ Ⓑ Ⓒ Ⓓ Ⓔ	49 Ⓐ Ⓑ Ⓒ Ⓓ Ⓔ	69 Ⓐ Ⓑ Ⓒ Ⓓ Ⓔ	89 Ⓐ Ⓑ Ⓒ Ⓓ Ⓔ	109 Ⓐ Ⓑ Ⓒ Ⓓ Ⓔ
10 Ⓐ Ⓑ Ⓒ Ⓓ Ⓔ	30 Ⓐ Ⓑ Ⓒ Ⓓ Ⓔ	50 Ⓐ Ⓑ Ⓒ Ⓓ Ⓔ	70 Ⓐ Ⓑ Ⓒ Ⓓ Ⓔ	90 Ⓐ Ⓑ Ⓒ Ⓓ Ⓔ	110 Ⓐ Ⓑ Ⓒ Ⓓ Ⓔ
11 Ⓐ Ⓑ Ⓒ Ⓓ Ⓔ	31 Ⓐ Ⓑ Ⓒ Ⓓ Ⓔ	51 Ⓐ Ⓑ Ⓒ Ⓓ Ⓔ	71 Ⓐ Ⓑ Ⓒ Ⓓ Ⓔ	91 Ⓐ Ⓑ Ⓒ Ⓓ Ⓔ	111 Ⓐ Ⓑ Ⓒ Ⓓ Ⓔ
12 Ⓐ Ⓑ Ⓒ Ⓓ Ⓔ	32 Ⓐ Ⓑ Ⓒ Ⓓ Ⓔ	52 Ⓐ Ⓑ Ⓒ Ⓓ Ⓔ	72 Ⓐ Ⓑ Ⓒ Ⓓ Ⓔ	92 Ⓐ Ⓑ Ⓒ Ⓓ Ⓔ	112 Ⓐ Ⓑ Ⓒ Ⓓ Ⓔ
13 Ⓐ Ⓑ Ⓒ Ⓓ Ⓔ	33 Ⓐ Ⓑ Ⓒ Ⓓ Ⓔ	53 Ⓐ Ⓑ Ⓒ Ⓓ Ⓔ	73 Ⓐ Ⓑ Ⓒ Ⓓ Ⓔ	93 Ⓐ Ⓑ Ⓒ Ⓓ Ⓔ	113 Ⓐ Ⓑ Ⓒ Ⓓ Ⓔ
14 Ⓐ Ⓑ Ⓒ Ⓓ Ⓔ	34 Ⓐ Ⓑ Ⓒ Ⓓ Ⓔ	54 Ⓐ Ⓑ Ⓒ Ⓓ Ⓔ	74 Ⓐ Ⓑ Ⓒ Ⓓ Ⓔ	94 Ⓐ Ⓑ Ⓒ Ⓓ Ⓔ	114 Ⓐ Ⓑ Ⓒ Ⓓ Ⓔ
15 Ⓐ Ⓑ Ⓒ Ⓓ Ⓔ	35 Ⓐ Ⓑ Ⓒ Ⓓ Ⓔ	55 Ⓐ Ⓑ Ⓒ Ⓓ Ⓔ	75 Ⓐ Ⓑ Ⓒ Ⓓ Ⓔ	95 Ⓐ Ⓑ Ⓒ Ⓓ Ⓔ	115 Ⓐ Ⓑ Ⓒ Ⓓ Ⓔ
16 Ⓐ Ⓑ Ⓒ Ⓓ Ⓔ	36 Ⓐ Ⓑ Ⓒ Ⓓ Ⓔ	56 Ⓐ Ⓑ Ⓒ Ⓓ Ⓔ	76 Ⓐ Ⓑ Ⓒ Ⓓ Ⓔ	96 Ⓐ Ⓑ Ⓒ Ⓓ Ⓔ	116 Ⓐ Ⓑ Ⓒ Ⓓ Ⓔ
17 Ⓐ Ⓑ Ⓒ Ⓓ Ⓔ	37 Ⓐ Ⓑ Ⓒ Ⓓ Ⓔ	57 Ⓐ Ⓑ Ⓒ Ⓓ Ⓔ	77 Ⓐ Ⓑ Ⓒ Ⓓ Ⓔ	97 Ⓐ Ⓑ Ⓒ Ⓓ Ⓔ	117 Ⓐ Ⓑ Ⓒ Ⓓ Ⓔ
18 Ⓐ Ⓑ Ⓒ Ⓓ Ⓔ	38 Ⓐ Ⓑ Ⓒ Ⓓ Ⓔ	58 Ⓐ Ⓑ Ⓒ Ⓓ Ⓔ	78 Ⓐ Ⓑ Ⓒ Ⓓ Ⓔ	98 Ⓐ Ⓑ Ⓒ Ⓓ Ⓔ	118 Ⓐ Ⓑ Ⓒ Ⓓ Ⓔ
19 Ⓐ Ⓑ Ⓒ Ⓓ Ⓔ	39 Ⓐ Ⓑ Ⓒ Ⓓ Ⓔ	59 Ⓐ Ⓑ Ⓒ Ⓓ Ⓔ	79 Ⓐ Ⓑ Ⓒ Ⓓ Ⓔ	99 Ⓐ Ⓑ Ⓒ Ⓓ Ⓔ	119 Ⓐ Ⓑ Ⓒ Ⓓ Ⓔ
20 Ⓐ Ⓑ Ⓒ Ⓓ Ⓔ	40 Ⓐ Ⓑ Ⓒ Ⓓ Ⓔ	60 Ⓐ Ⓑ Ⓒ Ⓓ Ⓔ	80 Ⓐ Ⓑ Ⓒ Ⓓ Ⓔ	100 Ⓐ Ⓑ Ⓒ Ⓓ Ⓔ	120 Ⓐ Ⓑ Ⓒ Ⓓ Ⓔ

NCS Trans-Optic F6292-54321

SIDE ONE

TM

BOARD OF REGISTRY

founded in 1928 by the
American Society of Clinical Pathologists

Representatives from:

American Society of Clinical Pathologists
Medical Technologists/Technicians
Pathologists
American Academy of Microbiology
American Association of Blood Banks
American Society of Cytology
National Registry in Clinical Chemistry
American Society of Hematology
National Society for Histotechnology

IMPORTANT DIRECTIONS FOR MARKING ANSWERS

- Use black lead pencil only (No. 2½ or softer).
- Do NOT use ink, felt tip or ballpoint pens.
- Erase cleanly any answer you wish to change.
- Make no stray marks on the answer sheet.
- Make heavy black marks that fill the circle completely.

EXAMPLES

WRONG: Fill in the circle completely.
1 (X) B C D E
2 A (✓) C D E
3 A B (partly filled) D E

WRONG: Make heavy black marks.
4 A B C (light fill) E

RIGHT: Make heavy black marks that fill in the circle completely.
5 A B C D (●)

121 A B C D E	141 A B C D E	161 A B C D E	181 A B C D E	201 A B C D E	221 A B C D E
122 A B C D E	142 A B C D E	162 A B C D E	182 A B C D E	202 A B C D E	222 A B C D E
123 A B C D E	143 A B C D E	163 A B C D E	183 A B C D E	203 A B C D E	223 A B C D E
124 A B C D E	144 A B C D E	164 A B C D E	184 A B C D E	204 A B C D E	224 A B C D E
125 A B C D E	145 A B C D E	165 A B C D E	185 A B C D E	205 A B C D E	225 A B C D E
126 A B C D E	146 A B C D E	166 A B C D E	186 A B C D E	206 A B C D E	226 A B C D E
127 A B C D E	147 A B C D E	167 A B C D E	187 A B C D E	207 A B C D E	227 A B C D E
128 A B C D E	148 A B C D E	168 A B C D E	188 A B C D E	208 A B C D E	228 A B C D E
129 A B C D E	149 A B C D E	169 A B C D E	189 A B C D E	209 A B C D E	229 A B C D E
130 A B C D E	150 A B C D E	170 A B C D E	190 A B C D E	210 A B C D E	230 A B C D E
131 A B C D E	151 A B C D E	171 A B C D E	191 A B C D E	211 A B C D E	231 A B C D E
132 A B C D E	152 A B C D E	172 A B C D E	192 A B C D E	212 A B C D E	232 A B C D E
133 A B C D E	153 A B C D E	173 A B C D E	193 A B C D E	213 A B C D E	233 A B C D E
134 A B C D E	154 A B C D E	174 A B C D E	194 A B C D E	214 A B C D E	234 A B C D E
135 A B C D E	155 A B C D E	175 A B C D E	195 A B C D E	215 A B C D E	235 A B C D E
136 A B C D E	156 A B C D E	176 A B C D E	196 A B C D E	216 A B C D E	236 A B C D E
137 A B C D E	157 A B C D E	177 A B C D E	197 A B C D E	217 A B C D E	237 A B C D E
138 A B C D E	158 A B C D E	178 A B C D E	198 A B C D E	218 A B C D E	238 A B C D E
139 A B C D E	159 A B C D E	179 A B C D E	199 A B C D E	219 A B C D E	239 A B C D E
140 A B C D E	160 A B C D E	180 A B C D E	200 A B C D E	220 A B C D E	240 A B C D E

BOARD OF REGISTRY

EXAM TYPE: ______________ DATE: ______________

IDENTIFICATION NUMBER									TYPE	
0	0	0	0	0	0	0	0	0	0	0
1	1	1	1	1	1	1	1	1	1	1
2	2	2	2	2	2	2	2	2	2	2
3	3	3	3	3	3	3	3	3	3	3
4	4	4	4	4	4	4	4	4	4	4
5	5	5	5	5	5	5	5	5	5	5
6	6	6	6	6	6	6	6	6	6	6
7	7	7	7	7	7	7	7	7	7	7
8	8	8	8	8	8	8	8	8	8	8
9	9	9	9	9	9	9	9	9	9	9

TEST BOOKLET NUMBER

IMPORTANT DIRECTIONS FOR MARKING ANSWERS

- Use black lead pencil only (No. 2½ or softer).
- Do NOT use ink, felt tip or ballpoint pens.
- Erase cleanly any answer you wish to change.
- Make no stray marks on the answer sheet.
- Make heavy black marks that fill the circle completely.

EXAMPLES

WRONG: Fill in the circle completely.

1 (A) (B) (C) (D) (E)

2 (A) (B) (C) (D) (E)

3 (A) (B) (C) (D) (E)

WRONG: Make heavy black marks.

4 (A) (B) (C) (D) (E)

RIGHT: Make heavy black marks that fill in the circle completely.

5 (A) (B) (C) (D) (E)

1 Ⓐ Ⓑ Ⓒ Ⓓ Ⓔ	21 Ⓐ Ⓑ Ⓒ Ⓓ Ⓔ	41 Ⓐ Ⓑ Ⓒ Ⓓ Ⓔ	61 Ⓐ Ⓑ Ⓒ Ⓓ Ⓔ	81 Ⓐ Ⓑ Ⓒ Ⓓ Ⓔ	101 Ⓐ Ⓑ Ⓒ Ⓓ Ⓔ
2 Ⓐ Ⓑ Ⓒ Ⓓ Ⓔ	22 Ⓐ Ⓑ Ⓒ Ⓓ Ⓔ	42 Ⓐ Ⓑ Ⓒ Ⓓ Ⓔ	62 Ⓐ Ⓑ Ⓒ Ⓓ Ⓔ	82 Ⓐ Ⓑ Ⓒ Ⓓ Ⓔ	102 Ⓐ Ⓑ Ⓒ Ⓓ Ⓔ
3 Ⓐ Ⓑ Ⓒ Ⓓ Ⓔ	23 Ⓐ Ⓑ Ⓒ Ⓓ Ⓔ	43 Ⓐ Ⓑ Ⓒ Ⓓ Ⓔ	63 Ⓐ Ⓑ Ⓒ Ⓓ Ⓔ	83 Ⓐ Ⓑ Ⓒ Ⓓ Ⓔ	103 Ⓐ Ⓑ Ⓒ Ⓓ Ⓔ
4 Ⓐ Ⓑ Ⓒ Ⓓ Ⓔ	24 Ⓐ Ⓑ Ⓒ Ⓓ Ⓔ	44 Ⓐ Ⓑ Ⓒ Ⓓ Ⓔ	64 Ⓐ Ⓑ Ⓒ Ⓓ Ⓔ	84 Ⓐ Ⓑ Ⓒ Ⓓ Ⓔ	104 Ⓐ Ⓑ Ⓒ Ⓓ Ⓔ
5 Ⓐ Ⓑ Ⓒ Ⓓ Ⓔ	25 Ⓐ Ⓑ Ⓒ Ⓓ Ⓔ	45 Ⓐ Ⓑ Ⓒ Ⓓ Ⓔ	65 Ⓐ Ⓑ Ⓒ Ⓓ Ⓔ	85 Ⓐ Ⓑ Ⓒ Ⓓ Ⓔ	105 Ⓐ Ⓑ Ⓒ Ⓓ Ⓔ
6 Ⓐ Ⓑ Ⓒ Ⓓ Ⓔ	26 Ⓐ Ⓑ Ⓒ Ⓓ Ⓔ	46 Ⓐ Ⓑ Ⓒ Ⓓ Ⓔ	66 Ⓐ Ⓑ Ⓒ Ⓓ Ⓔ	86 Ⓐ Ⓑ Ⓒ Ⓓ Ⓔ	106 Ⓐ Ⓑ Ⓒ Ⓓ Ⓔ
7 Ⓐ Ⓑ Ⓒ Ⓓ Ⓔ	27 Ⓐ Ⓑ Ⓒ Ⓓ Ⓔ	47 Ⓐ Ⓑ Ⓒ Ⓓ Ⓔ	67 Ⓐ Ⓑ Ⓒ Ⓓ Ⓔ	87 Ⓐ Ⓑ Ⓒ Ⓓ Ⓔ	107 Ⓐ Ⓑ Ⓒ Ⓓ Ⓔ
8 Ⓐ Ⓑ Ⓒ Ⓓ Ⓔ	28 Ⓐ Ⓑ Ⓒ Ⓓ Ⓔ	48 Ⓐ Ⓑ Ⓒ Ⓓ Ⓔ	68 Ⓐ Ⓑ Ⓒ Ⓓ Ⓔ	88 Ⓐ Ⓑ Ⓒ Ⓓ Ⓔ	108 Ⓐ Ⓑ Ⓒ Ⓓ Ⓔ
9 Ⓐ Ⓑ Ⓒ Ⓓ Ⓔ	29 Ⓐ Ⓑ Ⓒ Ⓓ Ⓔ	49 Ⓐ Ⓑ Ⓒ Ⓓ Ⓔ	69 Ⓐ Ⓑ Ⓒ Ⓓ Ⓔ	89 Ⓐ Ⓑ Ⓒ Ⓓ Ⓔ	109 Ⓐ Ⓑ Ⓒ Ⓓ Ⓔ
10 Ⓐ Ⓑ Ⓒ Ⓓ Ⓔ	30 Ⓐ Ⓑ Ⓒ Ⓓ Ⓔ	50 Ⓐ Ⓑ Ⓒ Ⓓ Ⓔ	70 Ⓐ Ⓑ Ⓒ Ⓓ Ⓔ	90 Ⓐ Ⓑ Ⓒ Ⓓ Ⓔ	110 Ⓐ Ⓑ Ⓒ Ⓓ Ⓔ
11 Ⓐ Ⓑ Ⓒ Ⓓ Ⓔ	31 Ⓐ Ⓑ Ⓒ Ⓓ Ⓔ	51 Ⓐ Ⓑ Ⓒ Ⓓ Ⓔ	71 Ⓐ Ⓑ Ⓒ Ⓓ Ⓔ	91 Ⓐ Ⓑ Ⓒ Ⓓ Ⓔ	111 Ⓐ Ⓑ Ⓒ Ⓓ Ⓔ
12 Ⓐ Ⓑ Ⓒ Ⓓ Ⓔ	32 Ⓐ Ⓑ Ⓒ Ⓓ Ⓔ	52 Ⓐ Ⓑ Ⓒ Ⓓ Ⓔ	72 Ⓐ Ⓑ Ⓒ Ⓓ Ⓔ	92 Ⓐ Ⓑ Ⓒ Ⓓ Ⓔ	112 Ⓐ Ⓑ Ⓒ Ⓓ Ⓔ
13 Ⓐ Ⓑ Ⓒ Ⓓ Ⓔ	33 Ⓐ Ⓑ Ⓒ Ⓓ Ⓔ	53 Ⓐ Ⓑ Ⓒ Ⓓ Ⓔ	73 Ⓐ Ⓑ Ⓒ Ⓓ Ⓔ	93 Ⓐ Ⓑ Ⓒ Ⓓ Ⓔ	113 Ⓐ Ⓑ Ⓒ Ⓓ Ⓔ
14 Ⓐ Ⓑ Ⓒ Ⓓ Ⓔ	34 Ⓐ Ⓑ Ⓒ Ⓓ Ⓔ	54 Ⓐ Ⓑ Ⓒ Ⓓ Ⓔ	74 Ⓐ Ⓑ Ⓒ Ⓓ Ⓔ	94 Ⓐ Ⓑ Ⓒ Ⓓ Ⓔ	114 Ⓐ Ⓑ Ⓒ Ⓓ Ⓔ
15 Ⓐ Ⓑ Ⓒ Ⓓ Ⓔ	35 Ⓐ Ⓑ Ⓒ Ⓓ Ⓔ	55 Ⓐ Ⓑ Ⓒ Ⓓ Ⓔ	75 Ⓐ Ⓑ Ⓒ Ⓓ Ⓔ	95 Ⓐ Ⓑ Ⓒ Ⓓ Ⓔ	115 Ⓐ Ⓑ Ⓒ Ⓓ Ⓔ
16 Ⓐ Ⓑ Ⓒ Ⓓ Ⓔ	36 Ⓐ Ⓑ Ⓒ Ⓓ Ⓔ	56 Ⓐ Ⓑ Ⓒ Ⓓ Ⓔ	76 Ⓐ Ⓑ Ⓒ Ⓓ Ⓔ	96 Ⓐ Ⓑ Ⓒ Ⓓ Ⓔ	116 Ⓐ Ⓑ Ⓒ Ⓓ Ⓔ
17 Ⓐ Ⓑ Ⓒ Ⓓ Ⓔ	37 Ⓐ Ⓑ Ⓒ Ⓓ Ⓔ	57 Ⓐ Ⓑ Ⓒ Ⓓ Ⓔ	77 Ⓐ Ⓑ Ⓒ Ⓓ Ⓔ	97 Ⓐ Ⓑ Ⓒ Ⓓ Ⓔ	117 Ⓐ Ⓑ Ⓒ Ⓓ Ⓔ
18 Ⓐ Ⓑ Ⓒ Ⓓ Ⓔ	38 Ⓐ Ⓑ Ⓒ Ⓓ Ⓔ	58 Ⓐ Ⓑ Ⓒ Ⓓ Ⓔ	78 Ⓐ Ⓑ Ⓒ Ⓓ Ⓔ	98 Ⓐ Ⓑ Ⓒ Ⓓ Ⓔ	118 Ⓐ Ⓑ Ⓒ Ⓓ Ⓔ
19 Ⓐ Ⓑ Ⓒ Ⓓ Ⓔ	39 Ⓐ Ⓑ Ⓒ Ⓓ Ⓔ	59 Ⓐ Ⓑ Ⓒ Ⓓ Ⓔ	79 Ⓐ Ⓑ Ⓒ Ⓓ Ⓔ	99 Ⓐ Ⓑ Ⓒ Ⓓ Ⓔ	119 Ⓐ Ⓑ Ⓒ Ⓓ Ⓔ
20 Ⓐ Ⓑ Ⓒ Ⓓ Ⓔ	40 Ⓐ Ⓑ Ⓒ Ⓓ Ⓔ	60 Ⓐ Ⓑ Ⓒ Ⓓ Ⓔ	80 Ⓐ Ⓑ Ⓒ Ⓓ Ⓔ	100 Ⓐ Ⓑ Ⓒ Ⓓ Ⓔ	120 Ⓐ Ⓑ Ⓒ Ⓓ Ⓔ

NCS Trans-Optic F6292-54321

TM

BOARD OF REGISTRY

founded in 1928 by the
American Society of Clinical Pathologists

Representatives from:

American Society of Clinical Pathologists
Medical Technologists/Technicians
Pathologists
American Academy of Microbiology
American Association of Blood Banks
American Society of Cytology
National Registry in Clinical Chemistry
American Society of Hematology
National Society for Histotechnology

IMPORTANT DIRECTIONS FOR MARKING ANSWERS

- Use black lead pencil only (No. 2½ or softer).
- Do NOT use ink, felt tip or ballpoint pens.
- Erase cleanly any answer you wish to change.
- Make no stray marks on the answer sheet.
- Make heavy black marks that fill the circle completely.

EXAMPLES

1 (A) (B) (C) (D) (E) WRONG: Fill in the circle completely.
2 (A) (B) (C) (D) (E)
3 (A) (B) (C) (D) (E)
4 (A) (B) (C) (D) (E) WRONG: Make heavy black marks.
5 (A) (B) (C) (D) (E) RIGHT: Make heavy black marks that fill in the circle completely.

121 (A) (B) (C) (D) (E)
122 (A) (B) (C) (D) (E)
123 (A) (B) (C) (D) (E)
124 (A) (B) (C) (D) (E)
125 (A) (B) (C) (D) (E)
126 (A) (B) (C) (D) (E)
127 (A) (B) (C) (D) (E)
128 (A) (B) (C) (D) (E)
129 (A) (B) (C) (D) (E)
130 (A) (B) (C) (D) (E)
131 (A) (B) (C) (D) (E)
132 (A) (B) (C) (D) (E)
133 (A) (B) (C) (D) (E)
134 (A) (B) (C) (D) (E)
135 (A) (B) (C) (D) (E)
136 (A) (B) (C) (D) (E)
137 (A) (B) (C) (D) (E)
138 (A) (B) (C) (D) (E)
139 (A) (B) (C) (D) (E)
140 (A) (B) (C) (D) (E)
141 (A) (B) (C) (D) (E)
142 (A) (B) (C) (D) (E)
143 (A) (B) (C) (D) (E)
144 (A) (B) (C) (D) (E)
145 (A) (B) (C) (D) (E)
146 (A) (B) (C) (D) (E)
147 (A) (B) (C) (D) (E)
148 (A) (B) (C) (D) (E)
149 (A) (B) (C) (D) (E)
150 (A) (B) (C) (D) (E)
151 (A) (B) (C) (D) (E)
152 (A) (B) (C) (D) (E)
153 (A) (B) (C) (D) (E)
154 (A) (B) (C) (D) (E)
155 (A) (B) (C) (D) (E)
156 (A) (B) (C) (D) (E)
157 (A) (B) (C) (D) (E)
158 (A) (B) (C) (D) (E)
159 (A) (B) (C) (D) (E)
160 (A) (B) (C) (D) (E)
161 (A) (B) (C) (D) (E)
162 (A) (B) (C) (D) (E)
163 (A) (B) (C) (D) (E)
164 (A) (B) (C) (D) (E)
165 (A) (B) (C) (D) (E)
166 (A) (B) (C) (D) (E)
167 (A) (B) (C) (D) (E)
168 (A) (B) (C) (D) (E)
169 (A) (B) (C) (D) (E)
170 (A) (B) (C) (D) (E)
171 (A) (B) (C) (D) (E)
172 (A) (B) (C) (D) (E)
173 (A) (B) (C) (D) (E)
174 (A) (B) (C) (D) (E)
175 (A) (B) (C) (D) (E)
176 (A) (B) (C) (D) (E)
177 (A) (B) (C) (D) (E)
178 (A) (B) (C) (D) (E)
179 (A) (B) (C) (D) (E)
180 (A) (B) (C) (D) (E)
181 (A) (B) (C) (D) (E)
182 (A) (B) (C) (D) (E)
183 (A) (B) (C) (D) (E)
184 (A) (B) (C) (D) (E)
185 (A) (B) (C) (D) (E)
186 (A) (B) (C) (D) (E)
187 (A) (B) (C) (D) (E)
188 (A) (B) (C) (D) (E)
189 (A) (B) (C) (D) (E)
190 (A) (B) (C) (D) (E)
191 (A) (B) (C) (D) (E)
192 (A) (B) (C) (D) (E)
193 (A) (B) (C) (D) (E)
194 (A) (B) (C) (D) (E)
195 (A) (B) (C) (D) (E)
196 (A) (B) (C) (D) (E)
197 (A) (B) (C) (D) (E)
198 (A) (B) (C) (D) (E)
199 (A) (B) (C) (D) (E)
200 (A) (B) (C) (D) (E)
201 (A) (B) (C) (D) (E)
202 (A) (B) (C) (D) (E)
203 (A) (B) (C) (D) (E)
204 (A) (B) (C) (D) (E)
205 (A) (B) (C) (D) (E)
206 (A) (B) (C) (D) (E)
207 (A) (B) (C) (D) (E)
208 (A) (B) (C) (D) (E)
209 (A) (B) (C) (D) (E)
210 (A) (B) (C) (D) (E)
211 (A) (B) (C) (D) (E)
212 (A) (B) (C) (D) (E)
213 (A) (B) (C) (D) (E)
214 (A) (B) (C) (D) (E)
215 (A) (B) (C) (D) (E)
216 (A) (B) (C) (D) (E)
217 (A) (B) (C) (D) (E)
218 (A) (B) (C) (D) (E)
219 (A) (B) (C) (D) (E)
220 (A) (B) (C) (D) (E)
221 (A) (B) (C) (D) (E)
222 (A) (B) (C) (D) (E)
223 (A) (B) (C) (D) (E)
224 (A) (B) (C) (D) (E)
225 (A) (B) (C) (D) (E)
226 (A) (B) (C) (D) (E)
227 (A) (B) (C) (D) (E)
228 (A) (B) (C) (D) (E)
229 (A) (B) (C) (D) (E)
230 (A) (B) (C) (D) (E)
231 (A) (B) (C) (D) (E)
232 (A) (B) (C) (D) (E)
233 (A) (B) (C) (D) (E)
234 (A) (B) (C) (D) (E)
235 (A) (B) (C) (D) (E)
236 (A) (B) (C) (D) (E)
237 (A) (B) (C) (D) (E)
238 (A) (B) (C) (D) (E)
239 (A) (B) (C) (D) (E)
240 (A) (B) (C) (D) (E)

BOARD OF REGISTRY

NAME: ______________________

EXAM TYPE: ______________ DATE: ______________

IDENTIFICATION NUMBER									EXAM TYPE	
0	0	0	0	0	0	0	0	0	0	0
1	1	1	1	1	1	1	1	1	1	1
2	2	2	2	2	2	2	2	2	2	2
3	3	3	3	3	3	3	3	3	3	3
4	4	4	4	4	4	4	4	4	4	4
5	5	5	5	5	5	5	5	5	5	5
6	6	6	6	6	6	6	6	6	6	6
7	7	7	7	7	7	7	7	7	7	7
8	8	8	8	8	8	8	8	8	8	8
9	9	9	9	9	9	9	9	9	9	9

TEST BOOKLET NUMBER				

IMPORTANT DIRECTIONS FOR MARKING ANSWERS

- Use black lead pencil only (No. 2½ or softer).
- Do NOT use ink, felt tip or ballpoint pens.
- Erase cleanly any answer you wish to change.
- Make no stray marks on the answer sheet.
- Make heavy black marks that fill the circle completely.

EXAMPLES

WRONG: Fill in the circle completely.

1 Ⓐ Ⓑ Ⓒ Ⓓ Ⓔ

2 Ⓐ Ⓑ Ⓒ Ⓓ Ⓔ

3 Ⓐ Ⓑ Ⓒ Ⓓ Ⓔ

WRONG: Make heavy black marks.

4 Ⓐ Ⓑ Ⓒ Ⓓ Ⓔ

RIGHT: Make heavy black marks that fill in the circle completely.

5 Ⓐ Ⓑ Ⓒ Ⓓ ●

1 Ⓐ Ⓑ Ⓒ Ⓓ Ⓔ	21 Ⓐ Ⓑ Ⓒ Ⓓ Ⓔ	41 Ⓐ Ⓑ Ⓒ Ⓓ Ⓔ	61 Ⓐ Ⓑ Ⓒ Ⓓ Ⓔ	81 Ⓐ Ⓑ Ⓒ Ⓓ Ⓔ	101 Ⓐ Ⓑ Ⓒ Ⓓ Ⓔ
2 Ⓐ Ⓑ Ⓒ Ⓓ Ⓔ	22 Ⓐ Ⓑ Ⓒ Ⓓ Ⓔ	42 Ⓐ Ⓑ Ⓒ Ⓓ Ⓔ	62 Ⓐ Ⓑ Ⓒ Ⓓ Ⓔ	82 Ⓐ Ⓑ Ⓒ Ⓓ Ⓔ	102 Ⓐ Ⓑ Ⓒ Ⓓ Ⓔ
3 Ⓐ Ⓑ Ⓒ Ⓓ Ⓔ	23 Ⓐ Ⓑ Ⓒ Ⓓ Ⓔ	43 Ⓐ Ⓑ Ⓒ Ⓓ Ⓔ	63 Ⓐ Ⓑ Ⓒ Ⓓ Ⓔ	83 Ⓐ Ⓑ Ⓒ Ⓓ Ⓔ	103 Ⓐ Ⓑ Ⓒ Ⓓ Ⓔ
4 Ⓐ Ⓑ Ⓒ Ⓓ Ⓔ	24 Ⓐ Ⓑ Ⓒ Ⓓ Ⓔ	44 Ⓐ Ⓑ Ⓒ Ⓓ Ⓔ	64 Ⓐ Ⓑ Ⓒ Ⓓ Ⓔ	84 Ⓐ Ⓑ Ⓒ Ⓓ Ⓔ	104 Ⓐ Ⓑ Ⓒ Ⓓ Ⓔ
5 Ⓐ Ⓑ Ⓒ Ⓓ Ⓔ	25 Ⓐ Ⓑ Ⓒ Ⓓ Ⓔ	45 Ⓐ Ⓑ Ⓒ Ⓓ Ⓔ	65 Ⓐ Ⓑ Ⓒ Ⓓ Ⓔ	85 Ⓐ Ⓑ Ⓒ Ⓓ Ⓔ	105 Ⓐ Ⓑ Ⓒ Ⓓ Ⓔ
6 Ⓐ Ⓑ Ⓒ Ⓓ Ⓔ	26 Ⓐ Ⓑ Ⓒ Ⓓ Ⓔ	46 Ⓐ Ⓑ Ⓒ Ⓓ Ⓔ	66 Ⓐ Ⓑ Ⓒ Ⓓ Ⓔ	86 Ⓐ Ⓑ Ⓒ Ⓓ Ⓔ	106 Ⓐ Ⓑ Ⓒ Ⓓ Ⓔ
7 Ⓐ Ⓑ Ⓒ Ⓓ Ⓔ	27 Ⓐ Ⓑ Ⓒ Ⓓ Ⓔ	47 Ⓐ Ⓑ Ⓒ Ⓓ Ⓔ	67 Ⓐ Ⓑ Ⓒ Ⓓ Ⓔ	87 Ⓐ Ⓑ Ⓒ Ⓓ Ⓔ	107 Ⓐ Ⓑ Ⓒ Ⓓ Ⓔ
8 Ⓐ Ⓑ Ⓒ Ⓓ Ⓔ	28 Ⓐ Ⓑ Ⓒ Ⓓ Ⓔ	48 Ⓐ Ⓑ Ⓒ Ⓓ Ⓔ	68 Ⓐ Ⓑ Ⓒ Ⓓ Ⓔ	88 Ⓐ Ⓑ Ⓒ Ⓓ Ⓔ	108 Ⓐ Ⓑ Ⓒ Ⓓ Ⓔ
9 Ⓐ Ⓑ Ⓒ Ⓓ Ⓔ	29 Ⓐ Ⓑ Ⓒ Ⓓ Ⓔ	49 Ⓐ Ⓑ Ⓒ Ⓓ Ⓔ	69 Ⓐ Ⓑ Ⓒ Ⓓ Ⓔ	89 Ⓐ Ⓑ Ⓒ Ⓓ Ⓔ	109 Ⓐ Ⓑ Ⓒ Ⓓ Ⓔ
10 Ⓐ Ⓑ Ⓒ Ⓓ Ⓔ	30 Ⓐ Ⓑ Ⓒ Ⓓ Ⓔ	50 Ⓐ Ⓑ Ⓒ Ⓓ Ⓔ	70 Ⓐ Ⓑ Ⓒ Ⓓ Ⓔ	90 Ⓐ Ⓑ Ⓒ Ⓓ Ⓔ	110 Ⓐ Ⓑ Ⓒ Ⓓ Ⓔ
11 Ⓐ Ⓑ Ⓒ Ⓓ Ⓔ	31 Ⓐ Ⓑ Ⓒ Ⓓ Ⓔ	51 Ⓐ Ⓑ Ⓒ Ⓓ Ⓔ	71 Ⓐ Ⓑ Ⓒ Ⓓ Ⓔ	91 Ⓐ Ⓑ Ⓒ Ⓓ Ⓔ	111 Ⓐ Ⓑ Ⓒ Ⓓ Ⓔ
12 Ⓐ Ⓑ Ⓒ Ⓓ Ⓔ	32 Ⓐ Ⓑ Ⓒ Ⓓ Ⓔ	52 Ⓐ Ⓑ Ⓒ Ⓓ Ⓔ	72 Ⓐ Ⓑ Ⓒ Ⓓ Ⓔ	92 Ⓐ Ⓑ Ⓒ Ⓓ Ⓔ	112 Ⓐ Ⓑ Ⓒ Ⓓ Ⓔ
13 Ⓐ Ⓑ Ⓒ Ⓓ Ⓔ	33 Ⓐ Ⓑ Ⓒ Ⓓ Ⓔ	53 Ⓐ Ⓑ Ⓒ Ⓓ Ⓔ	73 Ⓐ Ⓑ Ⓒ Ⓓ Ⓔ	93 Ⓐ Ⓑ Ⓒ Ⓓ Ⓔ	113 Ⓐ Ⓑ Ⓒ Ⓓ Ⓔ
14 Ⓐ Ⓑ Ⓒ Ⓓ Ⓔ	34 Ⓐ Ⓑ Ⓒ Ⓓ Ⓔ	54 Ⓐ Ⓑ Ⓒ Ⓓ Ⓔ	74 Ⓐ Ⓑ Ⓒ Ⓓ Ⓔ	94 Ⓐ Ⓑ Ⓒ Ⓓ Ⓔ	114 Ⓐ Ⓑ Ⓒ Ⓓ Ⓔ
15 Ⓐ Ⓑ Ⓒ Ⓓ Ⓔ	35 Ⓐ Ⓑ Ⓒ Ⓓ Ⓔ	55 Ⓐ Ⓑ Ⓒ Ⓓ Ⓔ	75 Ⓐ Ⓑ Ⓒ Ⓓ Ⓔ	95 Ⓐ Ⓑ Ⓒ Ⓓ Ⓔ	115 Ⓐ Ⓑ Ⓒ Ⓓ Ⓔ
16 Ⓐ Ⓑ Ⓒ Ⓓ Ⓔ	36 Ⓐ Ⓑ Ⓒ Ⓓ Ⓔ	56 Ⓐ Ⓑ Ⓒ Ⓓ Ⓔ	76 Ⓐ Ⓑ Ⓒ Ⓓ Ⓔ	96 Ⓐ Ⓑ Ⓒ Ⓓ Ⓔ	116 Ⓐ Ⓑ Ⓒ Ⓓ Ⓔ
17 Ⓐ Ⓑ Ⓒ Ⓓ Ⓔ	37 Ⓐ Ⓑ Ⓒ Ⓓ Ⓔ	57 Ⓐ Ⓑ Ⓒ Ⓓ Ⓔ	77 Ⓐ Ⓑ Ⓒ Ⓓ Ⓔ	97 Ⓐ Ⓑ Ⓒ Ⓓ Ⓔ	117 Ⓐ Ⓑ Ⓒ Ⓓ Ⓔ
18 Ⓐ Ⓑ Ⓒ Ⓓ Ⓔ	38 Ⓐ Ⓑ Ⓒ Ⓓ Ⓔ	58 Ⓐ Ⓑ Ⓒ Ⓓ Ⓔ	78 Ⓐ Ⓑ Ⓒ Ⓓ Ⓔ	98 Ⓐ Ⓑ Ⓒ Ⓓ Ⓔ	118 Ⓐ Ⓑ Ⓒ Ⓓ Ⓔ
19 Ⓐ Ⓑ Ⓒ Ⓓ Ⓔ	39 Ⓐ Ⓑ Ⓒ Ⓓ Ⓔ	59 Ⓐ Ⓑ Ⓒ Ⓓ Ⓔ	79 Ⓐ Ⓑ Ⓒ Ⓓ Ⓔ	99 Ⓐ Ⓑ Ⓒ Ⓓ Ⓔ	119 Ⓐ Ⓑ Ⓒ Ⓓ Ⓔ
20 Ⓐ Ⓑ Ⓒ Ⓓ Ⓔ	40 Ⓐ Ⓑ Ⓒ Ⓓ Ⓔ	60 Ⓐ Ⓑ Ⓒ Ⓓ Ⓔ	80 Ⓐ Ⓑ Ⓒ Ⓓ Ⓔ	100 Ⓐ Ⓑ Ⓒ Ⓓ Ⓔ	120 Ⓐ Ⓑ Ⓒ Ⓓ Ⓔ

NCS Trans-Optic F6292-54321 TM

SIDE ONE

BOARD OF REGISTRY

founded in 1928 by the
American Society of Clinical Pathologists

Representatives from:

American Society of Clinical Pathologists
Medical Technologists/Technicians
Pathologists
American Academy of Microbiology
American Association of Blood Banks
American Society of Cytology
National Registry in Clinical Chemistry
American Society of Hematology
National Society for Histotechnology

IMPORTANT DIRECTIONS FOR MARKING ANSWERS

- Use black lead pencil only (No. 2½ or softer).
- Do NOT use ink, felt tip or ballpoint pens.
- Erase cleanly any answer you wish to change.
- Make no stray marks on the answer sheet.
- Make heavy black marks that fill the circle completely.

EXAMPLES

1 A B C D E	WRONG: Fill in the circle completely.
2 A B C D E	
3 A B C D E	
4 A B C D E	WRONG: Make heavy black marks.
5 A B C D E	RIGHT: Make heavy black marks that fill in the circle completely.

121 A B C D E	141 A B C D E	161 A B C D E	181 A B C D E	201 A B C D E	221 A B C D E
122 A B C D E	142 A B C D E	162 A B C D E	182 A B C D E	202 A B C D E	222 A B C D E
123 A B C D E	143 A B C D E	163 A B C D E	183 A B C D E	203 A B C D E	223 A B C D E
124 A B C D E	144 A B C D E	164 A B C D E	184 A B C D E	204 A B C D E	224 A B C D E
125 A B C D E	145 A B C D E	165 A B C D E	185 A B C D E	205 A B C D E	225 A B C D E
126 A B C D E	146 A B C D E	166 A B C D E	186 A B C D E	206 A B C D E	226 A B C D E
127 A B C D E	147 A B C D E	167 A B C D E	187 A B C D E	207 A B C D E	227 A B C D E
128 A B C D E	148 A B C D E	168 A B C D E	188 A B C D E	208 A B C D E	228 A B C D E
129 A B C D E	149 A B C D E	169 A B C D E	189 A B C D E	209 A B C D E	229 A B C D E
130 A B C D E	150 A B C D E	170 A B C D E	190 A B C D E	210 A B C D E	230 A B C D E
131 A B C D E	151 A B C D E	171 A B C D E	191 A B C D E	211 A B C D E	231 A B C D E
132 A B C D E	152 A B C D E	172 A B C D E	192 A B C D E	212 A B C D E	232 A B C D E
133 A B C D E	153 A B C D E	173 A B C D E	193 A B C D E	213 A B C D E	233 A B C D E
134 A B C D E	154 A B C D E	174 A B C D E	194 A B C D E	214 A B C D E	234 A B C D E
135 A B C D E	155 A B C D E	175 A B C D E	195 A B C D E	215 A B C D E	235 A B C D E
136 A B C D E	156 A B C D E	176 A B C D E	196 A B C D E	216 A B C D E	236 A B C D E
137 A B C D E	157 A B C D E	177 A B C D E	197 A B C D E	217 A B C D E	237 A B C D E
138 A B C D E	158 A B C D E	178 A B C D E	198 A B C D E	218 A B C D E	238 A B C D E
139 A B C D E	159 A B C D E	179 A B C D E	199 A B C D E	219 A B C D E	239 A B C D E
140 A B C D E	160 A B C D E	180 A B C D E	200 A B C D E	220 A B C D E	240 A B C D E